Clinical Techniques in Otology

Clinical Techniques in Otology

Editor: Taliyah Hooper

AMERICAN
MEDICAL PUBLISHERS
www.americanmedicalpublishers.com

AMERICAN
MEDICAL PUBLISHERS
www.americanmedicalpublishers.com

Cataloging-in-Publication Data

Clinical techniques in otology / edited by Taliyah Hooper.
p. cm.
Includes bibliographical references and index.
ISBN 979-8-88740-012-9
1. Otology. 2. Ear--Diseases--Treatment--Technique. 3. Ear--Diseases--Diagnosis--Technique. I. Hooper, Taliyah.
RF121 .C55 2023
617.8--dc23

American Medical Publishers,
41 Flatbush Avenue,
1st Floor, New York,
NY 11217, USA

ISBN 979-8-88740-012-9 (Hardback)

Contents

Preface

In my initial years as a student, I used to run to the library at every possible instance to grab a book and learn something new. Books were my primary source of knowledge and I would not have come such a long way without all that I learnt from them. Thus, when I was approached to edit this book; I became understandably nostalgic. It was an absolute honor to be considered worthy of guiding the current generation as well as those to come. I put all my knowledge and hard work into making this book most beneficial for its readers.

Otology is a branch of medical science that deals with the diagnosis and treatment of diseases and disorders related to the ear. Some of the major pathologies associated with the ear include otitis, tinnitus, balance disorders, Usher syndrome, hearing loss and Meniere's disease. There are a number of different types of diagnostic tests performed to examine a patient. Audiogram is a common diagnostic test used to measure hearing sensitivity. Tympanogram test is performed to examine the function of the middle ear while vestibular test is done to measure inner ear function. Electronystagmogram, posturography, and videonystagmography are some other diagnostic tests performed within this field. Otological treatment is based on the specific type of ear disease or condition. Some common treatments for ear related conditions are surgery, hearing aids, cochlear implants, medication, and ear tubes. Surgery within otology generally involves the mastoid and middle ear. A few types of surgical procedures performed under this field are tympanoplasty, mastoidectomy and ossiculoplasty. This book includes some of the vital pieces of work being conducted across the world, on various topics related to clinical techniques in otology. It consists of contributions made by international experts. Researchers and students in the field of otology will be assisted by this book.

I wish to thank my publisher for supporting me at every step. I would also like to thank all the authors who have contributed their researches in this book. I hope this book will be a valuable contribution to the progress of the field.

Editor

1

Assessment of Cochlear Function during Cochlear Implantation by Extra- and Intracochlear Electrocochleography

Adrian Dalbert[1], Flurin Pfiffner[1], Marco Hoesli[1], Kanthaiah Koka[2], Dorothe Veraguth[1], Christof Roosli[1] and Alexander Huber[1]*

[1] Department of Otorhinolaryngology – Head and Neck Surgery, University of Zurich, University Hospital of Zurich, Zurich, Switzerland, [2] Department of Research and Technology, Advanced Bionics LLC, Valencia, CA, United States

Correspondence:
Adrian Dalbert
adrian.dalbert@usz.ch

Objective: The aims of this study were: (1) To investigate the correlation between electrophysiological changes during cochlear implantation and postoperative hearing loss, and (2) to detect the time points that electrophysiological changes occur during cochlear implantation.

Material and Methods: Extra- and intracochlear electrocochleography (ECoG) were used to detect electrophysiological changes during cochlear implantation. Extracochlear ECoG recordings were conducted through a needle electrode placed on the promontory; for intracochlear ECoG recordings, the most apical contact of the cochlear implant (CI) electrode itself was used as the recording electrode. Tone bursts at 250, 500, 750, and 1000 Hz were used as low-frequency acoustic stimuli and clicks as high-frequency acoustic stimuli. Changes of extracochlear ECoG recordings after full insertion of the CI electrode were correlated with pure-tone audiometric findings 4 weeks after surgery.

Results: Changes in extracochlear ECoG recordings correlated with postoperative hearing change ($r = -0.44$, $p = 0.055$, $n = 20$). Mean hearing loss in subjects without decrease or loss of extracochlear ECoG signals was 12 dB, compared to a mean hearing loss of 22 dB in subjects with a detectable decrease or a loss of ECoG signals ($p = 0.0058$, $n = 51$). In extracochlear ECoG recordings, a mean increase of the ECoG signal of 4.4 dB occurred after opening the cochlea. If a decrease of ECoG signals occurred during insertion of the CI electrode, the decrease was detectable during the second half of the insertion.

Conclusion: ECoG recordings allow detection of electrophysiological changes in the cochlea during cochlear implantation. Decrease of extracochlear ECoG recordings during surgery has a significant correlation with hearing loss 4 weeks after surgery. Trauma to cochlear structures seems to occur during the final phase of the CI electrode insertion. Baseline recordings for extracochlear ECoG recordings should be conducted after opening the cochlea. ECoG responses can be recorded from an intracochlear site using the CI electrode as recording electrode. This technique may prove useful for monitoring cochlear trauma intraoperatively in the future.

Keywords: cochlear implantation, cochlear implant, electrocochleography, residual hearing, hearing preservation, cochlear trauma

INTRODUCTION

Electrocochleography (ECoG) seems to be a promising method to assess cochlear trauma during cochlear implantation. In an animal model, changes in ECoG responses during insertion of an electrode into the cochlea correlated with histological trauma (Adunka et al., 2010; Campbell et al., 2010; Choudhury et al., 2011, 2014; Ahmad et al., 2012; DeMason et al., 2012). The feasibility of ECoG in human cochlear implant (CI) recipients has also been demonstrated (Choudhury et al., 2012; Mandalà et al., 2012; Radeloff et al., 2012; Calloway et al., 2014; Adunka et al., 2015; Campbell et al., 2015, 2016; Dalbert et al., 2015a,b, 2016). Recordings were performed from extracochlear sites (Choudhury et al., 2012; Mandalà et al., 2012; Radeloff et al., 2012; Adunka et al., 2015; Dalbert et al., 2015b, 2016) and from inside the cochlea using either customized recording electrodes (Calloway et al., 2014) or the contacts of the CI electrode itself as recording electrodes (Campbell et al., 2015, 2016; Dalbert et al., 2015a). Almost all human subjects showed some ECoG responses to sound despite substantial levels of hearing loss (Choudhury et al., 2012). Furthermore, some correlation between the assessment of cochlear trauma by ECoG and radiological findings could be demonstrated (Dalbert et al., 2016). However, the predictive value of ECoG changes during cochlear implantation regarding preservation of residual hearing is controversial. Although multiple studies demonstrated a correlation between hearing loss and ECoG changes during surgery for extra- (Mandalà et al., 2012; Radeloff et al., 2012; Dalbert et al., 2015b, 2016) as well as intracochlear recordings (Campbell et al., 2016), contradictory results have also been published (Adunka et al., 2015).

ECoG signals represent electrophysiological responses of the cochlea and the auditory nerve to sound and can provide information about the state of these structures. In CI recipients, these responses are generated by the remaining intact cochlear structures, which are the basis for residual hearing. The ECoG signal combines potentials of cochlear and neural origin. The cochlear microphonic (CM) is a hair cell potential, mainly produced by the outer hair cells. The auditory nerve neurophonic (ANN) and the compound action potential (CAP) are produced by the auditory nerve fibers. The summating potential (SP) most likely has hair cell as well as neural components (Sellick et al., 2003; Forgues et al., 2014).

For the assessment of cochlear trauma during cochlear implantation, the focus of most studies has been on the changes of the CM or the so called ongoing ECoG signal, composed of the CM and the ANN (Radeloff et al., 2012; Calloway et al., 2014; Adunka et al., 2015; Dalbert et al., 2015a,b; Campbell et al., 2016). The CAP has been investigated less extensively (Mandalà et al., 2012; Dalbert et al., 2016). The CM and the ongoing ECoG signal have three distinct advantages over the CAP: (1) Both signals are detectable in almost all CI recipients (Choudhury et al., 2012), (2) Animal studies have demonstrated a better correlation between cochlear trauma and changes of the CM than between cochlear trauma and changes of the CAP (Choudhury et al., 2014), and (3) Both signals show a linear growth up to high-intensity level stimulation (Dalbert et al., 2016). Due to the linear growth, threshold changes and changes of the amplitude near threshold reflect changes at higher intensities. This again allows to record at high intensities where clear ECoG signals are detectable and to avoid time-consuming threshold determinations during surgery.

On the other hand, the correlation between behavioral hearing tests and the amplitude or threshold of the CM or the ongoing ECoG signal is controversial (Campbell et al., 2015; Dalbert et al., 2015a; Koka et al., 2017). Most likely, changes in the CM or the ongoing ECoG signal cannot be directly translated into changes of residual hearing (Campbell et al., 2015; Dalbert et al., 2015a). This could be a reason in favor of using the CAP. It seems reasonable to assume that the purely neural CAP signal has a better correlation to behavioral hearing tests than signals representing hair cell activity, at least in part.

Nevertheless, based on animal studies, a pure hair cell potential would be the best electrophysiological marker to monitor trauma during insertion of an electrode into the cochlea, making the CM a natural choice (Choudhury et al., 2014). However, the often used assumption that the difference of two ECoG signals with alternating starting phases cancels out the neural contribution to the signal and only the CM remains, is not valid at low frequencies and high intensities (Forgues et al., 2014). Consequently, in human CI recipients, a separation of CM and ANN is difficult and to our knowledge, potentials labeled as CM in studies investigating ECoG in human CI recipients cannot be considered as pure hair cell potentials. Thus, the analysis of the ongoing ECoG signal seems to be more adequate as CM and ANN are combined. In this study, we analyzed the ongoing ECoG signal in the low and the CAP in the high frequencies.

This study aimed to accomplish the following: (1) Evaluation of the correlation between changes in extracochlear ECoG recordings at low and high frequencies immediately after insertion of the CI electrode with changes of residual hearing 4 weeks after surgery; (2) Determining electrophysiological changes at different time points during surgery by extra- and intracochlear ECoG.

MATERIALS AND METHODS

This study is part of a prospective, continuous enrollment study at the University Hospital of Zürich, Switzerland. Part of the data has been previously analyzed and published (Dalbert et al., 2015b, 2016). The study was performed in concordance with the Helsinki Declaration. The study protocol was approved by the Ethical Committee of Zurich (KEK-ZH-Nr. 2013-0317). The indication for cochlear implantation was given after standard evaluations in the CI Clinic of the University Hospital of Zurich, Switzerland. All subjects provided written informed consent before surgery. They were included between November 2013 and December 2016.

All surgeries were performed at the University Hospital of Zurich, Switzerland. A standard anterior mastoidectomy and a maximum size posterior tympanotomy were performed to allow for placement of the extracochlear recording electrode as described later. Then, an anterior-inferior cochleostomy, or an incision of the round window membrane, was conducted. The CI electrode was inserted, and after complete insertion, the site was sealed with soft tissue. Afterwards, the wound was closed in layers and CI telemetry performed. For a detailed description of the surgical procedure we refer to a previous publication (Dalbert et al., 2015b).

Pure-tone testing, performed according to ISO 8235-1, was conducted within 3 months prior to surgery and approximately 4 weeks after surgery. The pure-tone average (PTA) was calculated from the threshold values at 250, 500, 1,000, 2,000, and 4,000 Hz. Hearing loss after surgery was defined as the difference between the pre- and the postsurgical PTA. The maximum output of the audiometer plus 5 dB was used as a threshold value if no response was present at the maximum output of the audiometer.

Statistical analyses were conducted with Stata Statistical Software (Release 13, StataCorp LP, College Station, Texas, U.S.A.).

Extracochlear ECoG Recordings

The Navigator Pro stimulation/recording device and AEP software (Biologic Systems) were used for acoustic stimulation and recording. Before surgery, an insert earphone (Biologic Systems, Mundelein, IL, U.S.A.) was placed in the ear canal for acoustic stimulation. Tone bursts at 250, 500, 750, and 1,000 Hz were used as low-frequency acoustic stimuli, click stimuli as high-frequency acoustic stimuli. Responses to 400 tone bursts or 400 clicks with alternating starting phases were filtered and averaged. The high pass filter was set at 10 Hz, the low pass filter at 3000 Hz for acoustic stimuli at 250, 500, and 750 Hz, at 5,000 Hz for acoustic stimuli at 1,000 Hz, and at 1,500 Hz for acoustic click stimuli. The rise and fall time for tone bursts was 2 cycles shaped by a Blackman window. The plateau phase of tone bursts was 4 cycles at 250 Hz, 10 cycles at 500 Hz, 14 cycles at 750 Hz, and 20 cycles at 1,000 Hz. The recording window was 32 ms for tone bursts and 10.66 ms for click stimuli. The acoustic stimuli were presented at 80–85 dB nHL at 250 Hz, at 85–95 dB nHL at 500 Hz, and at 90–100 dB nHL at 750 and 1,000 Hz. Click stimuli were presented with an intensity of 95 dB nHL.

Standard needle electrodes (20 × 0.3 mm, Neurosign, Magstim Co., Wales, U.K.) were placed in the contralateral pre- or postauricular region (negative), on the forehead (ground), and after complete visualization of the round window on the promontory (positive). Impedances were below 10 kOhm on all electrodes for all ECoG recordings.

Data were exported from the AEP software using the AEP to ASCIII software from Biologic Systems. MATLAB (MathWorks Inc., Natick, MA, U.S.A.) and GraphPad Prism V5.04 (GraphPad Software Inc., La Jolla, CA, U.S.A.) were used for post-processing.

The data from condensation and rarefaction phases were stored separately. The average curve was determined by subtracting both responses and the sum curve by adding both responses. For analysis of the amplitude of the ongoing ECoG signal, the spectrum of each ECoG response was obtained. A time window was defined (9 to 23 ms), isolating the ongoing ECoG signal from the CAP, and a fast Fourier transform (FFT) conducted. The response amplitude at the frequency of the acoustic stimuli (first harmonic) and at the frequency of twice the acoustic stimuli (second harmonic) were determined and added. The sum was defined as the amplitude of the ongoing ECoG signal. An ongoing ECoG signal was considered valid if a response could be visually detected in the average and/or the sum curve and if the amplitude exceeded the mean noise floor plus 3 standard deviations. The mean noise floor and its standard deviation (SD) for each frequency were determined from 173 recordings without acoustic stimulation. To obtain the spectrum of each noise recording, an FFT was performed using the same time window as for all other recordings.

The repeatability of ECoG recordings was assessed by comparing the amplitude of ongoing ECoG signals. Sixty-four ECoG recordings (6 at 250 Hz, 37 at 500 Hz, 16 at 750 Hz, and 5 at 1,000 Hz) were repeated under unchanged conditions before insertion of the CI electrode. The mean amplitude difference was −0.2 dB (SD 0.1 dB).

As in a previous publication (Dalbert et al., 2015a), the sum of the amplitudes of valid ongoing ECoG signals at 250, 500, and 1,000 Hz was defined as the low-frequency ECoG response and taken as a measure of the cochlear function at low frequencies. In concordance with a previous publication (Dalbert et al., 2016), a difference of ≥3 dB between low-frequency ECoG responses was considered relevant. The low-frequency ECoG response was assessed together with the CAP in response to an acoustic click stimulus as high-frequency acoustic stimulus at two time points during surgery: (1) Before opening the cochlea and (2) after full insertion of the CI electrode and sealing of the insertion site with soft tissue. The CAP in response to acoustic click stimuli was assessed visually in the average curve.

In 11 subjects (S59–S62, S65, S66, S68, S69, S72–S74), ECoG recordings were conducted before opening the cochlea, after opening the cochlea, after halfway insertion of the CI electrode, and after full insertion and sealing of the insertion site with soft tissue. For these recordings, one frequency with a clear ECoG response before opening the cochlea was selected and changes of the ongoing ECoG signal at that frequency were analyzed. For the recording, the insertion of the CI electrode was paused and the CI electrode held in an unchanged position by the surgeon.

Intracochlear ECoG Recordings

Intracochlear ECoG recordings were conducted through the HiRes90K CI system (Advanced Bionics, Stafa, Switzerland). The Bionic Ear Data Collection System research software (BEDCS, Advanced Bionics, Stafa, Switzerland) was used. The BEDCS was connected to the CI through the Clarion Programming Interface (CPI, Advanced Bionics, Stafa, Switzerland) and the Platinum Series Speech Processor (Advanced Bionics, Stafa, Switzerland). The amplifier on the HiRes90K CI was configured to have a gain of 1000. The sampling rate was 9,280 Hz. The low pass filter was set at 5,000 Hz. The most apical contact of the HiFocus Mid-Scalar electrode array was used as the recording electrode, the ring electrode as reference electrode.

The acoustic stimulus was generated by a NI DAQ system (NI DAQ 6216, National Instruments Corporation, Austin, TX, U.S.A.) along with an audio amplifier (Sony PHA-2, Sony Corporation, New York, NY, U.S.A.). The sound was presented through ER-3A insert earphones (Etymotic Research Inc., Elk Grove Village, IL, U.S.A.). As acoustic stimulus, a sinusoidal tone burst at 500 Hz with a level of approximately 110 dB SPL was used. The CPI delivered an external trigger to synchronize stimulus generation and ECoG recording through the CI. The recordings were acquired either continuously (S77) or stepwise (S48, S52) during insertion of the CI electrode.

RESULTS

Extracochlear ECoG recordings were conducted in 22 subjects (**Figure 1**), intracochlear ECoG recordings in 3 subjects (S48, S52, S77). For further analyses, the data was combined with data from 36 additional subjects, which was published previously (Dalbert et al., 2015b, 2016). The demographic, audiometric and electrophysiological data are summarized in **Table 1**. Subjects included in the two previous publications are marked in **Table 1**.

Extracochlear ECoG Recordings after Insertion of the CI Electrode and Hearing Preservation

In 20 subjects, the low-frequency ECoG response was assessed before opening the cochlea and after full insertion and sealing of the round window with soft tissue. Changes in extracochlear ECoG recordings correlated with the postoperative hearing change (Pearson correlation coefficient, $r = -0.44$, $p = 0.055$, $n = 20$, **Figure 2**).

When the data from previous publications (Dalbert et al., 2015b, 2016) was included, a decrease of the low-frequency ECoG response of ≥3 dB occurred in 4/51 subjects (S15, S36, S44, S64) (**Figures 3A,B**). Subjects with a decrease of ≥3 dB in the low-frequency ECoG response after insertion of the CI electrode had a mean hearing loss of 24 dB at 4 weeks after surgery (SD 14 dB, mean presurgical PTA 94 dB HL); subjects with no relevant decrease in the low-frequency ECoG response, a mean hearing loss of 12 dB (SD 9 dB, mean presurgical PTA 92 dB HL).

A CAP in response to a high-frequency acoustic stimulus was detectable in 16 subjects. Including previously published data (Dalbert et al., 2015b, 2016), a decrease of the amplitude of the CAP or a complete loss of the CAP in response to an acoustic click stimulus after full insertion of the CI electrode was detectable in 6/24 subjects (**Figure 3C**). This was associated with a mean hearing loss of 21 dB (SD 13 dB, mean presurgical PTA 83 dB HL).

Overall, in subjects without a decrease or loss of ECoG signals in the high or low frequencies, the mean PTA was 91 dB HL (SD 15 dB) before surgery and 103 dB HL (SD 14 dB) 4 weeks after surgery. In subjects with detectable decrease or loss of ECoG signals, the mean PTA was 87 dB HL (SD 13 dB) before surgery and 109 dB HL (SD 15 dB) after surgery. Therefore, the mean hearing loss in subjects without decrease or loss of ECoG signals was 12 dB, compared to a mean hearing loss of 22 dB in subjects with a detectable decrease or loss of ECoG signals (Unpaired t-test, $p = 0.0058$, $n = 51$) (**Figure 4**).

Extracochlear ECoG Recordings during Insertion of CI Electrode

Different patterns occurred in extracochlear ECoG recordings during insertion of the CI electrode (**Figure 5**). After opening the cochlea, 5/11 subjects (S59, S60, S62, S69, S74) showed an increase of the amplitude of the ongoing ECoG signal of ≥3 dB. Six out of 11 subjects showed unchanged ongoing ECoG responses and no decrease occurred. On average, the amplitude of the ongoing ECoG signal increased by 4.4 dB after opening the cochlea.

During the first half of the insertion of the CI electrode, the ongoing ECoG signals remained unchanged in all subjects. The mean ECoG response amplitude was 29.2 dB re 0.1 uV (SD 6.8 dB) after opening the cochlea and 29.6 dB re 0.1 uV (SD 6.8 dB) after halfway insertion.

During the second half of the insertion, a decrease of the ongoing ECoG signal was detectable in 6/11 subjects (S59, S60, S62, S66, S68, S72). On average, the ECoG response amplitude was 26 dB re 0.1 uV (SD 12 dB) at the end of the insertion. In S72, no valid ECoG signal was detectable after full insertion (amplitude of the ongoing ECoG signal after halfway insertion was 28 dB re 0.1 uV).

Intracochlear ECoG Recordings during Insertion of the CI Electrode

The results of the intracochlear ECoG recordings are shown in **Figure 6**. Two out of 3 subjects (S52, S77) showed an increase of

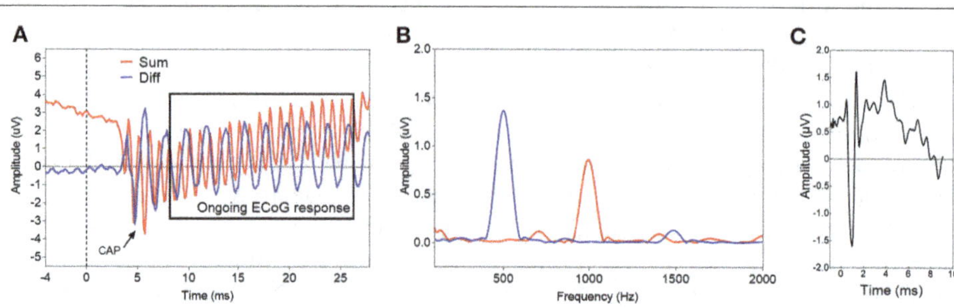

FIGURE 1 | Two examples of typical ECoG responses before insertion of the CI electrode. **(A,B)** show the time waveform **(A)** and the corresponding spectrum **(B)** of an ECoG signal in response to a sinusoidal tone burst with alternating starting phases at 500 Hz, 95 dB nHL (S54). The blue line represents the difference, the red line the average of the responses with alternating polarity. The black rectangle **(A)** marks the time window, used for the spectral analysis. **(C)** Displays an ECoG signal in response to an acoustic click stimulus at 95 dB nHL (S43). Only the average of the responses with alternating starting phases is shown. A clear CAP is visible.

TABLE 1 | Subject demographics, audiometric, and electrophysiological findings.

Subject no.	Age (Yr)	Cochlear implant	Round window insertion	Preoperative PTA (operated side) (dB HL)	Hearing change (operated side) (dB)	Hearing change (contralateral side) (dB)	Change in low-frequency ECoG response (dB)	Change in high-frequency ECoG response
S1*	43	Nucleus CI-512	No	112	Complete HL	2	0.7	–
S3*	52	Nucleus CI-422	Yes	70	9	4	−1.3	–
S4*	23	Nucleus CI-422	Yes	69	14	−2	−1.8	–
S5*	55	Nucleus CI-512	No	101	9	−2	0.6	–
S7*	38	HiRes90K HiFocus V	Yes	76	9	1	4.3	–
S8*	53	Nucleus CI-422	Yes	76	14	−2	0.6	–
S9*	72	HiRes90K HiFocus V	Yes	106	−1	2	−0.4	–
S10*	46	HiRes90K HiFocus V	Yes	71	19	No hearing	5	–
S11*	46	Nucleus CI-422	Yes	100	10	No hearing	1.9	–
S12*	66	HiRes90K HiFocus V	Yes	103	0	1	No response	–
S13*	38	HiRes90K HiFocus V	Yes	75	13	3	4	–
S14*	23	HiRes90K HiFocus V	Yes	102	11	−5	−1.6	–
S15*	64	Nucleus CI-422	Yes	76	Complete HL	−6	−3.8	–
S17*	78	Nucleus CI-422	Yes	94	18	1	No response	No response
S18*	61	HiRes90K HiFocus V	Yes	82	31	2	1.3	No decrease
S19*	59	HiRes90K HiFocus V	Yes	99	8	0	−2.4	–
S21*	55	HiRes90K HiFocus V	Yes	112	Complete HL	0	4.5	No response
S22*	67	Nucleus CI-422	Yes	101	Complete HL	7	No response	No response
S23*	67	Nucleus CI-422	Yes	89	Complete HL	0	−1.9	Loss
S24*	60	Nucleus CI-422	Yes	89	Complete HL	0	−0.4	No response
S25*	36	Nucleus CI-422	Yes	93	0	No hearing	3.3	Decrease
S26*	80	Nucleus CI-512	No	101	10	−7	0.4	No response
S27*	61	Nucleus CI-422	Yes	98	3	0	1.7	No decrease
S28*	71	Nucleus CI-422	Yes	76	24	3	4.4	No decrease
S29*	49	Nucleus CI-422	Yes	78	11	−1	13.5	No decrease
S30*	41	Nucleus CI-512	No	96	10	7	1.4	No response
S31*	55	Nucleus CI-512	Yes	97	Complete HL	4	No response	No response
S32*	30	Nucleus CI-512	No	102	10	1	7.4	No decrease
S34*	53	Nucleus CI-512	No	110	5	No hearing	0.9	No decrease
S35*	55	Nucleus CI-512	No	98	Complete HL	−1	No response	No response
S36*	76	Nucleus CI-512	No	103	15	−12	−6.6	No response
S37*	56	Nucleus CI-522	Yes	64	24	−1	3.8	Decrease
S38*	38	Nucleus CI-522	Yes	99	4	−1	7.6	No response
S39*	42	Nucleus CI-522	Yes	113	4	4	−2.9	No response
S41*	53	Nucleus CI-512	No	99	18	2	6.8	No response
S42*	53	HiRes90K HiFocus V	Yes	93	22	1	7.3	No decrease
S43	23	Nucleus CI-522	Yes	82	11	1	4.8	No decrease
S44	26	Nucleus CI-512	No	104	14	−1	−7.5	No response
S45	57	Nucleus CI-512	No	99	5	−3	2.5	No decrease
S48	73	HiRes90K HiFocus V	Yes	94	Complete HL	−1	Only intracochlear recordings	
S52	74	HiRes90K HiFocus V	Yes	79	10	−8	Only intracochlear recordings	
S53	56	Nucleus CI-522	Yes	100	15	7	3.5	No decrease
S54	31	HiRes90K HiFocus V	Yes	74	−1	−5	0.4	No response
S55	64	Nucleus CI-522	Yes	76	12	0	2	No decrease
S58	45	HiRes90K HiFocus V	Yes	103	Complete HL	−1	0.3	No response
S59	61	Nucleus CI-422	Yes	74	24	−7	11.4	No response
S60	60	Nucleus CI-512	No	94	Complete HL	−4	2.1	Loss
S61	43	Nucleus CI-512	No	104	Complete HL	–	−1.3	No decrease

(Continued)

TABLE 1 | Continued

Subject no.	Age (Yr)	Cochlear implant	Round window insertion	Preoperative PTA (operated side) (dB HL)	Hearing change (operated side) (dB)	Hearing change (contralateral side) (dB)	Change in low-frequency ECoG response (dB)	Change in high-frequency ECoG response
S62	70	Nucleus CI-522	Yes	86	8	−2	2.7	No decrease
S64	55	HiRes90K HiFocus V	No	102	Complete HL	5	−3.2	No response
S65	60	Nucleus CI-522	Yes	64	41	1	0.3	No decrease
S66	29	Nucleus CI-522	Yes	77	9	0	−0.3	Decrease
S67	62	HiRes90K HiFocus V	Yes	102	8	−3	2.3	No decrease
S68	19	Nucleus CI-512	Yes	94	7	−3	−0.9	No decrease
S69	27	Nucleus CI-522	Yes	104	9	−5	3.2	No response
S70	81	HiRes90K HiFocus V	Yes	72	13	0	2	No decrease
S71	72	HiRes90K HiFocus V	Yes	80	31	−4	0.4	Loss
S72	39	Nucleus CI-522	Yes	78	30	−1	Not applicable	
S73	52	Nucleus CI-522	Yes	91	−5	0	Not applicable	
S74	57	Nucleus CI-512	No	101	3	0	7.8	No decrease
S77	73	HiRes90K HiFocus V	Yes	89	9	0	Only intracochlear recordings	

*PTA indicates pure-tone average at 250, 500, 1,000, 2,000, and 4,000 Hz; ECoG, electrocochleography; HL, hearing loss; *previously published data (Dalbert et al., 2015a, 2016).*

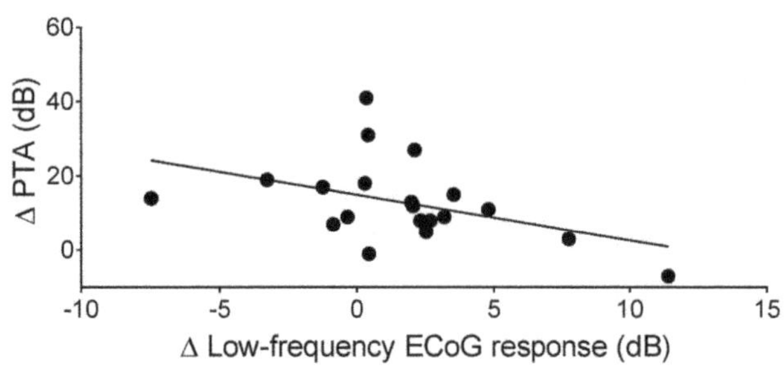

FIGURE 2 | Correlation between the change of the low-frequency ECoG response immediately after full insertion of the CI electrode array (Δ Low-frequency ECoG response) and the change of the pure-tone average 4 weeks after surgery (Δ PTA) (Pearson correlation coefficient, $r = -0.44$, $p = 0.055$, $n = 20$).

the amplitude of the ECoG signal until the last ECoG recording. In S77, one small, temporary decrease during insertion was detectable, whereas in S52, the ECoG responses continuously increased until full insertion. Subject S48 showed, after an initial increase of the ECoG signal, a decrease of 5.2 dB during the last fifth of the insertion.

DISCUSSION

As a correlation between histological trauma and a decrease of ECoG responses during insertion of an electrode into the cochlea could be demonstrated in animal studies (Adunka et al., 2010; Campbell et al., 2010; Choudhury et al., 2011, 2014; Ahmad et al., 2012; DeMason et al., 2012), it is plausible to assume that a decrease of ECoG responses in human CI recipients during insertion of the CI electrode represents trauma to cochlear structures. However, although the great potential of ECoG regarding monitoring cochlear trauma during cochlear implantation is generally accepted, the correlation between changes of ECoG signals during surgery and postoperative hearing loss—and therefore the clinical value of such recordings—has still to be proven. Therefore, the aim of this study was to further elucidate the correlation of ECoG changes during surgery and postoperative hearing loss. Furthermore, we aimed to describe at which points during cochlear implantation changes of ECoG signals occur.

Correlation between Changes of Extracochlear ECoG Responses after Insertion of the CI Electrode and Hearing Preservation

Changes in low-frequency ECoG responses correlated with the postoperative hearing change ($r = -0.44$, $p = 0.055$). Subjects with a decrease of high- or low-frequency ECoG signals immediately after insertion of the CI electrode, therefore assumed trauma to cochlear structures during CI surgery, showed a significantly greater hearing loss 4 weeks after surgery compared to subjects without decrease of ECoG signals (22 dB vs. 12 dB, $p = 0.0058$). Subjects with an atraumatic insertion, based on the ECoG recordings, showed a mean hearing loss of 12 dB, corresponding with the amount of hearing loss that is assumed to result from the mechanical changes caused by the insertion of an electrode into the cochlea (Gifford et al., 2008; Gantz et al., 2009; Podskarbi-Fayette et al., 2010). Overall, the presented findings show a significant relationship between trauma during cochlear implantation and loss of residual hearing after surgery. However, a lack of decrease in ECoG signals did not exclude hearing loss exceeding 12 dB or complete loss of residual hearing. This suggests that either postoperative mechanisms independent from cochlear trauma are responsible for postoperative hearing loss or that trauma to cochlear structures occurred but was not

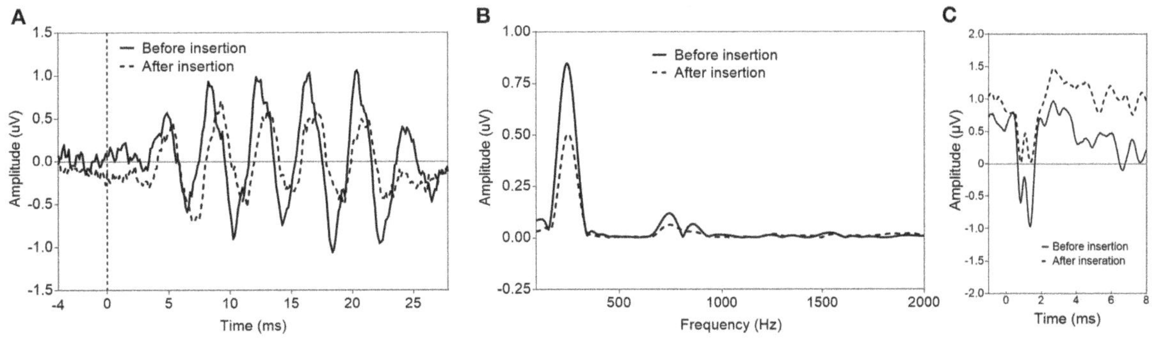

FIGURE 3 | Two examples of a decrease of ECoG signals after insertion of the CI electrode. **(A,B)** show the ECoG response (only the difference curve is shown) in response to a sinusoidal tone burst at 250 Hz, 85 dB nHL before and after insertion of the CI electrode. A decrease of the response amplitude after insertion is visible in the time waveform **(A)** and the corresponding spectrum **(B)** (S64). In S66 **(C)**, a decrease of the CAP amplitude in response to an acoustic click stimulus at 95 dB nHL was detectable after insertion of the CI electrode.

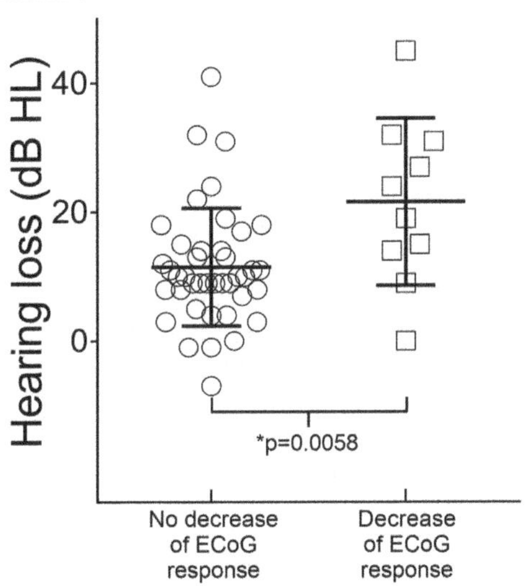

FIGURE 4 | Correlation of hearing loss 4 weeks after surgery with intraoperative ECoG findings. The mean postsurgical hearing loss was 12 dB (standard error of the mean 1.4 dB, $n = 41$) in subjects with no detectable decrease of ECoG signals after insertion of the CI electrode and 22 dB (standard error of the mean 4 dB, $n = 10$) in subjects with decrease of high- or low-frequency ECoG signals (Unpaired t-test, $p = 0.0058$).

detectable by extracochlear ECoG recordings. However, although a decrease of low-frequency ECoG signals seems to be associated with complete or almost complete loss of residual hearing in all cases, a decrease of high-frequency ECoG signals occurred without relevant postoperative hearing loss (S25, S66). In animal studies, changes in ECoG signals were also described when the inserted electrode only touched the basilar membrane but no histologically detectable trauma to cochlear structures resulted (Adunka et al., 2010). Such a mechanism could explain the decrease of high-frequency ECoG responses without relevant postoperative hearing loss.

The addition of high-frequency ECoG recordings, when responses can be detected, increases the information value of ECoG recordings regarding cochlear trauma. A decrease or loss of the high-frequency ECoG response without detectable changes in the low-frequency ECoG response (S23, S25, S37, S60, S66, S71) was associated with a mean hearing loss of 21 dB at 250, 500, and 1,000 Hz and therefore in a majority of cases—except S25 and S66—with a considerable postoperative hearing loss. Had we considered only low-frequency ECoG recordings, these insertions would have been considered atraumatic. Thus far, most studies investigating ECoG changes during cochlear implantation have focused on recordings in the low frequencies (Radeloff et al., 2012; Calloway et al., 2014; Adunka et al., 2015; Dalbert et al., 2015a,b; Campbell et al., 2016). This is an obvious choice, as most CI recipients primarily have low-frequency residual hearing and as hearing preservation is mainly attempted in the low frequencies. However, isolated trauma to high-frequency regions seems to affect hearing preservation in the low frequencies and remains undetected in low-frequency ECoG recordings. We hypothesize that such trauma limited to high-frequency regions triggers postoperative mechanisms that affect low-frequency residual hearing in the postoperative phase.

Changes of Extracochlear ECoG Responses during Insertion of the CI Electrode

The sequential extracochlear ECoG recordings during cochlear implantation showed that the previously described increase of ECoG responses (Adunka et al., 2015; Dalbert et al., 2015a,b, 2016) occurs after opening the cochlea. As discussed in a previous study (Dalbert et al., 2016), intracochlear pressure changes could explain the increase (Ruben et al., 1976). Alternatively, the increase could be caused by contact of the recording electrode with perilymph. As a consequence of this finding, future studies using extracochlear ECoG recordings should conduct baseline recordings after opening the cochlea as a decrease of ECoG signals during the following insertion could otherwise be concealed.

If a decrease of the ongoing ECoG signal occurred during the following insertion of the CI electrode, then the decrease

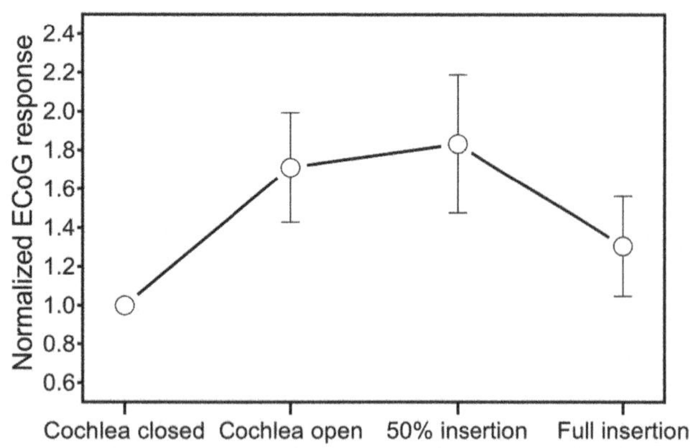

FIGURE 5 | Mean change of the ongoing ECoG signal in extracochlear ECoG recordings during insertion of the CI electrode.

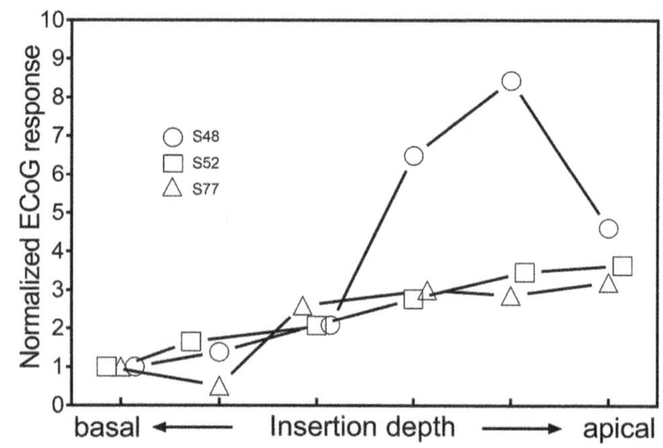

FIGURE 6 | Changes of ECoG signals in intracochlear ECoG recordings during insertion. The most apical contact of the CI electrode itself was used as recording electrode.

occurred during the second half of the insertion. As for these recordings, acoustic stimuli in the low frequencies were used, two explanations are possible: (1) Cochlear trauma during insertion of the CI electrode occurs mainly during the second half of the insertion and therefore mainly beyond the basal turn, or (2) Cochlear trauma can be detected by low-frequency ECoG recordings only when the CI electrode approaches the tonotopic regions of the acoustic stimulus.

Comparison of Extra- and Intracochlear ECoG Recordings

Extracochlear ECoG recordings are a reliable tool to assess electrophysiological changes during cochlear implantation. One distinct advantage over intracochlear ECoG recordings is that with the technique described in our study, the placement of the recording electrode remains stable for all recordings. In intracochlear ECoG recordings, the recording electrode moves along the cochlea during insertion, which itself causes a change of the ECoG signal as the relative placement toward the generators of the ECoG signals shifts.

In our study, the number of intracochlear ECoG recordings was not large enough to draw any conclusions. Nonetheless, the findings show the feasibility of this new technique for intraoperative ECoG recordings. Overall, we think intraoperative ECoG recordings using the CI electrode itself as recording electrode hold great promise for the future. The ECoG responses recorded from inside the cochlea are usually much larger and therefore more robust to background noise than extracochlear recordings (Calloway et al., 2014; Dalbert et al., 2015a). Additionally, the sometimes cumbersome placement of an extracochlear recording electrode is circumvented, which facilitates the procedure and makes widespread use in clinical practice more realistic. However, future studies have to investigate the correlation between extra- and intracochlear ECoG findings and thereby allow a more adequate interpretation of intracochlear ECoG recordings.

CONCLUSION

ECoG recordings allow for detection of electrophysiological changes in the cochlea during cochlear implantation. A decrease of extracochlear ECoG recordings has a significant correlation with hearing loss 4 weeks after surgery. Therefore, cochlear trauma detectable by extracochlear ECoG recordings seems to be associated with postoperative hearing loss. High-frequency ECoG recordings in addition to low-frequency ECoG recordings add valuable information regarding cochlear trauma. Multiple extracochlear ECoG recordings during surgery revealed a regular increase of ECoG responses after opening the cochlea. Consequently, baseline recordings for extracochlear ECoG recordings should be conducted after opening the cochlea. If a decrease of ECoG responses occurred, the decrease was detectable during the second half of the insertion of the CI electrode. This implies that trauma to cochlear structures occurs toward the end of the insertion of the CI electrode. Intracochlear ECoG recordings seem to be able to detect electrophysiological changes during cochlear implantation but further studies are needed to elucidate the implications of intraoperative findings.

AUTHOR CONTRIBUTIONS

AD was one of the leading investigators for this study, responsible for study planning, conducting recordings, data post-processing, and was the main author of manuscript. FP was responsible for study planning, conducting recordings, data post-processing, and for reviewing the manuscript. MH was responsible for conducting ECoG recordings and for data postprocessing. KK developed the technique to conduct intracochlear ECoG recordings using the cochlear implant and contributed to writing the manuscript. DV was responsible for study planning and reviewing the manuscript. CR was responsible for study planning, performing CI surgeries, and for contributing to writing the manuscript. AH was the initiator and leader of the study, he also participated in writing and reviewing the manuscript. All authors read and approved the final manuscript.

FUNDING

Forschungskredit of the University of Zurich, grant no. [FK-15-045].

ACKNOWLEDGMENTS

We would like to thank Patrick Boyle and Leo Litvak from Advanced Bionics for their continuous support throughout this project.

REFERENCES

Adunka, O. F., Giardina, C. K., Formeister, E. J., Choudhury, B., Buchman, C. A., and Fitzpatrick, D. C. (2015). Round window electrocochleography before and after cochlear implant electrode insertion. *Laryngoscope* 126, 1193–1200. doi: 10.1002/lary.25602

Adunka, O. F., Mlot, S., Suberman, T. A., Campbell, A. P., Surowitz, J., Buchman, C. A., et al. (2010). Intracochlear recordings of electrophysiological parameters indicating cochlear damage. *Otol. Neurotol.* 31, 1233–1241. doi: 10.1097/MAO.0b013e3181f1ffdf

Ahmad, F. I., Choudhury, B., De Mason, C. E., De Mason, C. E., Adunka, O. F., Finley, C. C., et al. (2012). Detection of intracochlear damage during cochlear implant electrode insertion using extracochlear measurements in the gerbil. *Laryngoscope* 122, 636–644. doi: 10.1002/lary.22488

Calloway, N. H., Fitzpatrick, D. C., Campbell, A. P., Iseli, C., Pulver, S., Buchman, C. A., et al. (2014). Intracochlear electrocochleography during cochlear implantation. *Otol. Neurotol.* 35, 1451–1457. doi: 10.1097/MAO.0000000000000451

Campbell, A. P., Suberman, T. A., Buchman, C. A., Fitzpatrick, D. C., and Adunka, O. F. (2010). Correlation of early auditory potentials and intracochlear electrode insertion properties: an animal model featuring near real-time monitoring. *Otol. Neurotol.* 31, 1391–1398. doi: 10.1097/MAO.0b013e3181f6c899

Campbell, L., Kaicer, A., Briggs, R., and O'Leary, S. (2015). Cochlear response telemetry: intracochlear electrocochleography via cochlear implant neural response telemetry pilot study results. *Otol. Neurotol.* 36, 399–405. doi: 10.1097/MAO.0000000000000678

Campbell, L., Kaicer, A., Sly, D., Iseli, C., Wei, B., and Briggs, R. (2016). Intraoperative real-time cochlear response telemetry predicts hearing preservation in cochlear implantation. *Otol. Neurotol.* 37, 332–338. doi: 10.1097/MAO.0000000000000972

Choudhury, B., Adunka, O. F., Awan, O., Pike, J. M., Buchman, C. A., and Fitzpatrick, D. C. (2014). Electrophysiologic consequences of flexible electrode insertions in gerbils with noise-induced hearing loss. *Otol. Neurotol.* 35, 519–525. doi: 10.1097/MAO.0b013e31829bdf2b

Choudhury, B., Adunka, O. F., Demason, C. E., Ahmad, F., Buchman, C. A., and Fitzpatrick, D. C. (2011). Detection of intracochlear damage with cochlear implantation in a gerbil model of hearing loss. *Otol. Neurotol.* 32, 1370–1378. doi: 10.1097/MAO.0b013e31822f09f2

Choudhury, B., Fitzpatrick, D. C., Buchman, C. A., Wei, B. P., Dillon, M. T., and He, S. (2012). Intraoperative round window recordings to acoustic stimuli from cochlear implant patients. *Otol. Neurotol.* 33, 1507–1515. doi: 10.1097/MAO.0b013e31826dbc80

Dalbert, A., Huber, A., Veraguth, D., Roosli, C., and Pfiffner, F. (2016). Assessment of cochlear trauma during cochlear implantation using electrocochleography and cone beam computed tomography. *Otol. Neurotol.* 37, 446–453. doi: 10.1097/MAO.0000000000000998

Dalbert, A., Pfiffner, F., Röösli, C., Thoele, K., Sim, J. H., and Gerig, R. (2015a). Extra- and intracochlear electrocochleography in cochlear implant recipients. *Audiol. Neurootol.* 20, 339–348. doi: 10.1159/000438742

Dalbert, A., Sim, J. H., Gerig, R., Pfiffner, F., Roosli, C., and Huber, A. (2015b). Correlation of electrophysiological properties and hearing preservation in cochlear implant patients. *Otol. Neurotol.* 36, 1172–1180. doi: 10.1097/MAO.0000000000000768

DeMason, C., Choudhury, B., Ahmad, F., Fitzpatrick, D. C., Wang, J., and Buchman, C. A. (2012). Electrophysiological properties of cochlear implantation in the gerbil using a flexible array. *Ear Hear* 33, 534–542. doi: 10.1097/AUD.0b013e3182498c28

Forgues, M., Koehn, H. A., Dunnon, A. K., Pulver, S. H., Buchman, C. A., and Adunka, O. F. (2014). Distinguishing hair cell from neural potentials recorded at the round window. *J. Neurophysiol.* 111, 580–593. doi: 10.1152/jn.00446.2013

Gantz, B. J., Hansen, M. R., Turner, C. W., Oleson, J. J., Reiss, L. A., and Parkinson, A. J. (2009). Hybrid 10 clinical trial: preliminary results. *Audiol. Neurootol.* 14(Suppl. 1), 32–38. doi: 10.1159/000206493

Gifford, R. H., Dorman, M. F., Spahr, A. J., Bacon, S. P., Skarzynski, H., and Lorens, A. (2008). Hearing preservation surgery: psychophysical estimates of cochlear damage in recipients of a short electrode array. *J. Acoust. Soc. Am.* 124, 2164–2173. doi: 10.1121/1.2967842

Koka, K., Saoji, A. A., and Litvak, L. M. (2017). Electrocochleography in cochlear implant recipients with residual hearing: comparison with audiometric thresholds. *Ear Hear.* 38, e161–e167. doi: 10.1097/AUD.0000000000000385

Mandalà, M., Colletti, L., Tonoli, G., and Colletti, V. (2012). Electrocochleography during cochlear implantation for hearing preservation. *Otolaryngol. Head Neck Surg.* 146, 774–781. doi: 10.1177/0194599811435895

Podskarbi-Fayette, R., Pilka, A., and Skarzynski, H. (2010). Electric stimulation complements functional residual hearing in partial deafness. *Acta Otolaryngol.* 130, 888–896. doi: 10.3109/00016480903567189

Radeloff, A., Shehata-Dieler, W., Scherzed, A., Rak, K., Harnisch, W., and Hagen, R. (2012). Intraoperative monitoring using cochlear microphonics in cochlear implant patients with residual hearing. *Otol. Neurotol.* 33, 348–354. doi: 10.1097/MAO.0b013e318248ea86

Ruben, R. J., Elberling, C., and Salomon, G. (1976). *In Electrocochleography.* Baltimore, MD: University Park Press.

Sellick, P., Patuzzi, R., and Robertson, D. (2003). Primary afferent and cochlear nucleus contributions to extracellular potentials during tone-bursts. *Hear. Res.* 176, 42–58. doi: 10.1016/S0378-5955(02)00716-5

2

Contralateral Inhibition of Click- and Chirp-Evoked Human Compound Action Potentials

Spencer B. Smith[1]*, Jeffery T. Lichtenhan[2] and Barbara K. Cone[1]

[1] Department of Speech, Language, and Hearing Sciences, University of Arizona, Tucson, AZ, USA, [2] Department of Otolaryngology, Washington University School of Medicine, St. Louis, MO, USA

***Correspondence:**
Spencer B. Smith
sbs1@email.arizona.edu

Cochlear outer hair cells (OHC) receive direct efferent feedback from the caudal auditory brainstem via the medial olivocochlear (MOC) bundle. This circuit provides the neural substrate for the MOC reflex, which inhibits cochlear amplifier gain and is believed to play a role in listening in noise and protection from acoustic overexposure. The human MOC reflex has been studied extensively using otoacoustic emissions (OAE) paradigms; however, these measurements are insensitive to subsequent "downstream" efferent effects on the neural ensembles that mediate hearing. In this experiment, click- and chirp-evoked auditory nerve compound action potential (CAP) amplitudes were measured electrocochleographically from the human eardrum without and with MOC reflex activation elicited by contralateral broadband noise. We hypothesized that the chirp would be a more optimal stimulus for measuring neural MOC effects because it synchronizes excitation along the entire length of the basilar membrane and thus evokes a more robust CAP than a click at low to moderate stimulus levels. Chirps produced larger CAPs than clicks at all stimulus intensities (50–80 dB ppeSPL). MOC reflex inhibition of CAPs was larger for chirps than clicks at low stimulus levels when quantified both in terms of amplitude reduction and effective attenuation. Effective attenuation was larger for chirp- and click-evoked CAPs than for click-evoked OAEs measured from the same subjects. Our results suggest that the chirp is an optimal stimulus for evoking CAPs at low stimulus intensities and for assessing MOC reflex effects on the auditory nerve. Further, our work supports previous findings that MOC reflex effects at the level of the auditory nerve are underestimated by measures of OAE inhibition.

Keywords: medial olivocochlear reflex, efferent auditory system, electrocochleography, compound action potential, chirps

INTRODUCTION

Cochlear outer hair cells (OHC) receive direct efferent feedback from the caudal auditory brainstem via the medial olivocochlear (MOC) nerve bundle. The MOC bundle inhibits OHC motility and indirectly modulates basilar membrane motion and inner hair cell (IHC) sensitivity—an effect termed the MOC reflex (Mountain, 1980; Siegel and Kim, 1982; Murugasu and Russell, 1996; Cooper and Guinan, 2003, 2006). Experiments in animal models have revealed that excitation of the MOC reflex "unmasks" signal representation in the auditory nerve by reducing mechano-electrical transduction of noise within the cochlea and therefore may play an active role in hearing in noise

(Kawase and Liberman, 1993; Kawase et al., 1993). The functional importance of the MOC reflex in human hearing, however, remains unclear.

Because otoacoustic emissions (OAEs) likely originate from mechanics associated with OHC motility (Liberman et al., 2002; Cheatham et al., 2004; Dallos et al., 2008), they are sensitive to MOC reflex-induced changes in OHC function and provide a non-invasive, albeit indirect, method to study efferent effects in humans. In the classic contralateral inhibition of OAEs paradigm, OAEs are measured without and with presentation of a contralateral acoustic stimulus (CAS; e.g., broadband noise, BBN), which activates the uncrossed MOC fibers of the reflex circuit. Magnitude and/or phase differences between OAEs recorded without and with CAS are then used to quantify MOC reflex-induced shifts in OHC function (Guinan, 2006). Such studies have quantified characteristics of human MOC reflex strength (e.g., Backus and Guinan, 2007; Marshall et al., 2014), tuning (e.g., Veuillet et al., 1991; Chéry-Croze et al., 1993; Lilaonitkul and Guinan, 2009; Zhao and Dhar, 2012), and laterality (e.g., Francis and Guinan, 2010; Garinis et al., 2011). However, OAEs are *pre-neural* measurements and are therefore less informative about the "downstream" MOC effects on IHC excitation and the subsequent neural ensembles that mediate hearing.

Few experiments have reported MOC reflex effects on evoked compound action potentials (CAPs) from the human auditory nerve (Folsom and Owsley, 1987; Kawase and Takasaka, 1995; Chabert et al., 2002; Lichtenhan et al., 2016; Najem et al., 2016). Both the dearth of research in this area and the wide range of reported inhibition with CAS (2–20 dB) may stem from technical issues related to CAP inhibition measurements. For example, OAE experiments have shown that the effect of MOC reflex inhibition on OHC activity is more potent at lower stimulus levels (e.g., Hood et al., 1996); however, clicks and tone bursts presented at these levels evoke less synchronized neural responses from a smaller population of auditory nerve fibers and therefore produce CAP waveforms with poorer morphology than higher stimulus levels. Without adequate response averaging, CAP waveforms evoked by low- to moderate-level clicks or tone bursts are highly variable with poor signal-to-noise ratios and "true" physiologic changes attributable to the MOC reflex (i.e., reduction in CAP amplitude) are difficult to separate from measurement variation.

Stimuli evoking more robust CAP responses than clicks or tone bursts, such as rising frequency chirps, may circumvent some of the technical issues related to neural MOC reflex measurements. Unlike a click, which initiates synchronized responses predominately from more basal auditory nerve fibers (Kiang, 1975; Abdala and Folsom, 1995), chirps synchronize auditory nerve fiber excitation along the length of the cochlear spiral by correcting for temporal delays associated with tonotopicity (Shore and Nuttall, 1985; Fobel and Dau, 2004). Recently, Chertoff et al. (2010) demonstrated that chirps optimized for eliciting human CAPs produced significantly larger amplitudes than those evoked by clicks in young, normal-hearing adults at moderate to high stimulus levels (75–125 pSPL). The improved signal-to-noise ratio of chirp-evoked CAPs, compared to those from clicks, may thus provide a higher fidelity response to assay CAS-induced MOC reflex effects on the auditory nerve. Additionally, MOC fibers innervate the length of the cochlear spiral with tuning similar to afferent auditory nerve fibers (Warr, 1992). Chirp-evoked CAPs may therefore be more sensitive to the summed CAS-induced MOC reflex effects along the entire length of the cochlea and thus show greater inhibition than click-evoked CAPs.

In this experiment, we tested two hypotheses: (1) That chirps evoke larger CAP amplitudes than clicks using low to moderate stimulus levels, which engage the cochlear amplifier and are thus more sensitive to MOC effects and (2) That MOC reflex inhibition of chirp-evoked CAPs is larger than for click-evoked CAPs due to the broader basilar membrane area represented in chirp responses. To relate our findings to more commonly used MOC reflex assays, we also compared average chirp- and click-evoked CAP inhibition to click evoked OAE (CEOAE) inhibition measured in the same subjects.

METHODS

Participants

The University of Arizona Human Subjects Protection Program approved the following methods which were carried out with written, informed consent from all subjects. Eighteen adult participants without history of neurologic or otologic disease were enrolled in the study; however, due to attrition, 14 subjects (average age 22.25 years; 10 females) completed all six testing sessions. Otoscopy examinations found that all ear canals were free of excess cerumen and that tympanic membranes (TMs) appeared healthy in all subjects. Participants had normal tympanograms bilaterally, defined as ear canal volume of 0.6–1.5 cc and peak-compensated static admittance between 0.3 and 1.4 mL (Margolis and Heller, 1987), and contralateral acoustic reflex thresholds to 1–10 kHz BBN $\geq$70 dB SPL, measured using conventional admittance methods (Sun, 2008). The latter requirement was to mitigate the possible involvement of middle ear muscle contractions during MOC inhibition measurements, although others have shown that acoustic reflex thresholds can be lower when measured using more sensitive techniques (e.g., Zhao and Dhar, 2010; Lichtenhan et al., 2016). Air conduction hearing thresholds from 0.25 to 8 kHz were within normal limits ($\leq$25 dB HL) bilaterally for all subjects.

Equipment and Procedures

Stimulus Generation and Calibration

A 100-μs click and 10-ms chirp were used to evoke CAPs. The click was created using the Intelligent Hearing Systems Smart-EP stimulus generator (Intelligent Hearing Systems, Miami, FL). The chirp was created in WAV file format in MATLAB (The Mathworks, Inc., Natick, MA, USA) using a modified "O-Chirp" from Fobel and Dau (2004), as implemented by Chertoff et al. (2010). The O-Chirp is a flat-spectrum stimulus relating frequency to basilar membrane delay using parameters from stimulus frequency OAEs. To optimize the O-Chirp for evoking CAPs, forward traveling wave delays were estimated from Eggermont's (1979) derived-band CAP latencies as opposed to stimulus frequency OAEs. The relationship between basilar membrane delay in milliseconds and frequency was expressed as:

$$\tau_{BM} = c^* f^{\alpha}$$

where 0.45 kHz $\leq f \leq$ 10 kHz and c (0.69) and α (−77) are constants. The chirp WAV file was converted into a stimulus file suitable for presentation by the Intelligent Hearing Systems Smart-EP program.

The click and chirp were presented through ER-3A insert earphones (Etymotic Research, Elk Grove Village, IL) to a 2-cc coupler and calibrated in units of *dB peak-to-peak equivalent sound pressure level* (ppeSPL) using a 1,000 Hz tone as a reference (Burkard, 2006). Click and chirp spectra were comparable with the exception that the chirp had 3–5 dB less energy below ~3.5–4 kHz (see Chertoff et al., 2010, **Figure 1**).

Behavioral thresholds for clicks and chirps were obtained from the right ears of 18 subjects using a modified Hughson-Westlake procedure. Stimuli were presented at a starting presentation level of 50 dB ppeSPL. Presentation level was decreased by 4 dB after every positive response and increased by 2 dB after each failure to respond. Threshold was defined as the lowest presentation level at which three positive responses occurred. These measurements were made without electrodes in the ear canal, as our previous work demonstrated that TM electrode contact with the eardrum can influence audiometric thresholds, particularly to low frequencies (Smith et al., 2016). Average behavioral thresholds were 32 dB ppeSPL and 30 dB ppeSPL for clicks and chirps, respectively. While we express stimulus levels in units of dB ppeSPL throughout this paper, behavioral thresholds to clicks and chirps can be subtracted from these values to convert from dB ppeSPL to normalized hearing level (nHL).

Tympanic Membrane Electrodes

Using a modified protocol by Ferraro and Durrant (2006), we assembled TM electrodes in our laboratory that were suitable for our evoked potentials recording system. The electrodes were constructed from 11.43-cm long sections of PFA-insulated silver wire (0.1 mm gauge) encased in 10.16-cm long pieces of flexible silastic medical tubing. The PFA-insulation was removed from the last 0.635 cm of each end of the wire. One uninsulated end was crimped with a female machine pin that was connected to an electrode cable interfacing with the bio-amplifier. The other uninsulated end was bent to form a hook around a 0.25 gram wisp of cotton, and the end of the hook was tucked back into the opening of the silastic medical tubing to ensure that it did not directly make contact with the eardrum when it was inserted. Prior to each recording session, the cotton-tipped end of a TM electrode was saturated with 1-cc of Synapse electrode cream (Kustomer Kinetics, Arcadia, CA) using a 27-gauge needle. TM electrodes were inserted into the right ear canal of each subject and advanced until the TM was contacted, which was verified by subject report of the occlusion effect and by monitoring electrode impedance changes until they were consistently ≤7 kΩ on the Intelligent Hearing Systems bio-amplifier (Ferraro, 2010). Further confirmation of electrode contact with the TM was indicated by areas of acute redness and accumulation of electrode gel observed otoscopically after TM electrodes were removed at the end of each testing session (see Smith et al., 2016, **Figure 1**). Each electrode was held in place throughout the session by a 13 mm ER3-14A foam ear tip coupled to the ER-3A insert earphone.

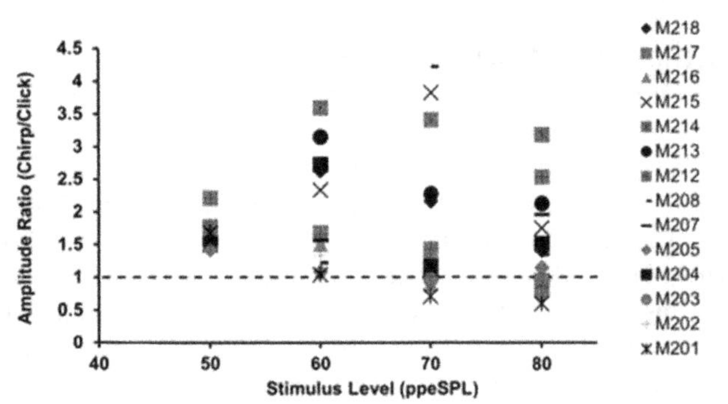

FIGURE 1 | Chirp-to-click CAP amplitude ratios for waveforms obtained without CAS. Each symbol represents a single subject. Symbols falling above the dotted line indicate larger chirp responses than clicks.

CAP Measurements and Amplitude Calculations

Each subject participated in six 2-h CAP recording sessions—three in which clicks were used to evoke CAPs and three in which chirps were used. The order in which subjects participated in click or chirp sessions was randomized. In every session, subjects were comfortably reclined in a lounge chair in an electromagnetically shielded sound booth and remained awake and alert throughout recordings. CAPs were acquired using a single-channel electrode montage: right TM electrode (+), left earlobe (−), and forehead (≟). Waveforms were sampled at a rate of 40 kHz over a 25.6 ms epoch, filtered from 0.1 to 3 kHz, and amplified by 150,000. Stimulus presentation rate was Gaussian distributed from 9.1/s to 13.1/s with a mean rate of 11.1/s. This relatively slow range of presentation rates was selected to ensure that the *stimuli* did not temporally summate to activate the MOC reflex, which has been shown to affect OAE measurements at stimulus presentation rates as low as 30/s–50/s (Veuillet et al., 1991; Francis and Guinan, 2010; Boothalingam and Purcell, 2015). A Gaussian-distributed (i.e., "temporally jittered") presentation rate was selected to facilitate subject alertness, as this may influence MOC reflex strength (Aedo et al., 2015).

CAP level-series measurements without and with CAS (1–10 kHz flat spectrum BBN at 60 dB SPL, delivered to left ears through an ER-2 earphone) were interleaved throughout the duration of each 2-h session with the exception that the first 20 min of the sixth session was devoted to CEOAE measurements (described in Section CEOAE Measurements). A 60 dB SPL CAS presentation level is commonly used for MOC reflex experiments, as it is the highest BBN level, on average, that elicits MOC reflex activity without triggering the middle ear muscle reflex (Guinan, 2006). CAP level-series were obtained using a chained stimulus paradigm (Hamill et al., 1991), which randomized stimulus levels from 50 to 80 dB ppeSPL using 10 dB steps. Each of the interleaved recording blocks automatically stopped after 2,048 averages were collected at each of the four stimulus levels and a 120 s break was inserted between each interleaved trial to allow subjects to reposition, etc. Advantages of using the chained paradigm in this context were that complete level-series functions could be obtained relatively quickly (~12 min) in a single testing block and that the effects of electrophysiologic or myogenic noise were randomly distributed across responses to all stimulus levels as opposed to one. In a typical recording session, three to four pairs of level-series functions without and with noise were obtained and averaged at the end of the session. Each recording session thus resulted in eight grand average waveforms (2 conditions × 4 stimulus levels) with each grand average waveform being comprised of ~6,144–8,192 sweeps. At the end of six recording sessions, there were 48 waveforms (2 conditions × 4 stimulus levels × 2 stimulus types × 3 sessions) for each subject.

The 48 CAP waveforms for each subject were saved as ASCII files and analyzed offline in MATLAB. CAP waveforms were grouped based on stimulus type (click or chirp), level (50–80 dB ppeSPL), and whether they were obtained without or with CAS. CAP amplitudes for each waveform were expressed in two different ways: (1) ***Raw amplitude*** was calculated as the μV difference between the pre-stimulus baseline average amplitude and the N1 peak, which was automatically selected as the largest waveform minimum within a restricted time epoch at each level based on normative click and chirp latency data from our laboratory. Responses were "not present" if the raw amplitude of a peak was less than one standard deviation of the pre-stimulus baseline amplitude. (2) ***Normalized amplitude*** expressed each CAP peak magnitude as a percentage of the maximum raw amplitude (either without or with CAS) in the level-series in which it was acquired:

$$\text{Normalized Amplitude} = \left(\frac{\text{Raw CAP Amplitude (uV)}}{\text{Single Session Level Series Maximum Amplitude (uV)}}\right) \times 100$$

Treating the data in this manner produced normalized level-series functions for each subject at the end of each recording session. We hypothesized two advantages to this approach. First, normalizing data obtained in each recording session would be expected to minimize differences in raw CAP amplitudes within subjects that were due to changes in electrode placement or orientation in the ear canal between visits, which can significantly influence raw amplitudes (e.g., Alhanada, 2012). Second, a normalized scale would be expected to make level-series functions between subjects more similar; because we analyzed group data in this experiment, it was imperative to reduce the effects of inter-subject differences in raw amplitude on our results.

CEOAE Measurements

Three pairs of CEOAE level-series functions (60-80 ppeSPL[1]) without and with CAS were obtained using a Mimosa Acoustics HearID System (Mimosa Acoustics, Inc. Champaign, IL). Responses were collected using "linear" clicks (i.e., consistent stimulus polarity and level across all presentations) presented at 11/s for 250 sweeps in each trial. CEOAEs were considered present if they were ≥6 dB above the noise floor and if emission waveform sub-averages from response bins A and B were ≥80% correlated. CEOAE files were saved and offline analyzed in MATLAB, which extracted the composite values representing total emission amplitude and noise floors for each level and CAS condition. All response amplitudes were converted from dB to a pressure scale in order express CEOAE level-series on a linear ordinate scale, as was done with CAPs.

Analyses

Chirp-to-Click CAP Amplitude Ratios and Amplitude Comparisons

Chirp-to-click CAP amplitude ratios were calculated for each stimulus level using grand-averaged chirp and click *raw amplitudes* obtained without CAS for each subject. The purpose of this analysis was to determine the relative amplitude advantage of the chirp at each stimulus level. Paired *t*-test comparisons between chirp and click raw amplitudes without CAS at each level were also conducted.

CAP Inhibition Measurements: Amplitude Reduction and Effective Attenuation

The first step in testing the hypothesis that chirp-evoked CAPs were more sensitive to MOC reflex inhibition than clicks was to determine whether level-series functions were less variable when expressed either in units of *raw amplitude* or *normalized amplitude*. While we expected that normalizing amplitudes for each recording session would decrease between-subject CAP amplitude variability and provide a better scale on which to analyze group data, this was tested empirically. Coefficients of variation, which allow for variability comparisons between data sets with different units (e.g., μV vs. %), were calculated at each level and compared for raw and normalized level-series functions for each stimulus type. The amplitude scale producing the smallest coefficients of variation at each stimulus level and across all stimulus levels was used in subsequent analyses of CAP inhibition under the assumption that the less variable scale would be more sensitive to "true" physiologic changes induced by the MOC reflex.

Group CAP inhibition for chirps and clicks was quantified using two measures reported in the literature: (1) ***Amplitude reduction*** was calculated as the average "vertical" (ordinate) difference in CAP amplitudes without and with CAS at each level of the level-series function. This method of quantifying MOC reflex strength is most commonly used in the OAE inhibition literature; (2) ***Effective attenuation*** of chirp and click CAPs was calculated as the "horizontal" (abscissa) difference between linear regression fits to level-series without and with CAS using all subject data. Effective attenuation expresses the amount of dB that the *stimulus* would need to be increased to overcome the effects of MOC reflex inhibition; it is therefore useful in quantifying inhibition in terms of input level, which allows for gross comparisons of pre-neural and neural responses on the same scale (e.g., Puria et al., 1996).

[1]CEOAE responses to clicks at 50 dB ppeSPL were absent in most subjects based on our criteria; therefore, CEOAE level-series measurements were made from 60 to 80 dB ppeSPL.

RESULTS

Amplitude Differences between Chirp- and Click- Evoked CAPs

With few exceptions, chirps produced larger raw peak amplitudes than clicks in individual ears, as evidenced by chirp-to-click CAP amplitude ratios (**Figure 1**). The size of the chirp/click amplitude ratio differed between subjects and showed a range of 0.76–4.22 across all stimulus levels. For most participants, the amplitude ratios decreased slightly as level was increased. Note that click-evoked responses at 50 dB ppeSPL were separable from the noise floor in all three test sessions in only 9 of the 14 participants; thus, amplitude ratios were calculated for only 9 participants at this level.

The mean *raw amplitudes* of chirp-evoked CAPs without CAS were larger than those for clicks at each level tested (**Figure 2**). Paired *t*-tests with Bonferroni corrections for multiple comparisons ($\alpha = 0.0125$) revealed that these differences were significant at 50 [$t_{(8)} = -2.85$, $p = 0.008$], 60 [$t_{(13)} = -7.19$, $p = 0.0009$], 70 [$t_{(13)} = -4.28$, $p = 0.001$], and 80 dB ppeSPL [$t_{(13)} = -2.57$, $p = 0.007$].

CAP Inhibition

Representative chirp- and click-evoked CAP waveforms without and with CAS from a randomly selected participant are plotted in **Figure 3**. This figure demonstrates three pertinent observations that were noted in most subjects including: (1) the overall amplitude advantage of chirps, especially at lower stimulus levels, (2) the small reductions in chirp- and click-evoked CAP amplitudes with CAS, and (3) the stability of pre-stimulus baselines prior to the N1 peak of the CAP.

Figure 4 displays chirp and click average level-series functions across all subjects and sessions without and with CAS. Level-series functions are expressed in both normalized and raw amplitudes for each stimulus type. For chirps, the average coefficient of variation across four stimulus levels and two noise conditions was 45% when expressed in raw amplitude and 20% when expressed in normalized amplitude; this mean difference was significant [$t_{(14)} = 3.46$, $p = 0.0038$]. For clicks, the average coefficient of variation was 47% when expressed in raw amplitude and 29% when expressed in normalized amplitude, which was also a significant mean difference [$t_{(14)} = 2.86$, $p = 0.013$]. Thus, we used the less-variable measurements expressed in *normalized amplitude* for subsequent MOC reflex inhibition of CAP analyses.

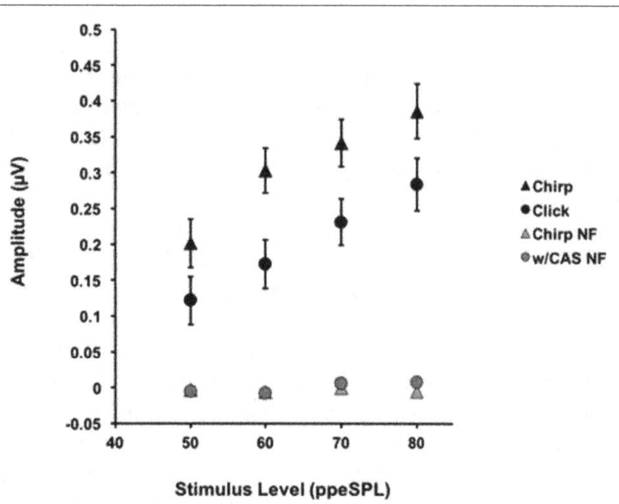

FIGURE 2 | The average amplitudes for CAPs in response to chirps (▲) and clicks (●) without CAS are shown as a function of level. Chirp raw amplitudes were significantly larger than click raw amplitudes at every level using a corrected alpha level for multiple comparisons ($\alpha = 0.0125$). Error bars = SEM; NF = Noise Floor.

Normalized CAP Amplitude Reductions

Average normalized amplitude inhibitions were largest for stimulus levels below 80 dB ppeSPL for both chirps and clicks (**Figure 5**). Normalized amplitude reduction with CAS was statistically significant only for chirp-evoked responses at 50 [$t_{(30)} = 3.55$, $p = 0.0006$] and 60 dB ppeSPL [$t_{(38)} = 4.18$, $p < 0.0001$], respectively, using an alpha level ($\alpha = 0.0125$) to account for multiple comparisons.

CAP Effective Attenuation

Separate linear regression models were fit to the normalized group level-series data[2] obtained without and with CAS for chirps ($y = 1.33x–11.96$, $R^2 = 0.47$; $y = 1.59x–33.22$, $R^2 = 0.57$) and clicks ($y = 1.77x–50.13$, $R^2 = 0.51$; $y = 1.86x–60.75$, $R^2 = 0.54$), respectively (**Figures 6A,B**). For both stimulus types, the models fit to CAP amplitudes without and with CAS diverged at low stimulus input levels and converged at higher stimulus input levels, indicating a greater effect of CAS on CAP amplitudes at low input levels. Regression coefficients as a function of condition (without or with CAS) were not significantly different for chirps ($t = 1.63$, $p = 0.103$) or clicks ($t = 0.45$, $p = 0.66$). Effective attenuation for each stimulus type was calculated as the difference in the abscissa between without and with CAS linear regression lines for equivalent ordinate values (**Figure 6D**). At the lowest stimulus level, effective attenuation was 5.07 dB for chirps and 3.02 dB for clicks (**Figure 6D**).

Comparison of CAP and CEOAE Effective Attenuation

Based on our findings that CAP amplitudes were less variable when expressed on a normalized scale (see Section CAP Inhibition), we only report CEOAE inhibition in terms of effective attenuation of normalized responses in the present experiment for comparison. CEOAE normalized level-series data from all subjects obtained without ($y = 2.84x–131.42$, $R^2 = 0.78$) and with CAS ($y = 2.92x–141.87$, $R^2 = 0.80$) were also fit with separate linear regression models (**Figure 6C**). The CEOAE models were better fit than CAP data, as normalized CEOAE amplitudes were less variable across subjects. The largest differences in without and with CAS models occurred at the lowest input level, as was observed in the CAP data. Regression

[2]Note that while normalizing CAP amplitudes to the maximum value in a subject's level-series function reduced amplitude variation across all levels, it also introduced heteroscedasticity; therefore, robust standard errors were used for each regression model, which allowed for the presence of heteroskedastic data by relaxing the assumptions that errors were independent and identically distributed (Hayes and Cai, 2007).

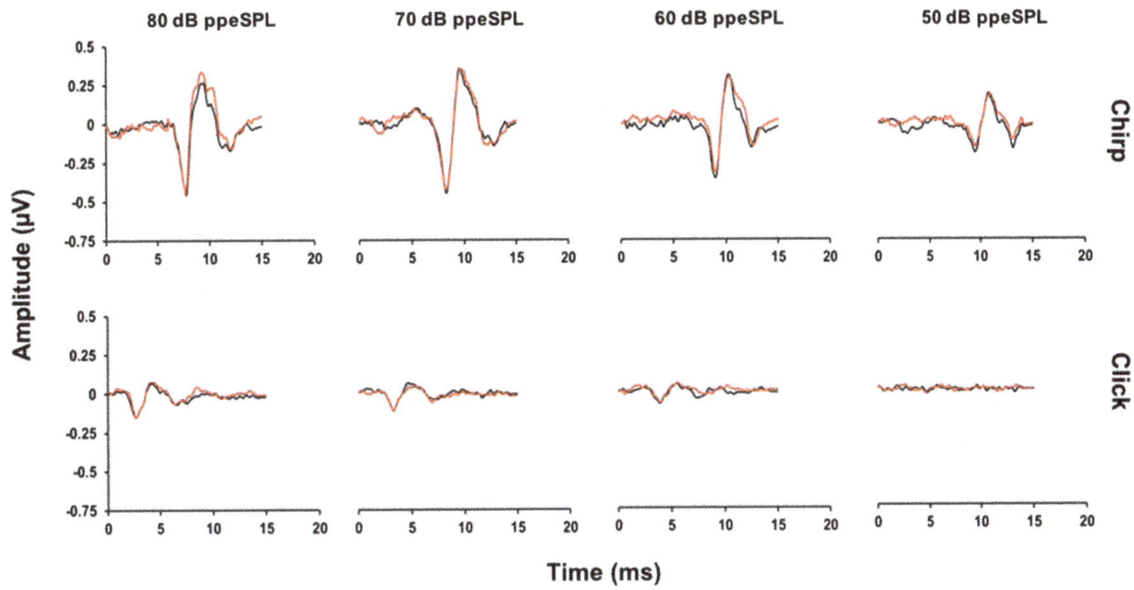

FIGURE 3 | Average CAP waveforms evoked by chirps (top) and clicks **(bottom)** for a representative subject. Small reductions in N1 peak amplitudes with CAS can be seen in the chirp-evoked CAP waveforms at lower stimulus levels, but not for the click at any level. Note that at 50 dB ppeSPL, a click-evoked CAP was not identified in this subject (Black = without CAS; Red = with CAS).

coefficients as a function of condition (without or with CAS) were not significantly different ($t = 0.43$, $p = 0.67$). Effective attenuation was calculated in the same manner as the CAP data. A comparison of chirp-evoked CAP, click-evoked CAP, and CEOAE effective attenuations at 60 dB ppeSPL revealed that inhibition was largest for chirps (3.42 dB), followed by click CAPs (2.49 dB) and CEOAEs (1.93 dB).

GENERAL DISCUSSION

The findings of this study were that: (1) Chirps evoked larger CAP amplitudes than clicks at low to moderate stimulus levels; (2) Normalized CAP amplitude reductions with CAS were largest at the group level using chirps at 50 and 60 dB ppeSPL (5.89 and 7.75%, respectively). These were the only statistically significant amplitude reductions observed; (3) Effective attenuation measurements were largest at the group level for chirp-evoked CAPs followed by click-evoked CAPs and CEOAEs, respectively, at the lowest stimulus levels where all three could be measured (i.e., 60 dB ppeSPL).

The Chirp Advantage

The chirp generated larger CAP amplitudes at each stimulus level in most subjects; however, the size of this advantage varied considerably across subjects. This finding is consistent with the observations of Chertoff et al. (2010; see **Figure 3**) who used higher presentation levels than the present study. Inter-subject differences in the chirp advantage may be related to multiple factors. First, the chirp used in the present study and by Chertoff et al. (2010) related frequency to basilar membrane delay using derived band CAP latencies from 15 normally hearing subjects reported by Eggermont (1979). Subject characteristics, such as sex, were not reported in that study, but it has been inferred that sex differences in cochlear length may affect basilar membrane delays and therefore the degree to which neural responses are synchronized (e.g., Don et al., 1993, 1994). With the current participant pool of 10 females and 4 males, it is possible that the chirp was not optimized for individual ears based on these differences. One way to quickly construct a CAP chirp that is more optimized for an individual ear than a click may be to use basilar membrane delay estimates from OAEs, as derived-band CAP masking procedures are time consuming. Secondly, some authors have encouraged the use of chirps that are optimized for different presentation levels (Elberling and Don, 2010; Elberling et al., 2010; Kristensen and Elberling, 2012), suggesting that cochlear frequency place maps do not scale simply with level. Our use of a chained stimulus paradigm, which allows for random level presentation of a *single* stimulus file, did not provide the flexibility to use multiple chirps optimized for different levels in this investigation.

The chirp advantage reported here and by Chertoff et al. (2010) suggests that chirps may also be a useful tool in studying animal and human synaptopathy—a pathology in which noise exposure predominately insults high threshold auditory nerve fibers but spares low threshold fibers and hair cells (Kujawa and Liberman, 2009). Synaptopathy has been postulated as the basis of severe hearing difficulties in patients with normal audiograms (i.e., "hidden hearing loss") and may also be involved in the generation of tinnitus (e.g., Schaette and McAlpine, 2011). The synaptopathy "phenotype" in animal models presents as significantly reduced CAP amplitudes evoked by suprathreshold sounds in the presence of normal

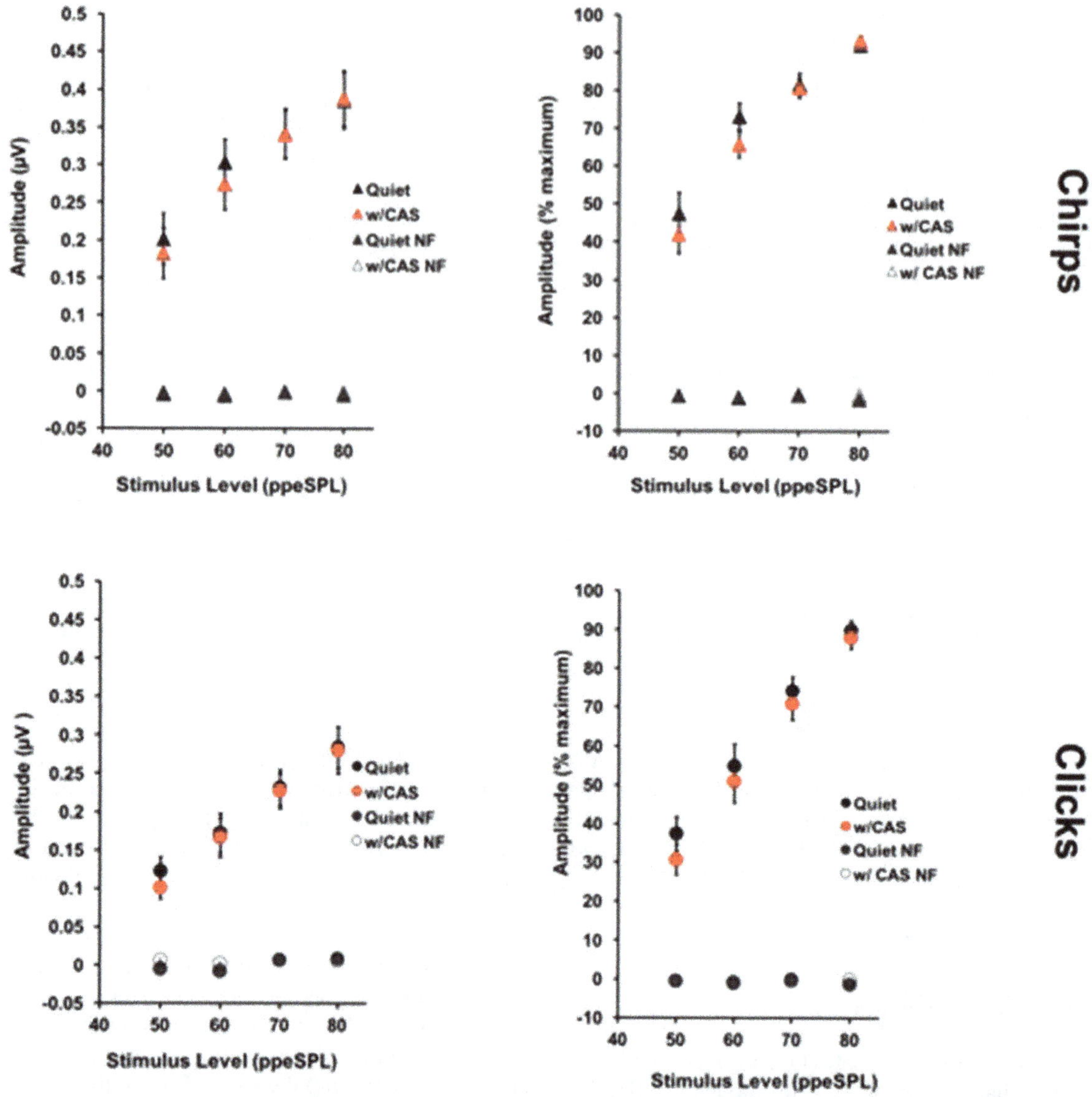

FIGURE 4 | Average level-series functions for chirps (top) and clicks **(bottom)** expressed in raw **(left)** and normalized **(right)** amplitudes. Response variability was smaller across all subjects when amplitudes were expressed on a normalized scale. Error Bars = SEM; NF = Noise Floor.

(electrophysiologic) audiometric thresholds and OAE responses. Because chirp-evoked CAPs are larger and represent the summed activity from auditory nerve fibers along the length of the basilar membrane, they may provide a more sensitive measure of synaptopathy. Further, narrowband chirps tailored to evoke CAPs may be even more sensitive to synaptopathy in distinct cochlear regions.

MOC Reflex Effects on CAPs

Our findings suggest that chirps may be more suitable than clicks in studying the neural consequences of MOC reflex inhibition for a few reasons. First, chirp-evoked CAPs were larger than clicks even at the lowest stimulus level, which allowed for more accurate N1 peak identification in quiet and with CAS conditions (e.g., compare 60 dB ppeSPL waveforms for chirps and clicks in **Figure 3**). Since OHCs are more potently inhibited by the MOC reflex at low input levels, using a chirp may allow for more accurate estimates of MOC effects in this range. Because chirp-evoked CAPs reflect the summed activity over broader cochlear regions, they may also be more sensitive to the summated effects of MOC fibers than click-evoked CAPs, which mainly reflect neural synchrony from fibers innervating the cochlear base (Don and Eggermont, 1978). Second, the variability of CAP inhibition for chirps was smaller relative to clicks on both amplitude reduction and effective attenuation measurement scales (**Figures 5, 6A,B**). This finding suggests that chirps may be more sensitive to "true" physiologic changes attributable to MOC reflex activation than clicks. It is important to note, however, that chirp and click CAP effective attenuation was calculated from relatively weak linear regression fits to *group* data, which may

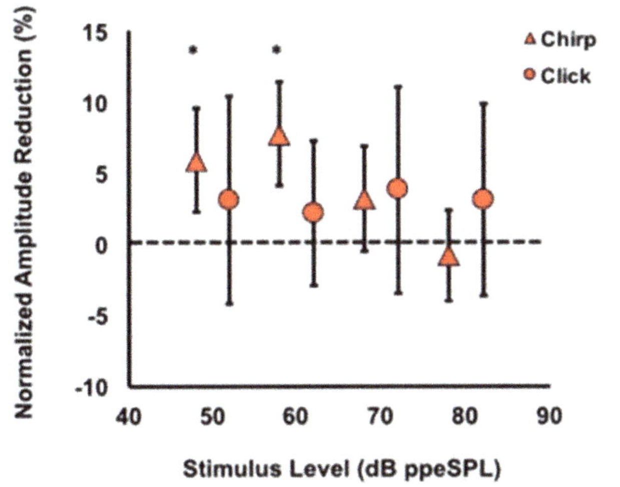

FIGURE 5 | Average normalized chirp and click amplitude reductions for all subjects. Asterisks indicate significant reductions ($p < 0.01$). Note that at every stimulus level, chirp inhibition was less variable than clicks, as indicated by the 95% confidence interval bars.

have been caused by individual differences in both level-series function contours and magnitude of inhibition. An analysis of individual data using the same method resulted in even poorer linear fits due to the fewer data points in the models. Thus, a limitation of our work is that we were unable to reliably resolve efferent inhibition of CAPs at the single-subject level, which is of interest in studying individual variation in MOC function and in understanding the predictive relationships between pre-neural and neural efferent assays. This issue may have been resolved by focusing recording time on obtaining more response averages to fewer low-intensity input levels (Lichtenhan et al., 2016); however, an advantage of acquiring a level-series function spanning 40 dB was that CAS effects on CAPs evoked by different stimulus levels could be evaluated.

Involvement of the middle ear muscle reflex is always a consideration in MOC reflex experiments, as CAS can activate both mechanisms. The observed CAP amplitude reductions with CAS were unlikely to be the consequence of "sub-threshold" middle ear compliance changes from activation of the middle ear acoustic reflex because such a change would be expected to reduce responses to *all* input levels of the level-series function. In contrast, the CAS-induced changes in our data were primarily at low input levels, which is suggestive of changes in OHC function. Nevertheless, the possibility of middle ear muscle involvement cannot be fully ruled out, as some reports indicate that standard measures of acoustic reflex threshold, like the one used in our screening protocol, may overestimate the level at which the stapedius muscle is activated by CAS (Feeney and Keefe, 2001; Zhao and Dhar, 2010).

CEOAE and CAP Effective Attenuation Comparisons

OAE measurements are used far more often as an indirect assay of MOC reflex effects than CAP amplitudes, as they require less time to collect and are less inherently variable than electrophysiologic techniques (see **Figure 6**). This difference is presumably because far-field CAP recordings are influenced by more sources of noise (e.g., background EEG, myogenic and electrical noise, high electrode impedance due to small surface area) than OAEs. Based on these technical differences, a compelling argument can be made for using OAE based assays of the MOC reflex in a clinical setting, for example. It is, however, of great importance to understand the relationships between pre-neural and neural inhibition because the latter reflects modulation of the auditory nerve signal mediating hearing, which cannot be assessed with OAEs. Pre-neural and neural inhibition comparisons must be made in light of evidence that there is not a one-to-one correspondence between changes in OHC function and modulation of IHC neurotransmitter release, which is the basis for auditory nerve fiber depolarization (Guinan, 2012). However, by expressing CEOAE and CAP inhibition in terms of effective attenuation, direct comparisons can be made between MOC reflex effects on each type of response.

Our observation that CEOAE effective attenuation *underestimated* chirp- and click-evoked CAP effective attenuation by up to ~1.5 dB at low stimulus levels was consistent with previous reports in animals and humans (e.g., Puria et al., 1996; Lichtenhan et al., 2016). The source of this consistently reported discrepancy is not clear. OHCs are postsynaptic only to MOC fibers, whereas the auditory nerve is postsynaptic to both MOC and lateral olivocochlear (LOC) fibers, which directly contact type I auditory nerve fibers (Warr and Guinan, 1979). This anatomical configuration suggests that CAP inhibition reflects the summation of MOC and LOC inhibition, whereas OAEs only reflect MOC inhibition. However, several lines of evidence appear to refute this suggestion. Gifford and Guinan (1987) measured CAP inhibition from cats while electrically stimulating different regions of the caudal brainstem. They observed that stimulating the floor of the fourth ventricle (which diffusely activates the OCB proper) is comparable to the combined inhibitory effects of directly stimulating MOC neurons. When LOC neurons were directly stimulated, no inhibitory effects on the CAP were observed. The investigators also documented that increases in cochlear microphonic amplitude were related to decreases in CAP amplitude during OCB stimulation, indicating that the same process (i.e., direct modulation of OHCs) likely mediates each effect. Brown et al. (1983) measured IHC receptor potential tuning curves (from the AC component) with and without fourth ventricle electrical stimulation and observed 9–24 dB of inhibition at the tuning curve "tips" (i.e., center frequency) with no change away from center frequencies. Basilar membrane displacement tuning curves show similar effects (Murugasu and Russell, 1996; Cooper and Guinan, 2003). While these measurements are pre-neural, they are remarkably similar to auditory nerve tuning curves using the same paradigm (Wiederhold and Kiang, 1970; Bonfils et al., 1986). Thus, there is strong evidence that the MOC system is the main effector of inhibition in both *pre-neural* and *neural* assays. In contrast,

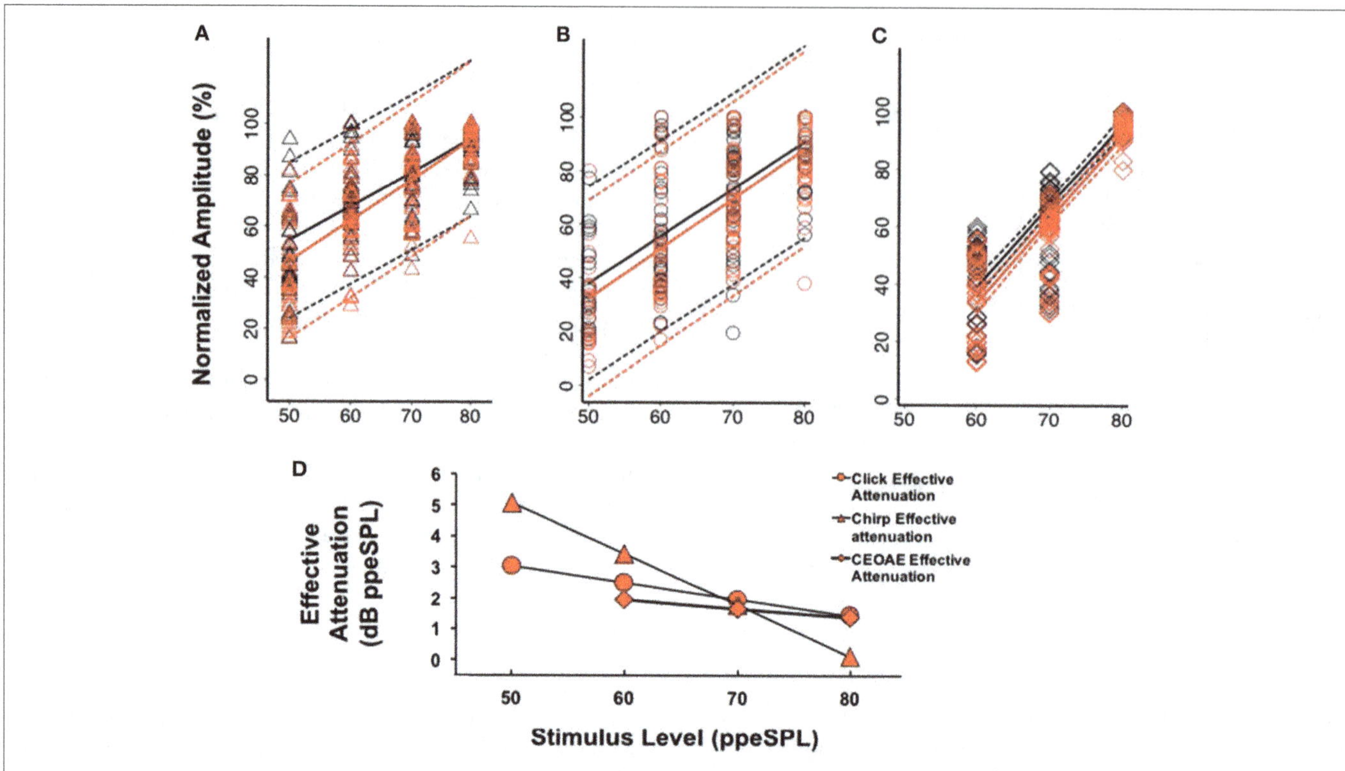

FIGURE 6 | Linear regression fits (with 95% CIs) to normalized chirp CAP (A), click CAP **(B)**, and CEOAE **(C)** level-series functions. Effective attenuation **(D)** was calculated as the abscissa (horizontal) difference between linear fits to without and with CAS group data.

there is no evidence that the LOC system can be excited with acoustic stimulation and its role in hearing remains poorly understood. The best available evidence suggests that the LOC system's influence on hearing is likely through slow "top-down" potentiation of auditory nerve activity (Sahley and Nodar, 1994; Groff and Liberman, 2003; Le Prell et al., 2005), which may protect auditory nerve fibers from acoustic trauma (e.g., Darrow et al., 2007).

If the MOC reflex accounts for inhibition measured from both OHCs and the auditory nerve, it may be expected that effective attenuation slopes of CEOAEs and CAPs would be parallel. We observed at the group level that the slopes of click CAP and CEOAE effective attenuation were similar to each other and quite different than chirp CAP effective attenuation (**Figure 6D**). Because we did not measure chirp-evoked OAEs, it is unclear if this difference is stimulus related or explained by some other mechanism. The temporal differences between clicks and chirps make the chirp a better stimulus for evoking synchronized *neural* responses, but these differences would not be expected to produce significantly dissimilar composite emission amplitudes evoked by each stimulus. Previous work has indicated that stimulus frequency OAEs (SFOAEs) and CEOAEs are generated in a nearly equivalent manner through coherent reflection when the spectral power within a bandwidth on the basilar membrane is equal (Neumann et al., 1994; Kalluri and Shera, 2007); if a chirp is conceptualized as a swept SFOAE, the effect of MOC reflex inhibition on chirp-evoked OAEs and CEOAEs would be expected to be similar. To our knowledge, there have been no experiments comparing MOC reflex inhibition of click- and chirp-evoked OAEs; therefore, the origin of the differences in effective attenuation slopes between chirp-evoked CAPs and pre-neural and neural measurements evoked with clicks in the group data is not clear.

CONCLUSIONS

The present study is the first in which a chirp was used to evoke CAPs from the human auditory nerve with and without MOC reflex activation. Our findings indicate that, at least at the group level, the chirp may be a more sensitive stimulus for evaluating *neural* efferent effects than a click because it evokes a larger response at lower stimulus intensities and may be more sensitive to summed efferent activity along the cochlear spiral. Additionally, our findings are consistent with previous work indicating that OAE assays of the MOC reflex underestimate neural inhibition (i.e., Puria et al., 1996; Lichtenhan et al., 2016). Future experiments which optimize chirp parameters for individual ears and allow for reliable within-subject neural measurements of MOC reflex inhibition are warranted.

AUTHOR CONTRIBUTIONS

SS developed the study, collected data, and ran analyses. JL supplied the script for generating the chirp stimulus and contributed to the theoretical development of the study. BC was also instrumental in study design and data analysis.

FUNDING

Financial disclosures: This research was funded by the National Institutes of Health, National Institute on Deafness and other Communication Disorders (F30 DC01418 and R01 DC014997).

REFERENCES

Abdala, C., and Folsom, R. C. (1995). Frequency contribution to the click-evoked auditory brain-stem response in human adults and infants. *J. Acoust. Soc. Am.* 97, 2394–2404. doi: 10.1121/1.411961

Aedo, C., Tapia, E., Pavez, E., Elgueda, D., Delano, P. H., and Robles, L. (2015). Stronger efferent suppression of cochlear neural potentials by contralateral acoustic stimulation in awake than in anesthetized chinchilla. *Front. Syst. Neurosci.* 9:21. doi: 10.3389/fnsys.2015.00021

Alhanada, M. R. (2012). *Electrocochleographic Recordings from the Eardrum: Variations and Effects of Electrode Location in Normal Subjects.* Doctoral dissertation, University of Kansas.

Backus, B. C., and Guinan, J. J. Jr. (2007). Measurement of the distribution of medial olivocochlear acoustic reflex strengths across normal-hearing individuals via otoacoustic emissions. *J. Assoc. Res. Otolaryngol.* 8, 484–496. doi: 10.1007/s10162-007-0100-0

Bonfils, P., Remond, M. C., and Pujol, R. (1986). Effects of section of the medial efferent tracts (crossed and uncrossed) on cochlear frequency selectivity. *Hear. Res.* 24, 285–287. doi: 10.1016/0378-5955(86)90027-4

Boothalingam, S., and Purcell, D. W. (2015). Influence of the stimulus presentation rate on medial olivocochlear system assays. *J. Acoust. Soc. Am.* 137, 724–732. doi: 10.1121/1.4906250

Brown, M. C., Nuttall, A. L., and Masta, R. I. (1983). Intracellular recordings from cochlear inner hair cells: effects of stimulation of the crossed olivocochlear efferents. *Science* 222, 69–72. doi: 10.1126/science.6623058

Burkard, R. (2006). Calibration of acoustic transients. *Brain Res.* 1091, 27–31. doi: 10.1016/j.brainres.2006.02.132

Chabert, R., Magnan, J., Lallemant, J. G., Uziel, A., and Puel, J. L. (2002). Contralateral sound stimulation suppresses the compound action potential from the auditory nerve in humans. *Otol Neurotol.* 23, 784–788. doi: 10.1097/00129492-200209000-00029

Cheatham, M. A., Huynh, K. H., Gao, J., Zuo, J., and Dallos, P. (2004). Cochlear function in Prestin knockout mice. *J. Physiol.* 560, 821–830. doi: 10.1113/jphysiol.2004.069559

Chertoff, M., Lichtenhan, J., and Willis, M. (2010). Click-and chirp-evoked human compound action potentials. *J. Acoust. Soc. Am.* 127, 2992–2996. doi: 10.1121/1.3372756

Chéry-Croze, S., Collet, L., and Morgon, A. (1993). Medial olivo-cochlear system and tinnitus. *Acta Otolaryngol.* 113, 285–290. doi: 10.3109/00016489309135810

Cooper, N. P., and Guinan, J. J. (2003). Separate mechanical processes underlie fast and slow effects of medial olivocochlear efferent activity. *J. Physiol.* 548, 307–312. doi: 10.1113/jphysiol.2003.039081

Cooper, N. P., and Guinan, J. J. (2006). Efferent-mediated control of basilar membrane motion. *J. Physiol.* 576, 49–54. doi: 10.1113/jphysiol.2006.114991

Dallos, P., Wu, X., Cheatham, M. A., Gao, J., Zheng, J., Anderson, C. T., et al. (2008). Prestin-based outer hair cell motility is necessary for mammalian cochlear amplification. *Neuron* 58, 333–339. doi: 10.1016/j.neuron.2008.02.028

Darrow, K. N., Maison, S. F., and Liberman, M. C. (2007). Selective removal of lateral olivocochlear efferents increases vulnerability to acute acoustic injury. *J. Neurophysiol.* 97, 1775–1785. doi: 10.1152/jn.00955.2006

Don, M., and Eggermont, J. J. (1978). Analysis of the click-evoked brainstem potentials in man using high-pass noise masking. *J. Acoust. Soc. Am.* 63, 1084–1092. doi: 10.1121/1.381816

Don, M., Ponton, C. W., Eggermont, J. J., and Masuda, A. (1993). Gender differences in cochlear response time: an explanation for gender amplitude differences in the unmasked auditory brain-stem response. *J. Acoust. Soc. Am.* 94, 2135–2148. doi: 10.1121/1.407485

Don, M., Ponton, C. W., Eggermont, J. J., and Masuda, A. (1994). Auditory brainstem response (ABR) peak amplitude variability reflects individual differences in cochlear response times. *J. Acoust. Soc. Am.* 96, 3476–3491. doi: 10.1121/1.410608

Eggermont, J. J. (1979). Narrow-band AP latencies in normal and recruiting human ears. *J. Acoust. Soc. Am.* 65, 463–470. doi: 10.1121/1.382345

Elberling, C., Callø, J., and Don, M. (2010). Evaluating auditory brainstem responses to different chirp stimuli at three levels of stimulation. *J. Acoust. Soc. Am.* 128, 215–223. doi: 10.1121/1.3397640

Elberling, C., and Don, M. (2010). A direct approach for the design of chirp stimuli used for the recording of auditory brainstem responses. *J. Acoust. Soc. Am.* 128, 2955–2964. doi: 10.1121/1.3489111

Feeney, M. P., and Keefe, D. H. (2001). Estimating the acoustic reflex threshold from wideband measures of reflectance, admittance, and power. *Ear Hear.* 22, 316–332. doi: 10.1097/00003446-200108000-00006

Ferraro, J. A. (2010). Electrocochleography: a review of recording approaches, clinical applications, and new findings in adults and children. *J. Am. Acad. Audiol.* 21, 145–152. doi: 10.3766/jaaa.21.3.2

Ferraro, J. A., and Durrant, J. D. (2006). Electrocochleography in the evaluation of patients with Meniere's disease/endolymphatic hydrops. *J. Am. Acad. Audiol.* 17, 45–68. doi: 10.3766/jaaa.17.1.6

Fobel, O., and Dau, T. (2004). Searching for the optimal stimulus eliciting auditory brainstem responses in humans. *J. Acoust. Soc. Am.* 116, 2213–2222. doi: 10.1121/1.1787523

Folsom, R. C., and Owsley, R. M. (1987). N1 action potentials in humans: influence of simultaneous contralateral stimulation. *Acta Oto-laryngol.* 103, 262–265. doi: 10.3109/00016488709107281

Francis, N. A., and Guinan, J. J. (2010). Acoustic stimulation of human medial olivocochlear efferents reduces stimulus-frequency and click-evoked otoacoustic emission delays: implications for cochlear filter bandwidths. *Hear. Res.* 267, 36–45. doi: 10.1016/j.heares.2010.04.009

Garinis, A. C., Glattke, T., and Cone, B. K. (2011). The MOC reflex during active listening to speech. *J. Speech Lang. Hear. Res.* 54, 1464–1476. doi: 10.1044/1092-4388(2011/10-0223)

Gifford, M. L., and Guinan, J. J. (1987). Effects of electrical stimulation of medial olivocochlear neurons on ipsilateral and contralateral cochlear responses. *Hear. Res.* 29, 179–194. doi: 10.1016/0378-5955(87)90166-3

Groff, J. A., and Liberman, M. C. (2003). Modulation of cochlear afferent response by the lateral olivocochlear system: activation via electrical stimulation of the inferior colliculus. *J. Neurophysiol.* 90, 3178–3200. doi: 10.1152/jn.00537.2003

Guinan, J. J. (2012). How are inner hair cells stimulated? Evidence for multiple mechanical drives. *Hear. Res.* 292, 35–50. doi: 10.1016/j.heares.2012.08.005

Guinan, J. J. Jr. (2006). Olivocochlear efferents: anatomy, physiology, function, and the measurement of efferent effects in humans. *Ear Hear.* 27, 589–607. doi: 10.1097/01.aud.0000240507.83072.e7

Hamill, T. A., Hussung, R. A., and Sammeth, C. A. (1991). Rapid threshold estimation using the" chained-stimuli" technique for auditory brain stem response measurement. *Ear Hear.* 12, 229–234. doi: 10.1097/00003446-199108000-00001

Hayes, A. F., and Cai, L. (2007). Using heteroskedasticity-consistent standard error estimators in OLS regression: an introduction and software implementation. *Behav. Res. Methods* 39, 709–722. doi: 10.3758/BF03192961

Hood, L. J., Berlin, C. I., Hurley, A., Cecola, R. P., and Bell, B. (1996). Contralateral suppression of transient-evoked otoacoustic emissions in humans: intensity effects. *Hear. Res.* 101, 113–118. doi: 10.1016/S0378-5955(96)00138-4

Kalluri, R., and Shera, C. A. (2007). Near equivalence of human click-evoked and stimulus-frequency otoacoustic emissions. *J. Acoust. Soc. Am.* 121, 2097–2110. doi: 10.1121/1.2435981

Kawase, T., Delgutte, B., and Liberman, M. C. (1993). Antimasking effects of the olivocochlear reflex. II. Enhancement of auditory-nerve response to masked tones. *J. Neurophysiol.* 70, 2533–2549.

Kawase, T., and Liberman, M. C. (1993). Antimasking effects of the olivocochlear reflex. I. Enhancement of compound action potentials to masked tones. *J. Neurophysiol.* 70, 2519–2532.

Kawase, T., and Takasaka, T. (1995). The effect of contralateral noise on masked compound action potential in humans. *Hear. Res.* 91, 1–6. doi: 10.1016/0378-5955(95)00145-X

Kiang, N. Y. S. (1975). "Stimulus representation in the discharge patterns of auditory neurons," in *The Nervous System, Vol. 3, Human Communication and Its Disorders*, ed D. B. Tower (New York, NY: Raven Press), 81–96.

Kristensen, S. G., and Elberling, C. (2012). Auditory brainstem responses to level-specific chirps in normal-hearing adults. *J. Am. Acad. Audiol.* 23, 712–721. doi: 10.3766/jaaa.23.9.5

Kujawa, S. G., and Liberman, M. C. (2009). Adding insult to injury: cochlear nerve degeneration after "temporary" noise-induced hearing loss. *J. Neurosci.* 29, 14077–14085. doi: 10.1523/JNEUROSCI.2845-09.2009

Le Prell, C. G., Halsey, K., Hughes, L. F., Dolan, D. F., and Bledsoe, S. C. Jr. (2005). Disruption of lateral olivocochlear neurons via a dopaminergic neurotoxin depresses sound-evoked auditory nerve activity. *J. Assoc. Res. Otolaryngol.* 6, 48–62. doi: 10.1007/s10162-004-5009-2

Liberman, M. C., Gao, J., He, D. Z., Wu, X., Jia, S., and Zuo, J. (2002). Prestin is required for electromotility of the outer hair cell and for the cochlear amplifier. *Nature* 419, 300–304. doi: 10.1038/nature01059

Lichtenhan, J. T., Wilson, U. S., Hancock, K. E., and Guinan, J. J. (2016). Medial olivocochlear efferent reflex inhibition of human cochlear nerve responses. *Hear. Res.* 333, 216–224. doi: 10.1016/j.heares.2015.09.001

Lilaonitkul, W., and Guinan, J. J. (2009). Reflex control of the human inner ear: a half-octave offset in medial efferent feedback that is consistent with an efferent role in the control of masking. *J. Neurophysiol.* 101, 1394–1406. doi: 10.1152/jn.90925.2008

Margolis, R. H., and Heller, J. W. (1987). Screening tympanometry: criteria for medical referral: original papers. *Audiology* 26, 197–208. doi: 10.3109/00206098709081549

Marshall, L., Miller, J. A. L., Guinan, J. J., Shera, C. A., Reed, C. M., Perez, Z. D., et al. (2014). Otoacoustic-emission-based medial-olivocochlear reflex assays for humans. *J. Acoust. Soc. Am.* 136, 2697–2713. doi: 10.1121/1.4896745

Mountain, D. C. (1980). Changes in endolymphatic potential and crossed olivocochlear bundle stimulation alter cochlear mechanics. *Science* 210, 71–72. doi: 10.1126/science.7414321

Murugasu, E., and Russell, I. J. (1996). The effect of efferent stimulation on basilar membrane displacement in the basal turn of the guinea pig cochlea. *J. Neurosci.* 16, 325–332.

Najem, F., Ferraro, J., and Chertoff, M. (2016). The effect of contralateral pure tones on the compound action potential in humans: efferent tuning curves. *J. Am. Acad. Audiol.* 27, 103–116. doi: 10.3766/jaaa.15002

Neumann, J., Uppenkamp, S., and Kollmeier, B. (1994). Chirp evoked otoacoustic emissions. *Hear. Res.* 79, 17–25. doi: 10.1016/0378-5955(94)90123-6

Puria, S., Guinan, J. J. Jr., and Liberman, M. C. (1996). Olivocochlear reflex assays: effects of contralateral sound on compound action potentials versus ear-canal distortion products. *J. Acoust. Soc. Am.* 99, 500–507. doi: 10.1121/1.414508

Sahley, T. L., and Nodar, R. H. (1994). Improvement in auditory function following pentazocine suggests a role for dynorphins in auditory sensitivity. *Ear Hear.* 15, 422–431. doi: 10.1097/00003446-199412000-00003

Schaette, R., and McAlpine, D. (2011). Tinnitus with a normal audiogram: physiological evidence for hidden hearing loss and computational model. *J. Neurosci.* 31, 13452–13457. doi: 10.1523/JNEUROSCI.2156-11.2011

Shore, S. E., and Nuttall, A. L. (1985). The effects of cochlear hypothermia on compound action potential tuning. *J. Acoust. Soc. Am.* 77, 590–598. doi: 10.1121/1.391877

Siegel, J. H., and Kim, D. O. (1982). Efferent neural control of cochlear mechanics? Olivocochlear bundle stimulation affects cochlear biomechanical nonlinearity. *Hear. Res.* 6, 171–182. doi: 10.1016/0378-5955(82)90052-1

Smith, S. B., Lichtenhan, J., and Cone, B. (2016). Behavioral pure-tone threshold shifts caused by tympanic membrane electrodes. *Ear Hear.* 37, e273–e275. doi: 10.1097/aud.0000000000000275

Sun, X. M. (2008). Contralateral suppression of distortion product otoacoustic emissions and the middle-ear muscle reflex in human ears. *Hear. Res.* 237, 66–75. doi: 10.1016/j.heares.2007.12.004

Veuillet, E., Collet, L., and Duclaux, R. (1991). Effect of contralateral acoustic stimulation on active cochlear micromechanical properties in human subjects: dependence on stimulus variables. *J. Neurophysiol.* 65, 724–735.

Warr, W. B. (1992). "Organization of olivocochlear efferent systems in mammals," in *The Mammalian Auditory Pathway: Neuroanatomy* (New York, NY: Springer), 410–448.

Warr, W. B., and Guinan, J. J. (1979). Efferent innervation of the organ of Corti: two separate systems. *Brain Res.* 173, 152–155. doi: 10.1016/0006-8993(79)91104-1

Wiederhold, M. L., and Kiang, N. Y. S. (1970). Effects of electric stimulation of the crossed olivocochlear bundle on single auditory-nerve fibers in the cat. *J. Acoust. Soc. Am.* 48, 950–965. doi: 10.1121/1.1912234

Zhao, W., and Dhar, S. (2010). The effect of contralateral acoustic stimulation on spontaneous otoacoustic emissions. *J. Assoc. Res. Otolaryngol.* 11, 53–67. doi: 10.1007/s10162-009-0189-4

Zhao, W., and Dhar, S. (2012). Frequency tuning of the contralateral medial olivocochlear reflex in humans. *J. Neurophysiol.* 108, 25–30. doi: 10.1152/jn.00051.2012

3

Tone Burst Electrocochleography for the Diagnosis of Clinically Certain Meniere's Disease

*Jeremy Hornibrook**

Department of Otolaryngology-Head and Neck Surgery, Christchurch Hospital, University of Canterbury and University of Otago, Christchurch, New Zealand

***Correspondence:**
Jeremy Hornibrook
jeremy@jhornibrook.com

The technique of transtympanic electrocochleography was initially developed as an objective hearing threshold test by Eggermont. Gibson et al. (1977) claimed that an enlarged direct current component of the action potential (AP) called the summating potential (SP) is an indication of endolymphatic hydrops, later confirmed by Coates who proposed an SP/AP ratio measure. This led to numerous publications using diagnostic ratios of 0.33–0.35. The insensitivity led to an eventual disenchantment with the test as a reliable objective test for Meniere's disease. It was further confused by audiologists employing remote canal or ear drum electrodes which give a response about one-fourth of the magnitude obtained by an electrode in contact with the cochlea. Subsequently Gibson stated that an SP/AP ratio of <0.5 is not diagnostic for hydrops. He then showed that a tone burst stimulus gave the test a significantly higher sensitivity and specificity, which has been supported by others. On MRI inner ear imaging with gadolinium hydrops can be seen, but the quality of images and what is seen may vary according to brand of scanner, settings, mode of gadolinium administration, and the possibility that gadolinium entry may favor the vestibule. Transtympanic tone burst electrocochleography is to date the simplest, cheapest and most sensitive technique for detecting cochlear endolymphatic hydrops to confirm a diagnosis of Meniere's disease.

Keywords: Meniere's disease, electrocochleography, tone bursts, transtympanic EcochG, clinically certain Meniere's disease

INTRODUCTION

Electrocochleography (EcochG) is a method of directly recording electrical activity of the cochlea and the acoustic nerve in response to acoustic stimulation. The three components measurable are the cochlear microphonic (CM), the action potential (AP), and the summating potential (SP). In contrast to the earliest studies, new computer averaging techniques have enabled routine testing of these components in humans.

This review will briefly summarize the useful components of the EcochG used in the diagnosis of Meniere's disease. The effects of electrode placement on the size of the AP and SP and the merits of tone burst stimuli will be discussed. New international criteria for the symptomatic diagnosis of Meniere's disease make no allowance for any diagnostic test for a disorder which always begins in the cochlea, even though objective testing can confirm or exclude it.

COCHLEAR MICROPHONIC

The CM, originally called the cochlear potential, was recorded in cats by Wever and Bray (1930). It is thought to be the summed microphonic from many hair cells recorded by a distant electrode. The lower the frequency of stimulation the larger the number of hair cells which will produce CMs in the same phase and the larger the CM will be. Although the CM has a number of new applications in auditory testing, its routine use is somewhat limited by the reduction in signal-to-noise ratio that occurs with a remote electrode.

ACTION POTENTIAL

The response from the acoustic nerve is the AP and was first demonstrated in the cochlear nerve and brainstem of cats by Saul and Davis (1932). Because of the concern that direct recording from the cochlea in individuals with normal hearing was dangerous, Ruben et al. (1961) measured APs in patients with hearing losses by a silver ball electrode placed in the round window niche after a typmanotomy and achieved the first intraoperative demonstration of hearing improvement during stapedectomy. In what was the first use of a remote electrode, Yoshie et al. (Yoshie, 1968) measured APs in normal hearing humans with a hypodermic needle shielded with a polyethylene tube inserted into the anesthetised posterior ear canal skin, about 5 mm from the annulus. In the same year Portmann (Portmann et al., 1967) demonstrated that it was safe to record from the round window niche with an electrode passed through the eardrum. In the USA fears of safety and litigation over transtympanic electrodes persist to this day.

A 100 ms click stimulus stimulates the whole basilar membrane. Frequency selective masking experiments suggest that the major contribution from a click is from the basal turn of the cochlea (Teas et al., 1962) from 10 to 4 kHz as the traveling wave is progressively damped as it travels toward the apex (Zwicker and Fast, 1972). Also the velocity of the traveling wave along the basilar membrane slows as it approaches the apex of the cochlea, resulting in a decrease in hair cells firing per unit time (Zerlin, 1969). This limitation is being addressed by the study of an alternative "Chirp" stimulus which has more low frequency energy occurring earlier in the stimulus (Chertoff et al., 2010).

The initial application of AP recordings was the objective determination of hearing thresholds. As the signal is generated so close to the recording electrode, masking of the opposite ear is not necessary.

SUMMATING POTENTIAL

The SP is a direct current component of the AP, described independently in guinea pigs by Davis et al. (1950) who assumed it was a post-synaptic response. von Bekesy (1952) considered it to be a shift of the CM. The CM was thought to be derived from the outer hair cells and the SP from the inner hair cells. However, it is present in pigeon ears which lack inner hair cells (Stopp and Whitfeild, 1964). The SP is now assumed to be a result of cochlear microphonic distortions (Dallos et al., 1972).

The maximum CM is recorded closest to maximum hair cell displacement, whereas the SP is maximum at a point where the summed effect from a large area of basilar membrane can be recorded. In endolymphatic hydrops the downward vibration of the basilar membrane is limited as it is being stretched, so the normal up-going asymmetry is enhanced, leading to a SP of increased amplitude (Gibson, 1978).

The SP became to be of interest as an indicator of endolymphatic hydrops, and therefore in the objective diagnosis of Meniere's disease.

SUMMATING POTENTIAL IN MENIERE'S DISEASE

Schmidt et al. (1974) noted that the SP in Meniere's disease from tone bursts is about five times larger than in patients with high frequency hearing loss. Eggermont (1979) found that short 4 kHz 4 ms tone pips elicit a small AP which limits their use for diagnosing Meniere's disease compared with a click stimulus (Gibson, 1978).

Gibson et al. (1977), using transtympanic EcochG with clicks, found a large DC potential causing a widening of SP/AP waveform that might be a useful indicator of Meniere's disease. There was a high correlation with the symptomatic likelihood of Meniere's disease. Moffat et al. (1978) achieved a decrease in the negative SP in 11/13 patients after oral glycerol dehydration, with no significant change in the pure tone audiogram or speech discrimination. This was suggested as being a useful indicator of prognosis in endolymphatic sac surgery.

Coats (1981a) found that Meniere's ears had a larger SP/AP ratio compared with non-Meniere's ears, when recorded using a canal electrode and a click stimulus. There was also a correlation between a large SP/AP ratio in ears with reduced caloric responses in comparison with a small SP/AP ratio in ears with normal caloric responses (Coats, 1981b).

A major issue of contention for the EcochG has been the magnitude and quality of responses depending on the type and placement of the active electrode.

ELECTRODE PLACEMENT

The majority of publications on click stimulus in Meniere's ears have been by audiologists using distant electrodes which, because of their distance, require more signal averaging to cancel out random noise, and produce far smaller responses.

Ferraro et al. (1986) compared the responses and comfort of three ear canal electrodes.

Of the three there was no difference in comfort. A disposable soft insulated ear canal foam plug electrode design with a central sound-conducting tube was the easiest to place and gave the best responses. Sohmer and Feinmesser (1967) recorded the AP in cats with silver ball electrode in the round window niche and the ear drum and from a subdermal needle and a clip on the ear lobe. He found that the AP recorded from the round window niche was 10–25 times larger than the AP recorded from the other three sites.

Roland et al. (1995) compared responses from a transtympanic electrode (TT) with an ear canal (EAC) electrode in 19 healthy volunteers. The click responses from a TT electrode were seven times the magnitude as those from a EAC electrode. In a further study 50 ear canal EcochG tracings interpreted by 10 different audiologists revealed statistically significant inter-interpreter differences between no response and very difficult to read SP/AP ratios (Roland and Roth, 1997). He emphasized the implications for diagnosis and its reliability in investigational studies.

CLICK SP/AP STUDIES IN MENIERE'S DISEASE

Gibson et al. (1983) performed click stimulus EcochG in 44 Meniere's ears and in 32 normal ears and 40 ears with sensorineural hearing loss. A SP/AP ratio of 0.30 clearly separated them, providing the loss exceeded an average of 40 dBHL.

The click SP/AP ratio as a diagnostic test for Meniere's disease became of world-wide interest and the basis of numerous publications, some of which are listed in **Table 1**. The highest sensitivity of 85% was achieved by Camilleri and Howarth (2001) with an SP/AP ratio of 0.33. In contrast Gibson et al. (Gibson, 2005) reported a 40% sensitivity with an SP/AP ratio of 0.47. The explanation for this will follow. In addition to a click SP/AP ratio Ferraro and Tibbils (1999) recorded the AP using an ET electrode. He advocated the addition of an SP/AP area ratio (Ferraro and Tibbils, 1999) to improve the sensitivity and specificity to 92 and 84%, respectively (Al-momani et al., 2009). However, Marcio et al. (transtympanic) (Marcio et al., 2006) and Ikino et al. (transtympanic) (Ikino and de Almeida, 2006) could not confirm it.

A significant advance in the EcochG sensitivity for diagnosing definite Meniere's disease has come from the use of tone burst stimuli.

TONE BURST STUDIES IN MENIERE'S DISEASE

In 1986 Dauman et al. (Dauman et al., 1986, 1998) measured the effect of glycerol on ears tested transtympanically with free field tone bursts of octave frequencies between 1 and 8 kZ at 90 dB HL, which produced a prolonged SP whose magnitude was measured in microvolts from its midpoint to the baseline. Long tone bursts in patients with Meniere's disease showed significantly larger SPs than in control subjects, with most Meniere's ears having an SP decrease observed after dehydration.

In 1990, at the Third International Symposium and Workshops on Surgery of the Inner Ear, Dauman and Aran (1991) expanded their experience, comparing clicks vs. 10 ms tone bursts. The responses to 1, 2, 4, and 8 Kz TBs are shown in **Figure 1**, with 8 kHz usually being positive. The mean amplitudes for those frequencies are shown in **Figure 2**, showing 1 and 2 kHz are the most sensitive for indicating hydrops.

TABLE 1 | SP/AP ratio criteria from extratympanic (ET) and transtympanic (TT) EcochG studies with a click stimulus.

Authors	Electrode	SP/AP criterion	Sensitivity (%)	Specificity (%)
Mori et al., 1987	ET	0.44	68	
Aso, 1991	TT	0.37	58	
Pou et al., 1996	ET	0.35	57	94
Filipo et al., 1997	TT	0.43	64	
		0.50	47	
Sass, 1998	TT	0.41	62	95
Ferraro and Tibbils, 1999	ET	0.41	60	
Camilleri and Howarth, 2001	TT	0.33	85	
Chung et al., 2004	ET	0.34	71	96
Gibson, 2005	TT	0.47	40	97
Marcio et al., 2006	TT	0.37	52	
Takeda and Kakigi, 2010	ET	0.40	56	
Claes et al., 2011	TT	0.35	56	

Gibson (1991) compared clicks with 1 kHz 12 ms tone bursts in 42 Meniere's ears and 48 normal sensorineural loss ears, with the symptomatic likelihood of Meniere's disease. At 90 dB HL a 1 kHz tone burst more negative than 3 mV separated the Meniere's ears very precisely from the normal and sensorineural ears. The false negatives for tone bursts were half those for clicks.

At The First International Conference on EcochG, Otoacoustic Emissions, and Intraoperative Monitoring Gibson (1993) expanded the comparison of clicks vs. tone bursts (12 ms) for the diagnosis of endolymphatic hydrops in 1,101 ears by transtympanic EcochG. The 0.5, 1, 2, 4, and 8 kHz tone burst diagnostic criteria are presented in **Table 2**.

Conlon and Gibson (2000) confirmed the superiority of tone bursts over clicks and with a 1 kHz tone burst found hydrops in 10% of contralateral ears in Meniere's patients (Conlon and Gibson, 1999). Claes et al. (2011) used a transtympanic technique with 100 dBHL tone bursts. He achieved a 91% sensitivity for implying hydrops in 91% of ears with an AAO-HNS definite diagnosis of Meniere's disease when the SP amplitude was more negative than −3 mV for 1 kHz or more negative than 2 mV in at least three tone burst frequencies.

Ferraro (Ferraro et al., 1994) found tone burst SPs measured with an extratympanic electrode were four times smaller compared with a transtympanic electrode. Bohlen et al. (1991) measured click and tone burst responses sequentially with an extratympanic and transtympanic electrode. In 90% of patients TT EcochG was equal to or more comfortable than for an ET electrode. Tone bursts with an ET electrode gave no response or were unreliably small.

In most EcochG studies on Meniere's ears the control ears have been Meniere's opposite ears or ears with normal hearing or ears with sensorineural hearing loss. To provide purer controls Gibson (2009) compared click and tone burst responses in 2,717 patients from Meniere's ears *with ears with equivalent hearing.* For a click SP/AP response there was no statistical difference between Meniere's ears and non-Meniere's ears. In a further analysis (Iseli and Gibson, 2010) a

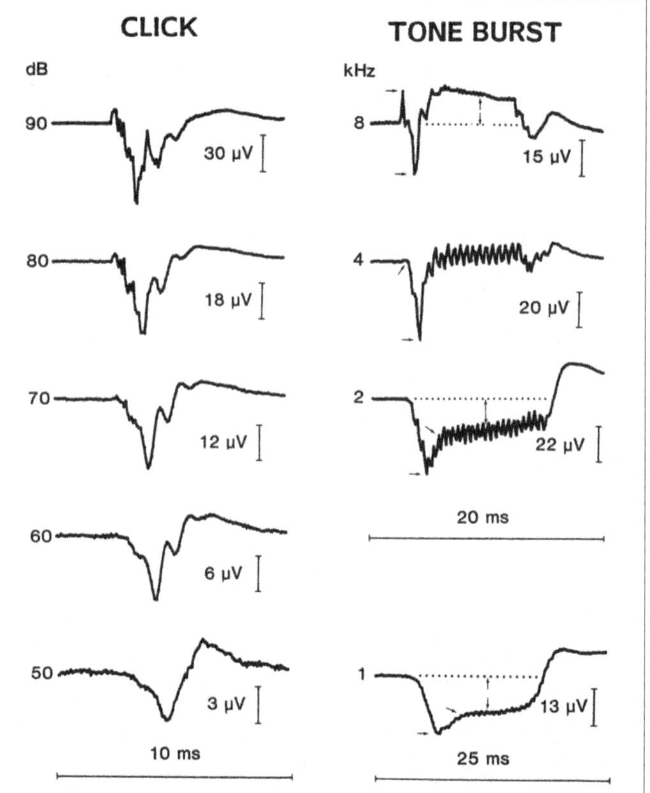

FIGURE 1 | Transtympanic SP responses to a 90 dB click and to 10 ms 1, 2, 4, and 8 kHz tone bursts with 8 kHz showing a reversed polarity. The magnitude is measured in microvolts from the midpoint of the prolonged SP to the baseline (Dauman and Aran, 1991). Reproduced from Dauman and Aran (1991).

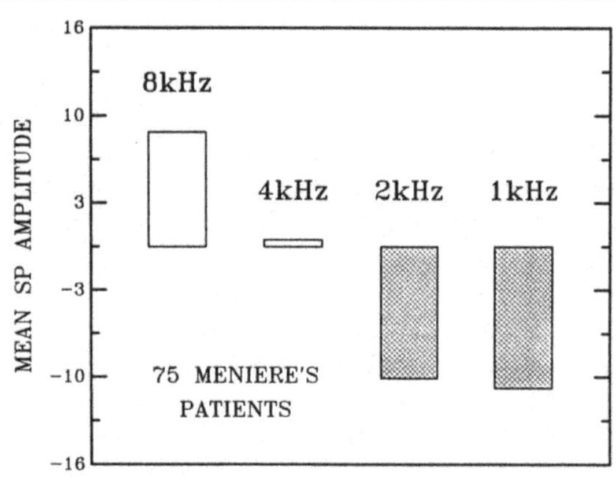

FIGURE 2 | The mean tone burst SP amplitudes (in mV) in 75 Meniere's patients at 1, 2, 4, and 8 kHz, respectively (Dauman and Aran, 1991). Reproduced from Dauman and Aran (1991).

click stimulus had diagnostic sensitivity of 35% and specificity of 91% for an SP/AP ratio of not <0.47, compared with and 95% sensitivity and 79% sensitivity for combination of 1 kHz tone burst thresholds and a tone burst SP/AP ratio.

TABLE 2 | Diagnostic level for tone bursts to diagnose hydrops (Gibson, 1993).

Hz of SP hearing level	dB HL	Diagnostic criterion (mV)
MORE NEGATIVE THAN		
500 HZ (85 dB HL)	under 25	−2
	20–35	−2
	40–55	−2
	60–75	−1
1 kHz (100 dB HL)	under 25	−6
	20–25	−6
	40–55	−6
	60–75	−3
2 kHz (100 dB HL)	under 25	−9
	20–35	−7
	40–55	−5
	60–75	−5
4 kHz (100dB HL)	under 25	−9
	20–35	−5
	40–55	−5
	60–75	−5
MORE POSITIVE THAN		
8 kHz (100 dB HL)	under 25	+6
	20–35	+6
	40–55	+6
	60–75	+6

The diagnostic level was chosen as the nearest whole figure to the level which provides a false rate of 5%.

Despite significant advances in the sensitivity of electrophysiological testing official diagnostic classifications for Meniere's disease remain symptom-based.

CURRENT DIAGNOSIS OF MENIERE'S DISEASE

Since Prosper Meniere's first descriptions of the disorder in 1861 there was no recognized symptomatic classification until 1972 (Barber et al., 1972). The Equilibrium Committee of the American Academy of Otolaryngology-Head and Neck Surgery (AAO-HNS) has produced three diagnostic definitions, the most recent one in 1995 (Monsell et al., 1995) used internationally until 2015 (**Table 3**). The four categories were possible, probable, definite, and certain. AAO-HNS definite has been a universal diagnostic criterion for numerous clinical studies. The definition of certain was histopathological confirmation from a post-mortem. The AAO-HNS has been and remains skeptical as to the reliability of any objective tests.

The Barany Society, an international vestibular disorders society based in Sweden, has embarked on a project to achieve worldwide agreement on precise definitions of vestibular symptoms and the symptomatic diagnosis of common vestibular disorders. To conform to The International Classification of Diseases the vestibular diagnoses are limited to probable and

TABLE 3 | AAO-HNS Committee on Hearing and Equilibrium 1995 diagnostic criteria for Meniere's disease (Monsell et al., 1995).

CERTAIN MENIERE'S DISEASE
Definite Meniere's disease, plus histopathologic confirmation
DEFINITE MENIERE'S DISEASE
Two or more definitive spontaneous episodes of vertigo of 20 min or longer
Audiometrically documented hearing loss on at last one occasion
Tinnitus or aural fullness in the treated ear
Other causes excluded
PROBABLE MENIERE'S DISEASE
One definite episode of vertigo
Audiometrically documented hearing loss on at least one occasion
Tinnitus or aural fullness in the treated ear
Other causes excluded
POSSIBLE MENIERE'S DISEASE
Episodic vertigo of the Meniere type without documented hearing loss, or
Sensorineural hearing loss, fluctuating, or fixed, with disequilibrium but without definitive episodes
Other causes excluded

TABLE 4 | The 2015 Barany Society diagnostic criteria for Meniere's disease (Lopez-Escamez et al., 2015).

DEFINITE MENIERE'S DISEASE
A. Two or more spontaneous episodes of vertigo, each lasting 20 min to 12 h
B. Audiometrically low-to-medium-frequency sensorinerual hearing loss in one ear, defining the affected ear on at least one occasion, during or after one of the episodes of vertigo
C. Fluctuating aural symptoms (hearing, tinnitus, or fullness) in the affected ear
D. Not better accounted for by another vestibular diagnosis
PROBABLE MENIERE'S DISEASE
A. Two or more episodes of vertigo or dizziness, each lasting 20 min to 24 h
B. Fluctuating aural symptoms (hearing, tinnitus, or fullness) in the affected ear
C. Not better accounted for by another vestibular diagnosis

definite. For definite Meniere's disease the new symptomatic criteria (Lopez-Escamez et al., 2015) are similar and a logical improvement on the AAO-HNS 1995 criteria (**Table 4**). Possible and certain no longer exist.

OPINION ON THE VALIDITY OF ECOCHG FOR THE DIAGNOSIS OF MENIERE'S DISEASE

Nguyen et al. (2010) conducted a survey among members of the American Otological Society and the American Neurotology Society as to their opinions on the usefulness of EcochG for diagnosing Meniere's disease. Approximately 70% employed an extratympanic electrode and 30% a transtympanic electrode. Eighty-three percent said they would discount a result that was contradictory to their clinical impression, with 57% preferring an ENG caloric test and VEMPs for 27%. Only 45% used EcochG. The overall conclusion was that EcochG is perceived to have low clinical use and reliability, and among those who use it there is little consensus on technique and stimulus modality.

Kim et al. (2005) conducted a click EcochG study with an extratympanic electrode and an SP/AP diagnostic ratio of >0.4 on 97 patients with suspected Meniere's disease. Of 60 patients with an AAO-HNS symptomatic diagnosis of Meniere's disease 67% with a definite diagnosis and 53% with a less-than-definite diagnosis had a positive test. They concluded that, because of its lack of sensitivity, EcochG should not play a decisive role in determining the presence or absence of Meniere's disease.

VESTIBULAR MENIERE'S DISEASE

The term vestibular Meniere's disease is sometimes used (Paparella, 1984a,b; Paparella and Mancini, 1985). It originated in the earliest iteration of the AAO-HNS diagnostic criteria (Barber et al., 1972), separating cochlear and vestibular forms, but abandoned in the 1995 criteria. Currently it has no official basis.

Dornhoffer and Arenberg (1993) studied 15 patients with recurrent vertigo attacks without fluctuating hearing they called vestibular Meniere's disease (or possible on the 1995 AAO-HNS criteria). On transtympanic tone burst EcochG at 1 and 2 kHz by their own criteria 6 were positive for hydrops, supporting a diagnosis of Meniere's disease.

With the abolition of the AAO-HNS certain Meniere's disease category (a post-mortem now rarely achievable) there is a need for alternative diagnostic certainty, particularly for investigational studies, and to unequivocally distinguish Meniere's disease from other causes of recurrent vertigo attacks.

CLINICALLY CERTAIN MENIERE'S DISEASE

The term clinically certain Meniere's disease can be defined as a diagnosis based on the 1995 AAO-HNS symptomatic criteria (Monsell et al., 1995) (or now probable and definite on the international Barany Society criteria (Lopez-Escamez et al., 2015) plus transtympanic electrocochleographic confirmation of endolymphatic hydrops, based on the most sensitive criteria for tone bursts and clicks.

Based on this definition Hornibrook (Hornibrook et al., 2010b, 2011; Johnson et al., 2016) and colleagues have conducted three studies on definite Meniere's disease patients in whom there was clinical certainty of the diagnosis. Objective proof of hydrops was established by transtympanic EcochG with tone bursts and clicks. The technique and settings are illustrated in **Figure 3**. The diagnostic tone burst criteria were at 1 and/or 2 kHz (**Table 2**; Gibson, 1993) and/or a click SP/AP ratio of >0.5.

Since the discovery that an abnormally low threshold cervical vestibular evoked potential (cVEMP) could confirm a diagnosis of superior canal dehiscence syndrome other diagnostic applications for VEMPs have been sought, including for Meniere's disease with numerous publications employing cVEMPS and ocular VEMPs (oVEMPs) to diagnose hydrops in the vestibule. These have produced conflicting interpretations as to the diagnostic sensitivity. In 18 patients with a clinically certain diagnosis in one ear, Johnson et al. (2016) measured cVEMP

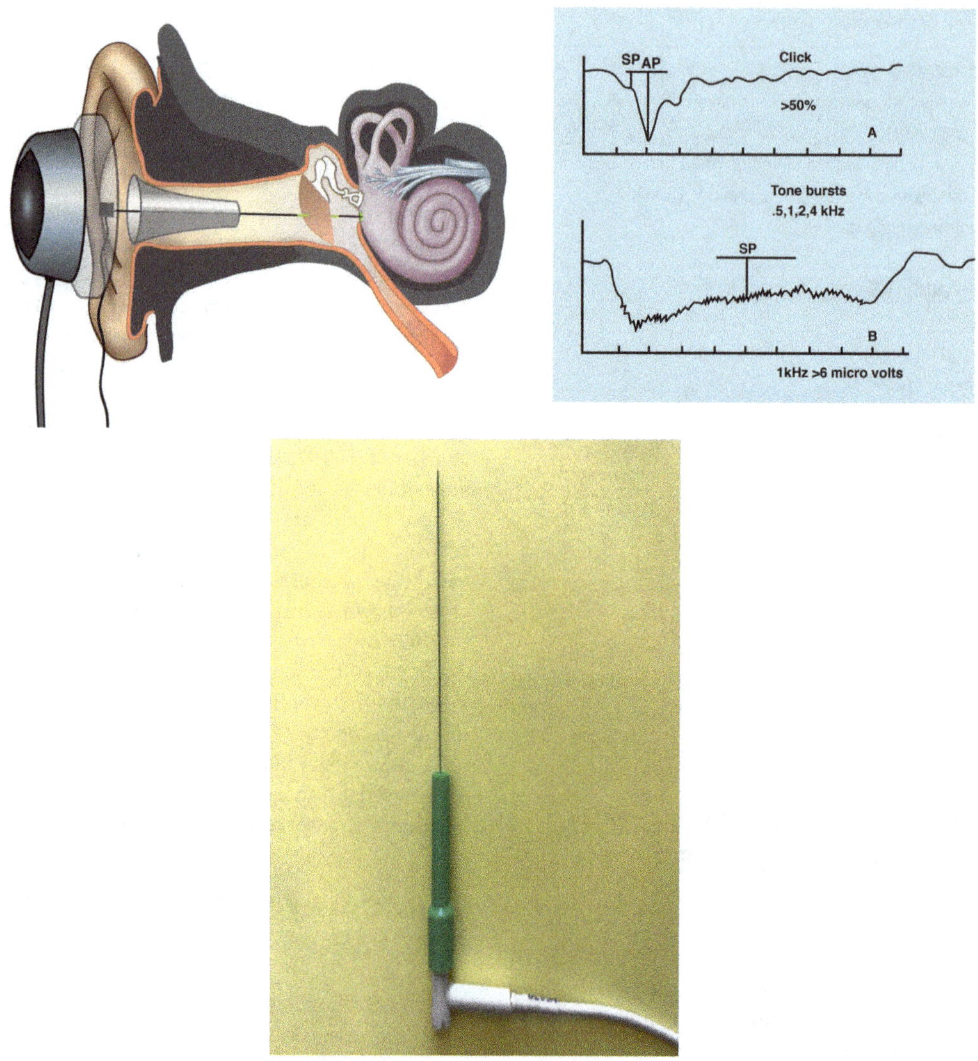

FIGURE 3 | Transtympanic EcochG for three studies on "clinically certain" Meniere's disease (Hornibrook et al., 2010b, 2011; Johnson et al., 2016). Local anesthesia is a tiny drop of phenol placed at 9 o'clock or 3 o'clock on the ear drum. An insulated needle is passed through the drum with its tip lying in the round window niche and secured by elastic bands to a circular bracket over the ear over which a headphone is placed. Stimuli were from an Amplaid mk15 diagnostic system. Clicks: 10 ms broadband alternating polarity clicks of 100 ms duration at 95 dB HL at repetition rate of 11.3/s with 100–200 repetitions. Tone bursts: 1 and 2 kHz 100 dB HL tone bursts with a 1 ms linear rise/fall and 14 ms plateau at a repetition rate of 30.1/s. The diagnostic criterion for clicks was an SP/AP ratio of >0.5, and for tone bursts criteria for 1 and 2 kHz as in **Table 2** (Gibson, 1991). From Hornibrook et al. (2012). **Inset:** TECA disposable monopolar needle 37 mm x 28 G (Natus Manufacturing Ltd., Gort, Galway, Ireland).

and oVEMP amplitude, latency and threshold in the Meniere's ear and their opposite ears and in the ears of 22 normal control ears. The overlap of results from the Meniere's patients compared with normal controls was such that VEMP abnormalities appear limited as a sole diagnostic test for Meniere's disease. As endolymphatic hydrops in Meniere's disease always starts in the cochlea (Pender, 2014) it would seem logical to employ the most sensitive test which confirms cochlear hydrops.

Confirmation of visible inner ear hydrops on MRI scanning with intratympanic gadolinium (Nakashima et al., 2009) has led to numerous MRI inner ear studies in the hope that a visible diagnosis of hydrops would be the standard by which other tests might be compared (Hornibrook et al., 2010a).

Hornibrook et al. (2015) compared the sensitivity of intratympanic gadolinium MRI with tone burst EcochG for diagnosing hydrops in 57 ears with AAO-HNS possible, probable, or definite Meniere's disease. In 30 patients with definite Meniere's disease the tone burst EcochG was positive in 83%, the click in 30%, and gadolinium MRI in 47%. Although adequate imaging was achieved in 90% of scans, with tone burst EcochG was a more sensitive test for definite Meniere's disease and therefore for cochlear hydrops. Tone burst EcochG was also more sensitive than MRI for probable and possible Meniere's disease and in some cases, with visible vestibular hydrops, more sensitive for confirming cochlear hydrops. Ziylan et al. (2016) reviewed and compared this study with three other

MRI/click-only EcochG studies with a low SP/AP diagnostic ratio of >0.33 which will have enhanced its apparent sensitivity. They concluded that there is a relative low sensitivity and predictive value for click stimulus EcochG compared with gadolinium inner ear MRI for detecting hydrops in Meniere's disease. Images and conclusions from MRI inner ear imaging appear confounded by variables such as scanner brand, head coil specifications, and the possibility that gadolinium entry may be variable and favor the vestibule (Hornibrook et al., 2016).

SUMMARY AND CONCLUSION

The initial promise of a click response SP/AP ratio as a sensitive test for endolymphatic hydrops has not been realized (Hornibrook et al., 2016). Although it can be measured by a ET electrode the responses are at least one quarter the magnitude of those obtained by a TT electrode.

ET electrodes are significantly inferior for measuring tone burst responses. Until the signal-to-noise ratio problem of ET electrodes is solved, TT recordings are of greater magnitude and accuracy.

An analysis of 128 Meniere's disease studies (Thorpe et al., 2003) found that the AAO-HNS 1995 definitions were misapplied in 50% of cases, implying that symptom-only criteria are unreliable and can result in underdiagnosis and overdiagnosis. Reliance on a symptom-only diagnosis, based on a pure tone audiogram, has the jeopardy that studies are likely to include patients who do not have the disorder, and to exclude some who do.

Of all investigative tests transtympanic tone burst EcochG remains the simplest, and most sensitive test to diagnose *cochlear* hydrops to confirm a diagnosis of Meniere's disease. There is agreement that a response of not < -3 mV is diagnostic for endolymphatic hydrops (Dauman and Aran, 1991; Gibson, 1991, 2005, 2009; Conlon and Gibson, 2000; Claes et al., 2011). Clear, reliable tone burst responses can only be achieved at 100 dbnHL, which cannot be achieved by newer model audiology evoked response systems.

As was once for electrocardiography there is an urgent need for universal agreement on equipment specifications (Hohmann et al., 1991; Arenberg et al., 1993; Wuyts et al., 1997), which for the EcochG should produce 100 dBnHL tone bursts.

AUTHOR CONTRIBUTIONS

The author confirms being the sole contributor of this work and approved it for publication.

REFERENCES

Al-momani, M. O., Ferraro, J. A., Gajewski, B. J., and Ator, G. (2009). Improved sensitivity of electrocochleography in the diagnosis of Meniere's disease. *Int. J. Audiol.* 48, 811–819. doi: 10.3109/14992020903019338

Arenberg, I. K., Gibson, W. P. R., Hohmann, D., and Mihalco, L. L. (1993). "International standards for transtympanic electrocochleography," in *ECoG, OAE and Intraoperative Monitoring*, ed D. Hohmann (Amsterdam; New York, NY: Kugler), 115–118.

Aso, S., Watanabe, Y., Mizukoshi, K. (1991). A clinical study of electrocochleography in Meniere's disease. *Acta Otolaryngol.* 111, 44–52.

Barber, H. O., Pennington, C., Pulec, J. L., Schuknecht, H. F., Tabor, J. R., and McCabe, B. F. (1972). Committee on Hearing and Equilibrium. Meniere's disease: criteria for diagnosis and evaluation of therapy for reporting. *Trans. Am. Acad. Opthalmol. Otolaryngol.* 76, 1462–1464.

Bohlen, H. K. H., Arenberg, I. K., and Gibson, W. P. R. (1991). "Diagnostic reliablility of electrocochleography for hydrops—ear canal/tympanic membrane versus transtympanic electrode placement," in *Surgery of the Inner Ear*, ed D. Hohmann (Amsterdam; New York: Kugler), 269–280.

Camilleri, A. E., and Howarth, K. L. (2001). Prognostic value of electrocochleography in patients with unilateral Meniere's disease undergoing saccus surgery. *Clin. Otolaryngol.* 26, 257–260. doi: 10.1046/j.0307-7772.2001.00468.x

Chertoff, M., Lichtenham, J., and Willis, M. (2010). Click- and chirp-evoked human compound action potentials. *J. Acoust. Soc. Am.* 127, 2992–2996. doi: 10.1121/1.3372756

Chung, W.-H., Cho, D.-Y., Choi, J.-Y., and Hong, S. H. (2004). Clinical usefulness of extratympanic electrocochleography in the diagnosis of Meniere's disease. *Otol. Neurotol.* 25, 144–149. doi: 10.1097/00129492-200403000-00011

Claes, G. M. E., De Valck, C. F., Van de Heyning, P., and Wuyts, F. L. (2011). The Meniere's disease index: and objective correlate of Meniere's disease, based on audiometric and electrocochleographic data. *Otol. Neurotol.* 32, 887–892. doi: 10.1097/MAO.0b013e318219ff9a

Coats, A. C. (1981a). The summating potential and Meniere's disease. I. Summating potential amplitude in Meniere's ears and non-Meniere's ears. *Arch. Otolaryngol.* 107, 199–208. doi: 10.1001/archotol.1981.00790400001001

Coats, A. C. (1981b). Meniere's disease and the summating potential. II. Vestibular test results. *Arch. Otolaryngol.* 107, 263–270. doi: 10.1001/archotol.1981.00790400001001

Conlon, B., and Gibson, W. P. R. (1999). Meniere's disease: the incidence of hydrops in the contralateral ear. *Laryngoscope* 109, 1800–1802. doi: 10.1097/00005537-199911000-00014

Conlon, B. J., and Gibson, W. P. R. (2000). Electrocochleography in the diagnosis of Meniere's disease. *Acta Otolaryngol.* 120, 480–483. doi: 10.1080/000164800750045965

Dallos, P., Schoeny, Z. G., and Cheatham, M. A. (1972). Cochlear summating potentials: descriptive aspects. *Acta Otolaryngol.* 302(Suppl.), 1–46.

Dauman, R., and Aran, J.-M. (1991). "Electrocochleography and the diagnosis of endolymphatic hydrops: clicks and tone bursts," in *Inner Ear Surgery*, ed I. K. Arenberg (Amsterdam; New York, NY: Kugler), 123–133.

Dauman, R., Aran, J. M., de Sauvage, C., and Portmann, M. (1998). Clinical significance of the summating potential in Meniere's disease. *Am. J. Otol.* 9, 31–38.

Dauman, R., Aran, J.-M., and Portmann, M. (1986). Summating potential and water balance in Meniere's disease. *Ann. Otol. Rhinol. Laryngol.* 95, 389–395. doi: 10.1177/000348948609500413

Davis, H., Fernandez, C., and McAuliffe, D. R. (1950). The excitatory process in the cochlea. *Proc. Natl. Acad. Sci. U.S.A.* 36, 580–587. doi: 10.1073/pnas.36.10.580

Dornhoffer, J. L., and Arenberg, I. K. (1993). Diagnosis of vestibular Meniere's disease with electrocochleography. *Am. J. Otol.* 14, 161–164.

Eggermont, J. J. (1979). Summating potentials in Meniere's disease. *Arch. Otorhinolaryngol.* 222, 63–75. doi: 10.1007/BF00456340

Ferraro, J. A., Thedinegr, B. S., Mediavilla, S. J., and Balckwell, W. L. (1994). Human summating potential to tone bursts: observations on tympanic membrane versus promonontory recordings in the same patients. *J. Am. Acad. Audiol.* 5, 24–29.

Ferraro, J. A., and Tibbils, P. (1999). SP/AP area ratio in the diagnosis of Meniere's disease. *Am. J. Audiol.* 8, 21–27. doi: 10.1044/1059-0889(1999/001)

Ferraro, Murphy, and Ruth, R. A. (1986). A comparative study of electrodes used in extratmp electrocohleography. *Semin. Hear.* 7, 279–286. doi: 10.1055/s-0028-1091464

Filipo, R., Cordier, M., Barbara, M., and Bertoli, G. A. (1997). Electrocochleographic findings: Menière's disease versus sudden sensorineural hearing loss. *Acta Otolaryngol. Suppl.* 526, 21–23.

Gibson, W. P. R. (1978). "Electrocochleography (EcochG)," in *Essentials of Clinical Electric Response Audiometry* (London: Churchill Livingtson), 69.

Gibson, W. P. R. (1991). "Electrocochleography: a comparison of clicks versus tone bursts in the diagnosis of endolymphatic hydrops," in *Inner Ear Surgery*, ed I. K. Arenberg (Amsterdam; New York, NY: Kugler), 281–285.

Gibson, W. P. R. (1993). "A comparison of clicks versus tone bursts in the diagnosis of endolymphatic hydrops," in *ECoG, OAE and Intraoperative Monitoring*, ed D. Hohmann (Amsterdam; New York, NY: Kugler), 55–59.

Gibson, W. P. R. (2005). "The role of transtympanic electrocochleography in the diagnosis of Meniere's disease: a comparison of and 1 kHz tone burst stimuli," in *Meniere's Disease and Inner Ear Homeostasis Disorders*, ed D. J. Lim (Los Angeles, CA: House Ear Institute), 140–142.

Gibson, W. P. R. (2009). A comparison of two methods of using transtympanic electrocochleography for the diagnosis of Meniere's disease: click summating potential/action potential ratio measurements and tone burst summating potential measurement. *Acta Otolaryngol.* 129, 38–42. doi: 10.1080/00016480902729843

Gibson, W. P. R., Moffat, D. A., and Ramsden, R. T. (1977). Clinical electrochleography in the diagnosis and management of Meniere's disorder. *Audiology* 16, 389–401. doi: 10.3109/00206097709071852

Gibson, W. P. R., Prasher, D. K., and Kilkenny, G. P. G. (1983). Diagnostic significance of transtympanic electrocochleography in Meniere's disease. *Ann. Otol. Rhinol. Laryngol.* 92, 155–159. doi: 10.1177/000348948309200212

Hohmann, D. H., Gibson, W. P. R., Arenberg, K. I., Dauman, R., and Bohlen, H. K. H. (1991). "International standards of transtympanic electrocochleography recordings," in *Inner Ear Surgery*, ed I. K. Arenberg (Amsterdam; New York, NY: Kugler), 249–252.

Hornibrook, J., Bird, P., Flook, E., and O'Beirne, G. A. (2016). Electrocochleography for the diagnosis of Ménière's disease: the wrong stimulus. *Otol. Neurotol.* 37, 1677–1678. doi: 10.1097/MAO.0000000000001206

Hornibrook, J., Coates, M., Goh, T., and Bird, P. (2010a). MRI inner ear imaging for Meniere's disease. *N. Z. Med. J.* 123, 64–68.

Hornibrook, J., Flook, E., Greig, S., Babbage, M., Goh, T., Coates, M., et al. (2015). MRI inner ear imaging and tone burst electrocochleography in the diagnosis of Meniere's disease. *Otol. Neurotol.* 36, 1109–1114. doi: 10.1097/MAO.0000000000000782

Hornibrook, J., George, P., and Gourley, J. (2010b). Vasopressin in definite Meniere's disease with positive eletrocochelographic findings. *Acta Otolaryngol.* 13, 613–617.

Hornibrook, J., George, P., Spellerberg, M., and Gourley, J. (2011). HSP70 antibodies in 80 patients with "clinically certain" Meniere's disease. *Ann. Otol. Rhinol. Laryngol.* 120, 651–655. doi: 10.1177/000348941112001004

Hornibrook, J., Kalin, C., Lin, E., O'Beirne, G. A., and Gourley, J. (2012). Transtympanic electrocochleography for the diagnosis of Ménière's disease. *Int. J. Otolaryngol.* 2012:852714. doi: 10.1155/2012/852714

Ikino, C. M. Y., and de Almeida, E. R. (2006). Summating potetntial-action potential waveform and width in the diagnosis of Meniere's disease. *Laryngoscope* 116, 1766–1769. doi: 10.1097/01.mlg.0000227976.43352.61

Iseli, C., and Gibson, W. P. R. (2010). A comparison of three methods of using transtympanic electrocochleography for the diagnosis of Meniere's disease: click summating potential measurements, tone burst summating potential measurements amplitude measures, and biasing of the summating potential with a low tone. *Acta Otolaryngol.* 130, 95–101. doi: 10.3109/00016480902858899

Johnson, S.-A., O'Beirne, G. A., Lin, E., Gourley, J., and Hornibrook, J. (2016). oVEMPs and cVEMPs in patienst with "clinically certain Meniere's disease." *Acta Otolaryngol.* 136, 1029–1034. doi: 10.1080/00016489.2016.1175663

Kim, H. H., Kumar, A. K., Battista, R. A., and Wiet, R. J. (2005). Electrocochleography in patients with Meniere's disease. *Am. J. Otolaryngol.* 26, 126–131. doi: 10.1016/j.amjoto.2004.11.005

Lopez-Escamez, J. A., Carey, J., Chung, W.-H., Goebel, J. A., Magnusson, M., Mandalà, M., et al. (2015). Diagnostic criteria for Menière's disease. *J. Vest. Res.* 25, 1–7. doi: 10.3233/VES-150549

Marcio, C., Ikino, Y., and de Almeida, R. (2006). Summating potential-action potential waveform amplitude and width in the diagnosis of Meniere's disease. *Laryngoscope* 116, 1766–1769. doi: 10.1097/01.mlg.0000227976.43352.61

Moffat, D. A., Gibson, W. P. R., Ramsden, A. W., and Booth, J. B. (1978). Transtympanic electrocochleography using glycerol dehydration. *Acta Otolaryngol.* 85, 158–166. doi: 10.3109/00016487809111922

Monsell, E. M., Balkany, T. A., Gates, G. A., Goldenberg, R. A., Meyerhoff, W. L., and House, J. W. (1995). Committee on hearing and equilibrium guidelines for the diagnosis and evaluation of therapy in Meniere's disease. *Otolaryngol. Head Neck Surg.* 113, 181–185. doi: 10.1016/S0194-5998(95)70102-8

Mori, N., Asai, H., and Matsunaga, T. (1987). Diagnostic value of extratympanic electrocochleography in Menière's disease. *Audiol.* 26, 103–110.

Nakashima, T., Naganawa, S., Katayama, N., Teranishi, M., Nakata S., Sugiura, M., et al. (2009). Clinical significance of endolympahtic imaging after intratympanic gadolinium injection. *Acta Otolaryngol.* 129, 9–14. doi: 10.1080/00016480902729801

Nguyen, L. T., Harris, J. P., and Nguyen, Q. T. (2010). Clinical utility of elctrocochleography in the diagnosis and management of Meniere's disease: AOS and ANS membership survey data. *Otol. Neurotol.* 31, 455–459. doi: 10.1097/MAO.0b013e3181d2779c

Paparella, M. M. (1984a). Pathogenesis of Meniere's disease and Meniere's syndrome. *Acta Otolaryngol.* 406(Suppl.), 10–25. doi: 10.1177/00034894840930S406

Paparella, M. M. (1984b). Pathology of Meniere's disease. *Ann. Otol. Rhinol. Laryngol. Suppl.* 112, 31–35. doi: 10.1177/00034894840930S406

Paparella, M. M., and Mancini, F. (1985). Vestibular Meniere's disease. *Otolaryngol. Head Neck Surg.* 93, 148–151. doi: 10.1177/019459988509300203

Pender, D. J. (2014). Endolymphatic hydrops and Meniere's disease: a lesion meta-analysis. *J. Laryngol. Otol.* 128, 859–865. doi: 10.1017/S0022215114001972

Portmann, M., Le Bert, G., and Aran, J. M. (1967). Potentiels cochleaires obtenus chez l'homme en dehors de toute intervention chirurgicale. *Rev. Laryngol. Otol.* 88, 157–164.

Pou, A. M., Hirsch, B. E., Durrant, J. D., Gold, S. R., and Kamerer, D. B. (1996). The efficacy of tympanic electrocochleography in the diagnosis of endolymphatic hydrops. *Am. J. Otol.* 17, 607–611.

Roland, P. S., and Roth, L. (1997). Interinterpreter variability in determining the SP/AP ratio in clinical electrocochleography. *Laryngoscope* 107, 1357–1361. doi: 10.1097/00005537-199710000-00012

Roland, P. S., Yellin, M. W., Meyerhoff, W. L., and Frank, T. F. (1995). Simultaneous comparison between transtympanic and extratympanic electrocochleography. *Am. J. Otol.* 16, 444–450.

Ruben, R. J., Bordley, J. E., and Lieberman, A. T. (1961). Cochlear potentials in man. *Laryngoscope* 71, 1141–1164. doi: 10.1288/00005537-196110000-00001

Sass, K. (1998). Sensitivity and specificity of transtympanic electrocochleography in Meniere's disease. *Acta Otolaryngol.* 118, 150–156. doi: 10.1080/00016489850154838

Saul, L. J., and Davis, H. A. (1932). Action currents in the central nervous system. I. Action currents of the auditory tracts. *Arch. Neurol Pyschol.* 28, 1104–1116. doi: 10.1001/archneurpsyc.1932.02240050140009

Schmidt, P. H., Eggermomt, J. J., and Odenthal, D. W. (1974). Study of Meneiere's disease by electrocochleography. *Acta Otolaryngol.* 36(Suppl.), 75–84. doi: 10.1080/16512251.1974.11675748

Sohmer, H., and Feinmesser, M. (1967). Cochlear action potentials recorded from the external ear in man. *Ann. Otol. Rinol. Laryngol.* 76, 427–435. doi: 10.1177/000348946707600211

Stopp, P. E., and Whitfeild, I. C. (1964). Summating potentials in the avian cochlea. *J. Physiol. (Lond).* 175, 45–46.

Takeda, T., and Kakigi, A. (2010). The clinical value of extratympanic electrocochleography in the diagnosis of Meniere's disease. *ORL J. Otorhinolaryngol. Relat. Spec.* 72, 196–204. doi: 10.1159/000315552

Teas, D. C., Eldrege, D. H., and Davis, H. (1962). Cochlear responses to acoustics transients: an interpretation of the whole action potentials. *J. Acoust. Soc. Am.* 34, 1438–1459. doi: 10.1121/1.1918366

Thorpe, M. A., Shehab, Z. P., Bance, M. L., and Rutka, J. A. (2003). The AAO-HNS Committee on Hearing and Equilibrium guidelines for the diagnosis and evaluation of therapy for Meniere's disease: have they been applied in the published literature in the last decade? *Clin. Otolaryngol.* 28, 173–176. doi: 10.1046/j.1365-2273.2003.00687.x

von Bekesy, G. (1952). D-C resting potentials in the cochlea partition. *J. Acoust. Soc. Am.* 24, 72–76. doi: 10.1121/1.1906851

Wever, E. G., and Bray, C. W. (1930). Action currents in the auditory nerve in response to acoustic stimulation. *Proc. Natl. Acad. Sci. U.S.A.* 16, 344–350. doi: 10.1073/pnas.16.5.344

Wuyts, F. L., Van de Heyning, P., Spaendonck, M. P., and Molenberghs, G. (1997). A review of electrocochleography: instrumental settings and meta-analysis or criteria for diagnosis of endolymphatic hydrops. *Acta Otolaryngol. Suppl.* 526, 14–20. doi: 10.3109/00016489709124014

Yoshie, N. (1968). Auditory action potentials to click in man. *Laryngoscope* 178, 198–215. doi: 10.1288/00005537-196802000-00002

Zerlin, S. (1969). Travelling-wave velocity in the human cochlea. *J. Acoust. Soc. Am.* 46, 1011–1016. doi: 10.1121/1.1911792

Ziylan, F., Smeeing, D. P. J., Stegeman, I., and Thomeer, H. G. (2016). Click stimulus electrocochleography versus MRI with intratympanic contrast in Meniere's disease: a systematic review. *Otol. Neurotol.* 37, 421–427. doi: 10.1097/MAO.0000000000001021

Zwicker, E., and Fast, L. (1972). On the development of the critical band. *J. Acoust. Soc. Am.* 52, 699–702. doi: 10.1121/1.1913161

4

Intracochlear Recordings of Acoustically and Electrically Evoked Potentials in Nucleus Hybrid L24 Cochlear Implant Users and their Relationship to Speech Perception

*Jae-Ryong Kim[1,2], Viral D. Tejani[1,3], Paul J. Abbas[1,3] and Carolyn J. Brown[1,3]**

[1] Department of Communication Sciences and Disorders, University of Iowa, Iowa City, IA, USA, [2] Department of Otolaryngology-Head and Neck Surgery, Inje University College of Medicine, Busan, South Korea, [3] Department of Otolaryngology-Head and Neck Surgery, University of Iowa Hospitals and Clinics, Iowa City, IA, USA

***Correspondence:**
Carolyn J. Brown
carolyn-brown@uiowa.edu

The Hybrid cochlear implant (CI) has been developed for individuals with high frequency hearing loss who retain good low frequency hearing. Outcomes have been encouraging but individual variability is high; the health of the cochlea and the auditory nerve may be important factors driving outcomes. Electrically evoked compound action potentials (ECAPs) reflect the response of the auditory nerve to electrical stimulation while electrocochleography (ECochG) reflects the response of the cochlear hair cells and auditory nerve to acoustic stimulation. In this study both ECAPs and ECochG responses were recorded from Nucleus Hybrid L24 CI users. Correlations between these two measures of peripheral auditory function and speech perception are reported. This retrospective study includes data from 25 L24 CI users. ECAPs and ECochG responses were recorded from an intracochlear electrode using stimuli presented at or near maximum acceptable loudness levels. Speech perception was assessed using Consonant-Nucleus-Consonant (CNC) word lists presented in quiet and AzBio sentences presented at a +5 dB signal-to-noise ratio in both the combined acoustic and electric (A+E) and electric (E) alone listening modes. Acoustic gain was calculated by subtracting these two scores. Correlations between these physiologic and speech perception measures were then computed. ECAP amplitudes recorded from the most apical electrode were significantly correlated with CNC scores measured in the E alone ($r = 0.56$) and A+E conditions ($r = 0.64$), but not with performance on the AzBio test. ECochG responses recorded using the most apical electrode in the intracochlear array but evoked using a 500 Hz tone burst were not correlated with either the scores on the CNC or AzBio tests. However, ECochG amplitude was correlated with a composite metric relating the additional benefit of acoustic gain in noise relative to quiet conditions ($r = 0.67$). Both measures can be recorded from Hybrid L24 CI users and both ECAP and ECochG measures may result in more complete characterization of speech perception outcomes than either measure alone.

Keywords: cochlear implant, auditory evoked potentials, electrocochleography, electrically evoked compound action potential, hybrid cochlear implant, neural response telemetry

INTRODUCTION

Since cochlear implants (CIs) were first introduced into clinical practice in the mid-1980s, CI technology has changed significantly. Those changes led to marked improvements in performance and today, CIs are considered to be the treatment of choice for individuals with bilateral profound sensorineural hearing loss (SNHL). Recently, and based in large part on the positive outcomes exhibited by standard CI users, candidacy criteria have been relaxed to include individuals with good low frequency hearing but severe-to-profound high frequency SNHL (Cohen, 2004; Lenarz et al., 2013; Roland et al., 2016). Hearing aids often provide only limited benefit for this population (Hornsby and Ricketts, 2006; Turner, 2006) making CIs an attractive alternative. However, insertion trauma associated with implanting a standard long electrode array often resulted in complete loss of residual acoustic hearing in the implanted ear. Hybrid CIs were developed specifically for this population and designed to help preserve residual acoustic hearing in the implanted ear (Gantz and Turner, 2003; Lenarz et al., 2009).

The original S8 Hybrid CI was manufactured by Cochlear Ltd. for investigational purposes and had a shorter electrode array (10 mm) and fewer intracochlear electrodes (6 electrodes) than the standard, long 22-electrode arrays offered by Cochlear Ltd. (Gantz and Turner, 2003). The goal was for the intracochlear electrode array to be inserted into the cochlea without adversely affecting residual low frequency acoustic hearing. Low frequency sounds were intended to be processed normally (with or occasionally without amplification). High frequency sounds were transmitted electrically, bypassing the damaged cochlear hair cells and stimulating the auditory nerve directly (Turner et al., 2008a). Preliminary results were promising (Turner et al., 2004; Gantz et al., 2009; Woodson et al., 2010). On average, speech perception scores measured in quiet and in background noise were significantly better when the listeners were allowed to combine both acoustic and electrical (A+E) input compared to when they were tested using either in the acoustic (A) alone or electrical (E) alone listening modes. Additionally, speech perception in noise was better for S8 Hybrid users compared to the standard 22-electrode implant users (Turner et al., 2004, 2008b). These findings led to the development of the commercially released Nucleus L24 Hybrid electrode array (described in more detail in "Materials and Methods"). Studies again showed good performance (Büchner et al., 2009; Lenarz et al., 2009, 2013; Roland et al., 2016), but individual variability remains high. Some Hybrid CI users (regardless of manufacturer and length of array) benefited tremendously from having access to both acoustic and electrical signals, while others did not (Kiefer et al., 2005; Reiss et al., 2008; Lenarz et al., 2013; Gantz et al., 2016; Roland et al., 2016).

Outcomes with a CI are a result of multiple factors (Lazard et al., 2012; Blamey et al., 2013; Holden et al., 2013; Shearer et al., 2017). Recent investigations have suggested that better outcomes with a traditional or Hybrid CI might be expected from individuals presenting with better overall "cochlear health" (Gantz et al., 2009; Kim et al., 2010; Fitzpatrick et al., 2013; Formeister et al., 2015). In other words, CI candidates who present with better hair cell and/or neural survival may have better outcomes. Cochlear health might be more important for Hybrid candidates with residual hearing than for traditional CI candidates. In this study, we use the Neural Response Telemetry (NRT) system to measure the response of the peripheral auditory system to both acoustic and electrical stimulation. Our goal is to explore the relationship between these objective measures of the status of the auditory periphery and speech perception.

Electrically evoked compound action potentials (ECAPs) are recordings of the synchronous response from a large number of auditory nerve fibers to the presentation of a brief electrical impulse. They are characterized by a negative peak (N1) that is recorded approximately 0.2–0.4 ms following the onset of the stimulus and is followed by a positive peak (P2) at 0.6–0.8 ms (Brown et al., 1998, 2000; Abbas et al., 1999). ECAPs are recorded routinely following cochlear implantation and do not require the presence of viable cochlear hair cells. As early as 1958, Goldstein and Kiang theorized that the amplitude of neural potentials should increase as the number of active neurons increased. Animal studies later showed that electrically evoked neural potentials are correlated with neural survival (Smith and Simmons, 1983; Hall, 1990; Miller et al., 1994; Prado-Guitierrez et al., 2006). One may theorize that stronger ECAPs or greater neural survival would reflect better CI outcomes (Kim et al., 2010; Seyyedi et al., 2014) but this has been somewhat difficult to prove. Kim et al. (2010) reported finding correlations between the slope of the ECAP amplitude growth functions and performance. That study included subjects who used both older generation devices (Nucleus CI24M standard implant and the 24M S8 Hybrid implant) and newer technology (Nucleus 24RE standard implant and the 24RE S8 Hybrid implant). The major difference between the older and newer implants was the lower noise floor of the amplifier on the newer devices. The noise floor of the measurement system could impact slope of the ECAP growth functions. Kim et al. (2010) reported that the slope of the ECAP growth functions measured using the newer technology implants was correlated with performance. This was not the case for the older generation of CIs.

Acoustically evoked neural responses can also be recorded from the auditory periphery. This measure is typically referred to as an electrocochleography (ECochG). ECochGs have traditionally been recorded using an electrode placed on the tympanic membrane or the promontory of the middle ear. They have played a role in diagnosing Meniere's disease (Gibson et al., 1977) and more recently have been used to explore the pathophysiology of a condition often described as "hidden hearing loss" where audiometric thresholds are normal but patients struggle to understand speech in background noise (Liberman et al., 2016). ECochGs have also been recorded using a round window electrode from individuals undergoing CI surgery. High level acoustic tone bursts that range in frequency from 250 to 4,000 Hz were presented. These responses were combined offline to generate a metric called the "total cochlear response" (Fitzpatrick et al., 2013; Formeister et al., 2015). Importantly, Fitzpatrick et al. (2013) and Formeister et al. (2015) reported a significant correlation between the magnitude of the ongoing

ECochG response across several frequencies and postoperative speech perception in adults and children using standard CIs.

Recently, several researchers described ECochG recordings obtained from CI users with residual hearing during the postoperative period (Dalbert et al., 2015; Abbas et al., 2017; Koka et al., 2017). Across these studies, acoustic stimuli were presented and ECochG recordings were obtained from an intracochlear electrode. Koka et al. (2017) and Abbas et al. (2017) used recording and analysis methods to emphasize contributions from either the cochlear hair cells or the auditory nerve. Significant correlations between the ECochG responses and audiometric thresholds were also reported. Results showed that acoustically generated ECochG responses could be used to monitor changes in hearing status following cochlear implantation.

In this study we propose to use a combination of both acoustic and electrical stimulation to more fully characterize the status of the auditory periphery in Hybrid L24 CI users. We argue that the two measures should provide a more complete profile of the status of the peripheral auditory system than either measure individually. Our goal is to determine the extent to which ECAP responses, which likely reflect the response primarily from the relatively basal region of the cochlea to electrical stimulation, and the acoustically evoked ECochG responses, which provide a measure of hair cell and neural responses from more apical regions of the cochlea, might be combined to more accurately characterize the status of the auditory periphery. We compare these measures to speech perception results obtained from a group of Hybrid L24 CI users to test the hypothesis that speech perception is related to the status of the auditory periphery. More specifically, we will assess if individuals with more robust (e.g., largest) ECAPs will exhibit better performance when testing is conducted in the electric only listening mode than individuals who have smaller amplitude ECAP responses. Additionally, we will assess if Hybrid CI recipients who enjoy the most benefit from use of acoustic stimulation are those who also present with the most robust (e.g., largest) acoustically evoked ECochG responses.

MATERIALS AND METHODS

This was a retrospective study. Records from individuals who received a Nucleus Hybrid L24 CI at the University of Iowa Hospitals and Clinics between 2010 and 2015 were reviewed and information about speech perception extracted. These results were then compared with ECAP and ECochG data also collected in our lab. The ECochG data was recently published (Abbas et al., 2017). That report focused on describing analysis techniques to emphasize contributions of hair cells and the auditory nerve to the ECochG response. In this report we focus on an alternative measure of ECochG magnitude. We also include measures of neural response to an electrical stimulus (ECAP) that were not included in the Abbas et al. (2017) study. All of the procedures used in this study were approved by the University of Iowa Institutional Review Board (IRB) and all subjects gave written informed consent in accordance with the Declaration of Helsinki.

Nucleus Hybrid L24 CI

The Nucleus Hybrid L24 CI is manufactured by Cochlear Ltd. The internal electrode array is 16 mm in total length and contains 22 electrode contacts. It is thinner than the previous generation CI24RE CI, and the electrode array is designed to rest against the lateral wall of the cochlea. The implanted electrode array spans approximately 270° of the basal turn of the cochlea with the most apical electrode lying at a place thought to correspond to approximately 1,500–2,000 Hz (Greenwood, 1990; Stakhovskaya et al., 2007; Lenarz et al., 2009, 2013; Jurawitz et al., 2014; Roland et al., 2016). The L24 array was approved by the Food and Drug Administration (FDA) for clinical use in March 2014; arrays implanted prior to that date were implanted under an FDA Investigational Device Exemption (IDE) status (IDE G070191 and G110089). The external processor used with this device includes both an electrical and acoustic component. It is designed to allow the user to integrate electric and acoustic information simultaneously and can be programmed to accommodate the extent and configuration of a recipient's acoustic hearing following surgery.

Subjects

Twenty-five adult Nucleus Hybrid L24 CI users participated in this study. **Table 1** shows demographic information about the study participants. Forty-four percent were male. Fifty-six percent were female. Approximately equal numbers of right and left ears were implanted. For the majority of study participants, the etiology of their hearing loss was unknown. Subjects ranged in age from 18 to 65 years at the time of surgery. Mean duration of hearing loss prior to CI surgery was 28 years ($SD = 16$ years) and mean duration of hearing aid use was 17 years ($SD = 12$ years). Preoperative Consonant-Nucleus-Consonant (CNC) word scores were, on average, 22% correct. Though for the purposes of this report, it was not necessary to compare preoperative and postoperative audiometric thresholds, we included this data for informative purposes (**Figure 1**). Postoperative thresholds were measured at the time ECAP, ECochG, and speech perception data were obtained. The majority of study participants had low frequency acoustic hearing (pure tone average of 250, 500, and 1,000 Hz) within 15 dB of their preoperative pure tone thresholds. Three subjects lost significant amounts of acoustic hearing post-operatively (>30 dB) and were also included in this report. Inclusion criteria required that the selected participants had stable residual hearing at the time of evoked potential and speech perception testing since, on occasion, testing occurred at two different points in time. Since ECochG responses in Hybrid users remain stable over time for those with stable residual hearing (Abbas et al., 2017), the different time periods of testing in some subjects was not concerning.

The 25 participants were part of a larger pool of individuals with hearing preservation implants who participated in earlier studies in our lab where post-operative ECochG and ECAP data were collected. Subjects were awake during the testing procedures. ECochG growth functions were collected using acoustic 500 Hz tone bursts and recorded using the most apical intracochlear electrode (Abbas et al., 2017). ECAP growth

TABLE 1 | Demographic and audiological history for study participants.

	n (%)		mean ± SD
Gender		Age at implantation (years)	50 ± 13
Male	11 (44%)		
Female	14 (56%)	Duration of HL (years)	28 ± 16
Ear implanted			
Right	13 (52%)	Duration of HA use (years)	17 ± 12
Left	12 (48%)		
Etiology		Preoperative PTA[§] (dB HL)	56 ± 13
Unknown	15 (60%)		
Hereditary	4 (16%)	Postoperative PTA[§] (dB HL)	70 ± 15
Noise exposure	4 (16%)		
Autoimmune	2 (8%)	Preoperative CNC word (%)	22 ± 16

[§] *Pure tone average of 0.25, 0.5, 1 kHz (No responses were converted to 120 dB HL). HL indicates hearing loss; HA, hearing aid; PTA, pure tone average; CNC, consonant-nucleus-consonant; SD, standard deviation.*

functions were collected from a subset of electrodes spaced across the array. Speech perception scores were extracted from the patient's clinical records. ECAP and ECochG data were generally collected at the same point in time (no earlier than 1 month post activation). Speech perception testing was conducted no earlier than 6 months post activation. All 25 study participants had been fit with and regularly used an acoustic component with their speech processor. The frequency boundary for acoustic-electric stimulation was defined as the highest audiometric frequency with an unaided audiometric threshold less than or equal to 70 dB HL (Cochlear Ltd., 2015). The acoustic component of the Hybrid system was programmed using the NAL-NL2 fitting formula (Keidser et al., 2011). In some instances, acoustic output was modified slightly to address problems with loudness tolerance. Frequencies higher than the acoustic-electric boundary were delivered via electrical stimulation.

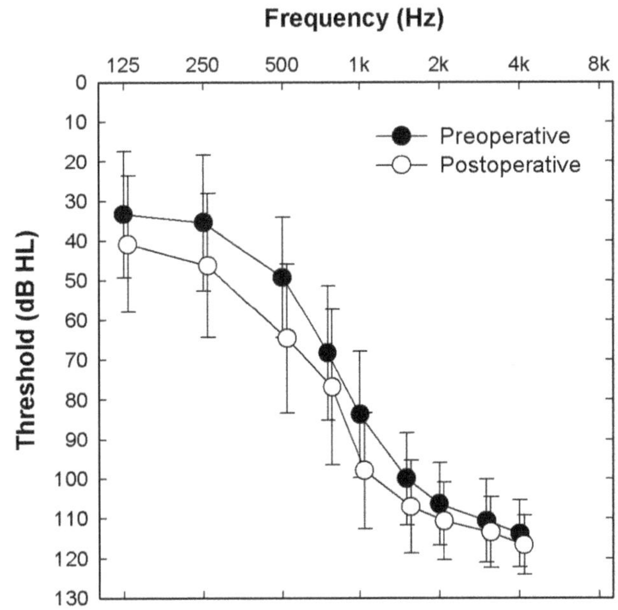

FIGURE 1 | Mean pre- and post-operative audiometric thresholds for the implanted ear of all 25 study participants. Error bars indicate ± 1 standard deviation.

Electrophysiologic Recordings: Electrical Stimulation

ECAPs were recorded using standard clinical software provided by Cochlear Ltd. (Custom Sound EP, version 4.3). Stimuli were biphasic current pulses presented in a monopolar stimulation mode at 80 Hz stimulation rate. Pulse durations were typically 25 μs/phase with a 7 μs interphase gap. Higher pulse durations (37 or 50 μs) were used in some cases to overcome voltage compliance limits. Three stimulating electrodes widely spaced across the electrode array were selected for testing. They included an apical electrode (20, 21, or 22), a middle electrode (12, 13, or 14), and a basal electrode (6, 7, or 8). Typically, an electrode located two electrodes apical relative to the stimulating electrode was used for recording. ECAPs were obtained at a 20 kHz sampling rate using the standard subtraction method detailed elsewhere (Brown et al., 1998, 2000; Abbas et al., 1999). Amplitude growth functions were obtained for these test electrodes. These functions were generated by a series of ECAPs that were recorded at probe levels that varied from just below the uncomfortable loudness level (UCL)—labeled here the maximum comfortable level (MCL) - to below the visual detection threshold. For the purposes of this retrospective review, only the ECAP amplitude recorded at MCL was used for correlational analysis.

ECAP waveforms consisted of an average of approximately 50–100 sweeps, and were analyzed offline using a custom MATLAB script. N1 and P2 peaks were selected manually and the ECAP amplitude for each waveform was defined as the voltage difference between the N1 and P2 peaks.

Electrophysiologic Recordings: Acoustic Stimulation

Acoustically evoked ECochG responses were recorded using Custom Sound EP (version 3.2). Details of the recording technique have been reported elsewhere (Abbas et al., 2017). Briefly, a research patch allowed Custom Sound EP to trigger an external acoustic stimulus. The stimulus was a 12 ms, 500 Hz tone burst that was shaped by a rectangular gating function and generated digitally at a 44.1 kHz sampling rate. The stimulus was presented to the implanted ear via an insert earphone at a 10 Hz stimulation rate. The level of the acoustic stimulus was varied from MCL down to visual ECochG threshold in 5–10 dB steps. ECochG responses were recorded using both positive and negative leading tone burst stimuli. For this study, only the ECochG response at MCL was examined. Electrode 22 (the most apical intracochlear electrode) was used as the recording electrode. Recording sampling rate was 20 kHz. Each response consisted of an average of 200 to 400 sweeps. Contamination due to system artifacts were minimized by obtaining an ECochG response when the acoustic probe was not placed in ear canal, but continued to deliver an acoustic stimulus at the highest test level.

This "no stimulus" recording of system artifact was subtracted from the ECochG recordings.

Responses recorded using initially positive and negative polarities were stored separately and analyzed in the frequency domain using a Fast Fourier Transform (FFT). The resolution of the FFT was 55.33 Hz/bin. These ECochG responses likely reflect activity generated at both the hair cell (i.e., cochlear microphonic) and the auditory nerve (i.e., auditory nerve neurophonic). The data from Abbas et al. (2017) were reanalyzed using different techniques. The magnitudes of the FFT responses recorded at the frequency corresponding to the first, second, and third harmonics of the tone burst were measured and were considered significant if the amplitude exceeded the noise plus three standard deviations. The noise and its standard deviation were calculated from 6 bins, 3 on each side of all harmonics, starting 2 bins away from the peak. Magnitude of ECochG was calculated as the sum of the magnitude of FFT responses at all significant harmonics in each polarity. For this study, the average of the magnitude of ECochG in each polarity was used for correlational analysis.

Speech Perception Measures

Two different measures of speech perception were obtained from the clinical records of each subject. Speech perception in quiet was measured using the CNC monosyllabic word test (Peterson and Lehiste, 1962). Speech perception in noise was assessed using the AzBio sentence test with the sentences presented at a +5 dB signal-to-noise ratio (SNR) (Spahr et al., 2012). The noise used for the AzBio sentence test was a 10-talker babble. For both tests, the speech signal was presented at 60 dBA via a loudspeaker located 1 meter away from the subject at 0 degrees azimuth. Noise was also presented from the same loudspeaker for the AzBio test. The CNC word test consists of 50 words in each list, and the AzBio sentence test is composed of 20 sentences in each list. Two lists were used for both tests. Results were reported in percentage of the total number of words correct.

Speech perception data obtained in the E alone (implant alone) and A+E (implant and ipsilateral hearing aid) listening conditions were extracted from the medical charts. To assess speech performance in the E alone mode, both ipsilateral and contralateral ear canals were occluded with foam earplugs and earmuffs. For performance in the A+E mode, only the contralateral ear canal was occluded. Pilot data collected from two normal hearing listeners revealed that use of plugs and muffs resulted in 25 to 40 dB of attenuation for frequencies between 125 and 1,000 Hz and 25 dB of attenuation for speech reception thresholds in the sound field. Clearly, we cannot argue that contribution from the non-test ear was eliminated; however, it should have been minimized based on these attenuation rates. Finally, we also calculated a metric we refer to as acoustic gain (A gain). A gain was computed by subtracting the E alone score from the A+E score. In theory, this subtracted response should reflect the benefit individual study participants receive from the use of their residual low frequency acoustic hearing.

RESULTS

Electrophysiologic Measures

ECAP recordings were obtained for 24 of the 25 study participants (96%). We attempted, but failed to record an ECAP for one participant. ECAP thresholds were possibly higher than MCL in this case. **Figure 2A** shows typical ECAP waveforms measured using stimulation of electrode 6 (basal), 14 (middle) and 20 (apical) for subject L4R. ECAP amplitude decreased as

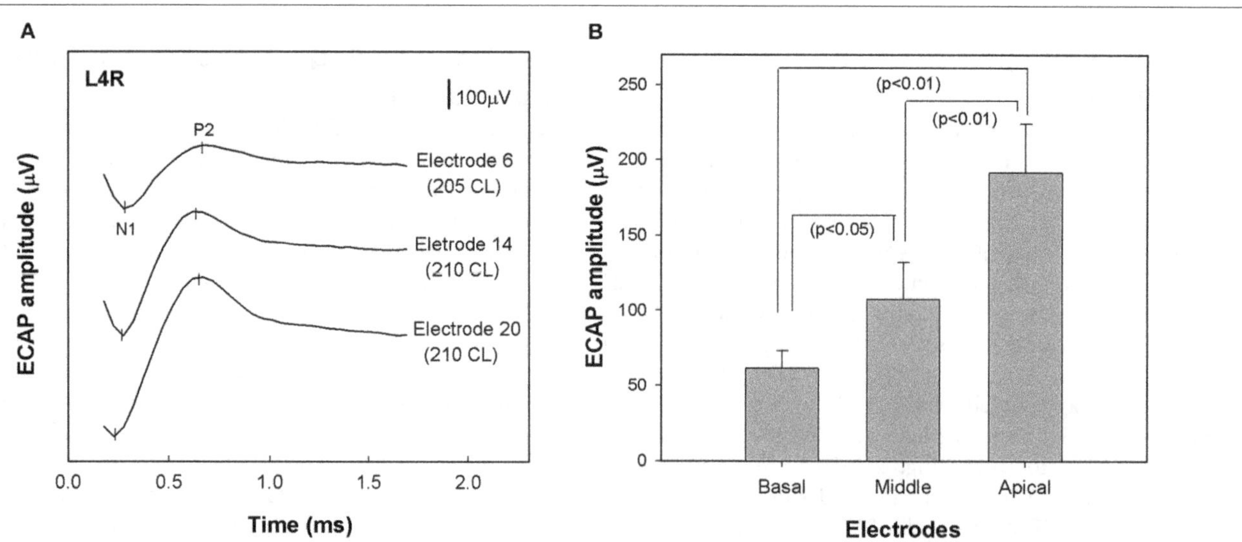

FIGURE 2 | (A) ECAP waveforms recorded from a single study participant (L4R) at three different stimulation sites: electrode 6 (basal), electrode 14 (middle), and electrode 20 (apical). Each waveform was recorded at the maximum acceptable loudness level. Stimulation level is specified in clinical programming units (CL). **(B)** Comparison of group mean ECAP amplitudes across stimulating electrode sites (basal, middle and apical) ($n = 24$). Error bars indicate ± 1 standard error around the mean. ECAP stands for electrically evoked compound action potential.

the stimulating electrode was changed from an apical to a more basal electrode.

Figure 2B shows the range of ECAP amplitudes recorded at each of the three stimulation sites. A repeated measures analysis of variance (ANOVA) was performed using stimulation site (apical, middle, and basal) as the within-subjects variable. The analysis revealed a significant effect of stimulation site [$F_{(1.482, 24)} = 19.461$, $p < 0.01$]. *Post-hoc* tests indicated that ECAP amplitudes became progressively larger as the stimulating electrode was moved toward the apex of the electrode array. Specifically, the ECAP amplitudes recorded with stimulation near the middle of the array were significantly greater than those recorded using a more basal stimulation site ($p < 0.05$) and were significantly smaller than those recorded using more apical stimulation ($p < 0.01$).

ECochG responses were recorded using 500 Hz tone bursts from all of the study participants. **Figure 3** shows example recordings obtained from two different subjects (L23R, L18R). The two panels on the left side of **Figure 3** show the pure tone audiogram for the implanted ear measured at the test session. 500 Hz audiometric thresholds were 40 dB HL for subject L23R and 85 dB HL for subject L18R. The center panels show ECochG waveforms recorded using 500 Hz tone bursts that were presented at MCL and in both polarities for each of the two subjects. The panels on the right side of **Figure 3** show the results of FFT analysis of ECochG recordings. Clear peaks in the FFT are apparent at 500 Hz and 1,000 Hz for subject L23R whose data is shown in the top row. For subject L18R, clear peaks in the FFT were evident at 500, 1,000, and 1,500 Hz. The frequencies correspond to the first, second and third harmonics of the 500 Hz stimulus. The circles indicate FFT responses where the specific harmonic was significantly above the noise floor of the measurement system. ECochG magnitude was calculated by averaging the sum of the magnitude of responses at all significant harmonics in each polarity. These values are indicated on the figure. Note that the magnitude of the ECochG response is larger for the subject with more residual hearing (L23R).

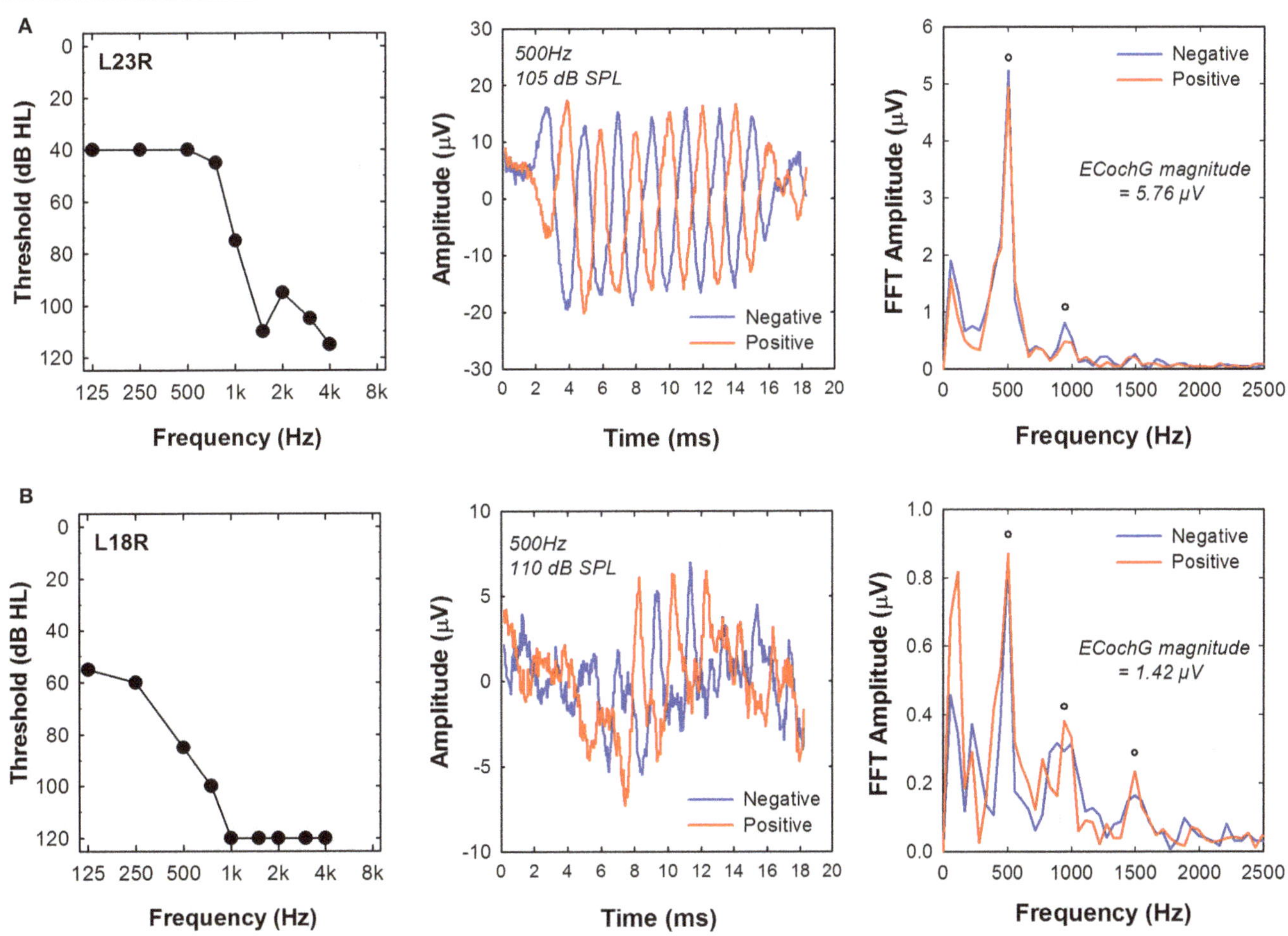

FIGURE 3 | Examples of ECochG responses recorded using a 500 Hz tone burst from two subjects, (A) L23R and **(B)** L18R. Left panels show the audiogram measured at the time of testing. Center panels show the time waveforms in response to positive and negative leading tone bursts. Right panels show the results of a FFT of the time waveforms. The circles indicate frequencies where the energy at the harmonic frequency was significantly above the noise floor of the measurement system. Note the different amplitude scales used for these two subjects. ECochG indicates electrocochleography; FFT, Fast Fourier Transform.

Speech Perception Measures

Figure 4 shows the effect of listening mode on speech perception measured in quiet (CNC word test) and in background noise (AzBio sentence test at +5 dB SNR). CNC scores were not available for two subjects and AzBio test results were not measured for three subjects in the E alone modes. For the CNC word test, mean scores were 74% in A+E mode and 54% in E alone mode. For the AzBio sentences test in noise, the mean scores were 53% in A+E condition and 26% in E alone condition. Performance in the A+E mode was significantly better than in E alone mode for both tests as shown by a paired samples *t*-test [CNC: $t_{(22)} = 9.12, p < 0.001$; AzBio: $t_{(21)} = 8.23, p < 0.001$].

This figure also shows that average performance in the E alone condition was greater when the task involved perception of speech in quiet (CNC test) compared to when the task required perception of speech in background noise (AzBio test). However, the benefit provided by having access to acoustic sound (A gain) is greater for speech perception in noise (AzBio test) compared to speech perception in quiet (CNC test). That is, the difference between the E alone and A gain scores is greater for the CNC test than for the AzBio test. While this may be due to differences in test materials (words vs. sentences), we suggest that it may also reflect that for speech stimuli presented in background noise, greater reliance on the acoustic signal is required for better performance.

In order to quantify the contribution of electric and acoustic stimulation to performance in the A+E listening mode, we computed two ratios for each subject. One ratio compared the speech perception score obtained in the E-alone condition to the A+E condition (E-alone/A+E). A second ratio compared speech perception score obtained using only acoustic stimulation (A gain) to the score obtained in the A+E listening mode (A gain/A+E). Paired t-tests revealed that the ratio of E alone/A+E was significantly larger for the CNC test compared to the AzBio test [$t_{(21)} = 6.75, p < 0.001$]. A similar analysis was performed comparing the ratio of A gain/A+E on the two speech perception tasks. Paired *t*-tests showed that the ratio of A gain/A+E was significantly larger for the AzBio test in noise than for the CNC test in quiet [$t_{(21)} = 4.59, p < 0.001$]. (Note that the sum of the E alone ratio and the A gain ratio will be 1, thus this analysis is complementary). We interpret these data to suggest that electric hearing may contribute more to the benefits of hybrid listening in quiet environments, while residual acoustic hearing is an important factor that may play a larger role in determining outcomes in noisy listening conditions.

Figure 5 shows correlations between performance on CNC word lists presented in quiet and AzBio sentences presented in noise. Linear regression analysis revealed significant correlation in scores for A+E ($r = 0.83$, $p < 0.0001$, $n = 25$), E alone ($r = 0.81, p < 0.0001, n = 22$) and A gain ($r = 0.85, p < 0.0001$, $n = 22$) conditions. Subjects who perform better on one speech perception test are likely to perform better on another measure of speech perception.

Correlations between Electrophysiologic Measures and Performance

The primary goal of this study was to characterize the relationship between electrically and acoustically evoked peripheral electrophysiologic measures and performance on speech perception tests in a representative group of Nucleus Hybrid L24 CI users. Hybrid CI users perceive high-frequency portions of the acoustic signal via electric hearing. Low frequency information in the acoustic signal is amplified and transmitted acoustically. Therefore, ECAP responses to electrical stimulation were compared to performance in E alone condition and ECochG responses to acoustic stimulation were compared to A gain. ECAP and ECochG responses were also compared to performance in A+E condition.

We hypothesized that performance on speech tests, particularly when testing is done in the E alone condition,

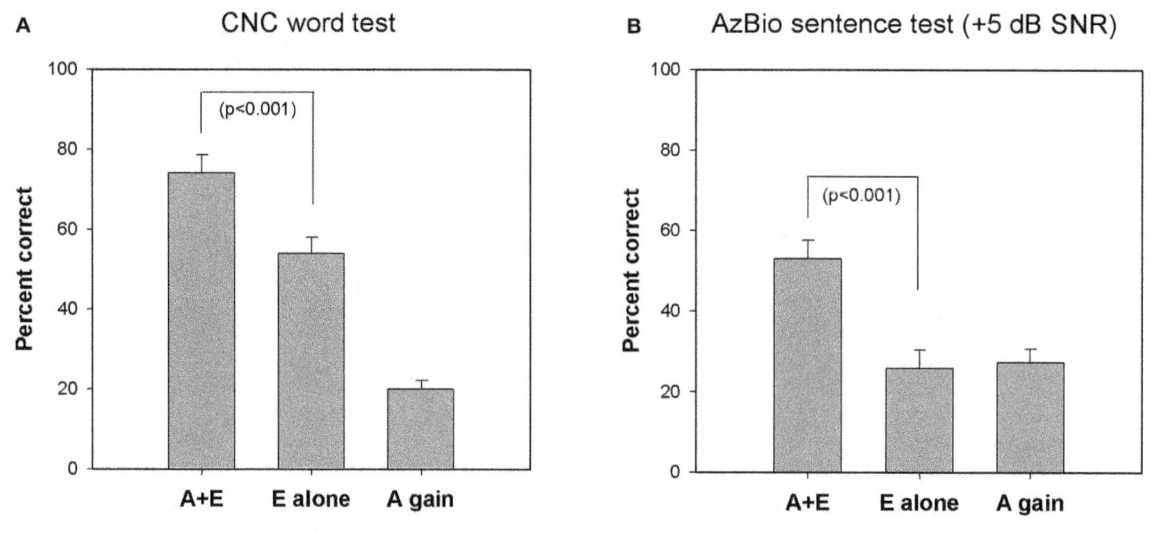

FIGURE 4 | Group mean speech perception scores in A+E, E alone, and A gain condition on (A) CNC word test in quiet ($n = 23$) and **(B)** AzBio sentence test at a +5 dB SNR ($n = 22$). Error bars are standard errors of means. CNC indicates consonant-nucleus-consonant; SNR, signal-to-noise ratio; A, acoustic; E, electric.

would correlate with electrically evoked responses. We found that the correlation between the amplitude of the ECAP recorded using stimulation of the most apical electrode in the intracochlear array and performance on the CNC word list administered in the E alone mode was, in fact, statistically significant ($r = 0.56$, $p < 0.01$). **Figure 6A** is a scatterplot that illustrates this relationship. No significant correlation between the ECAP amplitudes recorded from the middle or basal electrode and CNC performance were revealed nor were there significant correlations between ECAP amplitude and performance on the more challenging AzBio test when administered in the E alone mode.

We also hypothesized that speech perception in the A gain condition would be related to the acoustically evoked ECochG responses. We assumed that subjects who benefited most from the use of their residual acoustic hearing have more robust ECochG responses to a low frequency tone burst. However, no statistically significant correlations were found between the magnitude of the ECochG recorded using a 500 Hz tone burst and performance on either the CNC word lists or on the AzBio test in the A gain condition.

While correlations between the ECAP or ECochG and performance in the E alone and A gain conditions are informative, more important are correlations between these peripheral measures of auditory function and performance in the A+E listening mode. This is the condition where the subjects are most practiced and, from a clinical perspective, it is the most relevant test mode. The amplitude of the ECAP response

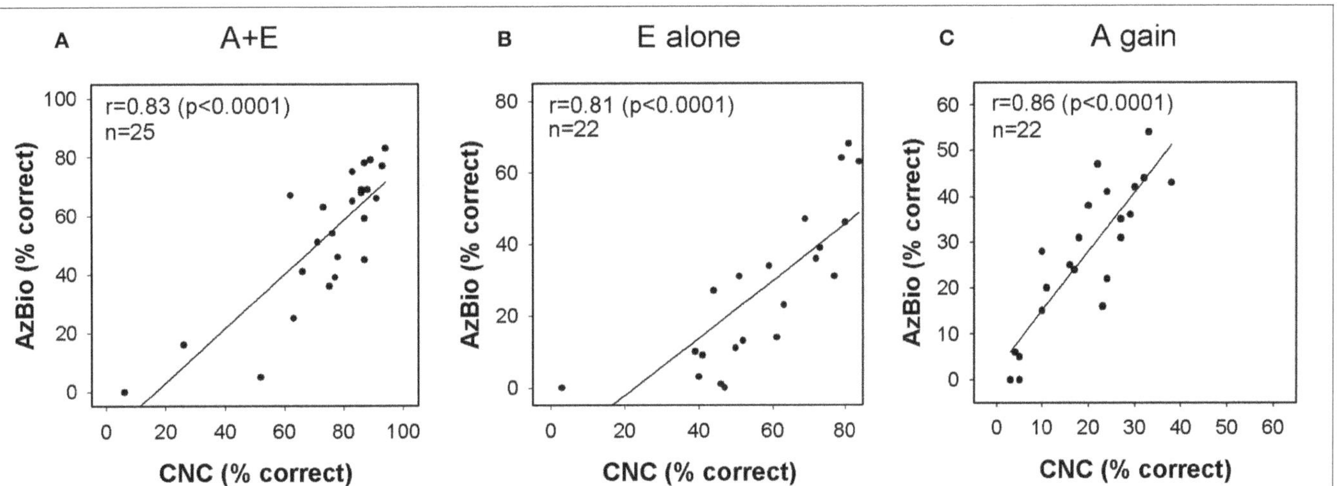

FIGURE 5 | Relationship between CNC and AzBio performance in (A) A+E, **(B)** E alone, and **(C)** A gain conditions. Each column plots the AzBio sentence scores as a function of CNC word scores. CNC indicates consonant-nucleus-consonant; A, acoustic; E, electric.

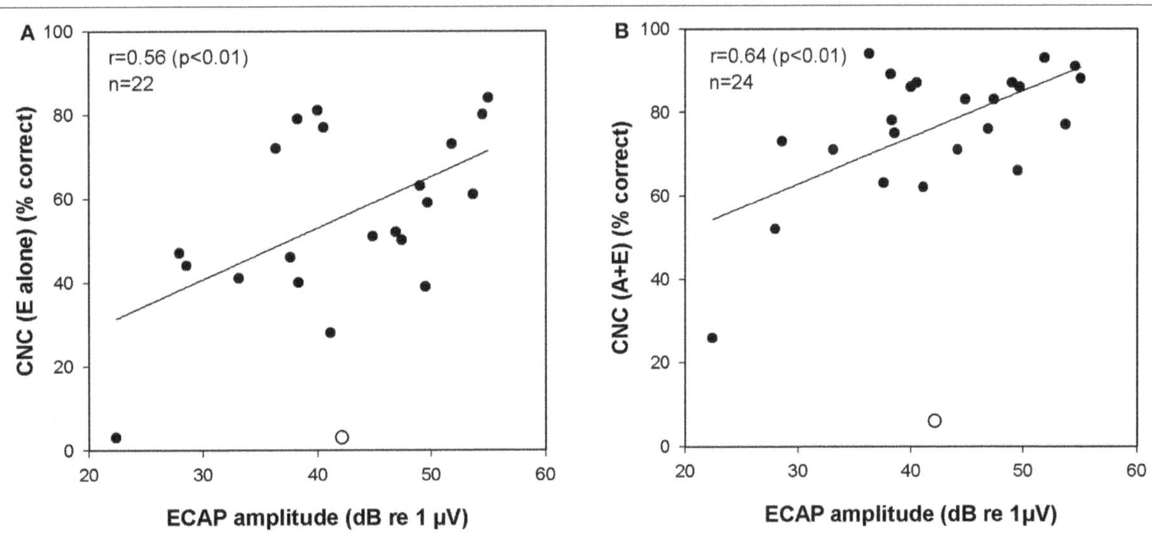

FIGURE 6 | (A) Correlation between ECAP amplitudes and CNC scores (E alone). **(B)** Correlation between ECAP amplitudes and CNC scores (A+E). One data point was identified as an outlier (studentized residual > 2.0). This data point is marked with an open circle and was excluded from correlation analysis. ECAP indicates electrically evoked compound action potential; CNC, consonant-nucleus-consonant; A, acoustic; E, electric.

recorded using stimulation of the most apical electrode was found to be significantly correlated with performance on the CNC word list when speech perception was measured in the A+E listening mode ($r = 0.64$, $p < 0.01$). **Figure 6B** is a scatterplot that illustrates this relationship. Significant correlations between the apical ECAP amplitude and performance on the AzBio test were not observed nor were significant correlations between the ECAP amplitudes recorded from middle or basal electrodes and speech performance revealed. The ECochG magnitudes were also compared to performance in A+E listening mode. However, there were no significant correlations between the ECochG magnitude and performance on CNC or AzBio tests.

Table 2 shows the summary of correlations between ECAP (recorded from an apical electrode) and ECochG responses to speech perception scores. No significant correlations were found for middle and basal electrodes; thus, for brevity, they were not included in **Table 2**.

We know that Hybrid CI users enjoy improved hearing in noise rather than in quiet relative to standard, long electrode CI users, likely due to the residual low frequency acoustic hearing (Turner et al., 2004; Gantz et al., 2009). In order to further investigate the relationship between the acoustically evoked ECochG measures and performance with the Hybrid implant, we computed a ratio of performance on speech perception in noise (AzBio test) relative to their ability to understand speech in quiet (CNC test). This was calculated as

$$A_{gain}\ Ratio = \frac{A_{gain\ (Noise)}}{A_{gain\ (Quiet)}} = \frac{AzBio_{A+E} - AzBio_{E\ alone}}{CNC_{A+E} - CNC_{E\ alone}}$$

We focused on the derived A gain scores, reasoning that these measures are the ones likely to be most sensitive to the status of the cochlea. **Figure 7** shows the results we observed when we made this comparison. The magnitude of the ECochG response to a 500 Hz tone burst was found to be correlated with speech perception as characterized using this ratio (A gain) of two different speech tests ($r = 0.67$, $p < 0.01$).

Lastly, we attempted a multiple regression analyses to look at the predictive values of both ECAP and ECochG metrics on speech perception scores. We performed it twice—one on CNC scores and once on AzBio scores. The analysis revealed that there was a significant correlation between the maximum amplitude of the ECAP (apical electrode) and performance of A+E ($F = 5.9851$, $p < 0.05$) on CNC words test. However, there was no significant correlation between ECochG and A+E scores on CNC words test nor was a statistically significant correlation found between performance on the AzBio test and either ECAP or ECochG magnitude.

TABLE 2 | Summary of correlation between peripheral electrophysiologic measures and speech performance.

EP measure	Speech perception measure	*n*	Pearson's *r*	*p*
ECAP	CNC word test			
	E alone	22†	0.56	0.009*
	A+E	24†	0.64	0.001*
	AzBio sentence test			
	E alone	21	0.35	0.118
	A+E	24	0.38	0.070
ECochG	CNC word test			
	A gain	23	0.06	0.780
	A+E	25	0.23	0.267
	AzBio sentence test			
	A gain	22	0.18	0.412
	A+E	25	0.20	0.343

Note that ECAPs listed in this table were measured from apical electrodes.
†One data identified as an outlier was excluded from correlation analysis.
**p < 0.05.*
EP indicates electrophysiologic; ECAP, electrically evoked compound action potential; ECochG, electrocochleography; CNC, consonant-nucleus-consonant; A, acoustic; E, electric.

DISCUSSION

The primary goal of this study was to determine the extent to which ECAPs recorded using electrical stimulation and ECochG responses recorded using acoustic stimulation were related with speech perception in Nucleus Hybrid L24 CI users. The reasoning is that ECAPs would reflect activity along different points of the electrode array, which is seated basally in the cochlea. ECochGs would reflect activity along more apical regions of the cochlea. Using both metrics may more fully characterize the status of the cochlea. To our knowledge, the present study is the first to investigate the relationship between post-operative peripheral electrophysiologic measures (specifically acoustically evoked potentials) and speech performance in hearing preservation implants. Prior studies have only demonstrated the feasibility

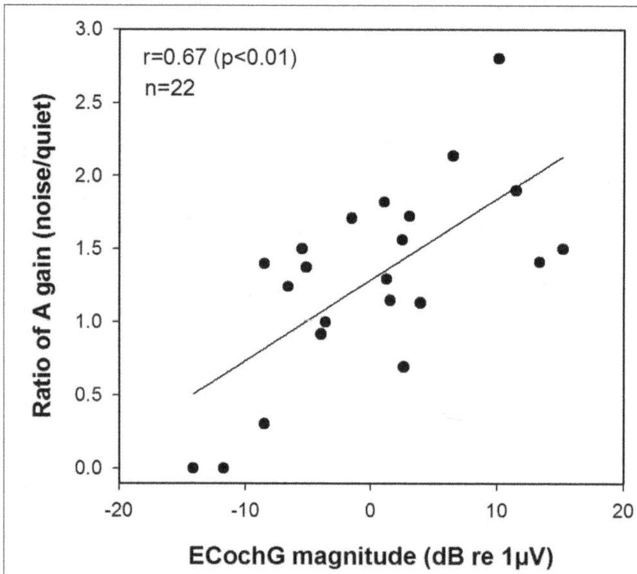

FIGURE 7 | Correlation between the magnitude of the ECochG response to a 500 Hz tone burst and the ratio of A gain scores on speech perception test in noise relative to quiet (AzBio/CNC). ECochG indicates electrocochleography; CNC, consonant-nucleus-consonant; A, acoustic.

of making such recordings (Dalbert et al., 2015; Abbas et al., 2017; Koka et al., 2017) but the clinical applicability of these measures need to be addressed beyond their ability to predict audiometric thresholds. It also extends previous studies that have found correlations between intraoperative ECochG measures in CI users and speech outcomes (Fitzpatrick et al., 2013; Formeister et al., 2015).

The Hybrid L24 CI does not extend along the full length of the cochlea. Additionally, neural survival is not likely to be uniform along the cochlear partition. Indeed, audiometric thresholds are better for low frequencies and poorer for high frequencies in our Hybrid CI users (see **Figure 1**). This observation suggests that neural survival is likely to be better closer to the apex than the base of the cochlea. ECAP recordings primarily reflect activity of neurons located along the relatively basal region of the cochlea (given that electrode arrays do not span the entire cochlea). We hypothesized that the position of the electrode array and the configuration of the hearing loss would result in larger ECAP responses for apical electrodes. That is, in fact, what we found (see **Figure 2**). ECAP amplitudes recorded from more apical electrodes are significantly larger than those recorded from more basal electrodes.

We assume that larger ECAP amplitudes may reflect better neural survival and that, in turn, may lead to better performance on tests of speech perception, particularly when the listening mode is E alone. Our results showed that the ECAP amplitudes recorded from apical electrodes are significantly correlated with speech perception as measured using CNC word tests (see **Figure 6A**). This finding is consistent with Kim et al. (2010) in which the slope of the ECAP amplitude growth function obtained from Nucleus Hybrid S8 (RE) and Standard CI24RE CI users were significantly correlated with speech perception. The slope metric was used as a marker of neural survival, similar to animal studies (Smith and Simmons, 1983; Hall, 1990; Miller et al., 1994; Prado-Guitierrez et al., 2006). The L24 Hybrid also has the same receiver-stimulator as the Hybrid S8 (RE) and standard 24RE, so results can be compared across devices. However, correlations are not often seen between electrophysiologic measures and speech perception in older devices (Abbas and Brown, 1991; Brown et al., 1995; for review see Van Eijl et al., 2017). Studies comparing post-mortem spiral ganglion neuron counts to speech outcomes don't often see correlations either (e.g., Nadol et al., 2001; Khan et al., 2005; Fayad and Linthicum, 2006; however, see Seyyedi et al., 2014). Mixed findings are not surprising; the ECAP is a peripheral response while speech perception requires peripheral and central processes, as well as cognitive resources. Both peripheral and central measures may be needed to increase the predictive power of electrophysiologic measures (Scheperle and Abbas, 2015). ECAP amplitudes recorded from middle or basal electrodes did not show correlations with CNC scores. ECAP responses were not as robust for these electrodes, possibly due to less neural survival, which may have precluded meaningful correlational analysis with speech outcomes.

No correlation between ECAP amplitude and performance on the AzBio sentence test in noise was obtained regardless of the stimulating electrode used. It may be that ECAP amplitudes do not reflect the spectral/spatial resolution needed for speech perception in noise. CI users require more electrodes for speech perception in noise relative to quiet, since more electrodes potentially provide better spectral/spatial resolution (Friesen et al., 2001). Experiments using vocoded speech have shown that only a few spectral bands are needed for adequate speech recognition in quiet (Shannon et al., 1995; Xu and Zheng, 2007), but more bands are needed for speech recognition in noise (Qin and Oxenham, 2003; Xu and Zheng, 2007), reflecting the contribution of increased spectral resolution to speech recognition in noise. Spatial resolution can be inferred from channel interaction measures made using ECAPs (Abbas et al., 2004), with a recent study demonstrating correlations between channel interaction measures and speech perception in noise (Scheperle and Abbas, 2015).

While ECAPs provide a measure of the response of the auditory nerve to electrical stimulation, ECochG responses include contributions from both cochlear hair cells and from the auditory nerve following acoustic stimulation. We know that use of a Hybrid CI improves speech understanding in part because it allows the listener to use his/her acoustic hearing to perceive low frequency cues in an acoustic signal and to use the electrical signal provided by the CI to perceive high frequency information (Turner et al., 2004; Ching, 2005; Brown and Bacon, 2009; Zhang et al., 2010). Our results also showed that performance in the A+E listening mode was significantly better than in E alone mode for both CNC and AzBio tests (see **Figure 4**) and demonstrate that preserving residual acoustic hearing was beneficial for our population of study participants. The ECochG recordings obtained using a 500 Hz tone burst provide a measure of how the auditory periphery responds to a low frequency acoustic stimulus. Here we suggest that ECochG recordings may provide a metric that reflects the overall "health" of at least the apical portion of the cochlea. We hypothesize that the ECochG magnitude measures might be more strongly correlated with A gain speech perception scores rather than results of tests conducted in the A+E or E alone listening modes. However, we found no significant correlations between ECochG responses and A gain scores on CNC words test nor on the AzBio sentences test. The lack of a correlation may be because A gain scores are not a direct measure of speech perception abilities in the A alone condition. We treated these measures as additive, assuming acoustic only scores plus electric only scores equals A+E score, which is not necessarily the case. Gifford et al. (2008a) tested S8 hybrid patients on word recognition in acoustic only, electric only, and A+E listening modes. None of those patients had A+E scores that were equal to A only + E only score. It seems equally likely, however, that in addition to cochlear health, other factors such as patient demographics, cognitive ability, and genetic variants may affect performance on speech perception tests, increase variance in our measures and reduce the correlations evident in this study (Lazard et al., 2012; Blamey et al., 2013; Holden et al., 2013; Shearer et al., 2017).

Compared to individuals who use standard CIs, Hybrid CI users perform better on tests of speech perception in background noise than in quiet. Several investigators have attributed this to residual low frequency acoustic hearing providing significant benefits—particularly when the task involves understanding speech in background noise (Turner et al., 2004, 2008b; Gantz et al., 2009; Zhang et al., 2010; Carroll et al., 2011). For example, Turner et al. (2004, 2008b) showed that Hybrid CI users outperformed standard CI users on tests of speech perception in background noise, even though these two groups had equivalent levels of speech perception in quiet. This advantage is primarily a result of the better frequency resolution provided by the residual acoustic hearing (Qin and Oxenham, 2003; Turner et al., 2004). We expect, therefore, that the benefits enjoyed by Hybrid CI users would be most evident in situations, such as speech perception in noise, where frequency resolution is important. Our results also suggested that acoustic hearing (A gain) plays a larger role in determining how well speech is perceived in noise (AzBio test) compared to quiet (CNC test), even though performance is better in the A+E mode compared to the E alone mode on both CNC and AzBio tests (see **Figure 4**). This is in general agreement with findings from other studies (Kiefer et al., 2005; Zhang et al., 2010). Therefore, we assumed that the benefits of acoustic hearing in noise relative to in quiet may be predicted by our ECochG data that has been proposed to serve as a measure of cochlear health. We did find that ECochG magnitude was significantly correlated with the ratio of the AzBio score and the CNC score when both were collected in the A gain condition (see **Figure 7**). This finding is consistent with an assumption that the magnitude of the ECochG response evoked using a 500 Hz tone burst may serve as an index to overall cochlear health at the apical region and at least partially explain benefit provided to the listener by their residual low frequency acoustic hearing. It could be argued, however, that the composite metric was made by using two different tests and may not accurately reflect the benefit of A gain in noisy situations. The CNC word test and the AzBio sentence test have differing cues, such as lexical, semantic, context, and acoustic cues, and could have differing distributions of speech scores amongst the patient population. However, Gifford et al. (2008b) reported a significant correlation between performance on CNC word lists and AzBio sentences presented in quiet ($r = 0.85$, $p < 0.0001$). Moreover, our results also revealed strong correlations between performance on the CNC word list presented in quiet and AzBio sentences presented in noise for each condition (A+E, E alone, and A gain) (see **Figure 5**).

This study also explored the correlation between the ECAP or ECochG and speech perception measured in the A+E listening mode. The ECAP amplitudes were significantly correlated with performance on CNC test (see **Figure 6B**), but not correlated with performance on AzBio test. We found that the ratios of E alone score to A gain score were approximately 7:3 and 5:5 for CNC word test presented in quiet and AzBio sentence test presented in noise, respectively (see **Figure 4**). That is, the high frequency portions of the speech signal conveyed electrically made a dominant contribution to speech perception in quiet as described in other studies (Kiefer et al., 2005; Turner et al., 2008a). This was not the case for speech perception in noise. Our results show that electrically evoked neural responses seems to be more predictive of performance when the task does not include background noise (e.g., the CNC test) and when testing is conducted in the A+E listening condition.

We assumed that the acoustically evoked ECochG magnitudes might serve as an index of overall cochlear health and as such might predict performance on speech perception tests. There was a tendency for magnitude of the ECochG responses evoked using the 500 Hz tone burst to be correlated with audiometric thresholds (e.g., see **Figure 3**). However, the ECochG measures we recorded were not correlated with outcome on either speech test when testing was conducted in the A+E listening modes. For example, despite differences in residual acoustic hearing and ECochG magnitude, speech perception results were similar for both subjects (L23R and L18R) whose data are shown in **Figure 3**. These results stand in contrast to data reported by Fitzpatrick et al. (2013) and Formeister et al. (2015) showing significant correlations between physiologic measures of "total cochlear response" (representing a sum of responses using 250 to 4,000 Hz tone bursts recorded using a round window electrode prior to insertion of the electrode array) and postoperative speech perception. In this study, we recorded ECochG responses from an intracochlear electrode rather than from the round window. Our recordings were also obtained post-operatively rather than prior to the insertion of the electrode array into the cochlea. We reasoned that an intracochlear recording electrode would be closer to the cochlear hair cells and auditory neurons and as such, could be more reflective of cochlear health than similar measures obtained from the round window. Therefore, we would have expected to find a better correlation between a postoperative electrophysiological measures and speech perception than had been reported previously. That was not the case. However, we used only one tone burst frequency to evoke the ECochG response, while Fitzpatrick et al. (2013) and Formeister et al. (2015) used several tone burst frequencies. Our results may, therefore, represent a measure of cochlear health from a more restricted region on the cochlea. We also assumed that insertion of the electrode array into the cochlea would be likely to affect cochlear function and as a result, post-implant measures would accurately predict outcome with a Hybrid CI than pre-operative measures. Our assumption may not have been valid. Animal studies show that it is possible to insert the electrode array into the cochlea and only transiently affect the ECochG (DeMason et al., 2012). If so, the impact on speech perception may not be significant and could also explain the difference between our results and those of Fitzpatrick et al. (2013) and Formeister et al. (2015). Perhaps recording the ECochG pre- and post-insertion could provide a more complete picture of overall cochlear health and the combination of those data with ECAP recordings may improve our ability to predict speech perception outcomes.

The results of the present study suggest that peripheral electrophysiologic responses to both acoustic and electric stimuli may be important to fully characterize the status of the cochlea for an individual Hybrid CI user and may be required to improve our ability to predict speech perception outcomes. While we did find correlations between ECAP or ECochG measures and speech perception, we acknowledge that there were fewer significant correlations than non-significant correlations and one might reasonably argue that the few significant correlations that were observed arose out of chance. A well-controlled prospective study design is needed to address the limitations of the current study.

This study has also some limitations due to the retrospective nature of the design. We tried to use similar metrics for both ECAP and ECochG data and focused on the amplitudes. Our ECAP growth functions had more data points, allowing us to visually determine the threshold and calculate slope. However, experimental limitations, as outlined in Abbas et al. (2017), prevented us from collecting many data points for a finely detailed growth function for ECochG responses. The ECochG thresholds from that study were calculated based on linear regression fits to the ECochG amplitude growth function rather than visual detection thresholds. Thus, we wanted to avoid using two different methodologies. Future prospective studies should collect ECochG amplitude growth functions with multiple levels, as well as at multiple frequencies. This would allow the use of visual detection thresholds, slopes, and amplitudes across different frequencies and levels to more fully characterize acoustic responses. Future studies can also use measurement and analysis techniques to emphasize responses from the hair cell and from the auditory nerve and correlate this to outcomes. Such studies might not only result in more accurate prediction of overall outcome with Hybrid CIs than have been available previously but also provide important clues as to the source of the cross-subject variance routinely observed in CI populations.

While Hybrid CI users currently are a small section of the CI population, there is increasingly more emphasis on the use of soft surgical techniques and electrode designs that may help reduce cochlear trauma. Multicenter trials have demonstrated hearing preservation is possible with both short (Gantz et al., 2009; Lenarz et al., 2013; Roland et al., 2016) and long electrode arrays (Santa Maria et al., 2013; Van Abel et al., 2015; Hunter et al., 2016). Our results show the relative contributions of acoustic and electric hearing to speech perception in quiet and noise. We would argue that if preservation of residual acoustic hearing in the implanted ear remains an important goal both for surgeons and CI manufacturers, methods to evaluate the contributions of residual acoustic hearing and electrical stimulation to speech perception will be necessary.

CONCLUSIONS

ECAPs reflect response of auditory neurons across the electrode array, seated at the relatively basal regions of the cochlea. ECochG responses provide a way to assess the response of the cochlear hair cells and auditory nerve for neurons innervating more apical regions of the cochlear partition. Both can be recorded from Hybrid L24 CI users. The results of this study suggest that outcomes with a Hybrid CI on tests of speech perception in quiet and/or in noise can be more accurately characterized by using both ECAP (recorded from an apical electrode) and ECochG measures rather than either metric alone.

AUTHOR CONTRIBUTIONS

JK, VT, PA, and CB: Substantial contributions to the conception or design of the work; Substantial contribution to the acquisition, analysis, or interpretation of data for the work; Drafting the work and revising it critically for important intellectual content; Final approval of the version to be published; Agreement to be accountable for all aspects of the work in ensuring that questions related to the accuracy or integrity of any part of the work are appropriately investigated and resolved.

FUNDING

This work was supported by grants from the NIH/NIDCD (P50 DC000242) and funding for a "research year" provided by Inje University in 2015.

ACKNOWLEDGMENTS

We would like to thank Rachel Scheperle, AuD, Ph.D. for her assistance with data acquisition and analysis. We also thank our patients for their continued efforts toward our research program.

REFERENCES

Abbas, P. J., and Brown, C. J. (1991). Electrically evoked auditory brainstem response: growth of response with current level. *Hear. Res.* 51, 123–137. doi: 10.1016/0378-5955(91)90011-W

Abbas, P. J., Brown, C. J., Shallop, J. K., Firszt, J. B., Hughes, M. L., Hong, S. H., et al. (1999). Summary of results using the Nucleus CI24M implant to record the electrically evoked compound action potential. *Ear Hear.* 20, 45–59. doi: 10.1097/00003446-199902000-00005

Abbas, P. J., Hughes, M. L., Brown, C. J., Miller, C. A., and South, H. (2004). Channel interaction in cochlear implant users evaluated using the electrically evoked compound action potential. *Audiol. Neurootol.* 9, 203–213. doi: 10.1159/000078390

Abbas, P. J., Tejani, V. D., Scheperle, R. A., and Brown, C. B. (2017). Using neural response telemetry to monitor physiological responses to acoustic stimulation in hybrid cochlear implant users. *Ear Hear.* doi: 10.1097/aud.0000000000000400. [Epub ahead of print].

Blamey, P., Artieres, F., Başkent, D., Bergeron, F., Beynon, A., Burke, E., et al. (2013). Factors affecting auditory performance of postlingually deaf adults using cochlear implants: an update with 2251 patients. *Audiol. Neurotol.* 18, 36–47. doi: 10.1159/000343189

Brown, C. A., and Bacon, S. P. (2009). Low-frequency speech cues and simulated electric-acoustic hearing. *J. Acoust. Soc. Am.* 125, 1658–1665. doi: 10.1121/1.3068441

Brown, C. J., Abbas, P. J., Bertschy, M., Tyler, R. S., Lowder, M., Takahashi, G., et al. (1995). Longitudinal assessment of physiological and psychophysical measures in cochlear implant users. *Ear. Hear.* 16, 439–449. doi: 10.1097/00003446-199510000-00001

Brown, C. J., Abbas, P. J., and Gantz, B. J. (1998). Preliminary experience with neural response telemetry in the Nucleus CI24M cochlear implant. *Am. J. Otol.* 19, 320–327.

Brown, C. J., Hughes, M. L., Luk, B., Abbas, P. J., Wolaver, A. A., and Gervais, J. P. (2000). The relationship between EAP and EABR thresholds and levels used to program the Nucleus 24 speech processor: data from adults. *Ear. Hear.* 21, 151–163. doi: 10.1097/00003446-200004000-00009

Büchner, A., Schüssler, M., Battmer, R. D., Stöver, T., Lesinski-Schiedat, A., and Lenarz, T. (2009). Impact of low-frequency hearing. *Audiol. Neurotol.* 14S, 8–13. doi: 10.1159/000206490

Carroll, J., Tiaden, S., and Zeng, F. G. (2011). Fundamental frequency is critical to speech perception in noise in combined acoustic and electric hearing. *J. Acoust. Soc. Am.* 130, 2054–2062. doi: 10.1121/1.3631563

Ching, T. (2005). The evidence calls for making binaural-bimodal fitting routine. *Hear. J.* 58, 32–41. doi: 10.1097/01.HJ.0000286404.64930.a8

Cohen, N. L. (2004). Cochlear implant candidacy and surgical considerations. *Audiol. Neurotol.* 9, 197–202. doi: 10.1159/000078389

Cochlear Ltd. (2015). *Cochlear TM Nucleus® Hybrid TM Hearing Solution: Desk Reference Guide*. Available online at: http://www.cochlear.com/wps/wcm/connect/1c88513a-7e5b-4cea-b6bf-cf3a3ff797c7/FUN1975+ISS3+JAN15+Hybrid+Reference+Guide.pdf?MOD=AJPERES&CONVERT_TO=url&CACHEID=1c88513a-7e5b-4cea-b6bf-cf3a3ff797c7

Dalbert, A., Pfiffner, F., Röösli, C., Thoele, K., Sim, J. H., Gerig, R., et al. (2015). Extra- and intracochelar electrocochleography in cochlear implant recipients. *Audiol. Neurotol.* 20, 339–348. doi: 10.1159/000438742

DeMason, C., Choudhury, B., Ahmad, F., Fitzpatrick, D. C., Wang, J., Buchman, C. A., et al. (2012). Electrophysiological properties of cochlear implantation in the gerbil using a flexible array. *Ear. Hear.* 33, 534–542. doi: 10.1097/AUD.0b013e3182498c28

Fayad, J. N., and Linthicum, F. H. Jr. (2006). Multichannel cochlear implants: relation of histopathology to performance. *Laryngoscope* 116, 1310–1320. doi: 10.1097/01.mlg.0000227176.09500.28

Fitzpatrick, D. C., Campbell, A. T., Choudhury, B., Dillon, M. P., Forgues, M., Buchman, C. A., et al. (2013). Round window electrocochleography just before cochlear implantation: relationship to word recognition outcomes in adults. *Otol. Neurotol.* 35, 64–71. doi: 10.1097/MAO.0000000000000219

Formeister, E. J., McClellan, J. H., Merwin, W. H. III, Iseli, C. E., Calloway, N. H., Teagle, H. F., et al. (2015). Intraoperative round window electrocochleography and speech perception outcomes in pediatric cochlear implant recipients. *Ear. Hear.* 36, 249–260. doi: 10.1097/AUD.0000000000000106

Friesen, L. M., Shannon, R. V., Baskent, D., and Wang, X. (2001). Speech recognition in noise as a function of the number of spectral channels: comparison of acoustic hearing and cochlear implants. *J. Acoust. Soc. Am.* 110, 1150–1163. doi: 10.1121/1.1381538

Gantz, B. J., Dunn, C., Oleson, J., Hansen, M., Parkinson, A., and Turner, C. (2016). Multicenter clinical trial of the Nucleus Hybrid S8 cochlear implant: final outcomes. *Laryngoscope* 126, 962–973. doi: 10.1002/lary.25572

Gantz, B. J., Hansen, M. R., Turner, C. W., Oleson, J. J., Reiss, L. A., and Parkinson, A. J. (2009). Hybrid 10 clinical trial: preliminary results. *Audiol. Neurotol.* 14S, 32–38. doi: 10.1159/000206493

Gantz, B. J., and Turner, C. W. (2003). Combining acoustic and electrical hearing. *Laryngoscope* 113, 1726–1730. doi: 10.1097/00005537-200310000-00012

Gibson, W. P., Moffat, D. A., and Ramsden, R. T. (1977). Clinical electrocochleography in the diagnosis and management of Ménière's disorder. *Audiology* 16, 389–401. doi: 10.3109/00206097709071852

Gifford, R. H., Dorman, M. F., Sphar, A. J., Bacon, S. P., Skarzynski, H., and Lorens, A. (2008a). Hearing preservation surgery: psychophysical estimates of cochlear damage in recipients of a short electrode array. *J. Acoust. Soc. Am.* 124, 2164–2173. doi: 10.1121/1.2967842

Gifford, R. H., Shallop, J. K., and Peterson, A. M. (2008b). Speech recognition materials and ceiling effects: considerations for cochlear implant programs. *Audiol. Neurotol.* 13, 193–205. doi: 10.1159/000113510

Goldstein, M. H. Jr., and Kiang, N. Y. S. (1958). Synchrony of neural activity in electric responses evoked by transient acoustic stimuli. *J. Acoust. Soc. Am.* 30, 107–114. doi: 10.1121/1.1909497

Greenwood, D. D. (1990). A cochlear frequency-position function for several species: 29 years later. *J. Acoust. Soc. Am.* 87, 2592–2605. doi: 10.1121/1.399052

Hall, R. D. (1990). Estimation of surviving spiral ganglion cells in the deaf rat using electrically evoked auditory brainstem response. *Hear. Res.* 49, 155–168. doi: 10.1016/0378-5955(90)90102-U

Holden, L. K., Finley, C. C., Firszt, J. B., Holden, T. A., Brenner, C., Potts, L. G., et al. (2013). Factors affecting open-set word recognition in adults with cochlear implants. *Ear. Hear.* 34, 342–360. doi: 10.1097/AUD.0b013e3182741aa7

Hornsby, B. W., and Ricketts, T. A. (2006). The effects of hearing loss on the contribution of high- and low-frequency speech information to speech understanding. II. Sloping hearing loss. *J. Acoust. Soc. Am.* 119, 1752–1763. doi: 10.1121/1.2161432

Hunter, J. B., Gifford, R. H., Wanna, G. B., Labadie, R. F., Bennett, M. L., Haynes, D. S., et al. (2016). Hearing preservation outcomes with a mid-scala electrode in cochlear implantation. *Otol. Neurotol.* 37, 235–240. doi: 10.1097/MAO.0000000000000963

Jurawitz, M. C., Büchner, A., Harpel, T., Schüssler, M., Majdani, O., Lesinski-Schiedat, A., et al. (2014). Hearing preservation outcomes with different cochlear implant electrodes: Nucleus® Hybrid^{TM}-L24 and Nucleus Freedom^{TM} CI422. *Audiol. Neurotol.* 19, 293–309. doi: 10.1159/000360601

Keidser, G., Dillon, H., Flax, M., Ching, T., and Brewer, S. (2011). The NAL-NL2 prescription procedure. *Audiol. Res.* 1:e24. doi: 10.4081/audiores.2011.e24

Khan, A. M., Handzel, O., Burgess, B. J., Damian, D., Eddington, D. K., and Nadol, J. B. Jr. (2005). Is word recognition correlated with the number of surviving spiral ganglion cells and electrode insertion depth in human subjects with cochlear implants? *Laryngoscope* 115, 672–677. doi: 10.1097/01.mlg.0000161335.62139.80

Kiefer, J., Pok, M., Adunka, O., Sturzbecher, E., Baumgartner, W., Schmidt, M., et al. (2005). Combined electric and acoustic stimulation of the auditory system: results of a clinical study. *Audiol. Neurotol.* 10, 134–144. doi: 10.1159/000084023

Kim, J. R., Abbas, P. J., Brown, C. J., Etler, C. P., O'Brien, S., and Kim, L. S. (2010). The relationship between electrically evoked compound action potential and speech perception: a study in cochlear implant users with short electrode array. *Otol. Neurotol.* 31, 1041–1048. doi: 10.1097/MAO.0b013e3181ec1d92

Koka, K., Saoji, A. A., and Litvak, L. M. (2017). Electrocochleography in cochlear implant recipients with residual hearing: comparison with audiometric thresholds. *Ear Hear.* doi: 10.1097/AUD.0000000000000385. [Epub ahead of print].

Lazard, D. S., Vincent, C., Venail, F., Van de Heyning, P., Truy, E., Sterkers, O., et al. (2012). Pre-, per- and postoperative factors affecting performance of postlinguistically deaf adults using cochlear implants: a new conceptual model over time. *PLoS ONE* 7:e48739. doi: 10.1371/journal.pone.0048739

Lenarz, T., James, C., Cuda, D., O'Connor, A. F., Frachet, B., Frijns, J. H. M., et al. (2013). European multi-centre study of the Nucleus Hybrid L24 cochlear implant. *Int. J. Audiol.* 52, 838–848. doi: 10.3109/14992027.2013.802032

Lenarz, T., Stöver, T., Buechner, A., Lesinski-Schiedat, A., Patrick, J., and Pesch, J. (2009). Hearing conservation surgery using the Hybrid-L electrode. Results from the first clinical trial at the Medical University of Hannover. *Audiol. Neurotol.* 14S, 22–31. doi: 10.1159/000206492

Liberman, M. C., Ebstein, M. J., Cleveland, S. S., Wang, H., and Maison, S. F. (2016). Toward a differential diagnosis of hidden hearing loss in humans. *PLoS ONE* 11:e0162726. doi: 10.1371/journal.pone.0162726

Miller, C. A., Abbas, P. J., and Robinson, B. K. (1994). The use of long-duration current pulses to assess neural survival. *Hear. Res.* 78, 11–26. doi: 10.1016/0378-5955(94)90039-6

Nadol, J. B. Jr., Shiao, J. Y., Burgess, B. J., Ketten, D. R., Eddington, D. K., Gantz, B. J., et al. (2001). Histopathology of cochlear implants in humans. *Ann. Otol. Rhinol. Laryngol.* 110, 883–891. doi: 10.1177/000348940111000914

Peterson, G. E., and Lehiste, I. (1962). Revised CNC lists for auditory tests. *J. Speech. Hear. Disord.* 27, 62–70. doi: 10.1044/jshd.2701.62

Prado-Guitierrez, P., Fewster, L. M., Heasman, J. M., McKay, C. M., and Shepherd, R. K. (2006). Effect of interphase gap and pulse duration on electrically evoked potentials is correlated with auditory nerve survival. *Hear. Res.* 215, 47–55. doi: 10.1016/j.heares.2006.03.006

Qin, M. K., and Oxenham, A. J. (2003). Effects of simulated cochlear implant processing on speech reception in fluctuating maskers. *J. Acoust. Soc. Am.* 114, 446–454. doi: 10.1121/1.1579009

Reiss, L. A., Gantz, B. J., and Turner, B. J. (2008). Cochlear implant speech processor frequency allocations may influence pitch perception. *Otol. Neurotol.* 29, 160–167. doi: 10.1097/mao.0b013e31815aedf4

Roland, J. T., Gantz, B. J., Waltzman, S. B., Parkinson, A. J., and Multicenter Clinical Trial Group (2016). United States multicenter clinical trial of the cochlear Nucleus Hybrid implant system. *Laryngoscope* 126, 175–181. doi: 10.1002/lary.25451

Santa Maria, P. L., Domville-Lewis, C., Sucher, C. M., Chester-Browne, R., and Atlas, M. D. (2013). Hearing preservation surgery for cochlear implantation–hearing and quality of life after 2 years. *Otol. Neurotol.* 34, 526–531. doi: 10.1097/MAO.0b013e318281e0c9

Scheperle, R. A., and Abbas, P. J. (2015). Relationships among peripheral and central electrophysiological measures of spatial and spectral selectivity and speech perception in cochlear implant users. *Ear Hear.* 36, 441–453. doi: 10.1097/AUD.0000000000000144

Seyyedi, M., Viana, L. M., Nadol, J. B. Jr. (2014). Within-subject comparison of word recognition and spiral ganglion cell count in bilateral cochlear implant recipients. *Otol. Neurotol.* 35, 1446–1450. doi: 10.1097/mao.0000000000000443

Shannon, R. V., Zeng, F. G., Kamath, V., Wygonski, J., and Ekelid, M. (1995). Speech recognition with primarily temporal cues. *Science* 270, 303–304. doi: 10.1126/science.270.5234.303

Shearer, A. E., Eppsteiner, R. W., Frees, K., Tejani, V. D., Sloan-Heggena, C. M., Brown, C. J., et al. (2017). Genetic variants in the peripheral auditory system significantly affect adult cochlear implant performance. *Hear. Res.* doi: 10.1016/j.heares.2017.02.008. [Epub ahead of print].

Smith, L., and Simmons, F. B. (1983). Estimating eighth nerve survival by electrical stimulation. *Ann. Otol. Rhinol. Laryngol.* 92, 19–23. doi: 10.1177/000348948309200105

Spahr, A. J., Dorman, M. F., Litvak, L. M., Van Wie, S., Gifford, R. H., Loizou, P. C., et al. (2012). Development and validation of the AzBio sentence lists. *Ear. Hear.* 33, 112–117. doi: 10.1097/AUD.0b013e31822c2549

Stakhovskaya, O., Sridhar, D., Bonham, B. H., and Leake, P. A. (2007). Frequency map for the human cochlear spiral ganglion: implications for cochlear implants. *J. Assoc. Res. Otolaryngol.* 8, 220–233. doi: 10.1007/s10162-007-0076-9

Turner, C. W. (2006). Hearing loss and the limits of amplification. *Audiol. Neurotol.* 11S, 2–5. doi: 10.1159/000095606

Turner, C. W., Gantz, B. J., and Reiss, L. A. (2008b). Integration of acoustic and electric hearing. *J. Rehab. Res. Develop.* 45, 769–778. doi: 10.1682/JRRD.2007.05.0065

Turner, C. W., Gantz, B. J., Vidal, C., Behrens, A., and Henry, B. A. (2004). Speech recognition in noise for cochlear implant listeners: benefits of residual acoustic hearing. *J. Acoust. Soc. Am.* 115, 1729–1735. doi: 10.1121/1.1687425

Turner, C. W., Reiss, L. A., and Gantz, B. J. (2008a). Combined acoustic and electric hearing: preserving residual acoustic hearing. *Hear. Res.* 242, 164–171. doi: 10.1016/j.heares.2007.11.008

Van Abel, K. M., Dunn, C. C., Sladen, D. P., Oleson, J. J., Beatty, C. W., Neff, B. A., et al. (2015). Hearing preservation among patients undergoing cochlear implantation. *Otol. Neurotol.* 36, 416–421. doi: 10.1097/MAO.0000000000000703

Van Eijl, R. H., Buitenhuis, P. J., Stegeman, I., Klis, S. F., and Grolman, W. (2017). Systemic review of compound action potentials as predictors for cochlear implant performance. *Laryngoscope* 127, 476–487. doi: 10.1002/lary.26154

Woodson, E. A., Reiss, L. A., Turner, C. W., Gfeller, K., and Gantz, B. J. (2010). The hybrid cochlear implant: a review. *Adv. Otorhinolaryngol.* 67, 125–134. doi: 10.1159/000262604

Xu, L., and Zheng, Y. (2007). Spectral and temporal cues for phoneme recognition in noise. *J. Acoust. Soc. Am.* 122, 1758. doi: 10.1121/1.2767000

Zhang, T., Dorman, M. F., and Spahr, A. J. (2010). Information from the voice fundamental frequency (F0) region accounts for the majority of the benefit when acoustic stimulation is added to electric stimulation. *Ear. Hear.* 31, 63–69. doi: 10.1097/AUD.0b013e3181b7190c

5

Assessment of Ipsilateral Efferent Effects in Human *via* ECochG

Eric Verschooten[1], Elizabeth A. Strickland[2], Nicolas Verhaert[3] and Philip X. Joris[1]*

[1] Laboratory of Auditory Neurophysiology, Department of Neurosciences, University of Leuven, Leuven, Belgium,
[2] Department of Speech, Language, and Hearing Sciences, Purdue University, West Lafayette, IN, United States, [3] ExpORL Research Group, Department of Neurosciences, University of Leuven, Leuven, Belgium

***Correspondence:**
Philip X. Joris
philip.joris@med.kuleuven.be

Development of electrophysiological means to assess the medial olivocochlear (MOC) system in humans is important to further our understanding of the function of that system and for the refinement and validation of psychoacoustical and otoacoustic emission methods which are thought to probe the MOC. Based on measurements in anesthetized animals it has been hypothesized that the MOC-reflex (MOCR) can enhance the response to signals in noise, and several lines of evidence support such a role in humans. A difficulty in these studies is the isolation of efferent effects. Efferent activation can be triggered by acoustic stimulation of the contralateral or ipsilateral ear, but ipsilateral stimulation is thought to be more effective. However, ipsilateral stimulation complicates interpretation of effects since these sounds can affect the perception of other ipsilateral sounds by mechanisms not involving olivocochlear efferents. We assessed the ipsilaterally evoked MOCR in human using a transtympanic procedure to record mass-potentials from the cochlear promontory or the niche of the round window. Averaged compound action potential (CAP) responses to masked probe tones of 4 kHz with and without a precursor (designed to activate the MOCR but not the stapedius reflex) were extracted with a polarity alternating paradigm. The masker was either a simultaneous narrow band noise masker or a short (20-ms) tonal ON- or OFF-frequency forward masker. The subjects were screened for normal hearing (audiogram, tympanogram, threshold stapedius reflex) and psychoacoustically tested for the presence of a precursor effect. We observed a clear reduction of CAP amplitude by the precursor, for different masking conditions. Even without an MOCR, this is expected because the precursor will affect the response to subsequent stimuli via neural adaptation. To determine whether the precursor also activated the efferent system, we measured the CAP over a range of masker levels, with or without precursor, and for different types of masker. The results show CAP reduction consistent with the type of gain reduction caused by the MOCR. These results generally support psychoacoustical paradigms designed to probe the efferent system as indeed activating the MOCR system, but not all observations are consistent with this mechanism.

Keywords: precursor, human, CAP, ipsilateral elicitor, efferent, medial olivocochlear system, MOC, ECochG

INTRODUCTION

An important property of the cochlea is the ability to "amplify" the mechanical vibrations at the basilar membrane (Dallos, 2008). This process is under the control of the medial olivocochlear (MOC) system via efferent fibers that innervate the outer hair cells. Activation of these efferents, called the MOC reflex (MOCR), hyperpolarizes the outer hair cells (Fuchs, 2002) and decreases the cochlear gain in anesthetized animals (Buno, 1978; Dolan and Nuttall, 1988; Liberman, 1989; Warren and Liberman, 1989; Kawase and Liberman, 1993; Guinan and Stankovic, 1996).

The role of the MOCR in auditory processing is not well-understood. Various proposals have been made, such as increased speech comprehension in noise (Giraud et al., 1997), protection against loud sounds (Kujawa and Liberman, 1997; Brown et al., 1998), and a possible role in the development of cochlear function (Walsh et al., 1998). Further elucidation of the role of the MOCR requires a combination of behavioral and physiological methods.

In humans, 3 basic approaches have been used to study the MOCR. Measurement of otoacoustic emissions while presenting contralateral sounds allows a rather direct probing of effects on outer hair cells (Guinan, 2006), but a drawback is that such measurements do not address effects on the cochlear neural output. This concern is alleviated by the measurement of acoustically evoked neural mass potentials while presenting contralateral stimuli (Folsom and Owsley, 1987; Kawase and Takasaka, 1995; Chabert et al., 2002; Lichtenhan et al., 2016), but in turn these techniques have other issues such as signal quality, state of arousal, and role of pathology in patients. Finally, a range of psychoacoustical paradigms have been developed to study efferent effects (see below). The challenge with behavioral paradigms is to know whether the effects observed indeed reflect the MOCR or whether they involve other neural pathways or phenomena. By probing cochlear neural potentials as directly as possible, in normal hearing subjects, and applying stimulus paradigms as used in psychoacoustical studies, we aim to tighten the interpretation of behavioral and physiological responses with respect to efferent function.

Although in physiological studies the MOCR may be elicited via direct electrical stimulation of the efferent pathway, the MOCR is more naturally activated by sounds to either ear (Gifford and Guinan, 1987). Use of acoustic stimulation of the contralateral ear to trigger efferent activity is appealing because of its technical and interpretational simplicity. However, anatomical and physiological evidence in cat and guinea pig (Liberman and Brown, 1986; Brown, 1989), indicates that the MOCR is more strongly activated by an ipsilateral elicitor than a contralateral one. While this suggests it is important to study ipsilateral elicitors of efferent activation, such elicitors introduce additional effects, such as cochlear suppression and neural adaptation, which complicate the interpretation of the results.

Under certain circumstances, neural responses to tones in noise may increase in amplitude when the MOCR is elicited. This is known as the anti-masking effect and is thought to reflect a decrease in masking due to a reduction in cochlear gain by the MOCR (Kawase and Liberman, 1993; Kawase et al., 1993). Various psychoacoustical paradigms have been developed to study the effect of the MOCR on masking. For example, in studies of the so-called overshoot or temporal effect (Zwicker, 1965), a precursor sound leads to effects which are qualitatively consistent with the neural anti-masking phenomenon (Strickland, 2001, 2004, 2008). The precursor sound is thought to lead to gain reduction by triggering the MOCR. To tease out the role of gain reduction against other cochlear phenomena (neural adaptation, suppression), psychoacoustic experimenters have developed forward masking paradigms in which masking by a short ON- or OFF-frequency masker is compared with and without a precursor (Roverud and Strickland, 2010). In contrast to the simultaneous masking condition, in forward masking the precursor increases signal threshold. However, the precursor increases signal threshold much more when the masker is well-below the signal frequency than when the masker is at the signal frequency, which would be consistent with a reduction in cochlear gain (Jennings et al., 2009; Jennings and Strickland, 2012; Yasin et al., 2014).

The interpretation of psychoacoustical results in terms of MOCR activity would be strengthened by linking psychoacoustical paradigms more directly with physiological measurements. Here, we attempt to electrophysiologically assess the mechanism by which a precursor affects the detection of a masked probe tone. Our stimulus paradigm is similar to the psychoacoustical studies, but modified to extract the compound action potential (CAP) from mass-potentials near the round window. The experiments were performed in two awake subjects. We first examine the impact of a precursor on a probe tone of 4 kHz and then explore the effect of an additional masker. Finally, we compare the results with predictions from simulations.

MATERIALS AND METHODS

This study (S56783) was carried out in accordance with the recommendations of good clinical practice (ICH/GCP), Medical Ethics Committee of the University of Leuven with written informed consent from all subjects. All subjects gave written informed consent in accordance with the Declaration of Helsinki. The protocol (ECochG-EF-P-2) was approved by the Medical Ethics Committee of the University of Leuven.

Subjects

We recruited volunteers between 20 and 30 years of age via an advertisement. Subjects were requested to avoid exposure to loud sounds such as rock concerts in the days preceding the experimental session. The day before or the morning of the experimental session, the subject's hearing was assessed including an inquiry for hearing problems, a pure tone audiogram (thresholds <20 dB nHL, 125 Hz–8 kHz), tympanometry to assess middle ear function, an otomicroscopy by an otolaryngologist, and the determination of the ipsilateral acoustically evoked middle ear reflex threshold for broadband noise and a 1 kHz tone (ZODIAC 901).

The duration of these experimental sessions varied between 1 and 4 h; subjects could end the session at any time. The experiments were conducted in a double-walled soundproofed and electrically shielded booth (Industrial Acoustics Company, Niederkrüchten, Germany). Subjects chose a comfortable reclined position on a bed and were asked to remain still during the recordings. When in the booth, subjects and experimenters were grounded to the booth via an antistatic wrist strap. During the actual experiment, an observer was present with the subject in the booth to monitor the status of the subject and to act as an intermediary with the experimenters outside the booth. Two female subjects participated in the electrophysiological experiments in this study.

Trans-Tympanic Procedure

A trans-tympanic procedure was used to record evoked mass responses from the human middle ear (Verschooten et al., 2013, 2015). For every subject, a custom silicone ear mold (Dentsply, Aquasil Ultra XLV regular) was made which contained two casted openings to hold tubes of 2 mm diameter for needle insertion, visualization, acoustic stimulation, and calibration. The complete acoustic system was calibrated *in situ* with a probe-microphone (Etymotic Research, ER-7C) close to the tympanic membrane. The earphone-speaker was connected to one of the openings of the ear mold via a plastic T-piece which also served as access port for a rigid endoscope with camera (R. WOLF, 8654.402 25 degree PANOVIEW; ILO electronic GmbH, XE50-eco X-TFT-USB) to visualize the ear canal and tympanic membrane. During the acoustic calibration all openings were sealed with Audalin acrylic impression compound (Microsonic); a tiny opening in one of the tubes prevented static pressure build-up. Before the needle-electrode was inserted, the tympanic membrane and ear canal were locally anesthetized with Bonain's solution (equal amounts of cocaine hydrochloride, phenol and menthol), which was aspirated after about 30 min. A short sterile plastic tube was inserted in the mold to accommodate the sterile needle-electrode. Ground and reference electrodes were connected to the equipment. The needle-electrode (TECA, sterile monopolar disposable, 75 mm × 26G, 902-DMG75-TP), was inserted and gently placed through the tympanic membrane on the cochlear promontory or in the niche of the round window under visual endoscopic control. To maintain its position and to ensure good electrical contact, the needle-electrode was maintained under slight tension with rubber bands supported by a custom frame, which was positioned over the external ear and fastened around the head with Velcro strips. Subjects usually had a short-lasting and vague sensation of touch during insertion of the electrode. The openings of the tubes were sealed with Audalin and the needle-electrode was connected to the preamplifier. The subject's right ear was studied: there was no experimental manipulation of the other ear. The session was terminated within 4 h or when the subject expressed the desire to stop. At the end of the experiment, the needle electrode and ear mold were removed and an otomicroscopic examination was performed. Subjects were requested to keep the ear dry for 10 days following the recording session. An otolaryngologyst was available during the weeks after the experiment to address any worries or for a second checkup.

Acoustical Stimulation

Stimuli were generated with custom software and a digital sound system (Tucker-Davis Technologies, system 2, sample rate: 125 kHz/channel) consisting of a digital-to-analog converter (PD1), a digitally controlled analog attenuator (PA5), a headphone driver (HB7) and an electromagnetically shielded earphone-speaker (Etymotic Research, ER2, 20 Hz–16 kHz) connected with plastic tubing to the ear mold. The stimuli were compensated for the *in situ* calibration.

Electrophysiological Recording

Auditory evoked potentials were measured using a low noise differential preamplifier (Stanford Research Systems, SR560). All contacts were made on the ipsilateral side to the recording: the signal input was connected to the needle-electrode; the reference input was connected to an earlobe clamp (with conductive gel) and the ground input was connected to a standard disposable surface electrode placed at the mastoid. For safety, the battery-operated preamplifier was galvanically isolated (A-M systems, Analog stimulus isolator Model 2200) from the mains-powered equipment outside the sound booth. Before the signal was recorded (TDT, RX8, ~100 kHz/channel, max. SNR 96 dB), stored and analyzed (MATLAB), the signal was further amplified (DAGAN, BVC-700A) and band pass filtered (30 Hz–30 kHz, cut-off slopes 12 dB/octave). All stimuli and recorded signals were monitored on-line (LeCroy, WaveSurfer 24Xs) during the session.

Analysis and Stimulus Paradigm

Human acoustically-evoked neural mass responses are smaller than those recorded in common laboratory animals. To improve the signal-to-noise ratio (SNR) of the response, the uncorrelated background noise was reduced by averaging the responses of many repetitions ($n = 200$). The averaged response was then de-noised (smoothed) with a non-causal low-pass filter using an RLOESS function (MATLAB). The RLOESS is a non-parametric robust local regression function using weighted linear squares and a 2nd degree polynomial model, which assigns lower weight to outliers in the regression (the weights are given by the bisquare function with zero weight for deviations greater than six mean absolute deviations). The span of the filter was chosen such that it corresponded to a low-pass cutoff of ~3 kHz, or ~1 kHz for CAP measurements with low SNR (i.e., heavily masked responses). The magnitude of the CAP was obtained between the first positive and first negative peak (P1-N1).

The recordings in the awake subjects occasionally contained artifacts due to sporadic head movements. These artifacts had a significant impact on the background noise and thus also on the SNR of the CAP. Single responses were selectively removed by measuring the individual contributions to the CAP (Jackknife method), and rejecting those that deviated in order to optimize the SNR. Note that the stimulus level of the precursor was kept below the subject's middle ear reflex threshold (90 dB SPL for subject 1 and 80 dB SPL for subject 2).

Our stimulus paradigm is designed to assess the mechanism by which a broadband noise precursor affects the detection of a tonal probe of 4 kHz. It is based on psychoacoustical paradigms, but modified to extract the CAP response from mass-potentials near the round window. A first modification is that we employ alternating stimulus polarity to cancel the cochlear microphonic (CM). Second, considerable attention was paid to remove masker artifacts—especially for simultaneous and strong forward maskers—and also to minimize drift between CAPs with different precursor conditions. Drift was expected due to the nature of the recording conditions (movements of awake subjects; varying state of arousal). **Figure 1** illustrates the two paradigms, for simultaneous masking (upper) and forward masking (lower). Only the first half presentation, to one stimulus polarity, is shown; the second half is the same, but with opposite polarity. The temporal sequence is such that each paradigm consists of 4 segments. The first segment (a) contains all 3 stimulus components: a probe with a masker and a precursor. The second segment (b) is the same as (a), but without a precursor. The third segment (c) is also the same as segment (a) but without the probe, and the last segment (d) contains only the masker. The duration of the precursor was 50 ms, which has been found to be the optimal length for maximizing gain reduction in psychoacoustic experiments (Roverud and Strickland, 2013). The probe and simultaneous masker were set at the same duration as the precursor. The forward masker was short (20 ms) in order to avoid activation of the MOCR, but long enough to mask the tone. The silent periods between the segments were chosen to be long enough (>500 ms) to allow the MOC-system to recover in between trials.

The probe was always a pure tone of 4 kHz, and the precursor was a Gaussian broadband noise (300–8,000 Hz). The masker was not fixed and changed over experiments and subjects. In the case of forward masking, the masker was either an ON- (4 kHz) or OFF-frequency (2.4 kHz) tone and for simultaneous masking, an OFF-frequency (2.4 kHz) tone or Gaussian narrowband noise (2–6 kHz). The level of the probe was 50, 60, or 70 dB SPL, dependent on subject and masker type. The level of the precursor was fixed to 50 dB SPL and below the subject's threshold of the acoustic reflex. The masker level was the independent variable, but did not exceed 95 dB SPL. Note that measurements with different masker levels were measured in blocks, where the masker level was changed across blocks in arbitrary order.

The rationale for the stimulus design (**Figure 1**) is as follows. The precursor is designed to activate the MOCR: comparison of segments (a) and (b) will therefore reveal the effect of this activation. Because the MOCR is hypothesized to reduce simultaneous masking, and to increase masking by an OFF-frequency masker more than for an ON-frequency masker, the effect of the precursor is assessed by examining the response to a masker-probe combination. More specifically, we are interested in the response to the probe, which should be reduced by the presence of a masker, and this reduction should change in the presence of a precursor. However, the response to the precursor-masker-probe combination (**Figure 1**, segment a) contains not only the CAP to the probe tone, but also an off- or on-set and ongoing response to the forward or simultaneous masker. Thus, to isolate the response to the probe, we add conditions in which there is no probe stimulus: a condition with precursor and masker (c) and one without precursor (d). To remove the masker response from (a) and (b), we subtract the responses to (c) and (d), respectively. A disadvantage of such a subtraction procedure is an increase in noise: the mathematical operation to remove the transient response increased the CAP's background noise by 3 dB (summation of two signals with independent background noise signals). For heavily masked responses, where the transient responses to the masker are the largest, we used as compensation the average of segment c and d, which was still satisfactory to suppress the masker's transient response but with less increase in background noise due to the averaging of the two independent background noises inside the compensation signals; the increase in background noise is only 1.6 instead of 3 dB.

We examined the effect of an ipsilateral precursor in simultaneous and forward masking paradigms, which have been used in previous physiological and psychoacoustical studies as

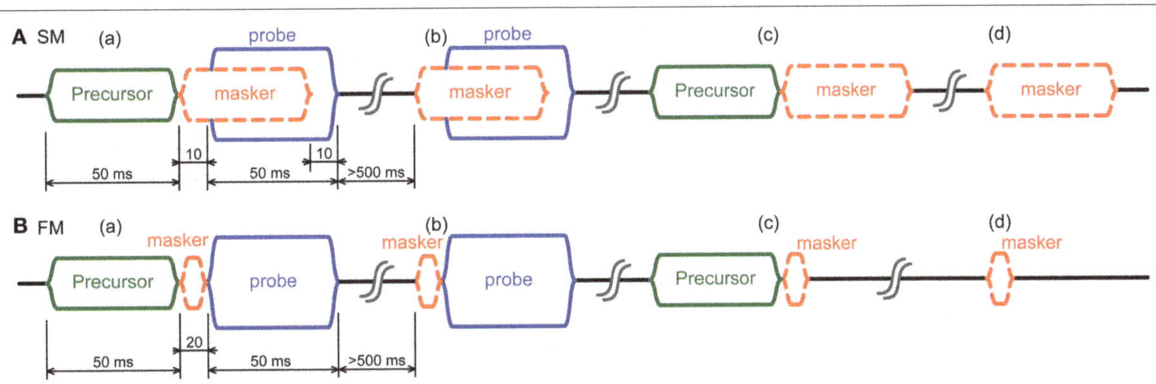

FIGURE 1 | Illustration of the first half presentation of the two stimulus paradigms used in this study. **(A)** paradigm with simultaneous masker and **(B)** with forward masker. Each presentation has 4 segments indicated by letters: **(a)** contains all 3 stimulus components: precursor, masker, and probe; **(b)** similar but without precursor; **(c)** similar but without probe; **(d)** masker only. The probe is always a tone of 4 kHz. The precursor is a broadband noise. The masker can be an ON-frequency (4 kHz) tone; a 2.4 kHz OFF-frequency tone; or a narrowband noise. The second half representation (not shown) is the same as the first, but with all stimuli presented in inverted polarity. A single "condition" consists of the half presentation shown here and the half with opposite polarity. The masker is drawn in dashed lines, indicating the possibility of a condition without masker.

described in the Introduction. In simultaneous masking, a release from masking (i.e., an increase in probe response) is expected following a precursor, based on previous physiological studies of the CAP (Kawase and Liberman, 1993) and psychoacoustical studies of overshoot (Zwicker, 1965). In forward masking with an OFF-frequency masker, the precursor will decrease the probe response but not the masker response: so more masking is expected for an OFF-frequency masker than for an on-frequency masker, based on previous psychoacoustical studies (Kawase et al., 2000; Jennings et al., 2009; Jennings and Strickland, 2012).

Forward masking paradigms have the advantage that the different stimulus components do not mutually interact (**Figure 1**) at the level of the cochlea, and do not induce additional cochlear suppression effects, such as two-tone suppression (e.g., Sachs and Kiang, 1968; Ruggero et al., 1992; van der Heijden and Joris, 2005), which complicate the interpretation of the results.

RESULTS

A total of five experiments were conducted: 3 in a single session with subject 1, and 2 in a single session with subject 2. The various stimulus conditions used in the two subjects are chronologically listed in **Table 1**. In all experiments, the masker level was parametrically varied. The first experiment (SM1n) studied masking of a tone in noise using a simultaneous masking paradigm (upper figure in **Figure 1**), while the other two experiments used OFF- (FM1off) and ON-frequency (FM1on) tonal maskers in a forward masking paradigm (lower figure in **Figure 1**). In the second session (subject 2), we used only OFF-frequency maskers and compared results with simultaneous (SM2off) and forward (FM2off) maskers. To facilitate comparison between different experiments, CAP responses are expressed as relative values (in %) with respect to the corresponding response without masker.

Effect of a Precursor without Masker

The precursor is the experimental variable that is intended to activate the MOCR. A difficulty in the study of ipsilateral effects is that the precursor may not only activate efferents but will also have "lingering" or history effects on responses of the same ear to subsequent stimuli even without efferent activation. For convenience, we group such non-efferent history effects (which may contain mechanical, hair cell, synaptic, and neural components) loosely under the term "neural adaptation." We first examine conditions, present in all experiments, in which there is no effective masker. This gives a first simple assessment of the effect of the precursor on the probe response. **Figure 2** shows CAP responses to 4 kHz tones with and without a precursor, from experiment FM2off. Two effects are visible. The CAP amplitude is reduced by the presence of the precursor. Expressing CAP amplitude as the difference in magnitude between the first positive peak P1 and the first negative peak N1, the precursor reduces the CAP magnitude by approximately 20%. Second, the presence of the precursor causes a small delay of 130 μs of N1.

Using the same precursor, experiments FM1off, FM1on and SM2off showed a very similar reduction of 20%, as shown in **Figure 3**. Curiously, the only exception is experiment SM1n, which shows a much greater reduction (35%) compared to the others, as well as smaller variability. Importantly, because **Figure 3** is for conditions in which there was no masker, and because the probe frequency and precursor were identical in all experiments, the only stimulus differences were in probe level and in the relative timing between precursor and probe. It appears that the high probe level in experiment SM1n somehow caused a larger effect.

Notwithstanding that the only experiment with somewhat different stimulus conditions gave a deviating result, it is reassuring that the other experiments—where the stimulus conditions were virtually identical—gave rise to very similar effects across experiments and across the two subjects. In the next session, a masker is added to attempt to tease out efferent vs. neural adaptation effects.

Effect of Masker

Anti-Masking

Figure 4 shows data for all experiments. We first discuss the overall effect of increasing masker levels, and then the influence of the precursor on that effect, while making abstraction of the different experimental conditions. The blue symbols and lines indicate the probe CAP responses without a precursor. A cursory look at **Figures 4A–E** shows that, as expected, for all masking configurations an increase in masker level caused a decrease in response to the probe. These curves, which we refer to as standard masking functions, show three regions—not distinct in all experiments. At low masker level there is a region without

TABLE 1 | Experimental conditions.

Experiment	Precursor 0.3–8 kHz BB-noise	Masker			Probe 4 kHz tone
SM1n	50 dB SPL	SM;	Quiet, 20, 30, ..., 60 dB SPL;	2-6 kHz noise	70 dB SPL
FM1off	50 dB SPL	FM;	Quiet, 50, 60, ..., 90 dB SPL;	2.4 kHz tone	50 dB SPL
FM1on	50 dB SPL	FM;	Quiet, 20, 30, ..., 60 dB SPL;	4.0 kHz tone	50 dB SPL
SM2off	50 dB SPL	SM;	Quiet, 40, ..., 80 dB SPL;	2.4 kHz tone	60 dB SPL
FM2off	50 dB SPL	FM;	Quiet, 50, ..., 95 dB SPL;	2.4 kHz tone	60 dB SPL

The names in the first column identify the experiments: the first two characters indicate whether simultaneous masking (SM) or forward masking (FM) was used; the subsequent number indicates the subject; the last characters indicate the stimulus type of the masker (noise or ON- or OFF-frequency masker).

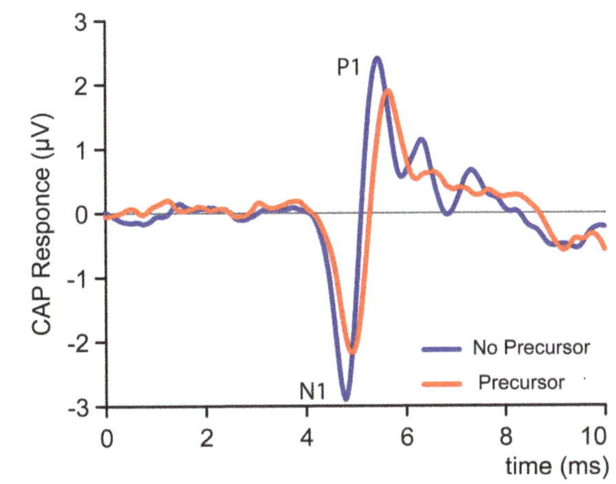

FIGURE 2 | An example of the effect of a broad-band noise precursor of 50 dB SPL on the amplitude and time-course of a human CAP response to a 4 kHz (50 dB SPL) tone, based on >600 averages. The CAP amplitude is measured between P1 and N1. Data is from experiment FM2off.

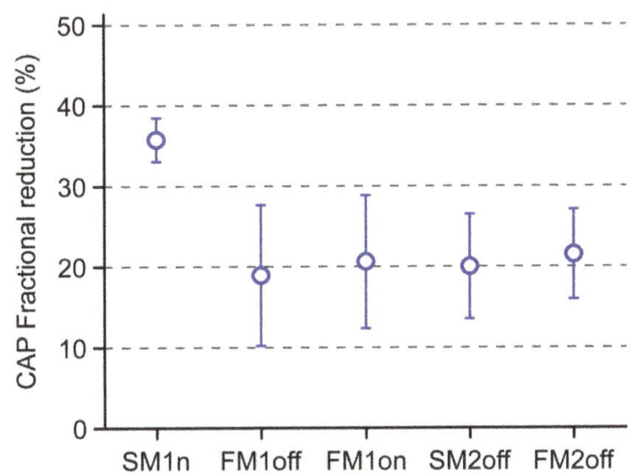

FIGURE 3 | Overview of CAP reduction by a precursor for the different experiments in this study. The error bars indicate propagated SEM obtained with bootstrapping.

masking; then a region of active masking where the response declines with masker level; then a region of saturation at high masker levels.

Given that there is masking of the probe response in all experimental conditions, we can look for anti-masking of CAP responses as was shown in anesthetized animals (Kawase and Liberman, 1993), using similar recordings. These investigators found efferent anti-masking effects on CAP responses to tones-in-noise with both forward and simultaneous maskers, which involved both the ipsi- and contra-driven efferent loops. If the noise precursor used here effectively activates the MOCR, the masked response could be larger in the presence of a precursor. This is however never the case (**Figures 4A–E**): none of the data pairs at any masker level exhibit an increase in response when there is a precursor, so that the red and blue lines and data never cross each other.

The absence of a simple anti-masking effect does not imply that there is no differential MOCR involvement between conditions with or without precursor. The data with a precursor have a similar course (red trendline) as the standard masking curves (blue trendline), but do not asymptote toward the same response values at high masker levels. At low masker levels there is the initial CAP reduction due to the presence of the precursor by itself (**Figure 3**). This reduction, relative to the condition without precursor, persists at active masker levels. Even at high masker levels, where there is a region of saturation, there remains a constant difference in CAP amplitude between conditions with and without precursor (only exception is at 60 dB for SM1n, **Figure 4A**, which we consider an outlier). This suggests that the effect of the precursor is not simply one of neural adaptation, because in that case the probe response at high, saturated masker levels would not be affected by the presence or absence of a precursor. We will return to this observation with a quantitative treatment in the final section and figure of Results.

Evidence for Gain Reduction

We now zoom in on a more detailed analysis and comparison of the results of the different experiments and exploit the differences in masker configurations to search for the presence of possible MOCR effects. With tonal ON-frequency maskers, cochlear gain changes due to the MOCR can affect both the probe and masker response. Tonal OFF-frequency maskers, of a frequency lower than the probe, perform masking in the tail of the masker's excitation pattern. Of course, with an OFF-frequency masker, higher masker levels are required to reach masking threshold. OFF-frequency maskers are of interest because they behave linearly with masker level, and, at the tonotopic location of the probe, are believed to be unaffected by the MOCR (Kawase et al., 2000; Cooper and Guinan, 2006). If the precursor indeed triggers the MOCR, this activation will cause a gain reduction for both ON-frequency masker and probe. However, with an OFF-frequency masker a gain reduction due to MOCR activation would only affect the probe and not the masker, effectively making the masker more potent. Thus, the expectation is that, when preceded by a precursor, ON-frequency maskers show a smaller response reduction than OFF-frequency maskers.

Figures 4C,E shows the effect of a precursor on the CAP response to a forward masked 4 kHz tone as a function of masker level. **Figure 4E** shows the results of the ON-frequency masker (experiment FM1on) and **Figure 4C** that of the OFF-frequency masker (experiment FM1off). Comparison of the two standard masking curves (blue lines, **Figures 4C,E**), shows, as expected, a rightward shift of ~40 dB for the OFF-frequency masker (value based on sigmoidal fits, explained in Section Predictions from a simple model). This rightward shift is simply due to the fact that it is only through the tail of its excitation pattern that the masker interferes with the probe. When compensated for this level shift, we observe that at active masker levels (i.e., 70, 80 dB SPL for the OFF-frequency masker and 30, 40 dB SPL for the ON-frequency masker) the CAP reduction by precursor is much larger for the OFF- than for ON-frequency maskers. This is illustrated in **Figure 5**, which shows the CAP reduction induced by the precursor for both experiments. At low masker levels, the

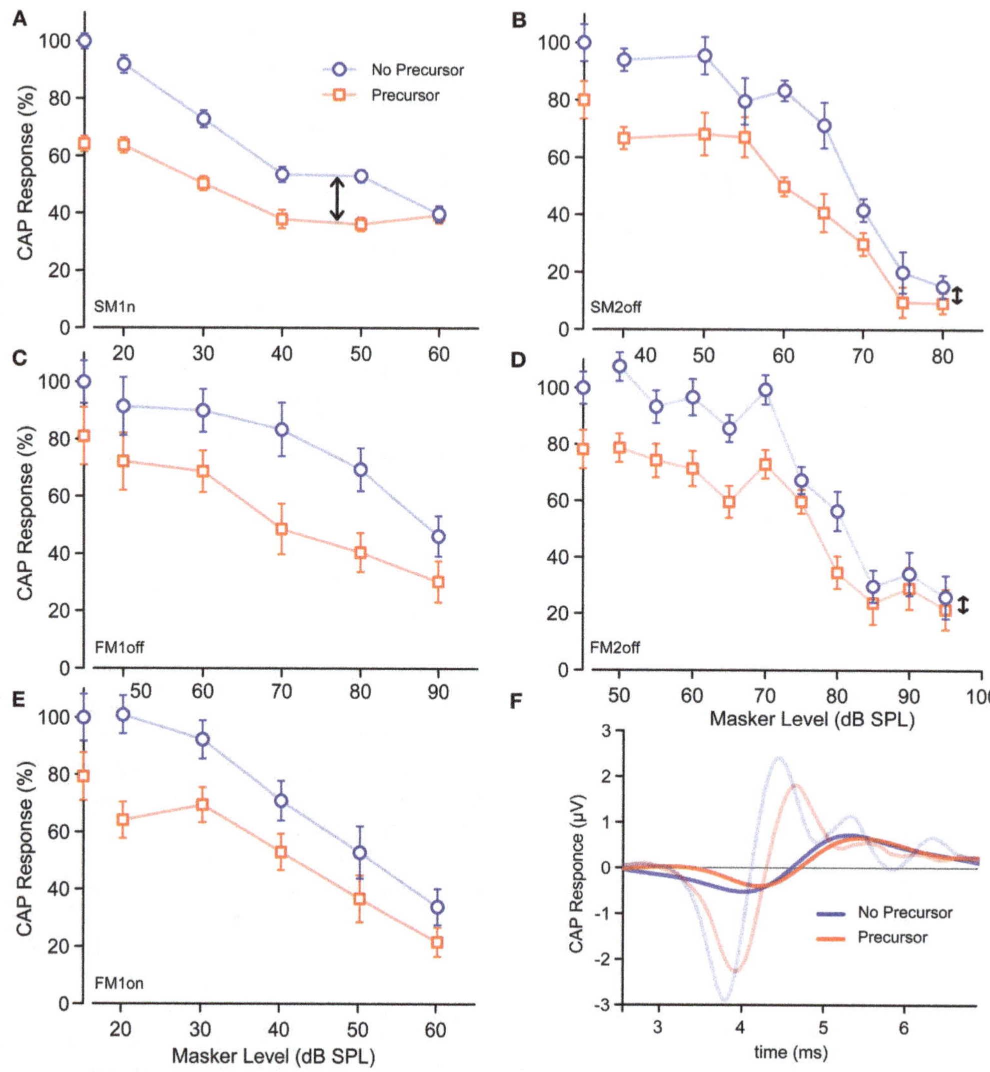

FIGURE 4 | (A–E) CAP responses of a 4 kHz masked tone as function of masker levels with (red symbols) and without (blue symbols) BBN precursor, for different experiments. Datapoints on Y-axis are those without masker. **(F)** CAP response at masking saturation of experiment FM2off, with and without precursor. Signals in background are from **Figure 2**.

same percentage of CAP reduction is observed for ON- and OFF-frequency maskers. At high masker levels, the percentage of CAP reduction is also similar, and presumably reflects gain reduction of the probe response due to the MOCR (see also **Figures 6I,J** and the final section of RESULTS). However, at masker levels in between, there is indeed a greater reduction by the precursor for the OFF-frequency masker than for the ON-frequency masker, consistent with a reduction in gain by activation of the MOCR (double arrow).

Residual Reduction at High Masker Levels

In our discussion of **Figure 4** (Section Anti-masking), we remarked that standard masking curves saturate to a certain asymptotic level. At these saturated masker levels, a further decrease in probe response is obtained when a precursor is present. We refer to this as a "residual reduction." This observation is important because it goes against the reasoning that any contribution by the precursor to neural adaptation can be overwhelmed by a stronger forward masker so that in the limit, at high masker levels, the curves with and without precursor should converge. The residual reduction at saturation suggests an MOCR effect. In the next section, we put this reasoning on a more quantitative footing.

The clearest examples of residual reduction are for Experiments SM2off and FM2off (**Figures 4B,D** double arrows). CAP responses for FM2off at saturation, with (red) or without (blue) precursor, are illustrated in **Figure 4F**. For comparison, overlaid in the background, are non-masked responses to these conditions. The masked responses exhibit the same precursor effects as the non-masked responses: a reduction in size and presence of a delay for N1 and P1 (red vs. blue traces). Note also the large delay accompanying the size reduction between

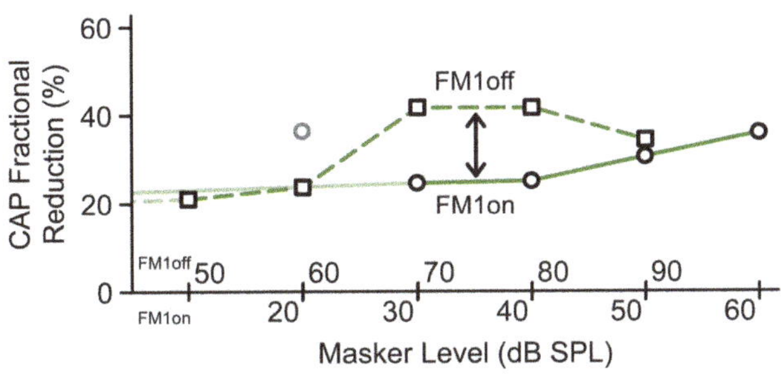

FIGURE 5 | Comparison of CAP response reductions by precursor as function of masker level for ON-and OFF-frequency forward maskers. The masker levels are horizontally offset by 40 dB, according to the midpoint of the masking curves. For each curve, the CAP reduction (in %) is calculated as (CAP response without precursor—CAP responses with precursor)/CAP response without precursor. The datapoint for FM1on at 20 dB is considered an outlier (see also **Figure 4E**).

non-masked and masked conditions (i.e., the delay between the two red curves and the delay between the two blue curves). Similar residual reductions are present at the highest masker levels in experiments SM1n, FM1off, and FM1on, but for these experiments saturation may not have been reached yet.

Examination of **Figure 4** suggests that the size of residual masking by the precursor is related to the size of the remaining response at saturation: the larger the response at saturation (i.e., the larger the blue datapoints at high masker levels), the larger the residual adaptation (i.e., the larger the length of the double arrows). More generally, at all masker levels, the reduction in CAP response between non-precursor and precursor conditions seems to be a constant fraction (between 20 and 30%) across experimental conditions. The observation that this fraction extends to saturated levels of masking suggests that the precursor triggers a constant attenuation of the probe response, consistent with a gain reduction by the MOCR. In **Figure 6**, we explore this with a phenomenological model and further analysis of the data.

Predictions from a Simple Model

Our model examines the effect of the precursor on the standard masking curve, which is fit by a function. For simplification, only the two most important mechanisms are considered, neural adaptation and reduction in gain. Two important assumptions we make are that the MOCR is modeled by an attenuation due to a reduction in gain; and both mechanisms (MOCR and neural adaptation) are assumed to be independent. We consider 3 situations: Case 1, a response reduction due to neural adaptation by the precursor; Case 2, a gain reduction by the MOCR which affects only the probe but not the masker (cf. OFF-frequency masker); and Case3, the same as Case2 but with an additional "masker release" due to the MOC i.e., an MOC effect on both probe and masker (cf. ON-frequency maskers).

Figures 6A–E shows the trend lines from the model, together with the data points. The blue traces are sigmoidal model fits through the standard masking curves, i.e., data points of the masked responses without a precursor (blue symbols). These fits are obtained with an automated fitting procedure using a modified logistic function (Equation 1).

$$R_{CAP}\left(L_{mask}\right)=\alpha\left(\frac{\left(R_{max}-R_{sat}\right)}{1+\exp\left(k\left(L_{mask}-L_{mid}\right)\right)}+R_{sat}\right) \quad (1)$$

Here, R_{CAP} is the masked response (in %), L_{mid} the level of the sigmoid midpoint (dB SPL), k determines the steepness of the sigmoid (dB SPL^{-1}), R_{max} is the unmasked CAP response (in %), R_{sat} is the response at masking saturation (in %), α is an attenuation factor determining the gain reduction by the MOC, and L_{mask} is the effective masker input level. For the automatic fitting procedure, MATLAB function "*fminsearch*" was used in search for the parameters (i.e., L_{mid}, R_{max}, R_{sat}, k) that minimized the RMS-error. Data points were weighted according to their SEM. The data point on the y-axis (**Figures 6A–E**) is the CAP response without masker (cf. **Figure 3**): for convenience these are inserted 20 dB below the lowest masker level.

For the standard masker curve, the attenuation (α) was set to 1. In general, the fit to the experimental data is good (**Figures 6A–E**, blue traces). Note that the data point at the highest masker level in SM1n (**Figure 6A**) is considered an outlier and was excluded from the dataset. In experiment FM1off (**Figure 6D**), there were not enough data points in the region of saturation for a proper automated fit, and parameter R_{sat} was manually chosen based on experiment FM1on.

The red dashed traces in **Figures 6A–E** represent the predicted trends with precursor for Case 1, thus only including neural adaptation. The same function and fitting parameters were used as for the standard masking curve (blue lines), but with recalculated effective masker input levels (L_m) to include neural masking by the precursor. Masking by the precursor is simply considered as an additional bias on the existing masking. The bias level was obtained from the standard masking curve as the masker level (L_{prec}) generating a CAP response of the same amplitude as a condition with precursor but without masker (R_{prec}; see **Figure 3**). L_{mask} was then recalculated as the square root of the power of L_{mask} and L_{prec}. This is illustrated by the gray dashed lines in **Figure 6A**. The R_{CAP} function so obtained (**Figures 6A–E**, dashed red line) matched the observed CAP values quite well for SM2off, but not in the other experiments. Clearly, neural adaptation is not adequate to model the effect of the precursor.

The red solid traces (**Figures 6A–E**) represent the predictions for Case 2, under the assumption that the MOCR induces a gain reduction of the probe only, matching the experimental conditions with OFF-frequency maskers. The same function and fitting parameters were used as for the standard masking curve (blue lines), but with an additional attenuation (α, constant within an experiment) equal to the initial reduction by the precursor, R_{prec}. This prediction clearly outperforms that of Case1 and gives a good fit to the masking data with precursor, except for experiment FM1off, where the predicted masking curve is too far to the right.

Finally, the red dashed-dotted traces (**Figures 6A–E**) represent the predictions of Case 3, where both masker and probe are affected by a gain reduction caused by the MOCR

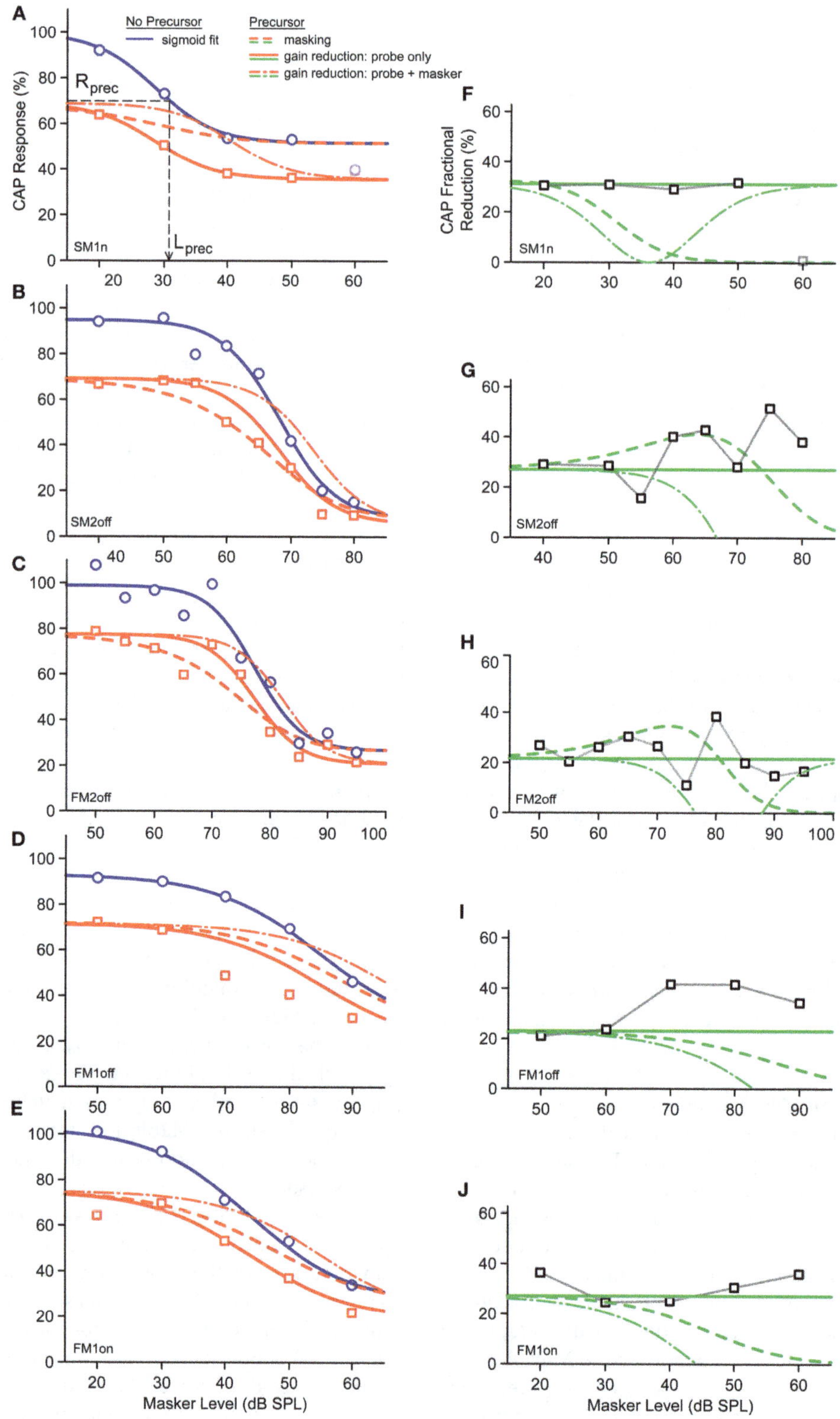

FIGURE 6 | (A–E) Predicted masked CAP responses in case the reduction by precursor is from masking (dashed red) or due to the activation of the MOCR (solid red). The data points of the masked responses with precursor are indicated by the red squares; those without precursor by the blue dots. These data points were fit by the blue curve, which was used for the predictions. The dashed gray lines indicated the bias level, Lprec. **(F–J)** Predicted response reductions obtained from the red and blue curves in **(A–E)**. Green dashed curve is for the prediction by masking; the solid green line is the predicted attenuation by the MOCR. The experimental data points are indicated by the black squares.

elicited by the precursor—the situation thought to arise with ON-frequency forward maskers. The same function and fitting parameters were used as for Case 2, but with an additional offset to the masker input level (L_{mask}) to incorporate a gain reduction by the MOC. The size of this additional offset is unknown: we estimate it based on the reduction of the CAP response by the precursor only, as follows. We first determine the maximal slope of the standard masking curve (at L_{mid} of solid blue line): this slope tells us how to translate a change in CAP response to a change in masker level. We then apply this slope to the reduction of the precursor only ($1 - R_{prec}$) as follows: offset = ($1 - R_{prec}$)/absmax(slope of the standard making curve). This offset is the masker threshold shift assuming similar gain reduction as for the probe. Note that—whatever the exact estimate of offset—a reduction in gain of the masker will always shift the masker curve to the right, to higher masker levels (**Figures 6A–E**, red dashed-dotted lines). A rightward shift actually brings the model prediction further from the observed datapoints than for Case2. Thus, whatever the estimated effect of a gain reduction on the masker, a combined reduction of both masker and probe (Case3) does not give better predictions than gain reduction just of the probe (Case2).

To illustrate the effect of the precursor more directly for these three cases, **Figures 6F–J** show the percent CAP reductions due to the precursor for the model and the data as a fractional change (% reduction with precursor − % reduction without precursor)/(% reduction without precursor). For Case2, the prediction is simply a horizontal line representing an attenuation or constant gain reduction. For the other two cases, the predicted reductions are strongly dependent on masker level. By and large, the horizontal trend of a constant gain reduction seems to best capture the data.

DISCUSSION

We assessed the ipsilateral sound-evoked MOCR in humans using CAPs recorded transtympanically in the middle ear using stimulus paradigms similar to previous MOC studies. We measured CAP responses to forward- or simultaneously-masked 4 kHz tones, preceded in some trials by a precursor designed to trigger the MOCR. Some, but not all, of the findings are consistent with MOCR effects as opposed to effects of neural adaptation. First, a noise precursor has a clear reducing effect on unmasked CAP responses (**Figures 2, 3**). The reduction observed does not seem entirely explainable in terms of neural adaptation. Second, we find residual masking at high masker levels, i.e., while masking saturates at high stimulus levels, a precursor causes further reduction in CAP responses (**Figure 4**). The behavior of this residual masking is consistent with a gain reduction due to MOCR activation (**Figure 6**). Third, a comparison between ON- and OFF-frequency maskers showed a clear difference in response reduction by the precursor, consistent with a gain reduction by the MOCR (**Figures 4, 5**).

Anti-Masking Effect

Previous CAP recordings in anesthetized animals show that the MOCR can produce an anti-masking effect, in the sense that CAP responses to a probe tone masked by ipsilateral noise increase in amplitude due to MOCR activation (Kawase and Liberman, 1993). In the latter study, involvement of efferents driven by the ipsilateral ear was detected by sectioning of the olivocochlear bundle which carries efferent fibers from the brainstem to the cochlea. A simple prediction for paradigms as employed in the present study, where the MOCR is triggered by a precursor in the ipsilateral ear, would be that masked CAP responses would increase when preceded by a precursor, relative to the responses without precursor. In the present study, such simple anti-masking effect was not found in any of the stimulus configurations (**Figure 4**): the datapoints with precursor (red) are always below the datapoints without precursor (blue). However, the absence of such simple anti-masking in the paradigms used in human but not in animals is not very informative and it is misleading to make this comparison. Cutting the olivocochlear bundle allows a clean comparison between responses of a system with and without efferents. The same is not true for the responses with and without precursor: the precursor can affect the responses by mechanisms which are separate from the efferent system. More specifically, the precursor also causes neural adaptation. A more pertinent question therefore is: does the presence of the precursor cause less reduction in masked responses than expected? Answering this question requires a means to disentangle effects of neural adaptation from effects of efferent activation.

Residual Reduction by Precursor

Perhaps the most convincing evidence of the presence of an MOCR triggered by the precursor, is the residual reduction of the CAP response at high masker levels. Our reasoning is that exhaustion of neural adaptation manifests itself as saturation of the masking curve at high masker levels (**Figure 4**). We refer to this as residual reduction, and argue that it is due to a triggering of the MOCR by the precursor. A concern is the reliability of the CAP measurements at high masker levels. Most of the saturated CAPs are quite small and have poor SNR (**Figure 4**). We took the peak-to-peak amplitude of the CAP to reduce contributions of the summating potential, and also observed that a reduction in amplitude was accompanied by a time delay (**Figures 2,4F**). Moreover, the presence of residual masking was quite consistent across experiments and across the two subjects. In summary, the data argue that the precursor triggers a process besides neural adaptation which reduces CAP responses.

Forward Masking

One technique used in psychoacoustical experiments to identify an efferent effect is to compare the effectiveness of ON- and OFF-frequency forward maskers. The underlying reasoning is that efferent activity maximally affects basilar membrane vibration near the cochlear location of maximal vibration (active region with gain), and less at more apical or more basal locations with a more linear behavior (Robles and Ruggero, 2001). Thus, while an ON-frequency masker will be rendered less effective by efferent activation, this is less the case for an OFF-frequency masker. We compared the two masker configurations (FM1on and FM1off). **Figure 5** shows indeed that the OFF-frequency masker is less affected (remains a stronger masker) by the precursor than for the ON-frequency masker, consistent with a gain reduction for the ON-frequency masker.

Nevertheless, review of the different experiments and quantitative comparisons with predictions from a simple model (**Figure 6**) reveals a pattern of results that is more complex than anticipated. If the precursor triggers the MOCR so that only the gain to the probe tone (and not to the masker) is affected, a constant CAP reduction is expected across masker levels (horizontal solid line in **Figures 6G–I**): this is the prediction for an OFF-frequency masker. There is however a tendency in the three experimental conditions with OFF-frequency maskers to display more reduction in fractional change with increasing masker level (i.e., datapoints above the solid horizontal lines in **Figures 6G–I**). Paradoxically, for the two experiments with ON-frequency maskers, the data very closely do follow the horizontal lines (**Figures 6F,J**), rather than the prediction for this condition (dash-dotted lines). To put it simply: the results for ON-frequency maskers look as expected for OFF-frequency maskers. The data therefore suggest that in all experiments there is an additional source of reduction of the probe response, which is not adequately modeled by a constant, MOCR-induced, reduction in gain at the probe frequency.

We surmise that a dependency exists between activation of the MOCR and masker level and/or masker type. For example, the shape of the masking curve with precursor might be influenced by the masker level *via* additional activation of the MOCR by the masker itself. In preliminary experiments (not shown) we have observed that efferent activation seems to be biased toward low-frequency stimuli. Although the short masker and slow MOCR activation make it unlikely, there is still a possibility that the presence of a low-frequency, OFF-frequency, masker increasingly contributes to activation of the MOCR with increasing masker level. This would cause additional reduction of the CAP response to the probe (note that the start of the masker always precedes that of the probe, **Figure 1**, even in the simultaneous masking paradigm). Such increased MOCR activation may explain why there tends to be more reduction of the CAP response with increasing masker level of OFF-frequency maskers (**Figures 6G–I**) than predicted by the model. With ON-frequency maskers (**Figures 6F,J**), we modeled the effect of the precursor as a constant attenuation of masker and probe by the MOCR, resulting in the dash-dotted lines, but again the data show more reduction in fractional change than the model. Increased MOCR activation by the increasing masker may be the cause of this additional reduction.

Other factors may add to the complexities of the results, which have more to do with technical aspects of the recorded signals. One issue is that, as masker level increases and CAP amplitude decreases, the nature of the recorded signal may change with a larger reflection of an IHC summating potential. A hint that this may be the case is that the masking curves do not always asymptote to the typically low values seen in animal experiment (Verschooten et al., 2012). Also, there is a possibility that a reflex contraction of the middle ear muscles (MEM) may have affected the recordings, even though the stimuli were below the clinical reflex threshold. We have several reasons to doubt that this was the case. First, muscle activity generates a large signal that is easily detected through the recording electrode, both during online visual and auditory monitoring of the recorded signal, and in the offline analysis (rejection of samples with artifacts). In another study (other subjects), where we used a more intense and longer broadband noise masker, we sometimes observed muscle activity at sound levels which were consistent with the reflex threshold measured with the clinical apparatus. However, in the subjects in this study, such sound-driven MEM artifacts were not observed. Second, another indicator for MEM activation is a significant and systematic decrease in CM amplitude, which is larger for low frequencies but still significantly present for mid and high frequencies (Pang and Guinan, 1997). In our data we did not find a consistent change in CM amplitude over any of the masker levels, including the highest levels at 95 dB SPL. Third, the masker is the stimulus component that reaches the highest levels, and it is present in all stimulus segments (see **Figure 1**). Considering the short duration of both the masker (20 ms) and its interval to the probe, and the slowness of MEM activation, it is improbable that MEM activation triggered by the masker would differentially affect the responses obtained with and without precursor. To conclude, we think there are sufficient arguments to rule out the possibility that the MEM-reflex rather than the MOCR underlies the effects observed.

Overshoot Effect?

Overshoot is a phenomenon observed in psychoacoustics, which refers to the enhanced detection of a simultaneously-masked pip-tone in the presence of a precursor. The most common hypotheses are that the overshoot is caused by a reduction in gain due to the MOCR (Strickland, 2004; Jennings et al., 2011; Fletcher et al., 2013) or by a reduction in masking due to the adaptive effect of the precursor (Fletcher et al., 2015). As already mentioned (Section Anti-masking effect), none of our electrophysiological experiments revealed an increase in response by the presence of a precursor. We subjected six subjects to a psychoacoustical experiment with a paradigm identical to SM1n, except that the probe tone was shortened to 6 ms. All subjects showed a clear psychoacoustical overshoot, with a consistent masker level increase of ~5 dB (not shown). The absence of an effect in the physiological recordings but not in the psychoacoustical testing does not provide support for the hypothesis that overshoot is caused by a simple gain reduction due to the MOCR, nor by an adaptive effect of the precursor. Rather, in line with conclusions based on psychoacoustical studies (Fletcher et al., 2013, 2015), it is possible that overshoot is a product of central auditory processing operating on peripheral changes that are not detected by our recording methods.

Effects on CAP Waveform

The CAP waveform reflects the summed synchronized discharge of a population of auditory nerve fibers (AN-fibers; Goldstein and Kiang, 1958; Kiang, 1984). Changes in acoustic input or in the processes leading up to the AN responses can affect this summed synchronized population discharge and thereby affect the waveform of the CAP. The most obvious example is the combined change in the waveform's amplitude and latency with input level (Eggermont, 1976; Chabert et al., 2002; Verschooten et al., 2012). In the present study, we focused on effects of the MOCR on CAP amplitude, but, as shown in **Figures 2,4F**, the precursor also affects latency and shape of the CAP. Particularly the difference in latency at high masker levels, between conditions with and without precursor, suggests that these temporal aspects of the response may help in disambiguating effects of forward masking vs. MOCR (**Figure 4F**).

The processes of gain reduction by the MOCR and of neural adaptation affect AN firing and consequently also the CAP waveform. The overall impact of neural adaptation on the CAP waveform is similar to a reduction in input level (Eggermont, 1979). The solid lines in **Figure 7A** show indeed that with increasing masker level, CAP amplitudes decrease and latencies increase. Formulating an expectation regarding the effect of an MOCR-induced gain reduction on latency, is more difficult. On the one hand, a reduction in gain is expected to cause a decrease in amplitude and an increase in latency similar to a reduction in input level. On the other hand, several studies report that efferent activation only causes a decrease in CAP amplitude but does not cause a change in latency (e.g., Desmedt et al., 1971; Chabert et al., 2002; Elgueda et al., 2011). In our data, the reduction in CAP amplitude caused by a precursor is accompanied by an increase in latency (**Figures 4F,7A**: compare solid and dashed lines for a given masker level). While this may at first sight suggest that the CAP reductions caused by the precursor do not reflect activation of the MOCR, but rather neural adaptation, it is important to note that other studies have demonstrated latency effects secondary to efferent activation (e.g., Liberman, 1989; Kawase and Liberman, 1993; Aedo et al., 2015). Possibly, these different outcomes in different studies are related to the type of CAP-evoking stimulus, where studies using clicks show no latency effects but studies using tones do. In any case, it is not clear that examination of the effects on latency allow a better disambiguation of effects of neural adaptation vs. effects of the MOCR.

Neural adaptation and gain reduction by the MOCR operate at different peripheral stages and affect AN-fibers differently. These differences may be reflected not only in amplitude and latency, but also in the precise shape of the CAP waveforms. To illustrate, **Figure 7B** shows an example of a masker-only (blue line) and precursor-only (red line) responses, that resulted in CAPs identical in amplitude and latency but not in exact waveform shape. The CAP without masker or precursor (dashed line) shows several late waves (e.g., N3,P3): such late features are present in the masker-only condition (blue line) but are more subtle in the precursor-only condition. Possibly, examination of such later features may help to reveal the presence of an MOCR, but a better SNR and availability of additional stimulus conditions would be required for such an effort.

General Considerations

Our expectation was to find an anti-masking effect in CAPs, similar to that observed in anesthetized cat by Kawase and Liberman (1993). Three further points merit consideration. First, especially regarding the comparison of our physiological recordings with psychoacoustical results, it should be remembered that the CAP response only captures a certain aspect of auditory nerve activity (synchronous onset responses). Changes in neural activity that are important for behavioral detection of a probe are not necessarily reflected in the CAP response to this probe. Second, there is a possibility that for some reason (e.g., related to the transtympanic procedure) the MOCR was continuously active during the recording sessions, and that the effect of the presence of the precursor cannot be equated to a simple on or off switching of the MOCR. Third, species differences may be important. In experimental animals, the ipsilateral MOC pathway and reflex is about double in size relative to the contralateral component (Warr, 1992; Guinan, 2011). Anatomical data support the existence of both a lateral and MOC system in humans (Arnesen, 1984; Moore et al., 1999) and, more generally, in primates (Bodian and Gucer, 1980; Thompson and Thompson, 1986), but there is

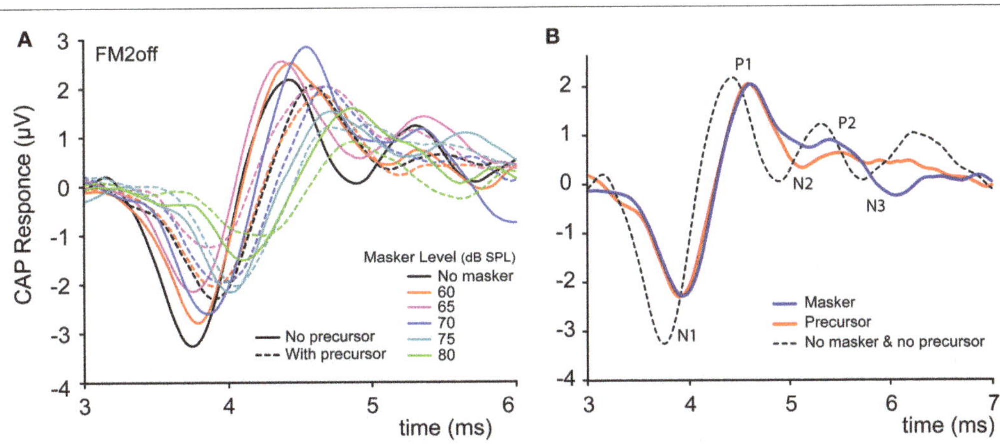

FIGURE 7 | CAP waveforms of experiment FM2off with and without precursor. **(A)** Different masker levels. **(B)** Comparison of CAP waveforms for different conditions: masker-only (blue), precursor-only (red), and without either (dashed). The waveform for the masking-only condition was obtained by interpolating the CAPs for masker levels 70 and 75 dB SPL, such that the CAP magnitude was equal to that of the precursor-only condition.

to our knowledge no human anatomical data that addresses anatomical size differences between ipsi- and contralateral MOC systems. Human OAE data suggest that there is little difference between the size of ipsilateral and contralateral MOC reflexes (Guinan, 2006), although more recent data show larger effects for ipsilateral elicitors under certain conditions (Lilaonitkul and Guinan, 2009, 2012).

CONCLUSION

It appears that the expected difference between reduction by neural masking and reduction in gain by the MOCR is more subtle and less clear than expected. However, we found several indications of MOC involvement, despite the absence of an anti-masking for tone in noise. Comparison between ON- and OFF-frequency maskers showed a larger reduction by a precursor for OFF than for ON-frequency, consistent with gain reduction. An inconsistency between our model and the data suggests a relationship between the masker level and gain reduction by the MOCR. The most convincing evidence of the presence of a MOCR is the residual response by the precursor at high masker levels.

To conclude, the results in this study show that the response reduction by the precursor is approximately 20–30%. We found that the reduction is fairly independent of masker type, masker level and probe level. These results support psychoacoustical paradigms that are designed to probe the efferent system as indeed activating that system.

AUTHOR CONTRIBUTIONS

EV, ES, and PJ designed the study; EV and NV performed the measurements; EV analyzed data; EV, ES, and PJ wrote the manuscript.

FUNDING

This work was supported by grants from BOF (OT-14-118 to PJ) and NIH (R01 grant DC008327 to ES).

ACKNOWLEDGMENTS

We would like to thank Iris Vlamings for her contributions to the experiments.

REFERENCES

Aedo, C., Tapia, E., Pavez, E., Elgueda, D., Delano, P. H., and Robles, L. (2015). Stronger efferent suppression of cochlear neural potentials by contralateral acoustic stimulation in awake than in anesthetized chinchilla. *Front. Syst. Neurosci.* 9:21. doi: 10.3389/fnsys.2015.00021

Arnesen, A. R. (1984). Fibre population of the vestibulocochlear anastomosis in humans. *Acta Otolaryngol.* 98, 501–518. doi: 10.3109/00016488409107591

Bodian, D., and Gucer, G. (1980). Denervation study of synapses of organ of Corti of old world monkeys. *J. Comp. Neurol.* 192, 785–796. doi: 10.1002/cne.901920411

Brown, M. C. (1989). Morphology and response properties of single olivocochlear fibers in the guinea pig. *Hear. Res.* 40, 93–109. doi: 10.1016/0378-5955(89)90103-2

Brown, M. C., Kujawa, S. G., and Liberman, M. C. (1998). Single olivocochlear neurons in the guinea pig. II. Response plasticity due to noise conditioning. *J. Neurophysiol.* 79, 3088–3097.

Buno, W. Jr. (1978). Auditory nerve fiber activity influenced by contralateral ear sound stimulation. *Exp. Neurol.* 59, 62–74. doi: 10.1016/0014-4886(78)90 201-7

Chabert, R., Magnan, J., Lallemant, J. G., Uziel, A., and Puel, J. L. (2002). Contralateral sound stimulation suppresses the compound action potential from the auditory nerve in humans. *Otol. Neurotol.* 23, 784–788. doi: 10.1097/00129492-200209000-00029

Cooper, N. P., and Guinan, J. J. Jr. (2006). Efferent-mediated control of basilar membrane motion. *J. Physiol.* 576, 49–54. doi: 10.1113/jphysiol.2006.114991

Dallos, P. (2008). Cochlear amplification, outer hair cells and prestin. *Curr. Opin. Neurobiol.* 18, 370–376. doi: 10.1016/j.conb.2008.08.016

Desmedt, J. E., La Grutta, V., and La Grutta, G. (1971). Contrasting effects of centrifugal olivo-cochlear inhibition and of middle ear muscle contraction on the response characteristics of the cat's auditory nerve. *Brain Res.* 30, 375–384. doi: 10.1016/0006-8993(71)90087-4

Dolan, D. F., and Nuttall, A. L. (1988). Masked cochlear whole-nerve response intensity functions altered by electrical stimulation of the crossed olivocochlear bundle. *J. Acoust. Soc. Am.* 83, 1081–1086. doi: 10.1121/1.396052

Eggermont, J. J. (1976). "Electrocochleography," in *Handbook of Sensory Physiology*, Vol. 5, Part 3, eds W. D. Keidel and W. D. Neff (New York, NY: Springer-Verlag), 626–705.

Eggermont, J. J. (1979). Compound action potentials: tuning curves and delay times. *Scand. Audiol. Suppl.* 129–139.

Elgueda, D., Delano, P. H., and Robles, L. (2011). Effects of electrical stimulation of olivocochlear fibers in cochlear potentials in the chinchilla. *J. Assoc. Res. Otolaryngol.* 12, 317–327. doi: 10.1007/s10162-011-0260-9

Fletcher, M., de Boer, J., and Krumbholz, K. (2013). Is overshoot caused by an efferent reduction in cochlear gain? *Adv. Exp. Med. Biol.* 787, 65–72. doi: 10.1007/978-1-4614-1590-9_8

Fletcher, M., de Boer, J., and Krumbholz, K. (2015). Is off-frequency overshoot caused by adaptation of suppression? *J. Assoc. Res. Otolaryngol.* 16, 241–253. doi: 10.1007/s10162-014-0498-0

Folsom, R. C., and Owsley, R. M. (1987). N1 action potentials in humans. Influence of simultaneous contralateral stimulation. *Acta Otolaryngol.* 103, 262–265. doi: 10.3109/00016488709107281

Fuchs, P. (2002). The synaptic physiology of cochlear hair cells. *Audiol. Neurootol.* 7, 40–44. doi: 10.1159/000046862

Gifford, M. L., Guinan, J. J. Jr. (1987). Effects of electrical stimulation of medial olivocochlear neurons on ipsilateral and contralateral cochlear responses. *Hear. Res.* 29, 179–194. doi: 10.1016/0378-5955(87)90166-3

Giraud, A. L., Garnier, S., Micheyl, C., Lina, G., Chays, A., and Chery-Croze, S. (1997). Auditory efferents involved in speech-in-noise intelligibility. *Neuroreport* 8, 1779–1783. doi: 10.1097/00001756-199705060-00042

Goldstein, M. H., and Kiang, N. Y. S. (1958). Synchrony of neural activity in electric responses evoked by transient acoustic stimuli. *J. Acoust. Soc. Am.* 30, 107–114. doi: 10.1121/1.1909497

Guinan, J. J. Jr., and Stankovic, K. M. (1996). Medial efferent inhibition produces the largest equivalent attenuations at moderate to high sound levels in cat auditory-nerve fibers. *J. Acoust. Soc. Am.* 100, 1680–1690. doi: 10.1121/1.416066

Guinan, J. J. Jr. (2006). Olivocochlear efferents, anatomy, physiology, function, and the measurement of efferent effects in humans. *Ear Hear.* 27, 589–607. doi: 10.1097/01.aud.0000240507.83072.e7

Guinan, J. J. Jr. (2011). "Physiology of the medial and lateral olivocochlear systems," in *Auditory and Vestibular Efferents*, eds D. K. Ryugo, R. R. Fay, and A. N. Popper (New York, NY: Springer Science), 39–81.

Jennings, S. G., and Strickland, E. A. (2012). Evaluating the effects of olivocochlear feedback on psychophysical measures of frequency selectivity. *J. Acoust. Soc. Am.* 132, 2483–2496. doi: 10.1121/1.4742723

Jennings, S. G., Heinz, M. G., and Strickland, E. A. (2011). Evaluating adaptation and olivocochlear efferent feedback as potential explanations of psychophysical overshoot. *J. Assoc. Res. Otolaryngol.* 12, 345–360. doi: 10.1007/s10162-011-0256-5

Jennings, S. G., Strickland, E. A., and Heinz, M. G. (2009). Precursor effects on behavioral estimates of frequency selectivity and gain in forward masking. *J. Acoust. Soc. Am.* 125, 2172–2181. doi: 10.1121/1.3081383

Kawase, T., and Liberman, M. C. (1993). Antimasking effects of the olivocochlear reflex. I. Enhancement of compound action potentials to masked tones. *J. Neurophysiol.* 70, 2519–2532.

Kawase, T., and Takasaka, T. (1995). The effects of contralateral noise on masked compound action potential in humans. *Hear Res.* 91, 1–6. doi, 10.1016/0378-5955(95)00145-X

Kawase, T., Delgutte, B., and Liberman, M. C. (1993). Antimasking effects of the olivocochlear reflex. II. Enhancement of auditory-nerve response to masked tones. *J. Neurophysiol.* 70, 2533–2549.

Kawase, T., Ogura, M., Hidaka, H., Sasaki, N., Suzuki, Y., and Takasaka, T. (2000). Effects of contralateral noise on measurement of the psychophysical tuning curve. *Hear. Res.* 142, 63–70. doi: 10.1016/S0378-5955(00)00010-1

Kiang, N. Y. S. (1984). "Peripheral neural processing of auditory information," in Handbook of Physiology, Vol. 3, eds J. M. Brookhart, V. B. Mountcastle (Bethesda, MD: American Physiological Society), 639–674.

Kujawa, S. G., and Liberman, M. C. (1997). Conditioning-related protection from acoustic injury: effects of chronic deefferentation and sham surgery. *J. Neurophysiol.* 78, 3095–3106.

Liberman, M. C. (1989). Rapid assessment of sound-evoked olivocochlear feedback: suppression of compound action potentials by contralateral sound. *Hear. Res.* 37, 47–122. doi: 10.1016/0378-5955(89)90127-5

Liberman, M. C., and Brown, M. C. (1986). Physiology and anatomy of single olivocochlear neurons in the cat. *Hear. Res.* 24, 17–36. doi: 10.1016/0378-5955(86)90003-1

Lichtenhan, J. T., Wilson, U. S., Hancock, K. E., and Guinan, Jr. J. J. (2016). Medial olivocochlear efferent reflex inhibition of human cochlear nerve responses. *Hear. Res.* 333, 216–224. doi: 10.1016/j.heares.2015.09.001

Lilaonitkul, W., and Guinan, Jr. J. J. (2009). Human medial olivocochlear reflex, effects as functions of contralateral, ipsilateral, and bilateral elicitor bandwidths. *J. Assoc. Res. Otolaryngol.* 10, 459–470. doi: 10.1007/s10162-009-0163-1

Lilaonitkul, W., and Guinan, Jr. J. J. (2012). Frequency tuning of medial-olivocochlear-efferent acoustic reflexes in humans as functions of probe frequency. *J. Neurophysiol.* 107, 1598–1611. doi: 10.1152/jn.00549.2011

Moore, J. K., Simmons, D. D., and Guan, Y. (1999). The human olivocochlear system: organization and development. *Audiol. Neurootol.* 4, 311–325. doi: 10.1159/000013855

Pang, X. D., and Guinan, J. J. Jr. (1997). Effects of stapedius-muscle contractions on the masking of auditory-nerve responses. *J. Acoust. Soc. Am.* 102, 3576–3586. doi: 10.1121/1.420399

Robles, L., and Ruggero, M. A. (2001). Mechanics of the mammalian cochlea. *Physiol. Rev.* 81, 1305–1352.

Roverud, E. M., and Strickland, E. A. (2013). Modeling effects of precursor duration on behavioral estimates of cochlear gain. *Adv. Exp. Med. Biol.* 787, 55–63. doi: 10.1007/978-1-4614-1590-9_7

Roverud, E., and Strickland, E. A. (2010). The time course of cochlear gain reduction measured using a more efficient psychophysical technique. *J. Acoust. Soc. Am.* 128, 1203–1214. doi: 10.1121/1.3473695

Ruggero, M. A., Robles, L., and Rich, N. C. (1992). Two-tone suppression in the basilar membrane of the cochlea: mechanical basis of auditory-nerve rate suppression. *J. Neurophysiol.* 68, 1087–1099.

Sachs, M. B., and Kiang, N. Y. (1968). Two-tone inhibition in auditory-nerve fibers. *J. Acoust. Soc. Am.* 43, 1120–1128. doi: 10.1121/1.1910947

Strickland, E. A. (2001). The relationship between frequency selectivity and overshoot. *J. Acoust. Soc. Am.* 109, 2062–2073. doi: 10.1121/1.1357811

Strickland, E. A. (2004). The temporal effect with notched-noise maskers: analysis in terms of input-output functions. *J. Acoust. Soc. Am.* 115, 2234–2245. doi: 10.1121/1.1691036

Strickland, E. A. (2008). The relationship between precursor level and the temporal effect. *J. Acoust. Soc. Am.* 123, 946–954. doi: 10.1121/1.2821977

Thompson, G. C., and Thompson, A. M. (1986). Olivocochlear neurons in the squirrel monkey brainstem. *J. Comp. Neurol.* 254, 246–258. doi: 10.1002/cne.902540208

van der Heijden, M., and Joris, P. X. (2005). The speed of auditory low-side suppression. *J. Neurophysiol.* 93, 201–209. doi: 10.1152/jn.00554.2004

Verschooten, E., Desloovere, C., and Joris, P. (2015). Human neural tuning estimated from compound action potentials in normal hearing human volunteersm," *Mechanics of Hearing: Protein to Perception,* eds K. D. Karavitaki and D. P. Corey (Melville, NY: American Institute of Physics), 070001.

Verschooten, E. (2013). *Assessment of Fundamental Cochlear Limits of Frequency Resolution and Phase-Locking in Humans and Animal Models.* Ph.D. thesis, KU Leuven.

Verschooten, E., Robles, L., Kovacic, D., and Joris, P. X. (2012). Auditory nerve frequency tuning measured with forward-masked compound action potentials. *J. Assoc. Res. Otolaryngol.* 13, 799–817. doi: 10.1007/s10162-012-0346-z

Walsh, E. J., McGee, J., McFadden, S. L., and Liberman, M. C. (1998). Long-term effects of sectioning the olivocochlear bundle in neonatal cats. *J. Neurosci.* 18, 3859–3869.

Warr, W. (1992). "Organization of olivocochlear efferent systems in mammals," in *Mammalian Auditory Pathway: Neuroanatomy,* eds D. B. Webster, A. N. Popper, and R. R. Fay (New York, NY: Springer-Verlag), 410–448.

Warren, E. H., and Liberman, M. C. (1989). Effects of contralateral sound on auditory-nerve responses. *I. Contributions of cochlear efferents. Hear Res.* 37, 89–104.

Yasin, I., Drga, V., and Plack, C. J. (2014). Effect of human auditory efferent feedback on cochlear gain and compression. *J. Neurosci.* 34, 15319–15326. doi: 10.1523/JNEUROSCI.1043-14.2014

Zwicker, E. (1965). Temporal effects in simultaneous masking and loudness. *J. Acoust. Soc. Am.* 38, 132–141. doi: 10.1121/1.1909588

6

Using Cochlear Microphonic Potentials to Localize Peripheral Hearing Loss

Karolina K. Charaziak[1, 2], Christopher A. Shera[1] and Jonathan H. Siegel[2]*

[1] Caruso Department of Otolaryngology, Keck School of Medicine, University of Southern California, Los Angeles, CA, USA, [2] Roxelyn and Richard Pepper Department of Communication Sciences and Disorders, Hugh Knowles Center, Northwestern University, Evanston, IL, USA

***Correspondence:** Karolina K. Charaziak karolina.charaziak@usc.edu*

The cochlear microphonic (CM) is created primarily by the receptor currents of outer hair cells (OHCs) and may therefore be useful for identifying cochlear regions with impaired OHCs. However, the CM measured across the frequency range with round-window or ear-canal electrodes lacks place-specificity as it is dominated by cellular sources located most proximal to the recording site (e.g., at the cochlear base). To overcome this limitation, we extract the "residual" CM (rCM), defined as the complex difference between the CM measured with and without an additional tone (saturating tone, ST). If the ST saturates receptor currents near the peak of its excitation pattern, then the rCM should reflect the activity of OHCs in that region. To test this idea, we measured round-window CMs in chinchillas in response to low-level probe tones presented alone or with an ST ranging from 1 to 2.6 times the probe frequency. CMs were measured both before and after inducing a local impairment in cochlear function (a 4-kHz notch-type acoustic trauma). Following the acoustic trauma, little change was observed in the probe-alone CM. In contrast, rCMs were reduced in a frequency-specific manner. When shifts in rCM levels were plotted vs. the ST frequency, they matched well the frequency range of shifts in neural thresholds. These results suggest that rCMs originate near the cochlear place tuned to the ST frequency and thus can be used to assess OHC function in that region. Our interpretation of the data is supported by predictions of a simple phenomenological model of CM generation and two-tone interactions. The model indicates that the sensitivity of rCM to acoustic trauma is governed by changes in cochlear response at the ST tonotopic place rather than at the probe place. The model also suggests that a combination of CM and rCM measurements could be used to assess both the site and etiology of sensory hearing loss in clinical applications.

Keywords: cochlear microphonic, electrophysiology, cochlea, acoustic trauma, hearing loss

INTRODUCTION

The practical application of anticipated pharmacological and genetic treatments for hearing loss will require diagnostic tests that can differentiate between sites and etiologies of the damage. Cochlear microphonic (CM) potentials could aid the diagnosis of sensory hearing loss by revealing cochlear regions with impaired outer hair cells (OHCs). Here, we use an animal model to test whether a new approach to CM measurements allows for detection of a notch-type sensitivity loss resulting from the disruption of OHC function (i.e., moderate acoustic trauma).

The CM is an alternating-current (AC) potential created primarily by the mass receptor currents of OHCs following basilar-membrane (BM) movement (e.g., Dallos and Cheatham, 1976). Conventionally, CM is measured in the steady state as a response to pure-tone stimulation. Despite the use of a tonal stimulus that reaches peak excitation at a specific cochlear location, the CM has poor spatial resolution, as it constitutes a complex sum of potentials produced by all the cells excited by the BM traveling wave. Due to the rapid phase variation of the BM displacement near the characteristic-frequency (CF) place of the tonal stimulus, the currents from OHCs located in that active region tend to cancel and contribute little to the measured CM. As a result, the CM is dominated by contributions from OHCs located in the passive tail region of the BM excitation, where the phase varies little with location and currents sum constructively (Dallos, 1973). Furthermore, the CM depends on the position of the recording electrode relative to the CM sources: both electrical attenuation of the cochlear potentials with distance from the source as well as the spiral shape and complex electroanatomy of the cochlea can affect the measured response (e.g., von Békésy, 1951; Chertoff et al., 2012). Together, these factors limit the CM's place-specificity (i.e., the ability to assess the function of OHCs located near the CF place of the stimulus). A dramatic demonstration of this limitation comes from a classic study by Patuzzi et al. (1989b) in guinea pig. In the study, the ablation of the apical turn of the cochlea had little effect on the CM measured at the round window (RW) in response to a low-frequency tone that would normally have peaked near the apical end. These limitations have hindered the clinical application of the CM, which now serves primarily as a gross indicator of OHC function across the cochlea (e.g., Gibson and Sanli, 2007; Radeloff et al., 2012).

We suggest that the poor sensitivity of the CM to local changes in OHC activity might be overcome by exploiting the properties of cochlear two-tone suppression. Two-tone suppression is observed in the BM responses of a healthy cochlea when the response to one tone (probe) is reduced by the presence of another (suppressor) tone (e.g., Ruggero et al., 1992). The suppressor is believed to act locally, near its own CF place, by saturating the receptor currents of nearby OHCs (Geisler et al., 1990). Two-tone interactions can be also detected in the CM, although, unlike for the single-location BM responses, the secondary tone can result in both reduction as well as enhancement of the probe-tone CM (Legouix et al., 1973; Cheatham and Dallos, 1982; Nuttall and Dolan, 1991; He et al., 2012). Thus, in the context of CM measurements, we refer to this secondary tone as a "saturating tone" (ST) to avoid the implicit assumption that, as in classic BM measurements, a secondary tone leads exclusively to a "suppressed" probe-tone response. The complex behavior of CM two-tone interactions has been explained as the result of changes in the spatial summation pattern of the voltage sources along the BM, which can produce CM enhancement (Nuttall and Dolan, 1991). However, near its own CF place, the ST presumably acts primarily as a "suppressor" of local CM sources (i.e., it saturates the transducer currents of nearby OHCs), as suggested by CM measurements from within the organ of Corti (Nuttall and Dolan, 1991). Thus, it may be possible to extract information about local OHC health by evaluating only the CM component(s) affected by the ST. In theory, this can be accomplished by deriving the complex difference between the probe-tone (PT) CMs obtained both with and without the ST; that is, by measuring the "residual CM" (rCM; Siegel, 2006). Ideally, the rCM represents contributions from the subpopulation of CM sources excited by the probe and suppressed by the ST near its CF place in the cochlea. It may therefore be possible to localize regions with malfunctioning hair cells by varying the probe and the ST frequencies together across the hearing range (e.g., at a constant ratio). In such a case, we expect the rCM to decrease in magnitude when the excitation pattern of the ST reaches the damaged region. A similar method has been successfully employed in otoacoustic emission (OAE) measurements for detecting local changes in cochlear sensitivity (e.g., Martin et al., 2010).

Here, we assess the ability of the rCM measured at the round window to detect a notch-type moderate loss of sensitivity in chinchillas. We induce the change in sensitivity via short exposure to an intense tone, as such trauma has been shown primarily to affect OHC function, resulting in diminished BM nonlinearity (e.g., Pickles et al., 1987; Puel et al., 1988; Davis et al., 1989; Ruggero et al., 1996; Nordmann et al., 2000; Chertoff et al., 2014). We test the hypothesis that rCM represents a response from sources located near the CF place of the ST in the cochlea by obtaining measurements at varying f_{ST}/f_{PT} ratios (ranging from $\sim$1 to 2.6) both before and after inducing the acoustic trauma. If rCM indeed represents responses from CM sources located near the ST place, rCM will drop in level when the ST frequency—but not necessarily the probe-tone frequency—matches the frequency of the sensitivity loss.

Lastly, to test the above prediction and to improve the interpretation of the data, we present a simple phenomenological model of CM generation and two-tone interactions based on published BM data from chinchillas. With this study, we aim to demonstrate that a new approach to CM measurements makes it possible to extract place-specific information about OHC function, thereby enhancing the diagnostic utility of electrocochleography.

METHODS

Animal Preparation

Most of our methods have been described previously (Charaziak and Siegel, 2014, 2015). Adult chinchillas were anesthetized with ketamine hydrochloride (20 mg/kg, injected subcutaneously), followed by Dial (diallylbarbituric acid) in urethane (initial doses 50 and 200 mg/kg, respectively) with additional doses (20% of the initial one) given as necessary. The animals were trachetomized, but forced ventilation was not used. The pinna and the lateral portion of the external auditory meatus were removed. The tip of the microphone probe system was placed near the tympanic membrane ($\sim$2 mm) and the probe was sealed with impression material. The bulla was opened, the tensor tympani was sectioned, and a silver-ball electrode was placed on the round window. The reference electrode was inserted in the skin of the contralateral ear, and the ground electrode was attached to the head holder. The rectal temperature was kept at ~37°C. The preparation was monitored via repeated recordings of distortion-product OAEs (not reported), CAP thresholds, and CMs throughout the duration of data collection (~9 h). The data collection involved experiments that were a part of another study (Charaziak and Siegel, 2015; Siegel and Charaziak, 2015). Experimental protocols were approved by the Animal Care and Use Committee of Northwestern University.

Instrumentation

All measurements were carried out in an electrically shielded sound-attenuating booth. Stimulus waveforms were generated and responses acquired and averaged digitally using 24-bit sound card (Card Deluxe-Digital Audio Labs; sampling rate 44.1 kHz) controlled with EMAV software ver. 3.24 (Neely and Liu, 2015). The round-window (RW) electrode signal was differentially amplified (40 dB), band-pass filtered (0.1–30 kHz), and corrected for the acoustic delay of the sound-delivery system, as well as for the delay of the preamplifier filter. The output of the probe microphone (Etymōtic ER-10A) was amplified (20 dB), high-pass filtered (0.15 kHz), and corrected for acoustic delays and mic sensitivity (Siegel, 2007). The stimuli were presented either via two modified Radio Shack RS-1377 Super Tweeters (for CAP/OAE/CM measurements) or via Fostex FT17H Horn Super Tweeter (for tonal overexposures) coupled via plastic tubing to the probe-microphone system. The speakers were grounded and shielded with heavy gauge steel boxes to minimize electrical and magnetic radiation. Potential contamination of the CM signals from the speakers was below the system's noise floor for all stimulus conditions. The stimulus levels were calibrated *in situ* to maintain a constant pressure level at the inlet of the probe microphone near the eardrum.

Measurements and Analyses

The RW signal was measured in response to stimulation with pure tone(s) (~1.57 s duration, including 10-ms onset/offset ramps). The stimuli were presented in recording blocks, each consisting of four conditions: probe tone (PT) alone, PT + near-probe-frequency saturating tone (ST), PT + high-frequency ST, PT + both STs (not reported). The four conditions were presented in sequence (with ~200 ms gaps in between conditions), and the ST and PT were always delivered via separate sound sources. Each condition was immediately repeated and the responses were stored in separate buffers (A and B). The two response buffers were averaged ($\frac{A+B}{2}$) and subtracted ($\frac{A-B}{2}$) from each other to obtain estimates of either the CM or the noise amplitude at the frequency of the probe (via Fast Fourier transform), respectively. In both cases, the first and the last 46.4 ms of the response buffer, were skipped to prevent contamination from responses to onset and offset transients (e.g., CAP). The probe tone (30 dB SPL, f_{PT}: 0.33–10 kHz in steps of 86 Hz), and near-probe ST (55 dB SPL, f_{PT}–43 Hz, $f_{ST}/f_{PT} \approx 1$) conditions were fixed, while a different, higher frequency ST (55 dB SPL, $f_{ST}/f_{PT} = 1.2, 1.4, 2.1,$ or 2.6) was used for each recording block (four in total). For the $f_{ST}/f_{PT} = 2.6$ condition, the value of f_{PT} was limited to 8 kHz to keep f_{ST} below the Nyquist frequency. For convenience, we abbreviate the various f_{ST}/f_{PT} ratio conditions as ST1, ST1.2, and so on, where the number gives the value of f_{ST}/f_{PT}. The rCMs were calculated as vector differences between RW responses to the PT alone and PT + ST presentations for any given PT (e.g., $rCM_{ST1} = CM_{PT}–CM_{PT+ST1}$). For comparison, the response to the PT alone (i.e., the "conventional" CM) was also evaluated. The same set of measurements was obtained before and after inducing the acoustic trauma. The PT alone and ST1 conditions were retested together with each higher-ST condition and were thus used to evaluate the stability of the preparation (in terms of CM and rCM_{ST1}). Unless stated otherwise, the probe-alone and ST1 data reported here were collected in the block of stimuli used to measure the ST2.1 condition.

Although CM measured at the RW may contain contributions from sources other than OHC receptor currents (see Discussion), we adhere to the terminology used previously in the literature and refer to the RW cochlear potential synchronized with the stimulus collectively as CM.

Tonal Overexposure

The acoustic trauma was induced by exposure to an intense 3-kHz tone (100–106 dB SPL) presented in 4-min time blocks until at least 30-dB sensitivity loss was achieved at and/or above 4 kHz as monitored with CAP thresholds (criterion response: 10 μV, see Charaziak and Siegel, 2015 for measurement details). Reaching the target CAP threshold elevation required total exposure durations ranging from 4 to 16 min across the animals ($n = 4$). When possible, CAP thresholds were re-measured at the termination of the experiment. Because the tone-pip-evoked CAP represents responses from auditory-nerve fibers innervating a region around the CF place of the stimulus (Teas et al., 1962; Özdamar and Dallos, 1978), changes in CAP thresholds faithfully reflect changes in local BM sensitivity following acoustic trauma (Ruggero et al., 1996). Thus, for the purposes of this study we equate the frequency-specific shifts in CAP thresholds with place-specific decreases in OHC-dependent gain.

RESULTS

In the following sections, we present data obtained in four chinchillas. In these four animals, the repeated measures of CM and rCM_{ST1} usually varied by <5 dB within pre- or post-exposure measurement blocks, except for run ST2.6 for animal E23 (last run in the post-exposure block; changes > 20 dB). Thus, the ST2.6 data for E23 were excluded from the analysis. Two out of four animals had initial notch-like elevations in their CAP thresholds that were either preexisting or induced by the surgery (~30 dB near 5.6 kHz for G03, and ~25 dB near 10 kHz for E23). The pre-existing threshold shift abolished neither the distortion-product OAEs evoked with low or moderate level tones nor the CM and rCM, suggesting that functioning OHCs were still present in the affected regions. Because we were interested in detecting changes in CM and rCM due to experimentally induced CAP threshold shifts, these animals were not excluded from the analysis.

Effect of the Acoustic Trauma on CM and rCM

Figure 1 shows examples of CM responses collected before and after the acoustic trauma for a representative animal (F13). Although the acoustic trauma had relatively little effect on CM levels (**Figure 1A**, dotted red vs. solid blue), rCM levels decreased by up to ~20 dB (B–F). The frequency range of the largest decreases in rCM level varied across the ST conditions, shifting toward lower probe frequencies at higher f_{ST}/f_{PT} ratios.

The group data are shown in **Figures 2A–D**, where trauma-induced changes in the CAP thresholds, and CM and rCM levels are plotted against the probe frequency for each animal. The corresponding average data are shown in **Figure 3A**. The exposure to an intense 3-kHz tone created a ~35 dB (32–50 dB range) notch-type sensitivity loss centered at 4 kHz (red) that could be attributed to malfunctioning OHCs (e.g., Saunders et al., 1991; Ruggero et al., 1996). Despite substantial loss of sensitivity, CM levels decreased on average by no more than ~7 dB (**Figure 3A**, black; 7–14 dB range, **Figures 2A–D**), with the largest change occurring at frequencies 0.6–0.7 octaves lower than the frequency of maximal shift in CAP thresholds. If the CM is dominated by potentials from OHCs located in the passive tail region of the BM excitation, the observed drop in CM level is consistent with decreased OHC transduction currents in the traumatized region (Patuzzi et al., 1989a; Nakajima et al., 2000). In contrast, for any ST condition tested, rCM level decreased on average by ~15 dB following the trauma. The range of affected probe frequencies varied systematically with the ratio f_{ST}/f_{PT}: The higher the ratio, the lower the frequency of the maximal shift (**Figures 2A–D**, **3A** also see inset). Typically, a 1 dB of CAP threshold shift resulted in ~0.6 dB of rCM level shift (see values of the scaling factor α in **Figures 2E–H**; see caption for details).

When the changes in rCM levels are plotted against the ST frequency (**Figures 2E–H**, **3B** also see inset), the range of affected frequencies coincides well with the range over which loss of sensitivity was observed (blue lines vs. red). This result supports our hypothesis that rCM originates predominately near the CF place of the ST, rather than the PT. Also note that if the rCM measures changes in OHC-related active amplification of the probe response, then the largest changes in rCM following the trauma should occur at the smallest f_{ST}/f_{PT} ratios. Instead, all rCM levels decreased by a similar amount, independent of the f_{ST}/f_{PT} ratio. These results suggest that rCM depends more heavily on the changes in active amplification of the ST (rather than the PT) response. In the next section, we explore this idea further using a phenomenological model of CM generation.

Modeling CM

Model Description

To explore the mechanisms underlying the sensitivity of rCM to acoustic trauma we developed a simple phenomenological model of CM generation in the chinchilla. In the model, the CM at

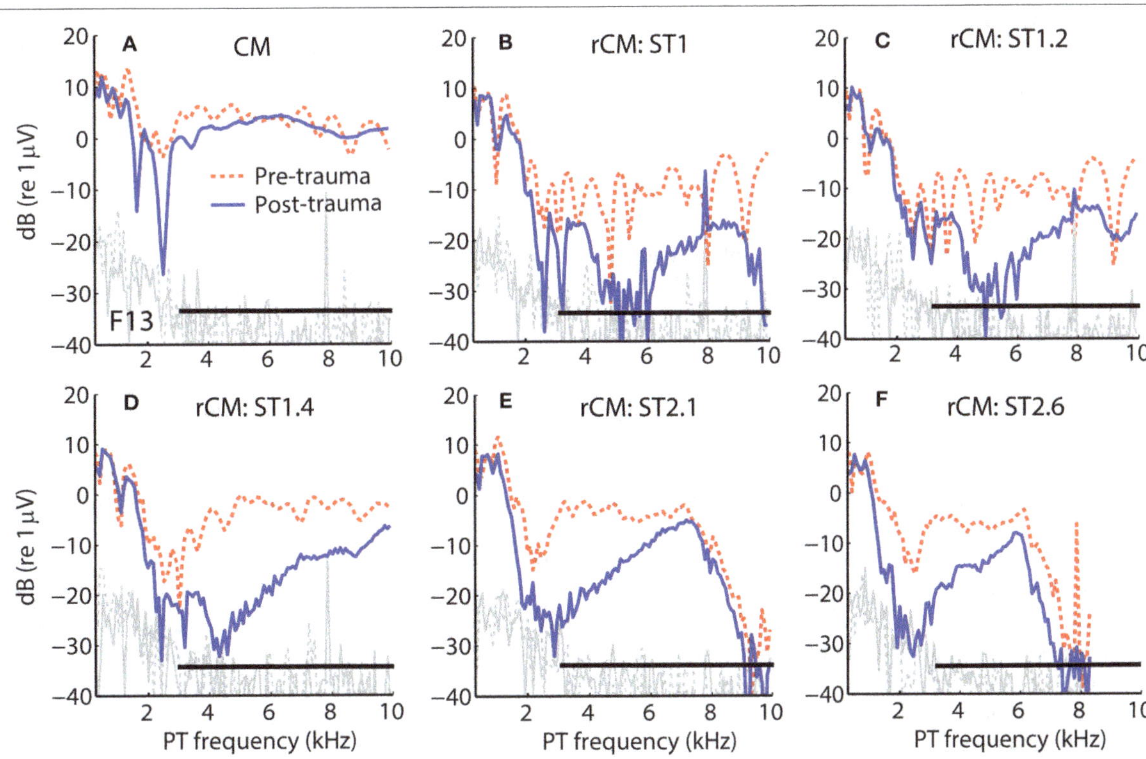

FIGURE 1 | Example of CM (A) and rCM **(B–F)** levels measured in a chinchilla before (dashed red) and after (solid blue) inducing an acoustic trauma. The black horizontal bar marks the frequency range with CAP sensitivity loss > 20 dB (3–11 kHz, with maximal shift at 6.3 kHz of 32 dB; also see **Figure 2B**). Noise floors are shown in gray.

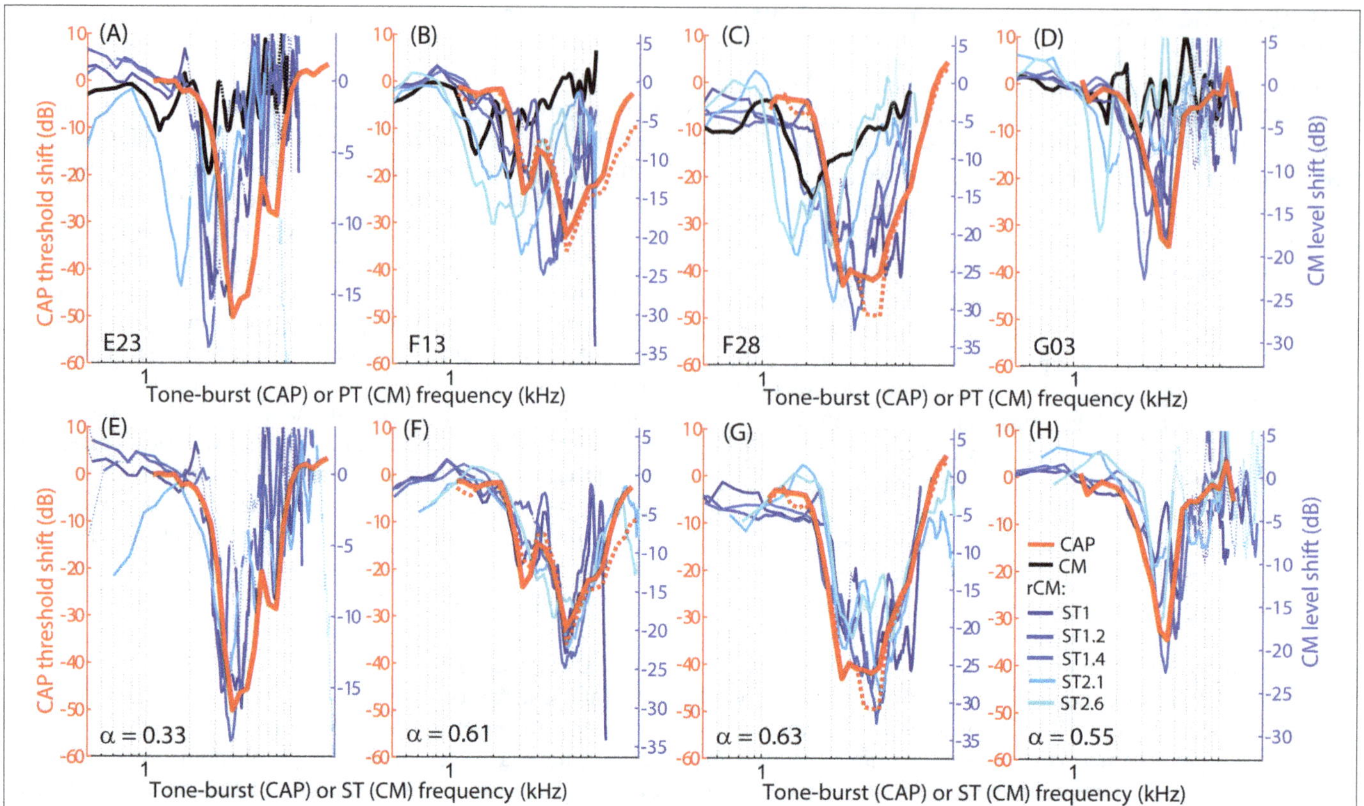

FIGURE 2 | Shifts in CM (black) and rCM levels (shades of blue, see legend in H) compared to shifts in CAP thresholds (red) resulting from an acoustic trauma in four chinchillas (columns). Note that CAP threshold shifts are plotted on left *y*-axes while CM and rCM changes are plotted on right *y*-axes. The CM *y*-axis was scaled for each animal in an iterative process until the root-mean-square error between rCM level shifts (plotted against ST frequency) and CAP shift was minimized. The scaling factors α are listed on the bottom panels (i.e., rCM or CM level shift equals to α x CAP shift in dB). Data with pre-exposure SNR < 6 dB are shown with dotted lines. The CM and rCM shifts were gently smoothed (moving average). In panels **(A–D)**, the rCM changes are plotted against the probe tone (PT) frequency and in **(E–H)** against the saturating tone (ST) frequency. For animals F13 and F28, CAP thresholds were re-measured at the end of the experiment to confirm the stability of the threshold shift (red dotted).

the round window is calculated as a vector sum of individual CM sources (i.e., hair cells) distributed along the BM. It is assumed that the source excitation is controlled by the local BM displacement via the hair-cell transducer function (He et al., 2004; Cheatham et al., 2011). Published BM data from four different chinchilla cochleae were used to introduce some realistic intersubject variability into the model predictions. For simplicity, the CM and rCMs were calculated for one PT frequency and two ST conditions (ST1 and ST2.1). The effects of acoustic trauma on CM responses at the probe frequency were simulated for two locations of damage: the first centered around the CF place of the PT and the second near the CF place of ST2.1 (i.e., basal to the probe tone CF place). Predicted changes in the CM, rCM_{ST1}, and $rCM_{ST2.1}$ due to acoustic trauma were compared with experimental data at the appropriate PT frequency.

Longitudinal BM displacement profiles were derived from published chinchilla data obtained at a single location (CFs from 6.6 to 10 kHz) under the assumption of scaling [data from Rhode (2007) for chinchillas N92 and N157, from Ruggero et al. (1997) for L113, and from Ruggero et al. (2000) for L208]. All derived displacement profiles (magnitudes and phases) were interpolated to a resolution of 2.4 μm over a BM length of 10 mm. (For comparison, the width of a single hair cell is about 10 μm.) The probe-tone displacement profiles derived from BM responses to 30 dB SPL tones were translated using the frequency-position map (Müller et al., 2010) so that they peaked at the 4-kHz CF place (i.e., at $x = 7.2$ mm, **Figure 4**, solid black). Although we fixed the probe-tone frequency at 4 kHz for simplicity, model predictions can be compared to data obtained at other frequencies using scaling. The ST displacement profiles, derived from the BM responses to 60 dB SPL tones, were translated to peak at the cochlear location tuned to either 4.4 kHz ($x = 6.8$ mm; to simulate the ST1 condition, **Figure 4** solid red) or 8.4 kHz ($x = 4.5$ mm; to simulate ST2.1 condition, solid blue). The instantaneous BM displacement at location *x* was calculated for a duration of 25.6 ms with sampling rate of 800 kHz as:

$$d_{PT}(x,t) = A_{PT}(x)\sin\left(2\pi f_{PT}t - \varphi_{PT}(x)\right), \qquad (1)$$

for the PT alone condition and as:

$$\begin{aligned} d_{PT+ST}(x,t) &= A_{PT}(x)\sin\left(2\pi f_{PT}t - \varphi_{PT}(x)\right) \\ &+ A_{ST}(x)\sin\left(2\pi f_{ST}t - \varphi_{ST}(x)\right), \end{aligned} \qquad (2)$$

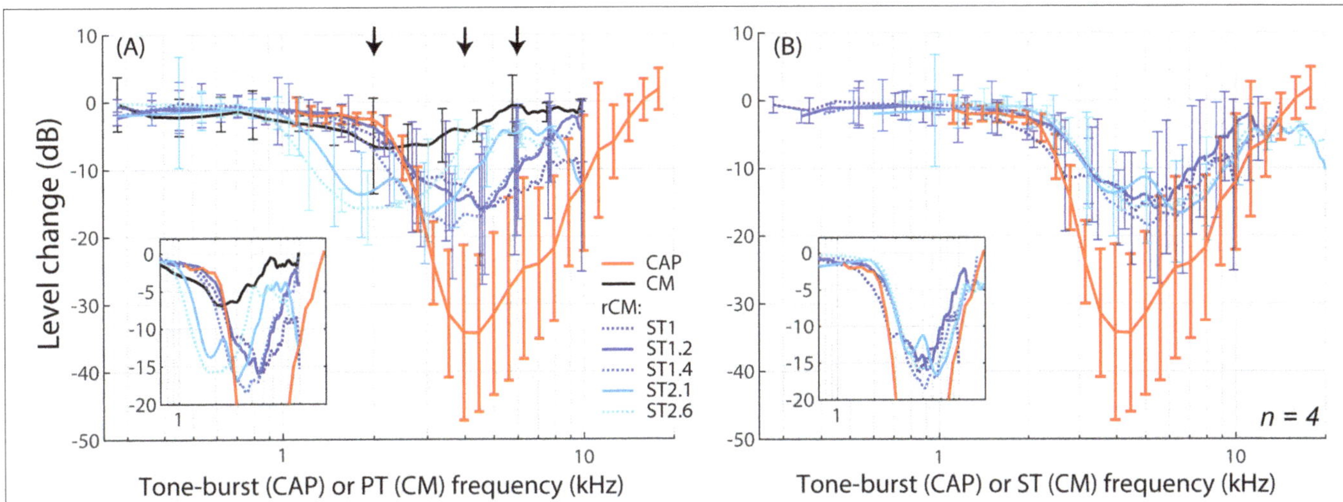

FIGURE 3 | Mean shifts in CM and rCM levels (shades of blue, see legend in A) compared to mean shifts in CAP thresholds (red) resulting from an acoustic trauma in four chinchillas. In panel **(A)** the rCM changes are plotted against the probe tone (PT) frequency and in **(B)** they are plotted against the saturating tone (ST) frequency. The error bars represent standard deviation of a mean (for the CM data error bars are shown every ~0.4 octave). Only data with pre-exposure SNR > 6 dB were included in the average (see solid lines in **Figure 2**), and the grand average was gently smoothed (moving average). The black arrows in A indicate frequencies at which data were compared to the model (**Figures 5**, **6**). The insets in each panel show the same data plotted with the error bars omitted to emphasize the alignment with the CAP data.

for the PT + ST conditions, where A and φ represent BM displacement amplitude and phase at location x in response to stimulation with PT (**Figure 4**, black) or ST (red or blue). Because the relationship between BM displacement and *in vivo* transducer nonlinearity is unknown in the chinchilla cochlea, we arbitrarily scaled the BM displacement profiles to a maximum value of 30 dB re 1 nm for the PT stimulus (**Figure 4A**, black). The scaling of the PT response was chosen so that it roughly matches the "threshold" of the transducer-function nonlinearity (Siegel, 2006), since a 30 dB SPL tone at CF usually corresponds to the onset of BM nonlinearity in chinchillas (i.e., for lower stimulus levels the responses typically scale linearly; Robles and Ruggero, 2001). Subsequently, the BM displacement profiles for STs were scaled to peak at 40 dB re 1 nm to reflect the compressive growth of the BM responses at the CF (assuming a growth rate of ~0.3 dB/dB; Robles and Ruggero, 2001). Additionally, we performed computations for the ST displacement profiles scaled to a maximum value of either 30 or 50 dB re 1 nm. The resulting rCMs were either lower or higher in level, respectively, but the best match with the data was obtained with STs scaled to peak at 40 dB re 1 nm (visual inspection).

The local BM responses (Equations 1, 2) were subsequently used as the input to an OHC transducer model to estimate the contribution of each "hair cell" to the CM (with an arbitrary scale). The transducer model is a second-order Boltzmann fit to experimentally measured transducer functions in mice:

$$\mathrm{cm}\,(x,t) \sim G\left[d\,(x,t)\right] = \frac{G_{max}}{1 + K_2\left[d\,(x,t)\right]\left(1 + K_1\left[d\,(x,t)\right]\right)}, \tag{3}$$

where G is the transducer conductance for input signal $d(x,t)$ (Equations 1, 2), G_{max} is the maximum conductance, and $\mathrm{cm}\,(x,t)$ is the local contribution of a hair cell's receptor current to the total CM in the time domain (Kros et al., 1995; Lukashkin and Russell, 1998; Siegel, 2006). The equilibrium constants K_1 and K_2 were set as in Siegel (2006), who used this model to describe properties of the CM and OAEs in chinchillas:

$$K = \mathrm{e}^{-\alpha\left(\frac{d(x,t)}{\beta} - 1\right)}, \tag{4}$$

where $\alpha_1 = 1.56$ (dimensionless), $\beta_1 = 24$ (nm) and $\alpha_2 = 0.656$, $\beta_2 = 42$ (nm) for K_1 and K_2, respectively.

The local CM source excitation at the probe-tone frequency, $\mathrm{CM}\left(x, f_{\mathrm{PT}}\right)$, was found by computing the probe-frequency Fourier component of $\mathrm{cm}\,(x,t)$ for a given stimulus condition (Equations 1, 2). An estimate of the conventional CM at the RW was then calculated as the vector sum of the local sources along the length of the BM in response to the probe-tone stimulus (Equations 1, 3):

$$\mathrm{CM}\left(f_{\mathrm{PT}}\right) = \Sigma w\,(x)\, \mathrm{CM}_{\mathrm{PT}}\left(x, f_{\mathrm{PT}}\right). \tag{5}$$

where, $w(x)$ is a weighting function that controls the electrical attenuation with distance from the source. We used $w\,(x) = e^{-x\frac{A}{20\log_{10}(e)}}$ with attenuation rate A in dB/mm. The rCM at the probe frequency was calculated as the vector difference between the summed CM source responses derived for the PT-alone and PT + ST conditions (Equations 2, 3):

$$\begin{aligned}\mathrm{rCM}\left(f_{\mathrm{PT}}\right) &= \Sigma w(x) \mathrm{CM}_{\mathrm{PT}}\left(x, f_{\mathrm{PT}}\right) \\ &- \Sigma w\,(x)\, \mathrm{CM}_{\mathrm{PT+ST}}\left(x, f_{\mathrm{PT}}\right).\end{aligned} \tag{6}$$

Because the probe frequency was fixed across all measurement conditions and only relative changes were evaluated (e.g., due

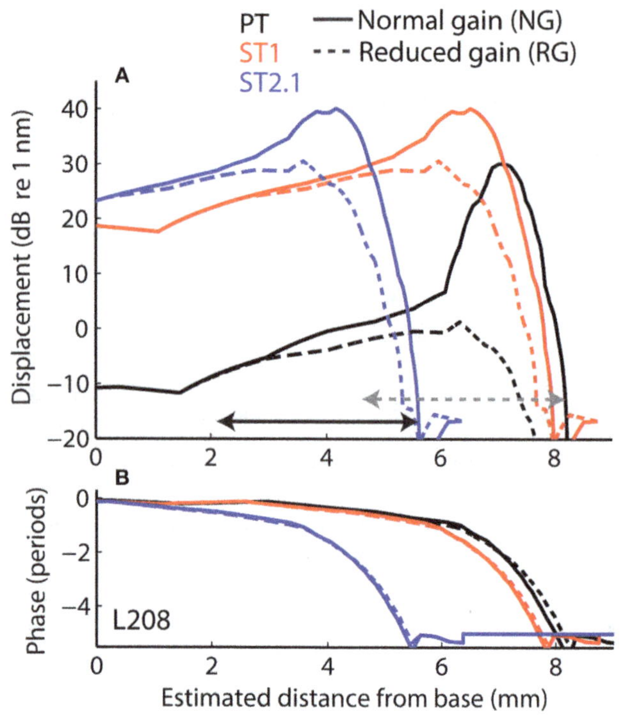

FIGURE 4 | Longitudinal basilar-membrane displacement profiles for probe tone (PT, black), ST1 (red), and ST2.1 (blue) derived from measurements in chinchilla L208 (Ruggero et al., 2000). The displacement profiles used to calculate CM responses for the normal cochlea are plotted with solid lines, while profiles with reduced mechanical gain are shown with dashed lines (magnitudes and phases are shown in **A** and **B**, respectively). The horizontal arrows span BM locations (1.4 octave range) where transduction was assumed damaged (in addition to gain reduction). The gray dotted arrow shows the region of damage centered at the CF place of the probe; the solid black arrow shows the damage located basal to the probe CF place (centered at ST2.1 CF place). The range of damaged locations was chosen to match the frequency range where average CAP thresholds were elevated by at least 20 dB (**Figure 3A**).

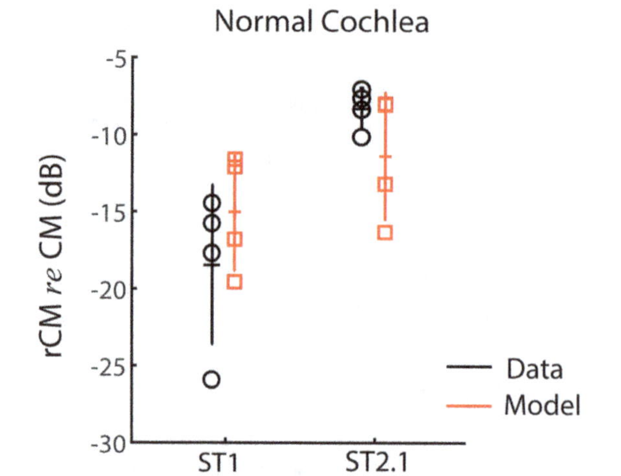

FIGURE 5 | The rCM levels (*re* CM) obtained for a probe tone of 4 kHz for the ST1 and ST2.1 conditions for four animals. Empirical data are shown in black and the results of CM modeling in red (normal gain, **Table 1**). The errors bars represent means and ± 1*SD*.

to loss of gain), we initially ignored any effects of electrical source attenuation with distance (i.e., $A = 0$ dB/mm; Section Model results). Because the electrical space constants in the chinchilla cochlea are unknown, we then evaluated attenuation effects separately using a range of hypothetical attenuation rates (Section Effects of Electrical Attenuation).

Acoustic trauma was modeled as a reduction of cochlear mechanical gain at the affected location, either with or without diminishing the transduction currents (Equation 3). While mechanical gain and OHC transduction are tightly linked in a living cochlea, we do not know the exact relationship between the two variables in the chinchilla ear, and we therefore modeled them independently. To simulate reductions of mechanical gain, the BM responses to 80 dB SPL tones (from the corresponding cochlea) were used to create scaled-down displacement profiles for the probe and ST stimuli (**Figure 4**, the dashed lines). In these cochleae, the mechanical gain decreased by 36 to 41 dB (mean 36.4 dB, SD 4.1 dB) with increasing stimulus levels from 30 to 80 dB SPL (Ruggero et al., 1997, 2000; Rhode, 2007), values that are similar to the loss of CAP sensitivity observed in our sample (**Figure 3**, red). To simulate changes in transduction following the trauma, we decreased the maximum conductance by either 50% ($G_{max} = G_{max}/2$ in Equation 3) or 100% ($G_{max} = 0$) in the affected region (see horizontal arrows in **Figure 4**), in addition to reducing the mechanical gain. The results were qualitatively similar, and thus only the results with $G_{max} = 0$ are discussed further.

The acoustic trauma was modeled to affect one of two cochlear locations: damage localized around the CF place of the probe tone and damage localized near the CF place of the ST2.1 (i.e., basal to the probe's CF place; see the horizontal arrows, dashed and solid, respectively, in **Figure 4**). In the first scenario, the BM responses to the PT and ST1 are reduced (black and red dashed lines in **Figure 4**) but the ST2.1 response remains unaffected (solid blue). In the second scenario, the BM response to the ST2.1 is reduced (dashed blue) while the gain of PT and ST1 responses are not changed (solid black and red). These conditions are summarized in **Table 1**. The simulations for damage at the probe CF place can be compared to the data measured for probe frequencies of 4–6 kHz where substantial loss of sensitivity was observed (**Figure 3**, red). The simulations for damage occurring basal to the CF place of the probe can be compared to the results obtained for probe frequencies of ~2 kHz, as the loss of sensitivity was centered at a location with CF about an octave above that of the probe frequency (**Figure 3**, red). Note that it was computationally easier to "move" the location of the damage relative to the probe CF place than it was to fix the location of the damage and compute various frequency conditions. In a scaling symmetric model, this distinction is irrelevant; in chinchillas, approximate scaling symmetry holds at CFs of 2 kHz and above (Temchin et al., 2008).

The model is derived from real cochlear data obtained in a group of animals different from the ones used in this study. Consequently, we did not attempt to optimize the model parameters to fit our data. Our goal was to evaluate whether a

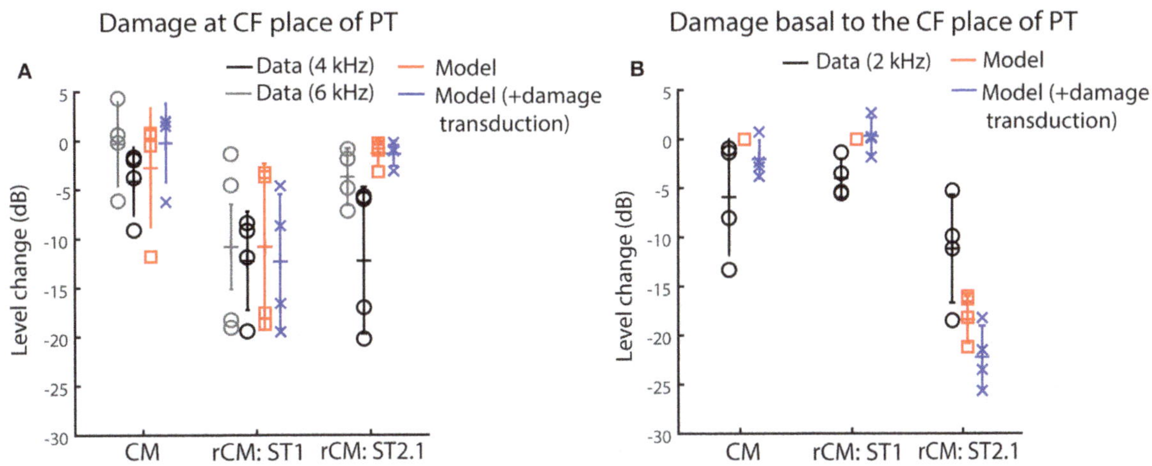

FIGURE 6 | Changes in the modeled CM and rCM (red) due to reduced cochlear gain at the probe CF place (A) or basal to it **(B)** compared to the measured responses at frequencies that fit the model assumptions best (black and gray, see legend and text). The acoustic trauma model was expanded to include the possible loss of transduction in the regions with reduced mechanical gain (in blue).

TABLE 1 | The BM displacement profiles used for calculating the CM and rCM (Equations 1–3, 5, and 6) responses across different modeling conditions.

	CM	rCM_{ST1}	$rCM_{ST2.1}$
Normal	PT: NG	PT: NG, ST1: NG	PT: NG, ST2.1: NG
Gain loss at the CF place	PT: RG	PT: RG, ST1: RG	PT: RG, ST2.1: NG
Gain loss basal to CF place	PT: NG	PT: NG, ST1: NG	PT: NG, ST2.1: RG

*The BM displacement profiles for PT and ST stimuli are listed using the same key as in **Figure 4**; e.g., the code "PT: NG, ST2.1: RG" indicates that a normal-gain BM profile for the probe stimulus and a reduced-gain BM profile for the ST2.1stimulus were used in the calculations.*

model derived from realistic cochlear responses can explain the data qualitatively. Thus, no statistical testing was performed.

Model Results

First, we evaluated whether the model captures basic properties of the CM and rCM in the normal cochlea. **Figure 5** shows modeled rCM levels (*re* conventional CM) for the ST1 and ST2.1 conditions (red squares) together with the CM data obtained in our sample of animals (black circles). The model correctly predicts that rCM levels for both ST conditions fall below the levels of conventional CM (i.e., note negative *y*-axis). In the model, the ST interacts only with a subpopulation of CM sources excited by the PT, and thus rCM is always lower in level than the conventional CM. Because the phase of the local CM sources excited by PT follows the phase of the BM displacement, the model also predicts that rCM_{ST1} tends to be lower in level than $rCM_{ST2.1}$ due to destructive interference between the CM sources located near the probe CF place (e.g., see **Figure 4B**, black curve).

Figure 5 shows the changes in modeled CM and rCMs resulting from different acoustic trauma conditions (red squares and blue crosses), together with corresponding chinchilla data (black and gray circles). When the gain of the BM displacement was reduced at the probe CF place (with transduction intact), the CM response either decreased or did not change much (**Figure 6A**, red), as the CM sources in that region tend to interfere destructively due to steep BM phase rotation (**Figure 4B**, black). This result agrees well with the data obtained at either the 4 or 6 kHz probe frequencies (black and gray), where at least 30 dB loss of sensitivity was observed (**Figure 3**, red, see the down pointing arrows). The modeled rCM_{ST1} response decreased in level following the gain reduction at the probe CF place, as also observed in the data (**Figure 6A**). On average 1 dB of BM gain loss produced ~0.3 dB shift in rCM_{ST1} (range 0.1–0.6 dB), similar, albeit less, than typically observed in the data (see α listed in **Figures 2E–H**). The shift in rCM_{ST1} level following the gain reduction at probe CF place is consistent with the ST1 interacting with a small population of sources in the affected region. However, it is not known whether the decrease in rCM_{ST1} level results from decreased BM response to the PT or ST1 or both. To tease these two factors apart, we performed additional simulations where only the gain of one or the other response was changed (e.g., PT: normal gain and ST1: reduced gain vs. PT: reduced gain and ST1: normal gain). There was a tendency for the reduced-gain ST1 only condition to cause a larger decrease in the rCM_{ST1} level compared to a reduced-gain PT only condition (by 1–5 dB), but neither resulted in changes as large as the combined condition (i.e., PT: RG and ST1: RG). This suggests that the change in the rCM_{ST1} due to trauma at the probe CF place depends on both the reduced BM responses to the probe and the ST1, although the latter appears to be more critical (i.e., the lower the ST response the less its ability to saturate the local CM sources).

In contrast to rCM_{ST1}, the modeled $rCM_{ST2.1}$ was relatively unaffected by the damage at the probe CF place (**Figure 6A**, red). This is expected if the ST interacts with the CM sources located near its own CF place. The data obtained for probe tone at 6 kHz (**Figure 6A**, gray) agree well with the model predictions. However, for the 4-kHz probe tone the $rCM_{ST2.1}$ (black) showed larger changes than predicted by the model (particularly so for the two animals, F13 and F28). This could be explained by the fact that in the model the reduction in gain was limited to the CF region of the probe tone, without affecting the CF place of the ST2.1 (**Figure 4**, dashed black and solid blue). In contrast, in the data the CAP thresholds were elevated over a broader frequency region affecting the ST2.1 frequency (8.4 kHz, **Figure 4**, red; in individual data for the F13 and F28 animals CAP shifts exceeded 20 dB, **Figures 2B,C**, respectively). Thus, the 4-kHz data do not match the model assumptions as well as the 6-kHz data where there was still a significant sensitivity loss at the PT frequency (~30 dB on average; **Figure 4**, red) but there was little change in the CAP thresholds at the ST2.1 frequency (12.6 kHz, ~5 dB on average). In conclusion, the model predicts correctly that the $rCM_{ST2.1}$ levels remain relatively unaffected when the loss of gain is localized to the probe CF region. Including the loss in transduction currents near the probe CF place in the simulations (**Figure 4A**, gray dashed arrow) did not affect the agreement between the model predictions and the data (**Figure 6A**, blue).

When the BM gain was reduced near the CF place of ST2.1 (e.g., basal to the probe CF place), the model predicted no change in either CM or rCM_{ST1} levels (**Figure 6B**, red, also see **Table 1**), unless the damage to transduction was added to the trauma simulations (blue). Decreased transduction in the basal region (**Figure 4A**, black horizontal arrow) produced no consistent change in the modeled CM and rCM_{ST1} (**Figure 6B**, blue), while either no change or decreases were predominately seen in the data (black). These results suggest either that our overexposure paradigm affected the transduction mechanism or that our simplified model does not capture the mechanism and/or the full extent of such damage (Patuzzi et al., 1989a; Nakajima et al., 2000). In contrast, the modeled $rCM_{ST2.1}$ levels decreased by ~20 dB following the gain reduction basal to the probe CF place (**Figure 6B**, red). Similar, albeit smaller, changes in the $rCM_{ST2.1}$ levels were observed in the data (**Figure 6B**, black). However, as seen in the data, 1 dB of BM gain loss produced ~0.5 dB shift in $rCM_{ST2.1}$ level (for the data see α listed in **Figures 2E–H**). Even larger decreases were observed when transduction was impaired as well (blue).

Altogether, our modeling results support the hypothesis that rCM is dominated by contributions from sources located near the CF place of the ST in the cochlea. Furthermore, the model implies that the sensitivity of the rCM to a local gain reduction is dictated predominantly by the decreased gain of the BM response to the ST rather than to the probe-tone stimulus. This is best demonstrated by the results for the ST2.1 condition: Even a small reduction in the BM response to ST2.1 (e.g., **Figure 4**, solid vs. dashed blue) diminishes the ability of the ST to drive the local CM sources into saturation. As a result, the $rCM_{ST2.1}$ decreases in level even though there is no change in the excitation of the sources evoked by the PT (**Figure 4B**, **Table 1**).

Effects of Electrical Attenuation

For a source at given cochlear location, the voltage recorded at the electrode decays approximately exponentially with distance between the source and the electrode (von Békésy, 1951). Thus, for an electrode placed on the RW, contributions from remote sources (i.e., at the cochlear apex) are attenuated relative to those from nearby sources (i.e., at the cochlear base). If the attenuation with distance is strong, the sensitivity of rCM to changes in cochlear gain at more apical locations may be reduced. We evaluate possible effects of electrical attenuation on rCM and CM in the model by weighting the source contributions along the cochlear length with an exponential decay function [$w(x)$ in Equations (5) and (6)]. Because electrical space constants in the chinchilla cochlea are unknown, we present modeling results for several plausible attenuation rates (varied from 0.5 to 10 dB/mm). The resulting weighting functions are shown in **Figure 7A** (dotted lines) together with illustrative spatial distributions of CM (black) and rCM (ST1: red; ST2.1: blue) sources (phase omitted). As an example, the figure can be interpreted as follows: for $A = 1$ dB/mm, a single CM source located at the CF place of the PT ($x = 7.2$ mm) is attenuated by an additional 7 dB compared to a source located at the base ($x = 0$ mm).

In a normal cochlea, increasing the attenuation rate decreases the levels of either rCM more rapidly than it decreases the CM level (red and blue vs. black in **Figure 7B**). Thus, for higher attenuation rates (e.g., 5 dB/mm) the model predicts that rCM levels fall 33 and 22 dB on average below the CM level for ST1 and ST2.1, respectively. This contrasts with our experimental data, where rCM_{ST1} and $rCM_{ST2.1}$ levels were only 18 and 8 dB lower on average than the CM level, respectively (**Figure 5**, black). Thus, the use of lower attenuation rates (i.e., less than ~2 dB/mm) results in more realistic model predictions. The complex electroanatomy of the cochlea likely resulted in an attenuation rate at the low end of this range.

In a damaged cochlea, the sensitivity of CM and rCM to gain reduction tends to decrease at attenuation rates above 2 dB/mm (**Figure 7C**). These effects are most prominent for rCM_{ST1} and damage at the CF place of PT (solid red) and for $rCM_{ST2.1}$ and damage basal to CF place of PT (dashed blue). For instance, on average the rCM_{ST1} level was little affected by the acoustic trauma when the sources were weighted using an attenuation rate of 5 dB/mm or greater (i.e., the sources near the CF place of PT were attenuated by additional 35 dB or more and contributed little to RW signal; **Figure 7A**). This contrasts with the experimental data where rCM_{ST1} level was reduced by 12 dB on average following the acoustic trauma (**Figure 6A**, black). For moderate attenuation rates (i.e., less than ~2 dB/mm), the model predictions are not altered much relative to the zero-attenuation case, consistent with our initial assumptions.

DISCUSSION

CM in Assessing the Functional State of the OHCS

Cochlear microphonic measurements have been used clinically mostly as an aid to differential diagnosis (e.g., in auditory neuropathy). However, CM could provide additional (e.g., place-specific) information on OHC health and function (Ponton et al., 1992; Chertoff et al., 2014). For instance, Chertoff and colleagues proposed a technique for detecting cochlear regions with missing OHCs by monitoring the level of CM evoked with a high-level 733-Hz tone-burst embedded in a high-pass masking noise. They hypothesized that the CM level should continue to

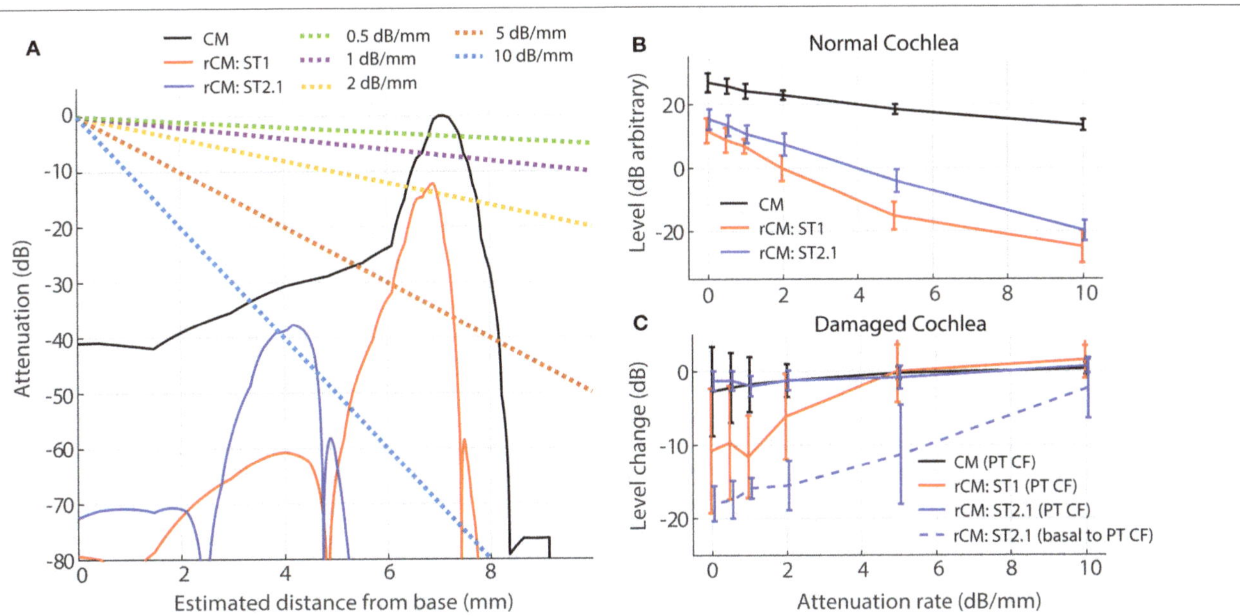

FIGURE 7 | Effects of electrical attenuation on modeled CM and rCM for a PT frequncy of 4 kHz. Panel **(A)** shows attenuation functions $w(x)$ for different attenuation rates (**A**, see the legend) using dashed lines, together with examples of spatial distrubutions of CM and rCM sources scaled *re* CM source strength at the CF place of the PT (solid lines; phase is not shown). The spatial source distributions were computed for normal-gain conditions based on the BM displacement shown in **Figure 4**. Panel **(B)** shows average levels ($\pm$ 1*SD*; $n = 4$,) of CM and rCM for varying attenuation constants (*x*-axis). In **(C)** the change in CM and rCM levels due to gain reduction either at the CF place of the PT (solid) or basal to it (dashed; CM, and rCM_{ST1} are not shown here, as neither is affected by basal damage; **Figure 6**, red squares).

increase as the cutoff frequency of the masker increased, until the noise frequency reached the region of missing OHCs. While this method is a promising approach for overcoming poor place-specificity of the CM, it does not appear sensitive enough to detect notch-type lesions in the middle cochlear turn or lesions in the apical end. Another approach for deriving place-specific information from CM was proposed by Ponton et al. (1992). In this study, a high-pass noise was used to mask basally located sources, ostensibly exposing the CM that originated at more apical locations. However, the assumptions of the method have not been validated experimentally, and it is not known whether the method provides a sensitive indicator of local damage to OHCs.

In the current study, we demonstrated that the residual CM (rCM) can successfully detect a frequency-specific elevation in neural thresholds most likely resulting from OHC impairment (**Figures 2E–H, 3B**). Our results suggest that rCM offers good place-specificity and sensitivity to changes in OHC-dependent cochlear gain, as measured using CAP thresholds. Importantly, though, CAP threshold measurements are not themselves free of limitations: the use of tone-burst stimuli and high levels of stimulation (necessary post-trauma) degrade the place-specificity of the CAP due to spectral splatter and spread of excitation, respectively (Özdamar and Dallos, 1978). Thus, it is likely that the CAP thresholds shifts underestimated the range and/or the degree of the cochlear sensitivity loss.

In theory, the place-specificity of the rCM is limited by the region of interaction between the PT and ST excitation patterns on the BM. The model indicates that a moderate level ST can effectively suppress sources near the peak of its own excitation pattern spanning the range of ~1–1.5 mm (i.e., ~0.4–0.6 octaves range; **Figure 4**; solid blue and red). In our sample, the CAP thresholds were elevated over a broader range of frequencies (**Figures 2A–C**, red), except for animal G03 (D) where the acoustic trauma created a sharp notch in the CAP thresholds ($\geq$ 20 dB elevation over ~0.6 octave range). Even in this case, the change in rCM levels matched the CAP threshold elevation well, particularly for higher f_{ST}/f_{PT} ratios (**Figure 2H**, lighter blue lines). The detection of a narrow notch in rCMs levels extracted with lower ratios (e.g., ST1 or ST1.2) can be obscured by the strong rippling pattern observed in the pre-exposure rCM levels (e.g., **Figures 1B,C**, dotted red). Nevertheless, the data from animal G03 suggest that rCM can detect sensitivity loss spanning a relatively narrow range of frequencies when moderate ST levels are used. The place-specificity of the rCM is likely to degrade at high ST levels due to spread of the ST excitation on the BM. In addition, place-specificity of the rCM may be diminished at low-ST frequencies due to the electrical source attenuation with distance (Section Effects of Electrical Attenuation).

Combining measurements of the rCM with conventional CM recordings may further expand the diagnostic utility of electrocochleography. Whereas, the rCM appears sensitive to changes in the active cochlear gain, the CM may be used to evaluate the state of transduction independently (e.g., Patuzzi et al., 1989a; Nakajima et al., 2000; Fridberger et al., 2002). For example, it may be possible to diagnose a loss of gain that does not depend on the OHC transduction (i.e., a mutation in the prestin protein—the motor behind the electromotility-dependent gain; Cheatham et al., 2011). Our model predicts a possible outcome of such a scenario: As illustrated in **Figure 6B** (red), when the acoustic trauma is simulated as a reduction in BM gain with the transduction apparatus intact, a large drop in $rCM_{ST2.1}$ level is produced without concomitant changes in CM levels. We speculate further that the combination of these two CM measures may help to understand the mechanisms underlying other OHC-dependent phenomena, such as medial olivocochlear reflex or recovery from temporary threshold shifts (TTS). For instance, it has been suggested that recovery from TTS may involve up-regulation of the prestin protein in surviving cells as a means to compensate for the loss in gain from missing OHCs (Xia et al., 2013). In such a case, one might expect to see large changes in rCM during the recovery period with little change in CM levels. In summary, our measurements and model predictions suggest that rCM provides a unique and insightful window on the health and function of the OHCs.

Optimal Parameters for rCM Measurements

The sensitivity of rCM to local changes in OHC function may depend on the stimulus parameters. In the current study, we varied one important aspect of the stimulus parameter space: the f_{ST}/f_{PT} ratio. We found that rCMs mapped the frequency-range of sensitivity loss well (independent of the f_{ST}/f_{PT} ratio; **Figures 2E–H, 3B**). However, our modeling results suggest that changes in rCMs obtained with the ST fixed at a frequency considerably higher than the PT are easier to interpret due to the spatial separation of their respective CF places in the cochlea. Using a high-frequency ST also provides the benefit of a better SNR in the mid-frequency range (at least in chinchillas; e.g., **Figure 1**), which may be crucial for measurements obtained using less invasive techniques (e.g., with the electrode placed on the eardrum rather than on the RW). The use of steady-state tonal stimuli, coupled with time-domain averaging and spectral analysis, presumably allows the extraction of very small signals from the noise. Our model also suggests that the sensitivity of rCM to changes in cochlear gain stems primarily from its effects on the intracochlear response to the ST rather than to the probe tone. Thus, an ST of a moderate level should be used; that is, the ST level should be high enough to saturate the local CM sources but low enough that it is still within the nonlinear range of BM processing (e.g., in chinchillas ~55–80 dB SPL; Robles and Ruggero, 2001; Siegel, 2006). The use of high-level STs is also expected to diminish the place-specificity of the rCM (Section CM in assessing the functional state of the OHCs).

Although our simple model appears to match the trends observed in the data, a more realistic model that captures the interplay between OHC transduction and its effects on amplified BM motion might improve the interpretation of our results. Furthermore, modeling the whole cochlear length with propagating BM traveling waves may be crucial for assessing whether any non-local and dynamic interactions between responses to the probe tone and ST must be considered in interpreting the origin and behavior of rCM (Versteegh and van der Heijden, 2013).

Contamination by Neural Responses

At low frequencies, the RW electrode signal contains phase-locked auditory-nerve action potentials (auditory neurophonics) as well as hair-cell potentials (e.g., Henry, 1995; He et al., 2012; Lichtenhan et al., 2013). Interference between the long-delay neurophonic and the short-delay CM might explain the pattern of irregular sharp peaks and notches in CM levels at low frequencies (< 2 kHz, e.g., **Figure 1A**; note that at higher frequencies the CM microstructure appeared smoother and nearly periodic). The significant contribution of the neurophonic to the RW potential can also be demonstrated by evaluating the phase of the response. For instance, He et al. (2012) showed that in gerbils a steep phase slope of the CM at low frequencies can be abolished by application of the neurotoxin tetrodotoxin. In our sample, similar steep phase slopes were observed in the CM responses at frequencies below ~1.5–2 kHz (data not shown), suggesting significant contamination from the neurophonic. At higher frequencies, however, the CM phase was shallow, suggesting little or no contamination from the neurophonic, as expected due to the low-pass nature of neural phase-locking (Johnson, 1980; Weiss and Rose, 1988). Thus, it seems unlikely that the neurophonic contributed to the sensitivity of rCM to the acoustic trauma centered at ~4 kHz. However, to monitor OHC function at lower frequencies, it may be necessary to separate the CM and neurophonic responses (Forgues et al., 2014; Verschooten and Joris, 2014). The use of high f_{ST}/f_{PT} ratios for rCM measurements may avoid the contamination from the neurophonic, given that the neurophonic originates primarily in neurons innervating the CF place of the probe tone (Henry, 1997; Lichtenhan et al., 2014).

Electrical Attenuation with Distance

Due to electrical attenuation with distance, CM sources more distant from the recording electrode contribute less to the measured response than proximal ones. Thus, for an electrode placed at the RW, contributions from more apical sources are deemphasized relative to those near the base, an effect that can compromise the place-specificity of the CM (Patuzzi et al., 1989b). The use of rCM overcomes some of the limitations of poor place-specificity of the CM. Although our modeling results confirm that strong attenuation can diminish rCM sensitivity to local change in gain (**Figure 7C**), our data (e.g., **Figure 3B**) suggest that the electrical attenuation in chinchilla is not strong enough to conceal contributions from the 4-kHz CF place (~7.2 mm away from the RW). Determining whether the rCM will prove equally successful at detecting damage to more apical cochlear locations requires further research.

Although the rate of electrical attenuation with distance in the chinchilla cochlea is unknown, our modeling results suggests that the attenuation rates are relatively small (i.e., <2 dB/mm). In contrast, intracochlear measurements of electrical space constants in other species, while varying widely across studies (from 0.042 to 2 mm), all indicate considerably higher attenuation rates (i.e., ~9–200 dB/mm; von Békésy, 1951;

Misrahy et al., 1958; Johnstone et al., 1966; Fridberger et al., 2004; Dong and Olson, 2013). Our data suggest that these intracochlear measurements fail to capture actual CM attenuation rates seen from the RW. For instance, if one assumes a nominal 10 dB/mm attenuation rate, CM sources at the 4-kHz place would be attenuated by 72 dB, implying that rCM_{ST1} would be small (perhaps even undetectable) and unlikely to reveal acoustic trauma at the probe CF place—contrary to our experimental results (e.g., **Figure 6A**, black and gray). Similarly, Chertoff et al. (2012) concluded that attenuation rates of ~9 dB/mm are too rapid to accurately predict the growth rates of the RW CM with increasing cutoff frequency of the high-pass noise in gerbil. Perhaps the attenuation rate seen at the RW differs from the rate observed intracochlearly because of the different positions of the recording and/or the reference electrodes. Although these relationships are challenging to test experimentally, models that incorporate realistic cochlear dimensions and material properties (e.g., Teal and Ni, 2016) may provide insight on how attenuation is affected by electrode position.

CONCLUSIONS

We demonstrated that remote (e.g., RW) measurements of cochlear-microphonic potentials may serve as sensitive indicators of the reduction in OHC-dependent cochlear gain induced by acoustic trauma. By measuring the residual CM (rCM), which represents the contributions to CM potentials from hair-cell sources located near the CF place of an additional, saturating tone (ST), it appears possible to overcome the limitations of RW recordings, which are otherwise heavily weighted by contributions from sources proximal to the electrode (i.e., at the cochlear base). Our phenomenological model of CM generation and two-tone interactions indicates that the sensitivity of rCM levels to decreased cochlear gain depends on nonlinearity at the CF place of the ST rather than of the probe. This implies that using STs of high levels, so that they do not depend on cochlear nonlinearity, may yield rCMs that are largely insensitive to the loss of gain, especially for high f_{ST}/f_{PT} ratios. Thus, moderate level STs may be preferred in practice. Although all rCMs, independent of the ST condition, showed similar sensitivity to acoustic trauma, in practice, higher-frequency STs (e.g., the ST2.1) offered better SNR, possibly less contamination of rCM from the neurophonic, and easier interpretation of the data (as suggested by the model). This study demonstrates the potential for using rCM to monitor the health of the OHCs.

AUTHOR CONTRIBUTIONS

KC contributed to the design of the experiment; to the acquisition, analysis, modeling, and interpretation of the data; and drafted the manuscript. JS contributed to the design of the experiment, to the acquisition and interpretation of the data, and to the final version of the manuscript. CS contributed to the analysis, modeling, and interpretation of the data, and to the final version of the manuscript.

ACKNOWLEDGMENTS

Supported by NIH grants R01 DC00419 (to M. Ruggero) and R01 DC003687 (to CS) and by Northwestern University. Parts of this report were presented at 39th ARO MidWinter Meeting, San Diego, CA.

REFERENCES

Charaziak, K. K., and Siegel, J. H. (2014). Estimating cochlear frequency selectivity with stimulus-frequency otoacoustic emissions in chinchillas. *J. Assoc. Res. Otolaryngol.* 15, 883–896. doi: 10.1007/s10162-014-0487-3

Charaziak, K. K., and Siegel, J. H. (2015). Low-frequency tone-pip-evoked otoacoustic emissions originate over a broad cochlear region in chinchillas. *AIP Conf. Proc.* 1703, 090016. doi: 10.1063/1.4939414

Cheatham, M. A., and Dallos, P. (1982). Two-tone interactions in the cochlear microphonic. *Hear. Res.* 8, 29–48. doi: 10.1016/0378-5955(82)90032-6

Cheatham, M. A., Naik, K., and Dallos, P. (2011). Using the cochlear microphonic as a tool to evaluate cochlear function in mouse models of hearing. *J. Assoc. Res. Otolaryngol.* 12, 113–125. doi: 10.1007/s10162-010-0240-5

Chertoff, M. E., Earl, B. R., Diaz, F. J., and Sorensen, J. L. (2012). Analysis of the cochlear microphonic to a low-frequency tone embedded in filtered noise. *J. Acoust. Soc. Am.* 132, 3351–3362. doi: 10.1121/1.4757746

Chertoff, M. E., Earl, B. R., Diaz, F. J., Sorensen, J. L., Thomas, M. L., Kamerer, A. M., et al. (2014). Predicting the location of missing outer hair cells using the electrical signal recorded at the round window. *J. Acoust. Soc. Am.* 136, 1212. doi: 10.1121/1.4890641

Dallos, P. (1973). *The Auditory Periphery: Biophysics and Physiology*. New York, NY: Academic Press.

Dallos, P., and Cheatham, M. A. (1976). Production of cochlear potentials by inner and outer hair cells. *J. Acoust. Soc. Am.* 60, 510–512. doi: 10.1121/1.381086

Davis, R. I., Ahroon, W. A., and Hamernik, R. P. (1989). The relation among hearing loss, sensory cell loss and tuning characteristics in the chinchilla. *Hear. Res.* 41, 1–14. doi: 10.1016/0378-5955(89)90173-1

Dong, W., and Olson, E. S. (2013). Detection of Cochlear amplification and its activation. *Biophys. J.* 105, 1067–1078. doi: 10.1016/j.bpj.2013.06.049

Forgues, M., Koehn, H. A., Dunnon, A. K., Pulver, S. H., Buchman, C. A., Adunka, O. F., et al. (2014). Distinguishing hair cell from neural potentials recorded at the round window. *J. Neurophys.* 111, 580–593. doi: 10.1152/jn.00446.2013

Fridberger, A., de Monvel, J. B., Zheng, J., Hu, N., Zou, Y., Ren, T., et al. (2004). Organ of Corti potentials and the motion of the basilar membrane. *J. Neurosci.* 24, 10057–10063. doi: 10.1523/JNEUROSCI.2711-04.2004

Fridberger, A., Zheng, J., Parthasarathi, A., Ren, T., and Nuttall, A. (2002). Loud sound-induced changes in cochlear mechanics. *J. Neurophys.* 88, 2341–2348. doi: 10.1152/jn.00192.2002

Geisler, C. D., Yates, G. K., Patuzzi, R. B., and Johnstone, B. M. (1990). Saturation of outer hair cell receptor currents causes two-tone suppression. *Hear. Res.* 44, 241–256. doi: 10.1016/0378-5955(90)90084-3

Gibson, W. P., and Sanli, H. (2007). Auditory neuropathy: an update. *Ear Hear.* 28(Suppl. 2), 102S–106S. doi: 10.1097/aud.0b013e3180315392

He, D. Z., Jia, S., and Dallos, P. (2004). Mechanoelectrical transduction of adult outer hair cells studied in a gerbil hemicochlea. *Nature* 429, 766–770. doi: 10.1038/nature02591

He, W., Porsov, E., Kemp, D., Nuttall, A. L., and Ren, T. (2012). The group delay and suppression pattern of the cochlear microphonic potential recorded at the round window. *PLoS ONE* 7:e34356. doi: 10.1371/journal.pone.0034356

Henry, K. R. (1995). Auditory nerve neurophonic recorded from the round window of the *Mongolian gerbil*. *Hear. Res.* 90, 176–184. doi: 10.1016/0378-5955(95)00162-6

Henry, K. R. (1997). Auditory nerve neurophonic tuning curves produced by masking of round window responses. *Hear. Res.* 104, 167–176. doi: 10.1016/S0378-5955(96)00195-5

Johnson, D. H. (1980). The relationship between spike rate and synchrony in responses of auditory-nerve fibers to single tones. *J. Acoust. Soc. Am.* 68, 1115–1122. doi: 10.1121/1.384982

Johnstone, B. M., Johnstone, J. R., and Pugsley, I. D. (1966). Membrane resistance in endolymphatic walls of the first turn of the guinea-pig cochlea. *J. Acoust. Soc. Am.* 40, 1398–1404. doi: 10.1121/1.1910239

Kros, C. J., Lennan, G. W. T., and Richardson, G. P. (1995). "Voltage dependence of transducer currents in outer hair cells of neonatal mice," in *Active Hearing*, ed A. Flock *(Oxford: Elsevier Science)*, 113–125.

Legouix, J. P., Remond, M. C., and Greenbaum, H. B. (1973). Interference and two-tone inhibition. *J. Acoust. Soc. Am.* 53, 409–419. doi: 10.1121/1.1913337

Lichtenhan, J. T., Cooper, N. P., and Guinan, J. J. Jr. (2013). A new auditory threshold estimation technique for low frequencies: proof of concept. *Ear Hear.* 34, 42–51. doi: 10.1097/AUD.0b013e31825f9bd3

Lichtenhan, J. T., Hartsock, J. J., Gill, R. M., Guinan, J. J. Jr., and Salt, A. N. (2014). The auditory nerve overlapped waveform (ANOW) originates in the cochlear apex. *J. Assoc. Res. Otolaryngol.* 15, 395–411. doi: 10.1007/s10162-014-0447-y

Lukashkin, A. N., and Russell, I. J. (1998). A descriptive model of the receptor potential nonlinearities generated by the hair cell mechanoelectrical transducer. *J. Acoust. Soc. Am.* 103, 973–980. doi: 10.1121/1.421214

Martin, G. K., Stagner, B. B., and Lonsbury-Martin, B. L. (2010). Evidence for basal distortion-product otoacoustic emission components. *J. Acoust. Soc. Am.* 127, 2955–2972. doi: 10.1121/1.3353121

Misrahy, G. A., Hildreth, K. M., Shinabarger, E. W., and Gannon, W. J. (1958). Electrical properties of wall of endolymphatic space of the cochlea (guinea pig). *Am. J. Physiol.* 194, 396–402.

Müller, M., Hoidis, S., and Smolders, J. W. (2010). A physiological frequency-position map of the chinchilla cochlea. *Hear. Res.* 268, 184–193. doi: 10.1016/j.heares.2010.05.021

Nakajima, H. H., Hubbard, A. E., and Mountain, D. C. (2000). Effects of acoustic trauma on acoustic enhancement of electrically evoked otoacoustic emissions. *J. Acoust. Soc. Am.* 107(5 Pt 1), 2603–2614. doi: 10.1121/1.428647

Neely, S., and Liu, Z. (2015). *EMAV: Otoacoustic Emission Averager. Technical Memorandum 17.* Omaha, NE: Boys Town National Research Hospital.

Nordmann, A. S., Bohne, B. A., and Harding, G. W. (2000). Histopathological differences between temporary and permanent threshold shift. *Hear. Res.* 139, 13–30. doi: 10.1016/S0378-5955(99)00163-X

Nuttall, A. L., and Dolan, D. F. (1991). Cochlear microphonic enhancement in two tone interactions. *Hear. Res.* 51, 235–245. doi: 10.1016/0378-5955(91)90040-G

Özdamar, Ö., and Dallos, P. (1978). Synchronous responses of the primary auditory fibers to the onset of tone burst and their relation to compound action potentials. *Brain Res.* 155, 169–175. doi: 10.1016/0006-8993(78)90320-7

Patuzzi, R. B., Yates, G. K., and Johnstone, B. M. (1989a). Changes in cochlear microphonic and neural sensitivity produced by acoustic trauma. *Hear. Res.* 39, 189–202. doi: 10.1016/0378-5955(89)90090-7

Patuzzi, R. B., Yates, G. K., and Johnstone, B. M. (1989b). The origin of the low-frequency microphonic in the first cochlear turn of guinea-pig. *Hear. Res.* 39, 177–188. doi: 10.1016/0378-5955(89)90089-0

Pickles, J. O., Osborne, M. P., and Comis, S. D. (1987). Vulnerability of tip links between stereocilia to acoustic trauma in the guinea pig. *Hear. Res.* 25, 173–183. doi: 10.1016/0378-5955(87)90089-X

Ponton, C. W., Don, M., and Eggermont, J. J. (1992). Place-specific derived cochlear microphonics from human ears. *Scand. Audiol.* 21, 131–141. doi: 10.3109/01050399209045993

Puel, J. L., Bobbin, R. P., and Fallon, M. (1988). The active process is affected first by intense sound exposure. *Hear. Res.* 37, 53–63. doi: 10.1016/0378-5955(88)90077-9

Radeloff, A., Shehata-Dieler, W., Scherzed, A., Rak, K., Harnisch, W., Hagen, R., et al. (2012). Intraoperative monitoring using cochlear microphonics in cochlear implant patients with residual hearing. *Otol. Neurotol.* 33, 348–354. doi: 10.1097/MAO.0b013e318248ea86

Rhode, W. S. (2007). Basilar membrane mechanics in the 6-9 kHz region of sensitive chinchilla cochleae. *J. Acoust. Soc. Am.* 121(5 Pt 1), 2792–2804. doi: 10.1121/1.2718397

Robles, L., and Ruggero, M. A. (2001). Mechanics of the mammalian cochlea. *Physiol. Rev.* 81, 1305–1352. Available online at: http://physrev.physiology.org/content/81/3/1305

Ruggero, M. A., Narayan, S. S., Temchin, A. N., and Recio, A. (2000). Mechanical bases of frequency tuning and neural excitation at the base of the cochlea: comparison of basilar-membrane vibrations and auditory-nerve-fiber responses in chinchilla. *Proc. Natl. Acad. Sci. U.S.A.* 97, 11744–11750. doi: 10.1073/pnas.97.22.11744

Ruggero, M. A., Rich, N. C., and Recio, A. (1996). The effect of intense acoustic stimulation on basilar-membrane vibrations. *Aud. Neurosci.* 2, 329–345.

Ruggero, M. A., Rich, N. C., Recio, A., Narayan, S. S., and Robles, L. (1997). Basilar-membrane responses to tones at the base of the chinchilla cochlea. *J. Acoust. Soc. Am.* 101, 2151–2163. doi: 10.1121/1.418265

Ruggero, M. A., Robles, L., and Rich, N. C. (1992). Two-tone suppression in the basilar membrane of the cochlea: mechanical basis of auditory-nerve rate suppression. *J. Neurophysiol.* 68, 1087–1099.

Saunders, J. C., Cohen, Y. E., and Szymko, Y. M. (1991). The structural and functional consequences of acoustic injury in the cochlea and peripheral auditory system: a five year update. *J. Acoust. Soc. Am.* 90, 136–146. doi: 10.1121/1.401307

Siegel, J. H. (2006). "The biophysical origin of otoacoustic emissions," in *Auditory Mechanisms: Processes and Models*, eds A. L. Nuttall, T. Ren, P. Gillespie, K. Grosh, and E. de Boer (Singapore: World Scientific), 361–367.

Siegel, J. H. (2007). "Calibration of otoacoustic emission probes," in *Otoacoustic Emissions: Clinical Applications, 3rd Edn.* eds *M. S. Robinette, and T. J. Glattke (New York, NY: Thieme)*, 403–429.

Siegel, J. H., and Charaziak, K. K. (2015). High-frequency tone-pip-evoked otoacoustic emissions in chinchillas. *AIP Conf. Proc.* 1703:090002. doi: 10.1063/1.4939400

Teal, P. D., and Ni, G. (2016). Finite element modelling of cochlear electrical coupling. *J. Acoust. Soc. Am.* 140, 2769–2779. doi: 10.1121/1.4964897

Teas, D. C., Eldredge, D. H., and Davis, H. (1962). Cochlear responses to acoustic transients: an interpretation of whole-nerve action potentials. *J. Acoust. Soc. Am.* 34, 1438–1459. doi: 10.1121/1.1918366

Temchin, A. N., Rich, N. C., and Ruggero, M. A. (2008). Threshold tuning curves of chinchilla auditory-nerve fibers. *I. Dependence on characteristic frequency and relation to the magnitudes of cochlear vibrations. J. Neurophysiol.* 100, 2889–2898. doi: 10.1152/jn.90637.2008

Verschooten, E., and Joris, P. X. (2014). Estimation of neural phase locking from stimulus-evoked potentials. *J. Assoc. Res. Otolaryngol.* 15, 767–787. doi: 10.1007/s10162-014-0465-9

Versteegh, C. P., and van der Heijden, M. (2013). The spatial buildup of compression and suppression in the mammalian cochlea. *J. Assoc. Res. Otolaryngol.* 14, 523–545. doi: 10.1007/s10162-013-0393-0

von Békésy, G. (1951). The coarse pattern of the electrical resistance in the cochlea of the guinea pig (electroanatomy of the cochlea). *J. Acoust. Soc. Am.* 23, 18–28. doi: 10.1121/1.1906721

Weiss, T. F., and Rose, C. (1988). A comparison of synchronization filters in different auditory receptor organs. *Hear. Res.* 33, 175–179. doi: 10.1016/0378-5955(88)90030-5

Xia, A., Song, Y., Wang, R., Gao, S. S., Clifton, W., Raphael, P., et al. (2013). Prestin regulation and function in residual outer hair cells after noise-induced hearing loss. *PLoS ONE* 8:e82602. doi: 10.1371/journal.pone.0082602

7

The Electrically Evoked Compound Action Potential: From Laboratory to Clinic

Shuman He[1], Holly F. B. Teagle[2] and Craig A. Buchman[3]*

[1] Center for Hearing Research, Boys Town National Research Hospital, Omaha, NE, United States, [2] Department of Otolaryngology—Head and Neck Surgery, University of North Carolina at Chapel Hill, Chapel Hill, NC, United States, [3] Department of Otolaryngology—Head and Neck Surgery, Washington University, St. Louis, MO, United States

***Correspondence:**
Shuman He
Shuman.He@boystown.org

The electrically evoked compound action potential (eCAP) represents the synchronous firing of a population of electrically stimulated auditory nerve fibers. It can be directly recorded on a surgically exposed nerve trunk in animals or from an intra-cochlear electrode of a cochlear implant. In the past two decades, the eCAP has been widely recorded in both animals and clinical patient populations using different testing paradigms. This paper provides an overview of recording methodologies and response characteristics of the eCAP, as well as its potential applications in research and clinical situations. Relevant studies are reviewed and implications for clinicians are discussed.

Keywords: electrically evoked compound action potential, stimulating paradigm, clinical application, auditory nerve, cochlear implant outcome

INTRODUCTION

The electrically evoked compound action potential (eCAP) represents a synchronized response generated by a group of electrically activated auditory nerve fibers. Current cochlear implants (CI) incorporate a "reverse" telemetry capability that allows near-field recordings of the eCAP using intra-cochlear electrodes. Compared with other electrophysiological measures, the eCAP offers several advantages that make it of great value to hearing scientists and audiologists. First, measuring the eCAP in CI patients does not require extra equipment, special software, or an external recording electrode other than the standard equipment for clinical programming. It can be done through the telemetry function implemented in the CI and the commercial software provided by the manufacture. Second, it requires minimal patient cooperation and is not affected by patient's arousal status, which is an important advantage for working with pediatric CI users. Additionally, it is known to be a stable measure overtime in typical CI recipients and therefore can be a reliable indicator of change.

Electrical stimuli delivered by the CI are first encoded by the auditory nerve, and subsequently transmitted to higher auditory neural structures. Theoretically, the ability of the auditory nerve to faithfully encode and process electrical stimuli should be important for CI outcomes. Results of several studies suggest that the physiological status (i.e., number and responsiveness of neurons) of the auditory nerve may be important for CI outcomes (e.g., Kim et al., 2010; Kirby and Middlebrooks, 2010, 2012; Garadat et al., 2012, 2013; Long et al., 2014; Pfingst et al., 2015a,b). The eCAP is a direct measurement of neural responses generated by auditory nerve fibers, which makes it feasible to exclusively evaluate the physiological status of the auditory nerve. Many studies have focused on evaluating the feasibility of using the eCAP to determine stimulus levels for individual electrodes in CI patients (e.g., Brown et al., 2000; Hughes et al., 2000; Thai-Van et al., 2001; Gordon et al., 2002, 2004; Eisen and Franck, 2004).

Over the past 10 years, there has been a steady increase in the number of studies using the eCAP to assess different aspects of responsiveness of the auditory nerve and their associations with CI outcomes in both adult and pediatric CI users (e.g., Botros and Psarros, 2010; Hughes et al., 2012; Lee et al., 2012; He et al., 2016a). This article provides an overview of these studies, with an emphasis on several potential applications of the eCAP in research and clinical situations in human CI users.

GENERAL OVERVIEW

Brief History

Even though the acoustically evoked compound action potential (CAP) has been widely used in basic and clinical studies for more than six decades (Goldstein and Kiang, 1958), the feasibility of measuring the eCAP in animals or human listeners was not established until late 1980s (van de Honert and Stypulkowski, 1986; Game et al., 1987; Miyamoto and Brown, 1987; Abbas and Brown, 1988). The delay is primarily due to the lack of technique for recognizing and minimizing contamination of stimulus artifact on the recorded response. In 1990, Brown et al. developed a forward-masking technique for measuring the eCAP from an intra-cochlear electrode in human CI patients (Brown et al., 1990). This technique can successfully minimize stimulus artifact and allow artifact-free eCAPs to be recorded. Telemetry function became commercially available for eCAP recording in 1998, when Cochlear™ Limited (Sydney, Australia) incorporated two-way telemetry in the Nucleus® CI24 CI (Neural Response Telemetry [NRT]). In 2001, Advanced Bionics (Valencia, California) followed by including telemetry capability in their devices (Neural Response Imaging [NRI]). MED-EL's (Innsbruck, Austria) version of telemetry (Auditory Response Telemetry [ART]) was commercially approved in the United States in 2007.

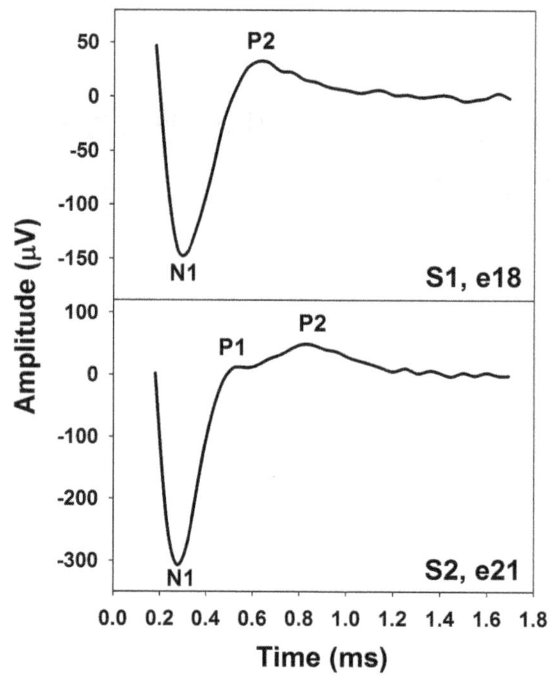

FIGURE 1 | The eCAP with one (**Upper**) or two positive peaks (**Lower**). These responses were recorded using intra-cochlear electrodes in pediatric Cochlear Nucleus CI users with prelingual deafness. Subject and electrode number are labeled in both panels.

eCAP Morphology

The eCAP recorded using an intra-cochlear electrode in human CI users typically shows a biphasic morphology. The upper panel of **Figure 1** shows an example of an eCAP recorded in one pediatric Cochlear 24RE CI user with prelingual deafness. The biphasic eCAP consists of one negative peak (N1) within a time window of 0.2–0.4 ms after stimulus onset followed by a positive peak (P2) occurring around 0.6–0.8 ms (Brown and Abbas, 1990; Brown et al., 1990, 1998; Abbas et al., 1999). This single-peak eCAP accounts for more than 80% of all measurable eCAPs (Lai and Dillier, 2000; Cafarelli Dees et al., 2005; Miller et al., 2008b).

In addition to the single-peak response, eCAPs with two positive peaks (P1 and P2) have been observed (Stypulkowski and van den Honert, 1984; Lai and Dillier, 2000; van de Heyning et al., 2016). This type of response has been referred to as a double-peak or a Type II nerve response (Lai and Dillier, 2000). For this type of eCAP response, the P1 typically occurs around 0.4–0.5 ms and the P2 typically occurs around 0.6–0.7 ms (Lai and Dillier, 2000; van de Heyning et al., 2016). The incidence of the Type II response is around 10–20% (Lai and Dillier, 2000; van de Heyning et al., 2016). The lower panel of **Figure 1** shows an example of a Type II response measured in a prelingually deaf child with a Cochlear N5 CI. Based on results recorded in cats, Stypulkowski and van den Honert (1984) proposed that the P1 and the P2 peak arise from action potentials generated by the axonal and the dendritic processes, respectively. Latency differences between these two peaks might reflect the time of spike propagation along the dendrite and across the spiral ganglion cell body. This "two-component" hypothesis is supported by simulation results of a mathematical model including a liner combination of responses generated by axons and dendrites (Lai and Dillier, 2000).

The eCAP amplitude can be as large as 1–2 mV. Due to its large amplitude, the eCAP is relatively resistant to contamination of myogenic activity. In addition, due to its peripheral neural origin, the eCAP is not affected by maturation of the central auditory system. As a result, morphological characteristics of eCAPs recorded in adult and pediatric CI users are similar (e.g., Brown et al., 1990; Eisen and Franck, 2004; Gordon et al., 2004) and show little or no change as the duration of CI use increases (Brown et al., 2010). Nevertheless, amplitude and peak latency of the eCAP recorded in human CI users are affected by extrinsic factors, including stimulation level, intra-cochlear test electrode location, the separation between stimulating and recording electrodes, stimulus polarity, etc. For example, eCAP amplitude increases as the stimulation level increases. The speed of the increase can be quantified by the slope of an eCAP input-output (I/O) function. In addition, eCAPs recoded at the apical electrodes tend to have larger amplitudes than those recorded at the basal electrodes at an equal stimulus or loudness level (e.g., Frijns et al., 2002; Polak et al., 2004; Brill et al., 2009; van de Heyning et al., 2016; Tejani et al., 2017). Potential factors accounting for the increase in eCAP amplitude toward the apical region include better neural survival and shorter distance between the test electrode and the stimulated neural structure at the apex. As the separation between stimulating and recoding electrodes increases, the eCAP latency may decrease (Finley et al., 2013; Kashio et al., 2016) due to potential changes in the site of action potential initiation (Kashio et al., 2016). Finally, the eCAP evoked by the anodic-leading biphasic pulse has a larger amplitude and shorter latency than that evoked by the cathodic-leading biphasic pulse at the same stimulus level (e.g., Macherey et al., 2006, 2008; Undurraga et al., 2010, 2012; Baudhuin et al., 2016). The proposed underlying neurophysiological mechanism is that auditory nerve fibers with degenerated or unmyelinated peripheral processes are more sensitive to anodic than to cathodic stimulation (Rattay, 1999; Rattay et al., 2001; Macherey et al., 2008; Undurraga et al., 2010, 2012). Details of this mechanism are described later in the Polarity Sensitivity section.

Artifact Rejection Methods

Ideally, the eCAP is recorded from the same intra-cochlear electrode that delivers electrical stimulus. However, this is not feasible due to residual decaying charges of the electrical stimulus (i.e., artifact). This artifact is often large enough to saturate the recording amplifier. Once the amplifier is saturated, no response can be recorded before it recovers, which is problematic for measuring the eCAP due to its short latency. In practice, the stimulating and recording electrodes used for intra-cochlear eCAP measures are typically separated by one or two electrodes. Unfortunately, the physical separation between the stimulating and recording electrodes cannot completely eliminate the distortion introduced by the stimulus artifact. Additional artifact reduction techniques are typically needed for measuring the artifact-free eCAP. Each method is described as follows.

Figure 2 shows schematic illustrations of the three most commonly used artifact reduction techniques for measuring the intra-cochlear eCAP: alternating polarity (**Figure 2a**), subthreshold template subtraction (**Figure 2b**), and two-pulse forward-masking paradigm (**Figure 2c**). Alternating polarity method is used in Advanced Bionics' NRI and MED-EL's ART programs. All three methods are offered as options in Cochlear's NRT software.

In the alternating polarity method, responses (including the artifact and the eCAP) evoked by the cathodic-leading (trace A) and the anodic-leading (trace B) biphasic pulse are recorded. The polarity of the stimulus artifact in these two traces is reversed. In contrast, the polarity of the eCAP remains the same. The stimulus artifact is eliminated or minimized and the eCAP is derived by averaging the responses of both polarities (i.e., (A+B)/2). While simple in theory, the success of this method depends on the underlying assumption that eCAPs evoked by cathodic- or anodic-leading biphasic pulses are identical. Unfortunately, this assumption is not valid. Results of recent studies have shown that human auditory nerve fibers are more sensitive to anodic-leading than cathodic-leading biphasic pulses (e.g., Macherey et al., 2006, 2008; Undurraga et al., 2010). As a result, eCAPs in response to stimuli with reversed polarities differ in amplitude and latency (Frijns et al., 2002; Macherey et al., 2006, 2008; Undurraga et al., 2010; Baudhuin et al., 2016). Therefore, using the alternating polarity artifact reduction method may result in distorted eCAP responses (Frijns et al., 2002; Baudhuin et al., 2016).

The subthreshold template subtraction method (**Figure 2b**) was first proposed by Miller et al. (1998) in their animal studies. In this method, a response evoked by a biphasic pulse that is below neural threshold is recorded (trace A). This trace contains only stimulus artifact, which serves as the template. Trace B contains the stimulus artifact and the eCAP evoked by a supra-threshold biphasic pulse. The template is then scaled up to match the magnitude of stimulus artifact in trace B. The eCAP is derived by subtracting the scaled template from trace B. Successfully implementing this paradigm requires a precise and unerring recording system with a linear recording amplifier, a low level of ambient noise, and the capability of accurately sampling stimulus artifact. As a result, the subthreshold template subtraction method is used less frequently than the other two methods in studies with human CI users.

The two-pulse forward masking paradigm (**Figure 2c**) takes advantage of refractory properties of the auditory nerve (Brown et al., 1990). In this paradigm, responses are recorded in four stimulation conditions. In the first condition (trace A), a response evoked by a single biphasic pulse (i.e., the probe) is recorded. This response includes the stimulus artifact and the eCAP evoked by the probe. In the second condition (trace B), two biphasic pulses are presented sequentially with a relatively short inter-pulse interval. The first pulse (i.e., the masker) is typically higher in stimulation level than the second pulse (i.e., the probe). When the masker-probe-interval (MPI) is sufficiently short (~350–400 μs), the response to the masker is assumed to leave the nerve in a refractory state such that it is unable to generate a neural response to the probe. Therefore, the trace recorded in this condition includes artifacts evoked by the masker and the probe and the eCAP evoked by the masker. In the third condition (trace C), only the masker is presented and the recorded response includes the artifact and the eCAP evoked by the masker. The fourth condition (not shown in this illustration) is used to control for power-up artifact of the recording system. The eCAP elicited by the probe can be derived by subtracting artifact evoked by the probe (i.e., B-C) from the response evoked by the probe alone (i.e., A-(B-C)). The success of this paradigm depends on the absence of neural response evoked by the probe in trace B. Unintended neural response to the probe will be evoked if the masking effect induced by the masker is insufficient in cases where the MPI is too long/short or the level of the masker is too low.

APPLICATIONS

Potential clinical application of the eCAP has been extensively studied. Despite that many studies were done in patients with Cochlear Nucleus devices, general knowledge gained from these

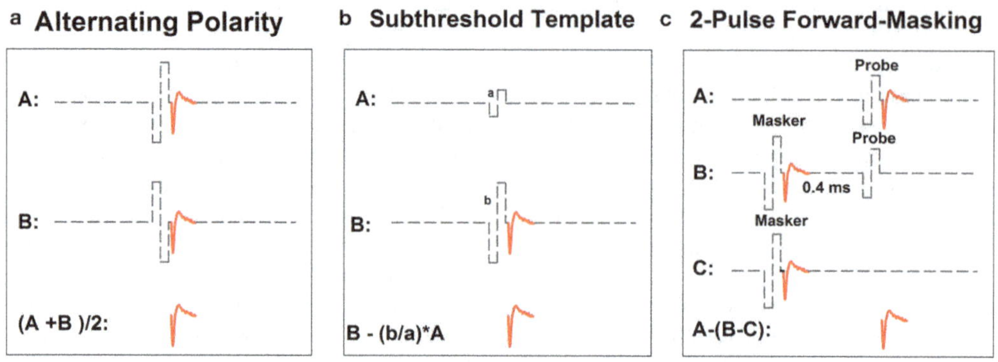

FIGURE 2 | Schematic illustration of three methods for minimizing contamination of stimulus artifact in eCAP recordings: alternating-polarity **(a)**, subthreshold template **(b)** and 2-pulse forward masking paradigm **(c)**. Gray dashed lines and red solid lines indicate biphasic electrical pulses and eCAP responses, respectively.

studies applies to any CI users. Much of the early literature on this topic focused on using the eCAP to determine program levels for individual CI electrodes (e.g., Brown et al., 1998, 2000; Abbas et al., 1999; Hughes et al., 2000; Franck and Norton, 2001; Gordon et al., 2002, 2004; Smoorenburg et al., 2002; Eisen and Franck, 2004; Thai-Van et al., 2004; McKay et al., 2005, 2013; Potts et al., 2007). Accumulating evidence suggests that the status of the auditory nerve may be important for CI outcomes (e.g., Garadat et al., 2012, 2013; Kirby and Middlebrooks, 2012; Pfingst et al., 2015a,b). In addition, eCAPs have been shown to be sensitive to electrode placement and the health status of auditory nerve fibers near the recording electrode (Shepherd et al., 1993; Miller et al., 2008a). Therefore, recent literature has been focusing on using the eCAP to evaluate neural survival (e.g., Botros and Psarros, 2010; Kim et al., 2010; Pfingst et al., 2015a) and spectral and temporal encoding of electrical stimulus at the level of the auditory nerve and their associations with auditory perception in CI users (e.g., Hughes and Abbas, 2006; Hughes and Stille, 2008; Hughes et al., 2012; Snel-Bongers et al., 2012; Carlyon and Deeks, 2015; Scheperle and Abbas, 2015a,b; DeVries et al., 2016; He et al., 2016a; Tejani et al., 2017). The following section summarizes studies investigating potential applications of the eCAP in each of these areas.

Clinical Programming

Clinical programming of a CI speech processor requires estimations of the lowest level that patients can detect (T level) and the upper limit of the level that patients determine to be comfortable (C or M level) for multiple stimulating electrodes. Optimal C level allows accessing loud sound without causing discomfort. Accurate T level has been shown to be critical for understanding low-level speech and speech presented in noise (e.g., Skinner et al., 1997, 1999, 2002; James et al., 2003; Firszt et al., 2004; Dawson et al., 2007; Holden et al., 2007, 2011; Spahr et al., 2007; Davidson et al., 2009; Baudhuin et al., 2012; van der Beek et al., 2015). Measuring T and C levels for multiple stimulating electrodes is time consuming and requires a significant amount of attention and effort to accomplish. Further complicating programming efforts is the fact that some CI users have limited abilities to provide reliable behavioral responses due to their young age or other comorbidities. Having objective tools for determining stimulus levels can potentially accelerate the programming process and be especially useful for managing patients who cannot perform behavioral tasks.

The feasibility of using the eCAP evoked by a single biphasic pulse to estimate T and C levels has been extensively evaluated in both adult and pediatric CI users (Brown et al., 1998, 2000; Abbas et al., 1999; Hughes et al., 2000; Franck and Norton, 2001; Gordon et al., 2002, 2004; Smoorenburg et al., 2002; Eisen and Franck, 2004; Thai-Van et al., 2004; Han et al., 2005; McKay et al., 2005; Potts et al., 2007; Wolfe and Kasulis, 2008; Holstad et al., 2009; Jeon et al., 2010). Overall, results of these studies suggest that stimulus at the level of eCAP threshold is always audible to CI patients. However, there is only a weak to moderate correlation between eCAP thresholds and behavioral T or C levels in both adult and pediatric CI users. The reported correlation coefficients vary across studies. For the correlation between eCAP thresholds and T levels, the reported coefficients range from 0.5 to 0.9. For the correlation between eCAP thresholds and C levels, the reported coefficients range from 0.1 to 0.9. The correlation between eCAP thresholds and T and C levels appears to be stronger at the apical compared to the basal electrodes (Eisen and Franck, 2004; Wolfe and Kasulis, 2008). Even though the eCAP threshold typically falls between behavioral T and C levels, there are substantial variations among patients, as well as across CI electrodes within individual patients. It is common for the eCAP threshold to exceed C level, especially at high stimulation rates (Eisen and Franck, 2004; Han et al., 2005; Jeon et al., 2010).

It has been proposed that the difference in stimulus used for eCAP measures (a single pulse presented at 80 Hz or lower) and behavioral procedures [a train of pulses with pulse rates of 250 pulses per second (pps) or higher] could, at least partially, account for the lack of robust correlation between these two measures (McKay et al., 2005). Specifically, the eCAP to a single biphasic pulse is relatively independent of the history of prior neural activity and mainly reflects the inherent excitability of the electro-neural interface. In contrast, behavioral T and C levels measured using a train of pulses are affected by additional peripheral and central factors. For example, responsiveness of the auditory nerve to the pulse-train stimuli is affected by many neural response properties, including peri-stimulus neural refractoriness and adaptation, as well as recovery from refractoriness and adaptation induced by prior stimulation. In addition, auditory perception of a pulse train is affected by auditory temporal integration that is generally believed to occur at the central auditory system (Viemeister and Wakefield, 1991; McKay and McDermott, 1998). Therefore, several studies have tried to address this caveat by using similar stimuli for eCAP and behavioral measures. The correlation between eCAP threshold and behavioral T and C levels improves when low rate pulses (e.g., 80 Hz or lower) are used in both measures (Brown et al., 1996, 1998; Zimmerling and Hochmair, 2002). Nevertheless, substantial inter- and intra-subject variations in the relationship between these two measures still exist. McKay et al. (2013) explored the feasibility of using eCAP evoked by trains of biphasic pulses at different pulse rates to predict behavioral T and C levels in both adult and pediatric CI users. Unfortunately, their results revealed insufficient predictive power of eCAP measure for setting program levels for individual patients.

Several methods have been proposed for improving the correlation between eCAP threshold and behavioral T and C levels. For example, Brown et al. (2000) and Hughes et al. (2000) plotted eCAP thresholds as a function of the electrode location. This function was then shifted up and down based on the difference in stimulus level between eCAP threshold and behavioral T and C levels that was measured for one electrode. This method improves overall correlations between eCAP threshold and behavioral T and C levels in both adult and pediatric CI users. However, it does not work well for patients whose behavioral T and C levels vs. electrode contours are different from eCAP threshold vs. electrode contours (Miller et al., 2008a). In addition, programming maps created using this method do not lead to improved speech understanding in CI patients (Seyle and Brown, 2002; Smoorenburg et al., 2002). Combining eCAP threshold with the slope of the eCAP amplitude growth function has been shown to improve the correlation between eCAP threshold and behavioral C levels (Franck and Norton, 2001). The "tilt" of the eCAP threshold vs. electrode contour is more strongly correlated with behavioral T levels than the absolute eCAP threshold (Smoorenburg et al., 2002). Therefore, varying the "tilt/curvature" in addition to shifting the contour up and down has also been recommended (Smoorenburg et al., 2002). Nevertheless, it remains unknown whether these two additional methods would result in optimal program levels for CI outcomes.

In summary, eCAP threshold can provide information to clinicians about the function of the internal device and its interface with neural elements. In addition, it can provide an initial estimation of program levels, which is important for working with patients who cannot provide reliable behavioral responses. However, the poor predictive power of eCAP threshold for behavioral T and C levels prevents it from being used as a sole indicator for setting the program levels for individual patients. Accurate behavioral T and C levels are still warranted for optimal programming settings.

Spectral Resolution

Compared to normal hearing listeners, CI users are known to have impaired spectral resolution (e.g., Fu et al., 1998; Friesen et al., 2001; Loizou and Poroy, 2001; Henry and Turner, 2003; Jeon et al., 2015; Winn and Litovsky, 2015), and the severity of this deficits correlates with their speech perception capabilities (Fu et al., 1998; Friesen et al., 2001; Henry and Turner, 2003; Fu and Nogaki, 2004; Henry et al., 2005; Litvak et al., 2007; Won et al., 2007; Winn et al., 2016). The number of individual electrodes that provides perceptually distinct spectral information (i.e., effective spectral channels) has been proposed to be an important factor for spectral resolution in CI users (Friesen et al., 2001; Jones et al., 2013). The electrical current delivered by each CI electrode creates an electric field that stimulates the surrounding neural tissue. The electrical fields created by different electrodes typically overlap with each other, resulting in channel interactions wherein the same neural population is excited by more than one stimulating electrode. The lack of across-fiber independence reduces the number of "effective spectral channels" of a multichannel CI, which compromises speech perception in implanted patients (Zwolan et al., 1997; Throckmorton and Collins, 1999; Dawson et al., 2000; Henry et al., 2000; Friesen et al., 2001; Noble et al., 2013).

Electrophysiological measures of the eCAP can be used to assess channel interaction at the electrode-neural interface (i.e., spread of excitation or SOE). The amount of SOE can be estimated based on eCAP amplitudes measured at different spatial separations between the masker- and the probe-electrode (e.g., Miller et al., 2001; Cohen et al., 2003; Abbas et al., 2004; Eisen and Franck, 2005; Hughes and Abbas, 2006; Hughes, 2008; Hughes and Stille, 2008; Hughes and Goulson, 2011; Snel-Bongers et al., 2012; Undurraga et al., 2012; van der Beek et al., 2012; Won et al., 2014; Scheperle and Abbas, 2015a,b). To evaluate SOE, the eCAP can be measured using either a two-pulse forward-masking/channel-interaction paradigm (e.g., Eisen and Franck, 2005; Hughes and Abbas, 2006; Hughes, 2008; Hughes and Stille, 2008; Hughes and Goulson, 2011; Snel-Bongers et al., 2012; Undurraga et al., 2012; van der Beek et al., 2012; Won et al., 2014) or a modified template subtraction method (Cohen et al., 2003; Abbas et al., 2004). In both methods, the probe-electrode is typically fixed and the masker-electrode is varied across the electrode array.

Figures 3a,c,e show schematic illustrations of relationships between electrode-spatial separations and neural populations activated by the probe and the masker. **Figures 3b,d,f** show schematic illustrations of measured eCAPs in these stimulation conditions using the two-pulse forward-masking/channel-interaction paradigm. In **Figure 3a**, the masker and the probe are presented on the same stimulating electrode (black open circle). Electrical fields (red circle) created by these two pulses are completely overlapped, which leads to activating only one group of neurons. Coupled with a short masker-probe-interval (MPI), all neurons that respond to the probe (trace A) are set into the refractory stage by the masker, which results in no neural response evoked by the probe in trace B in **Figure 3b**. The derived eCAP (the bottom trace of panel [b]) has the

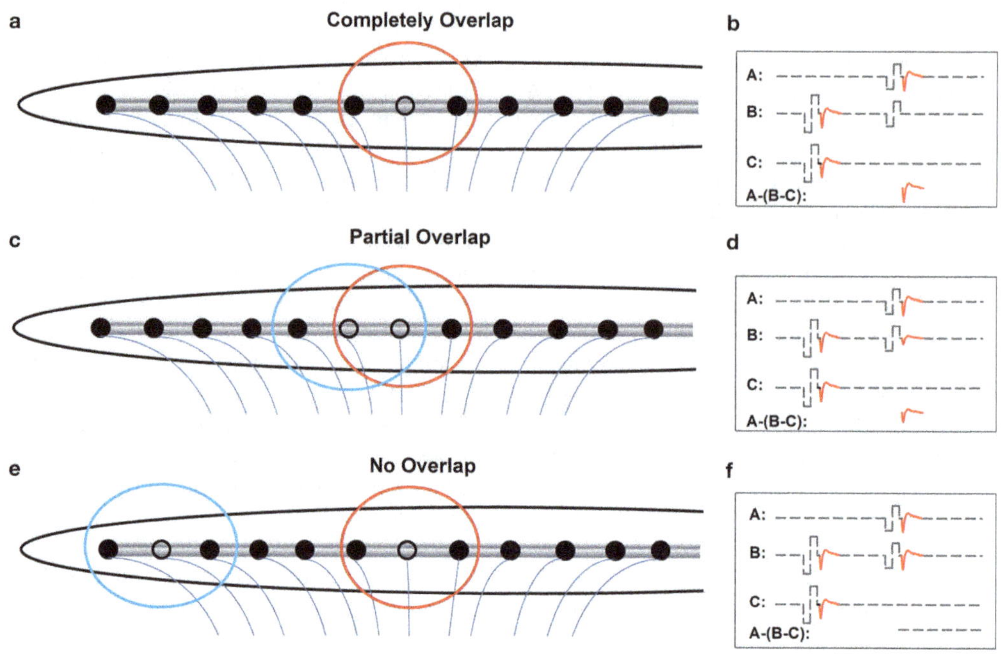

FIGURE 3 | Schematic illustration of effects of increasing distance between the masker- and the probe-electrode on recorded eCAP response. Blue and red circles indicate electrode field evoked by the masker and the probe pulse, respectively. **(a, b)** Illustrate the condition where the masker pulse and the probe pulse are delivered to the same electrode. **(c, d)** Illustrate cases where the masker- and the probe-electrode are close to each other, which yields partially overlapped electrode fields. **(e, f)** Illustrate conditions where there is a large separation in distance between the masker- and the probe-electrode, which results in two separated electrical fields.

largest amplitude among all conditions shown in **Figure 3**. **Figure 3c**, the masker and the probe are presented on two adjacent electrodes. The electrical field created by the masker (blue circle) partially overlaps with that created by the probe (red circle), which leaves a subgroup of neurons that are unaffected by the masker pulse and thus can be activated by the probe. Consequently, trace B of **Figure 3d** contains a small response generated by these neurons in response to the probe, leading to a small eCAP in the subtracted trace (A-[B-C]). In **Figure 3e**, the masker and the probe are presented to two electrodes that are spatially separated by a large distance. There is no overlap between electrical fields created by these two pulses. The neural population that responds to the probe is unaffected by the masker. As a result, the eCAP evoked by the probe is recorded in trace B of **Figure 3f**. No eCAP is obtained after the subtraction (bottom trace of **Figure 3f**). Therefore, eCAP amplitudes as a function of spatial separations between the masker- and the probe-electrode provide an indication of the degree of overlap in the stimulated neural populations. This can be use used to quantify channel interaction occurring at the peripheral auditory system.

Compared with the two-pulse forward-masking/channel interaction paradigm, the modified template subtraction method is less commonly used and is not implemented in current telemetry capabilities by any CI manufacture. Details of this method have been described in Abbas et al. (2004). Briefly, the artifact evoked by the probe pulse is derived by subtracting trace C from trace B in cases where the masker and the probe are presented on the same electrode (**Figure 3b**), which serves as the "artifact template." Contamination of stimulus artifact on recorded eCAPs is then removed or minimized by subtracting this "artifact template" from subtracted trace (B-C) recorded when the masker is presented on different electrodes. The template subtraction method results in the smallest eCAP when the neuronal overlap is greatest and vice versa.

The top panel of **Figure 4** shows an example of one series of eCAP waveforms measured using the two-pulse forward-masking/channel-interaction paradigm in one pediatric Cochlear N5 CI user. The probe-electrode was fixed at electrode 9, and the masker-electrode location was systematically moved from electrode 2 to electrode 22. It is apparent that smaller spatial separations between the probe- and the masker- electrode result in larger eCAPs. The bottom panel shows eCAP amplitudes plotted as a function of masker-electrode locations (i.e., SOE function) measured at two stimulus levels. The function measured at 709 μA (open circles) is wider than that measured at 648 μA (solid circles). For this subject, the functions measured at both levels are asymmetrical, with more spread of neural excitation occurring at more apical masker electrodes. This asymmetry in excitation pattern is consistent with results reported in previous studies (Cohen et al., 2003; Abbas et al., 2004; Hughes and Stille, 2008; Hughes and Goulson, 2011; Scheperle and Abbas, 2015a,b). SOE functions vary in the overall amplitude, the width, and the shape among patients, as well as across electrode locations within individual CI users. Factors accounting for these variations

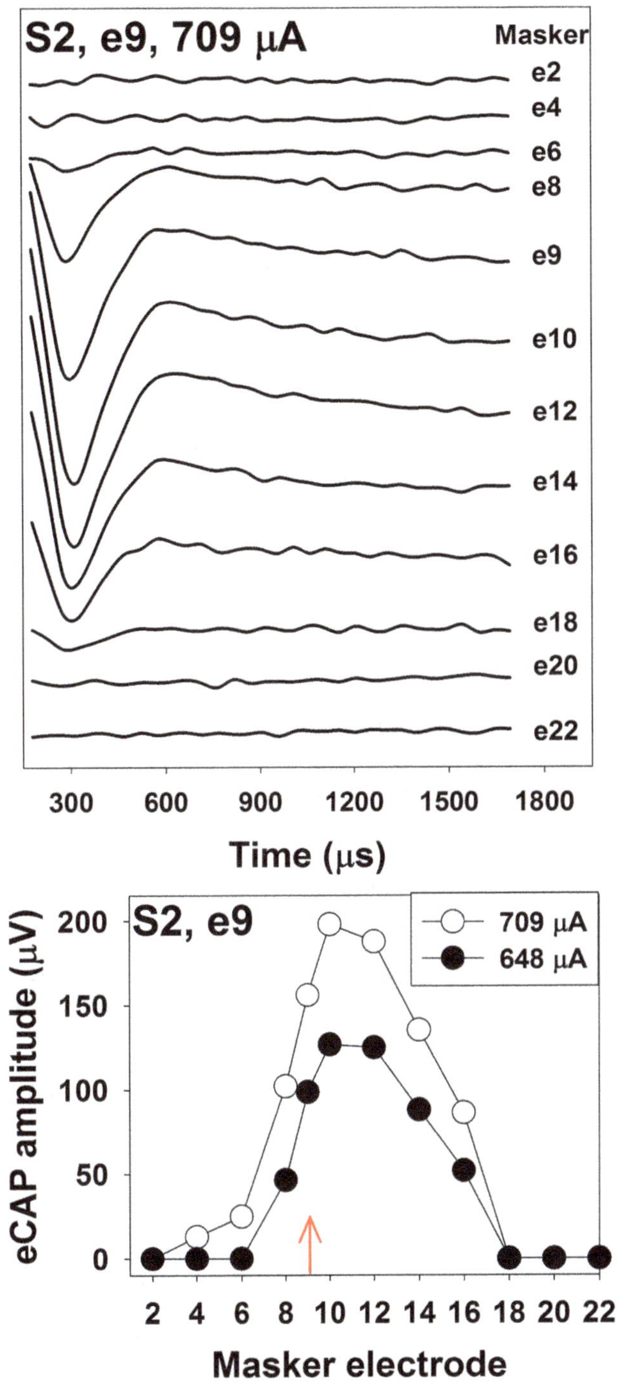

FIGURE 4 | The top panel shows eCAP response series used to generate a channel-interaction function in S2. Each waveform is the derived eCAP measured for a probe pulse presented to electrode 9 at 709 μA. Masker electrode number is labeled for each trace. The bottom panel shows channel-interaction functions measured at 709 μA (open symbols) and 648 μA (filled symbols) in for the probe electrode 9 (red arrow) in S2.

include the stimulus level, the degree and pattern of neural survival, the electrode position relative to the stimulable neurons, the orientation of the electrodes and the resulting electrical field, and the impedance pathway for electrical current spread. To quantitatively compare the eCAP SOE function, eCAP amplitudes are typically normalized to the amplitude of the eCAP measured when the masker and the probe are presented on the same electrode.

Studies evaluating the association between eCAP SOE function, electrode pitch ranking and speech perception reveal mixed results. While most of these studies found no association between results of eCAP and behavioral measures (Cohen et al., 2003; Hughes and Abbas, 2006; Snel-Bongers et al., 2012; van der Beek et al., 2012), other studies reported that eCAP SOE functions were associated with electrode pitch ranking (Hughes, 2008) and speech perception in CI users (Won et al., 2014; Scheperle and Abbas, 2015a,b). Differences in the methodology used in these studies might account for the discrepancy in their results. For example, Hughes and Abbas (2006) measured the width of the eCAP SOE function at 75% of the normalized amplitude, and assessed its association with electrode pitch ranking ability and speech perception performance in CI users. Their results revealed no association among results of these measures. However, Hughes (2008) re-analyzed the same set of data by using the eCAP channel-separation index (CSI) to quantify SOE functions. Results showed a significant correlation between the eCAP SOE function and electrode pitch ranking ability, with less overlap of eCAP SOE functions associated with greater accuracy of electrode pitch ranking performance. Compared with the eCAP SOE width, the CSI is more sensitive to differences in locations and overall shapes of eCAP SOE functions. In addition, it provides a way for quantifying non-overlapped SOE functions. Therefore, it has been used in many recent studies (e.g., Abbas and Brown, 2015; Scheperle and Abbas, 2015a,b). For details of CSI calculation, please see Hughes (2008). The number of electrode locations tested may be another important factor to consider (Scheperle and Abbas, 2015b). Measuring the eCAP SOE function at few stimulating electrode locations may not capture the likely variability of SOE along the cochlea, which might partially account for the lack of correlation between eCAP SOE functions and speech perception reported in some studies (Cohen et al., 2003; van der Beek et al., 2012).

In summary, electrophysiological measures of the eCAP can be used to assess SOE pattern occurring at the electrode-neural interface. The CSI is a better parameter than the function width for quantifying the eCAP SOE function. Even though earlier literature showed no association between eCAP SOE function and behavioral measures of pitch ranking or speech perception, recent studies using the improved quantification method and more stimulating electrodes along the cochlea reported significant correlations among these measures. Nevertheless, the eCAP is generated by the auditory nerve. It does not provide information of auditory processing at the central auditory system that is important for speech perception. Scheperle and Abbas (2015a) found that eCAP SOE functions could only account for part of the variance observed in neural encoding of spectral information at the central auditory system. Therefore, the eCAP SOE function should not be used as the sole objective measure for predicting speech perception or electrode discrimination in CI users. However, this measure may provide useful information

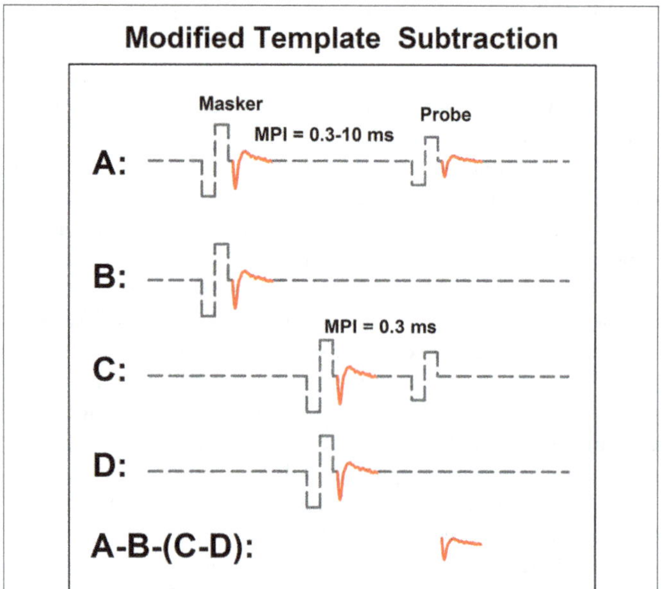

FIGURE 5 | A schematic illustration of the modified template subtraction method for measuring the eCAP refractory recovery function. Gray dashed lines and red solid lines indicate biphasic electrical pulses and eCAP responses, respectively.

about channel interaction occurring at the electrode-neural interface, which leaves the possibility for new applications. For example, it can potentially be used to guard against tip fold-over electrode array during surgery. Further studies are warranted to test this speculation.

Temporal Responsiveness

Temporal information is important for speech perception in CI users, as minimal spectral cues are available to these patients. Temporal cues, especially rapid spectral and amplitude changes or acoustic onsets, are represented in the discharge patterns of the auditory nerve (Delgutte, 1980; Delgutte and Kiang, 1984). Evidence from recent studies suggests that temporal responsiveness of the auditory nerve plays an important role in encoding speech envelope cues (e.g., Kirby and Middlebrooks, 2012; Tejani et al., 2017). By using different stimulation paradigms, results of eCAP measures can provide information about many aspects of temporal response properties of the auditory nerve, including refractory recovery, neural adaptation, adaptation recovery, capability of encoding of amplitude modulation cues, etc. This section describes these eCAP stimulation paradigms and reviews related studies in human CI users.

Refractoriness and Recovery

Refractoriness refers to a status in which neurons are incapable of generating an action potential immediately after a previous stimulation. It is a fundamental temporal property of the auditory nerve that enhances spike timing precision (Avissar et al., 2013). The time during which an action potential cannot be generated regardless of the magnitude of the stimulus is defined as the absolute refractory period (ARP). The ARP is followed by a relative refractory period (RRP) during which time the neuron can be activated by a strong stimulus. It has been shown that refractory properties have a significant effect on neural encoding of electrical pulse trains delivered by the CI at the level of the auditory nerve (Wilson et al., 1997).

In human CI users, the ARP and the RRP can be estimated based on the eCAP refractory recovery function (RRF). The eCAP RRF is typically measured with two biphasic, charge-balanced, electrical pulses using a modified template subtraction method (Miller et al., 2000). A schematic illustration of this method is shown in **Figure 5**. In this paradigm, traces evoked by two masker-probe pairs are measured. The masker-probe-interval (MPI) of the first masker-probe pair systematically varies from 300 to 10,000 μs (trace A). As the MPI increases, the auditory nerve gradually recovers from the refractoriness induced by the masker, which results in larger eCAPs at longer MPIs in trace A. Subtracting trace "B" from trace "A" (i.e., A-B) yields the artifact and the eCAP evoked by the probe. The MPI of the second masker-probe pair is typically around 300 μs, which minimizes the neural response evoked by the probe (trace C) (Morsnowski et al., 2006). Subtracting trace "D" from trace "C" (i.e., C-D) results in the artifact evoked by the probe. The difference between these two derived traces (i.e., A-B-[C-D]) is the eCAP evoked by the first probe. The eCAP RRF is obtained by plotting (normalized) eCAP amplitudes as a function of MPIs.

The top panel of **Figure 6** shows a series of eCAP waveforms measured at different MPIs for electrode 12 in one pediatric CI user. MPIs used to measure these responses are labeled for these traces. These data clearly show that the eCAP becomes larger as the MPI increases. In this case, the eCAP amplitude was normalized to the amplitude of the eCAP measured at the MPI of 10 ms. The eCAP RRF was obtained by plotting the normalized eCAP amplitude (red symbol) as a function of MPIs, which is shown in the bottom panel of **Figure 6**. The eCAP RRF is typically modeled by an exponential decay function (e.g., Morsnowski et al., 2006; Botros and Psarros, 2010; Fulmer et al., 2011; He et al., 2017) of the form

$$eCAP_N = A\left[1 - e^{\frac{-(MPI-t_0)}{\tau}}\right], \qquad (1)$$

where $eCAP_N$ represents the normalized eCAP amplitude, t_0 is aligned with the ARP, τ is a measure of the speed of recovery from relative refractoriness (i.e., the RRP), and A represents the maximum eCAP amplitude evoked by the probe after a sufficiently long MPI. The line in the bottom panel of **Figure 6** shows results of data fitting using this exponential decay function. Estimated t_0 and τ are shown in the low right corner of this panel.

The speed of recovery from refractoriness is affected by stimulus level, with faster recovery at higher levels (Finley et al., 1997; Pesch et al., 2005). Medians/means of the ARP and the RRP measured at C level in "typical" CI users range from around 276 to 645 μs and from around 600 to 1350 μs, respectively (Pesch et al., 2005; Morsnowski et al., 2006; Hughes et al., 2012; Wiemes et al., 2016). Refractoriness measured for virtual vs. physical channels are comparable (Hughes and Goulson, 2011). Several

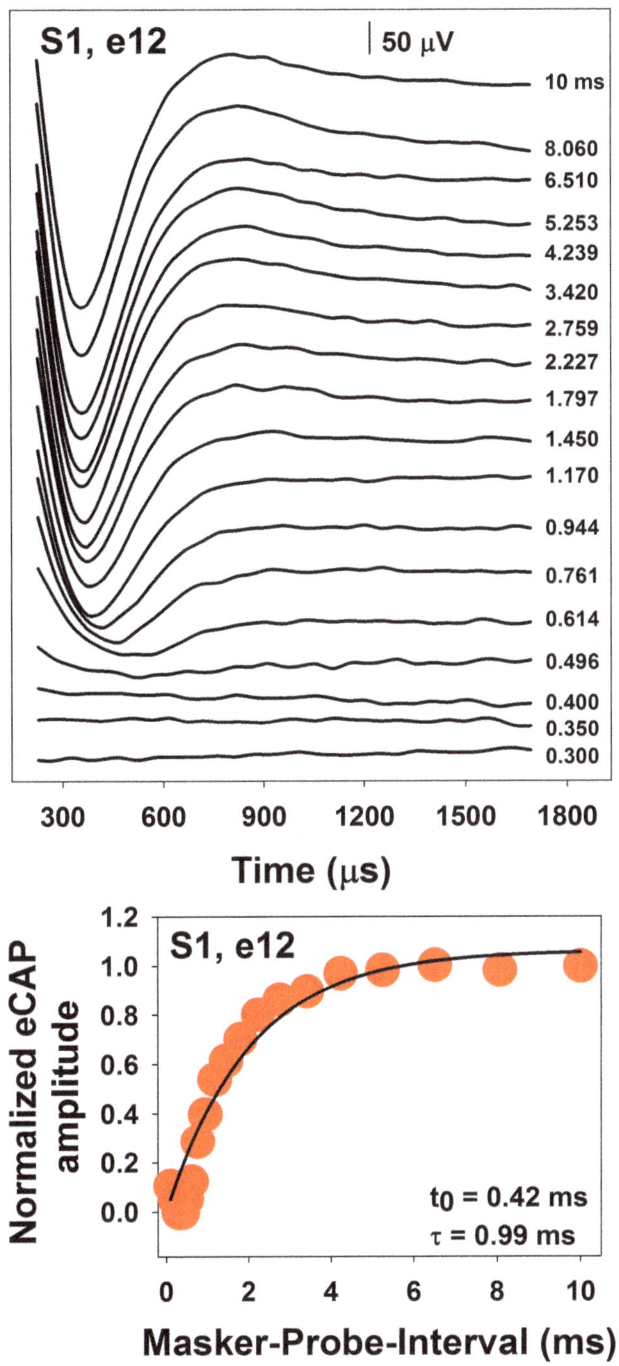

FIGURE 6 | A series of eCAP waveforms (**Top**) and the derived eCAP refractory recovery function (**Bottom**) measured at electrode 12 in S1.

studies have investigated refractory properties of the auditory nerve in some special patient populations, including children with auditory neuropathy spectrum disorder (ANSD) (Fulmer et al., 2011), elderly CI users (Lee et al., 2012), and children with cochlea nerve deficiency (CND) (He et al., 2017). Results of these studies showed that children with ANSD had similar refractory recovery time constants compared with children with typical sensorineural hearing loss (SNHL) (Fulmer et al., 2011). There is no association between refractory recovery time constants and chronological age (Lee et al., 2012). However, the RRP tends to prolong in patients with longer duration of hearing loss (Botros and Psarros, 2010; Lee et al., 2012). Compared with implanted children with normal-size auditory nerves, implanted children with CND have prolonged ARPs but similar RRPs (He et al., 2017).

Studies that investigated potential clinical applications of the eCAP RRF in optimizing programming rates and predicting CI outcomes reported inconsistent results (Brown et al., 1990; Abbas and Brown, 1991; Gantz et al., 1994; Kiefer et al., 2001; Shpak et al., 2004; Shpak, 2005; Fulmer et al., 2011; Lee et al., 2012). Shpak et al. (2004) reported a positive correlation between refractory recovery time constants and preferred programming rates. This finding was not replicated in a subsequent study by the same investigators (Shpak, 2005). Faster recovery from refractoriness has been reported to correlate with better speech perception scores in some studies (Brown et al., 1990; Kiefer et al., 2001; Fulmer et al., 2011). However, this association is not observed in other studies (Finley et al., 1997; Turner et al., 2002; Battmer et al., 2005; Lee et al., 2012). Factors accounting for these inconsistencies are unclear. One possibility is that the eCAP RRF may be affected by factors other than temporal responsiveness of the auditory nerve. For example, it has been proposed that refractory recovery time constants are affected by the size of neuron population. Specifically, prolonged ARP has been shown to be associated with reduced auditory nerve fiber density in rats (Shepherd et al., 2004). These results are consistent with prolonged ARPs estimated in children with CND (He et al., 2017). Based on simulation results of a computational model, Botros and Psarros (2010) proposed that longer RRPs were associated with better neural survival in CI patients. However, this theory is not supported by the relatively normal RRPs measured in children with CND who presumably have reduced number of neurons (He et al., 2017). Other factors, like difference in stimulation mode (bipolar vs. monopolar) and sample size, might also attribute to the inconsistent findings among these studies.

In summary, the ARP and the RRP of the electrically-stimulated auditory nerve can be estimated based on the eCAP RRF. To date, potential clinical application of the eCAP RRF is unclear due to limited research findings. Further studies with large sample sizes are warranted.

Neural Adaptation and Adaptation Recovery

The firing rate of the auditory nerve rapidly increases to the maximum at the onset of sustained stimulation followed by a gradual decay in firing rate (i.e., neural adaptation); neural activity and responsiveness to subsequent stimulation are reduced for a brief period following the cessation of the initial stimulation, resulting in forward masking effects (e.g., Smith, 1977). Neural adaptation plays important roles in speech encoding at the level of the auditory nerve (Delgutte, 1997). Fast neural adaptation and recovery from prior stimulation have been proposed to be important for producing peaks in the discharge rate of the auditory nerve that serve to enhance acoustic onsets in the speech waveform (Delgutte, 1997). Abnormal neural adaptation patterns, excessive adaptation and/or slow recovery from adaptation could potentially cause poor representation of temporal envelopes at the auditory nerve (Jeng et al., 2009), and might contribute to poor speech perception in some CI users (Wilson et al., 1994; Nelson and Donaldson, 2002).

In implanted patients, neural adaptation of the auditory nerve can be evaluated by measuring eCAP amplitudes in response to individual pulses in a constant-amplitude pulse train using a modified forward-masking paradigm (Brown et al., 1990; Finley et al., 1997; Wilson et al., 1997; Rubinstein et al., 1999; Miller et al., 2000; Hay-McCutcheon et al., 2005; Hughes et al., 2012, 2014; McKay et al., 2013; He et al., 2016a). **Figure 7** shows a schematic illustration of this paradigm. The left side of **Figure 7** illustrates the classic two-pulse forward-masking paradigm (Brown et al., 1990). Subtracting trace C from trace B yields a template of the probe artifact. To derive eCAPs to each of the other pulses in a pulse train, a modification of the forward-masking technique is needed and shown schematically on the right side of **Figure 7**. In this paradigm, the MPI is adjusted to correspond to the period of the pulse rate minus the duration of one biphasic pulse. For example, the MPI is 1,943 μs if the pulse rate is 500 pps (period = 2,000 μs) and the pulse duration is 57 μs. With this increased MPI duration, coupled with the constant level pulses, some neural response is expected to be evoked by each successive pulse due to partial recovery from refractoriness. In an iterative process, the number of pulses comprising the masker is increased by one, with the final pulse in the pulse train always designated as the probe. For each iteration, the response to the final probe pulse is derived as (Bn-Cn)-(B1-C1), as shown on the right panel of **Figure 7**. One caveat is that the success of this method depends on one underlying assumption: the probe artifact stays constant during pulse train stimulation. However, this assumption may be invalid in some cases (He et al., 2016a; Tejani et al., 2017), which results in incomplete artifact removal. A careful inspection of derived eCAP waveforms is highly recommended for any study using this stimulation paradigm in order to identify cases where residual artifact exists. Unfortunately, there is still no method that can be used to overcome this technical challenge.

Figure 8 shows eCAP amplitudes in response to individual pulses of a train of 32 pulses measured at electrode 3 in one implanted child with SNHL (S7). Results are shown for four pulse rates, ranging from 500 to 2,400 pps. These data show that eCAP amplitudes measured at 500 pps (black symbols) rapidly decrease in the first few milliseconds after stimulus onset followed by a more gradual decline. It should be noted that this decline in eCAP amplitude typically does not occur for pulse rates of 200 pps or lower (Wilson et al., 1997), which suggests that the excitability of auditory nerve fibers fully recovers in these conditions between any two pulsatile stimulations (Wilson et al., 1997; Matsuoka et al., 2000a). At 900 pps (red symbols), eCAP amplitudes as a function of pulse numbers starts to show an alternating response pattern, with eCAPs to odd-numbered pulses having larger amplitudes than those evoked by even-numbered pulses. This alternating pattern typically occurs at pulse rates of 400–2,400 pps (Wilson et al., 1997; Hughes et al., 2012) and is believed to be a result of the refractory properties of auditory neurons (Finley et al., 1997; Wilson et al., 1997; Matsuoka et al., 2000b; Abbas et al., 2001). Theoretically, all neurons in the electrical field generated by the first pulse are available for activation at the maximum excitability. While these neurons are in their refractory phase, they will be unresponsive or have reduced excitability to the second pulse if the time period between these pulses is less than 3 or 4 ms (i.e., refractory period). At the time of the third pulse, many of these neurons will now be sufficiently recovered to be excited by the third pulse. Consequently, eCAP amplitude to the third pulse will be larger than that to the second pulse. This recovery-refractory process occurs during the entire process of pulse-train stimulation, which results in this alternating pattern (Wilson et al., 1997). The alternation in eCAP amplitude becomes more robust at 1,800 pps (blue symbols) in this case, as evidenced by a larger difference in amplitude between eCAPs evoked by the odd- vs. even-numbered pulses. The rate at which the maximum alternation occurs is typically around 900–1,800 pps (Hughes et al., 2012; He et al., 2016a), which presumably "resonate" with the RRP of the stimulated auditory nerve fibers (Matsuoka et al., 2000a; Hughes et al., 2012). In addition to this simple alternating pattern, complex alternating patterns, ranging from triplet to sextuplets patterns (i.e., increase and decrease in amplitude repeated every three–six responses) have been described in some studies (Wilson et al., 1997; Hughes et al., 2012; He et al., 2016a). The underlying mechanism of the complex alternating pattern or its clinical association with CI outcomes or programming settings remains unknown. Further increases in stimulation rate to 2,400 pps (yellow symbols in **Figure 8**) diminish the alternating pattern of eCAP amplitude due to stochastic independence among auditory nerve fibers. This stochastic state is caused by the combined effects of incomplete refractory recovery, increased neural adaptation, and increased temporal jitter (Hay-McCutcheon et al., 2005; Mino and Rubinstein, 2006). The rate at which the stochastic state occurs is typically at 2,000 pps or higher (Wilson et al., 1997; Rubinstein et al., 1999; Hughes et al., 2012). Even though high pulse rates are initially recommended due to its capability of inducing a stochastic state in which "pseudo-spontaneous" neural discharges occur, inconsistent results have been reported in terms of whether high pulse rates are beneficial for speech perception in CI users (e.g., Fu and Shannon, 2000; Loizou et al., 2000; Vandali et al., 2000; Friesen et al., 2005; Weber et al., 2007). Despite well-reported basic properties of eCAPs evoked by pulse train stimuli, it still remains unknown whether/how these eCAP response patterns are associated with speech and language outcomes or whether they can be used to select the optimal programming rate for individual CI patients.

Data shown in **Figure 8** clearly demonstrate that eCAP amplitude decreases as the pulse rate increases. The amount of reduction in eCAP amplitude (i.e., adaptation) can be quantified by comparing amplitudes of eCAPs elicited by pulses occurring later in the pulse train to eCAP amplitudes elicited by early pulses (Hay-McCutcheon et al., 2005; Hughes et al., 2012, 2014; Zhang et al., 2013; He et al., 2016a). Although several studies have used

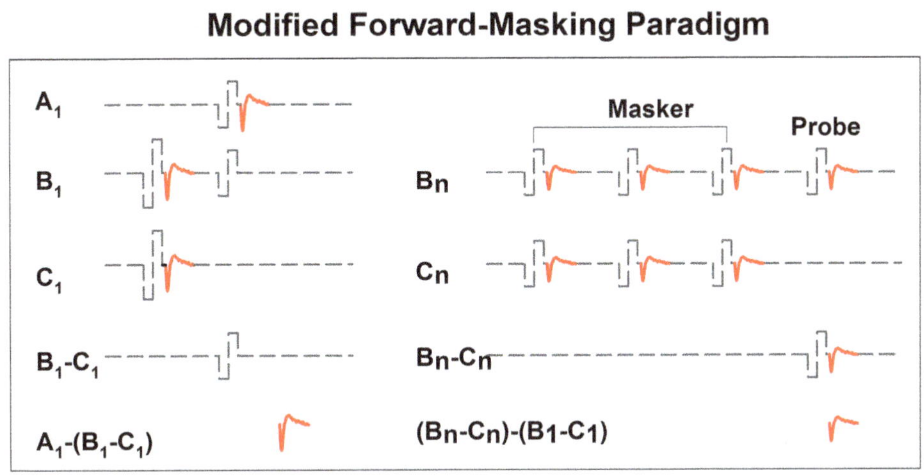

FIGURE 7 | A schematic illustration of the modified forward-masking paradigm that can be used to measure eCAPs evoked by individual pulses in a pulse train. Gray dashed lines and red solid lines indicate biphasic electrical pulses and eCAP responses, respectively.

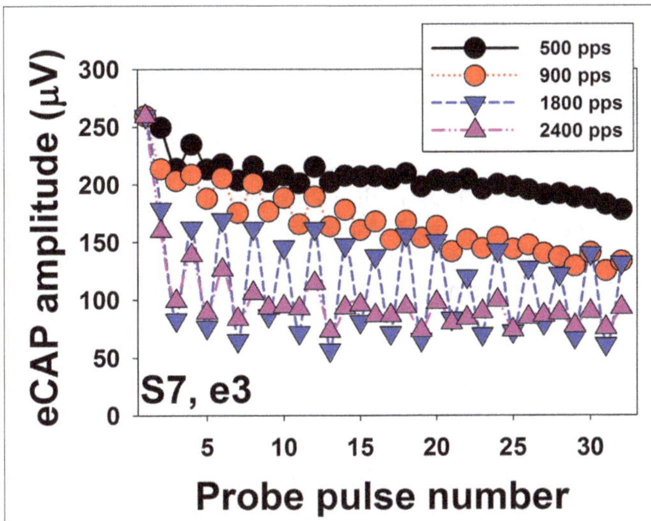

FIGURE 8 | Amplitudes of eCAPs measured for individual pulses in a train of 32 pulses. Results measured at different pulse rates are indicated using different symbols and colors.

eCAPs to measure the amount of neural adaptation in human CI users (Finley et al., 1997; Wilson et al., 1997; Rubinstein et al., 1999; Hay-McCutcheon et al., 2005; Hughes et al., 2012, 2014; McKay et al., 2013; He et al., 2016a), comparing results among these studies is challenging due to differences in duration of pulse train (ranging from 13 to 50 ms), pulse rate tested (ranging from 250 to 5,000 pps), and the time point used to calculate the amount of neural adaptation. To date, the association between neural adaptation of the auditory nerve and auditory perception in human CI users has only been evaluated in one study (Zhang et al., 2013). In this study, Zhang and colleague measured the neural adaptation of the audtory neve induced by a 50-ms pulse train with a pulse rate of 1,000 pps at one electrode in 14 post-lingually deaf adult CI users. For each subject, they also measured behavioral gap detectoin threshold (GDT) and speech perception scores. Their results showed no assocation between the amount of neural adapation of the auditory nerve and GDTs or speech perception scores. However, these results need to be interpreted with caution since only one electrode site was tested for adaptation of the auditory nerve in each subject despite the fact that adaptation varies across stimulation sites within individual patients (Hughes et al., 2012; He et al., 2016a). In contrast, behavioral GDTs and speech perception were evaluated through the speech processor using sound-field presentation at relatively high stimulation levels. As a consequence, results of Zhang et al. (2013) did not provide direct evidence for the effect of adaptation of the auditory nerve on perceptual sensivitiy to temporal gaps or speech perception capabilities in CI users. To date, it remains unknown to what extent neural adaptation of the auditory nerve affects auditory temporal processing and speech perception capabilities in CI users. Further studies are warranted in order to fill in these gaps in knowledge.

Recovery from neural adaptation at the level of the auditory nerve can be evaluated by measuring eCAP amplitude in response to the probe pulse at different time points after the masker-pulse-train ceases. Two stimulation paradigms have been used for this purpose (Dhuldhoya, 2013; He et al., 2016b; Adel et al., 2017). A schematic illustration of the first paradigm is shown in **Figure 9**. This paradigm is very similar to the modified forward-masking paradigm shown in **Figure 7** except for the varied MPI between the probe and the masker-pulse-train (right panel of **Figure 9**). As the MPI increases, the eCAP evoked by the probe pulse (i.e., [B'-C']-[B-C]) gradually recover from the neural adaptation induced by the masker-pulse-train. The adaptation recovery function (ARF) can be obtained by plotting eCAP amplitudes as a function of MPIs. In addition to this paradigm, the modified alternating polarity paradigm has recently been used to derive ARFs in human CI users. For details of this paradigm, please see Adel et al. (2017).

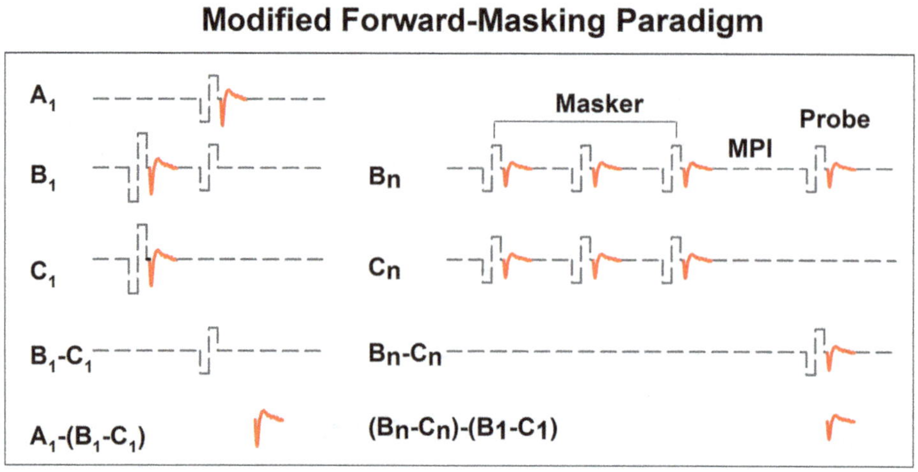

FIGURE 9 | A schematic illustration of the modified forward-masking paradigm that can be used to evaluate recovery from neural adaptation introduced by a pulse train using eCAP recordings. Gray dashed lines and red solid lines indicate biphasic electrical pulses and eCAP responses, respectively.

The top panel of **Figure 10** shows a series of eCAP waveforms measured at various MPIs at electrode 20 in S3. The masker was a 100-ms pulse train with a pulse rate of 2,400 pps presented at the C level. The MPIs used to measure these eCAPs ranged from 2 to 256 ms and are labeled for these traces. These data show that eCAP amplitudes are larger at longer MPIs. The bottom panel shows ARFs measured at four pulse rates ranging from 500 to 2,400 pps at the same electrode. These ARFs follow exponential distributions. eCAP amplitudes reach a plateau at longer MPIs for faster pulse rates, which suggests slower adaption recovery at faster pulse rates. As a result, ARFs measured at faster rates (green and blue symbols) appear to be flatter than those measured at slower rates (black and red symbols).

The literature related to recovery from neural adaptation of the auditory nerve in CI users is relatively scarce. To date, only three studies have evaluated this specific issue (Dhuldhoya, 2013; He et al., 2016b; Adel et al., 2017). Overall, these studies showed that ARFs could consist of up to three components with an initial rapid increase (fast recovery) followed by a rapid decrease (adaptation enhancement) and a second slower increase (slow recovery) in eCAP amplitude (Dhuldhoya, 2013; He et al., 2016b). An example of the ARF with all three components is shown in **Figure 11**. In this example, the fast recovery is observed for MPIs of 1–2 ms, followed by the adaptation enhancement occurring at MPIs of 2–8 ms. The slow recovery is observed for MPIs of 16–256 ms. This example represents the most complicated ARF observed in human CI users. Not all reported ARFs have all three components. The slow recovery is the most commonly observed component in CI users (Dhuldhoya, 2013; He et al., 2016b). It has been proposed that the fast recovery is due to increased neural synchrony of auditory nerve fibers (Nourski et al., 2007), and the adaptation enhancement possibly results from the loss of current integration at the neural membrane due to long MPIs (Miller et al., 2011). The slow recovery is believed to reflect recovery from neural adaptation (Nourski et al., 2007; Miller et al., 2011). However, these interpretations may be oversimplified. High masker level or low probe level yields longer adaptation recovery in both adult and pediatric CI users (Dhuldhoya, 2013). At a fixed current level, increasing pulse rate yields long recovery from neural adaptation (He et al., 2016b; Adel et al., 2017). Preliminary data reported by He et al. (2016b) indicated that auditory nerve fibers in older CI users might have slower adaptation recovery than those of young CI patients. To date, our understanding of adaptation recovery of the electrically-stimulated auditory nerve in human listeners is still very limited. As a result, the potential clinical implication of the eCAP ARF is unclear.

Amplitude Modulation Encoding

Neural encoding of amplitude modulation cues at the level of the auditory nerve can be evaluated by measuring eCAPs evoked by individual pulses in an amplitude-modulated (AM) pulse train using a stimulation paradigm shown in **Figure 12**. This paradigm is the same as the modified forward-masking paradigm shown in **Figure 7** with two important exceptions. First, the pulse train (right panel) is amplitude modulated. Second, the probe level used in the two-pulse forward masking paradigm (left panel) needs to be the same as that of the probe pulse in the AM pulse train (right panel). The eCAP evoked by individual pulses of the AM pulse train is derived by the subtraction of (B'-C')-(B-C).

Figure 13A shows a series of eCAP waveforms evoked by a 200-ms pulse train with a carrier pulse rate of 2,000 pps that was sinusoidally amplitude modulated (SAM) at 40 Hz at electrode 20 (e20) in one adult CI user (S10). These eCAP recordings span one SAM cycle. These responses show a periodical change in amplitude, which tends to follow the SAM of the stimulus. **Figure 13B** shows amplitudes of eCAPs to pulse trains with SAM rate of 20 Hz (red symbols) and 200 Hz (blue symbols) plotted as a function of time measured at e20 in S10 and S11 (top and bottom, respectively). Both subjects are post-lingually deaf adult CI users. Amplitudes of eCAPs evoked by single pulses at each of the probe levels used in the AM pulse train are indicated in black. These results show that the auditory nerve near e20 in both subjects can robustly encode AM cues delivered by single-pulse stimulation. However, AM cues delivered by pulse-train stimulation are better transmitted by the auditory nerve in S10 than in S11 at both AM rates, as indicated by greater modulation depth of eCAP amplitudes measured in S10 than those recorded in S11. For both subjects, there is a phase shift (lead) in eCAP responses evoked by the pulse train relative to eCAPs evoked by the single pulse. These data are consistent with results reported in human CI users (Wilson et al., 1997; Tejani et al., 2017) and acutely deafened guinea pigs (Abbas et al., 1998; Jeng et al., 2009). This phase shift has been proposed to be due to non-linear growth of the eCAP amplitude and a combined effect of refractoriness, adaptation, and facilitation (Jeng et al., 2009).

The association between how the auditory nerve responds to AM stimuli and auditory perception in human CI users is the least understood feature among all topics covered in this review. Even though the feasibility of measuring eCAPs using SAM pulse trains has been established for almost 20 years (Wilson et al., 1997), this feature has only been investigated in human CI users in two studies (Carlyon and Deeks, 2015; Tejani et al., 2017). Carlyon and Deeks (2015) assessed the association between AM neural encoding as evaluated by eCAP measures and temporal pitch perception in CI users. Their results showed that the ability of the auditory nerve to faithfully encode and transmit AM cues might be important for pitch perception. Factors accounting for limitation of pulse-rate discrimination were beyond the auditory nerve. Tejani et al. (2017) evaluated how well the auditory nerve encoded SAM cues by measuring eCAPs in response to a SAM pulse train with a carrier rate of 4,000 pps and AM rates of 125, 250, 500, and 1,000 Hz in adult CI users. In addition, they examined the association between eCAP results and psychophysical measures of amplitude modulation detection threshold (AMDT) at these AM rates in these patients. Their results showed that amplitudes of eCAPs in response to SAM pulse trains reflected the overall periodicity of the stimuli. The amount of variation in eCAP amplitude correlated with AMDT at SAM rates up to 500 Hz, with larger variations associated with lower AMDTs. However, the association between results of eCAP and behavioral measures was not observed at the SAM rate of 1,000 Hz, which was proposed to indicate the limitation of central auditory encoding and processing of AM cues at high rates (Tejani et al., 2017). The extent of modulation in eCAP amplitude is affected by the modulation depth in stimulus and the electrode location (Carlyon and Deeks, 2015; Tejani et al., 2017). It has been shown that stronger modulations in eCAP amplitude are evoked by stimuli with larger modulation depths (Carlyon and Deeks, 2015; Tejani et al., 2017). At the fixed modulation depth, eCAPs recorded at the apical electrodes demonstrate stronger modulation in amplitude (Tejani et al., 2017).

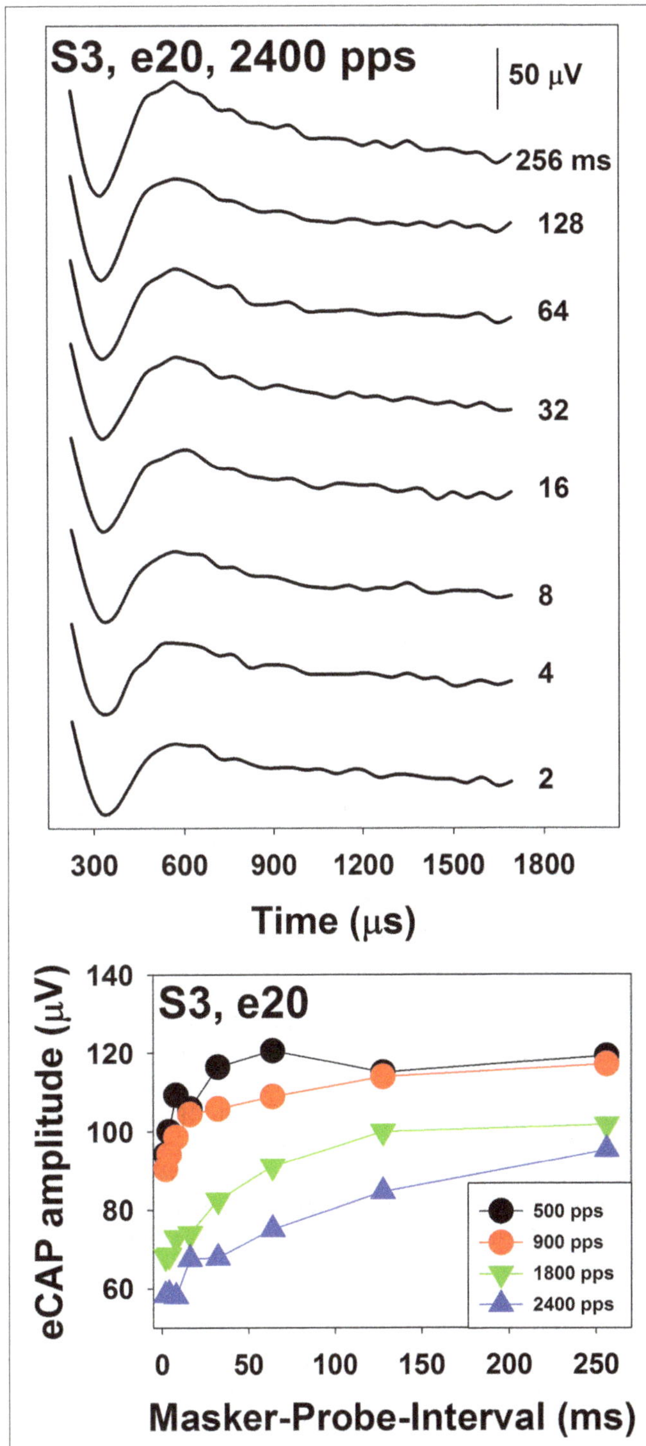

FIGURE 10 | Neural adaptation recovery function measured at four pulse rates in S3. These results were measured for electrode 20 in a Cochlear CI user. Results recorded at different rates are indicated using different symbols.

Neural Survival

Due to the compromised functional status of the auditory system, hearing impaired patients presumably have less channels that provide useful information for auditory perception than normal-hearing listeners. The number of available "functional channels" should, in theory, associate with speech and language outcomes in CI patients. At the peripheral auditory system, the pattern and degree of neural survival of auditory fibers may be an important factor for the number of available "functional channels." Developing tools for estimating the

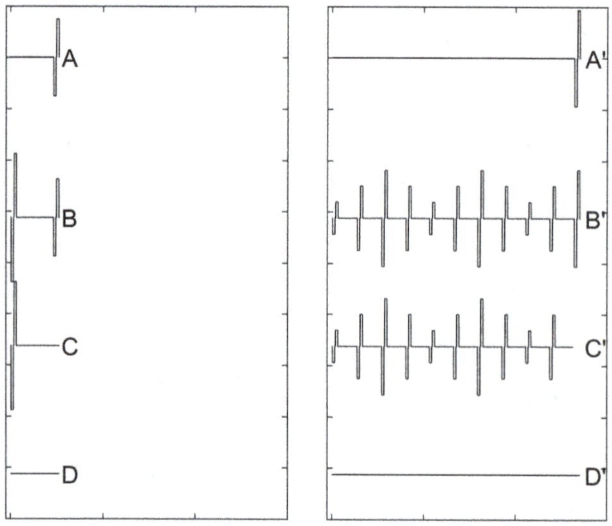

FIGURE 11 | A schematic illustration of the stimulation paradigm that can be used to measure eCAPs evoked by individual pulses of a sinusoidally amplitude-modulated pulse train. This figure is courtesy of Viral D. Tejani at The University of Iowa.

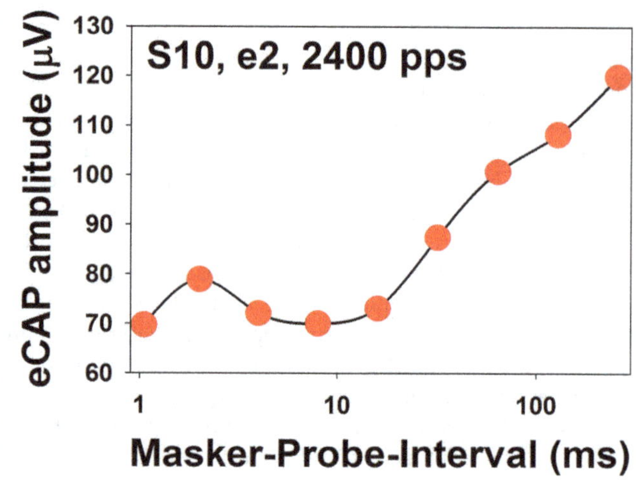

FIGURE 12 | eCAP amplitudes measured at different MPIs for electrode 2 in one adult CI patient (S10). The stimulus was a 100-ms constant-amplitude pulse train with a pulse rate of 2,400 pps presented at the maximum comfortable level. MPIs are shown in a logarithmic scale.

number of survival auditory fibers and predicting CI outcomes for individual patients has been a research topic for many years. There has been an increased interest in using the eCAP to estimate neural survival of auditory nerve fibers. However, a direct comparison between eCAP responses and spiral ganglion cell density in human listeners is not feasible. Therefore, animal models are used to identify eCAP measures that are sensitive to neural survivals (e.g., Miller et al., 1994; Prado-Guitierrez et al., 2006; Ramekers et al., 2014). These measures have been subsequently used in human CI users to evaluate their correlations with behavioral measures of auditory perception and/or speech perception (e.g., Brown et al., 1990; Gantz et al., 1994; Kim et al., 2010; Pfingst et al., 2015a; Schvartz-Leyzac and Pfingst, 2016). This section reviews studies related to one eCAP measure that has been studied for many years (i.e., slope of the eCAP I/O function) and the three most recently developed eCAP measures (sensitivity to inter-phase-gap, phase duration and pulse polarity).

Slope of the eCAP I/O Function

In animal models, sleeper slopes of eCAP I/O functions have been found to be generally associated with higher spiral ganglion density (e.g., Miller et al., 1994; Pfingst et al., 2014, 2015a,b). However, the spiral ganglion density only accounted for 50% of the variance in the slope of eCAP I/O function (Pfingst et al., 2014). In human CI users, flatter slopes have been found to be associated with longer duration of hearing loss (e.g., Schvartz-Leyzac and Pfingst, 2016). Studies evaluating the association between the slope of eCAP I/O function and speech perception scores in human CI users show inconsistent results. Whereas, some studies reported better speech perception scores measured in CI users with sleeper slopes (Brown et al., 1990; Kim et al., 2010), other studies found no association between these two measures (Franck and Norton, 2001; Turner et al., 2002). Factors accounting for the inconsistency include, but are not limited to, relative small sample size, limited test electrode location, and heterogeneity of patients tested in these studies.

Inter-Phase-Gap and Phase Duration

In guinea pigs, sensitivity of the eCAP to changes in interphase gap (IPG) and phase duration (PD) of a biphasic pulse have been shown to be correlated with auditory nerve survival (Prado-Guitierrez et al., 2006; Ramekers et al., 2014). Results of these animal studies showed that increasing IPG and/or PD reduced threshold and increased amplitude of the eCAP, presumably due to current integration occurring at the cell membrane. Poor spiral ganglion survival reduces the magnitude of IPG and PD. To date, the effect of increasing IPG on eCAP responses in human CI users has been only examined in one study. Schvartz-Leyzac and Pfingst (2016) studied the effect of increasing IPG from 7 to 30 μs on eCAP amplitude and slope of I/O function in human CI users. Their results showed that increasing IPG generally yielded increased eCAP amplitude and steeper slopes of I/O function. However, this effect varied across subjects and electrode locations. It remains unknown whether variations in sensitivity to IPG affect auditory perception or CI outcomes. The effect of PD has not been investigated in human CI users.

Polarity Sensitivity

The charge-balanced biphasic pulse used in current CI consists of a cathodic phase followed by an anodic phase. Both cathodic and anodic stimuli can generate spikes in auditory nerve fibers (e.g., van den Honert and Stypulkowski, 1984; Miller et al., 1998, 2004; Shepherd and Javel, 1999). Simulation results using biophysical models suggested that the site of spike generation differs for anodic and cathodic stimuli (Rubinstein,

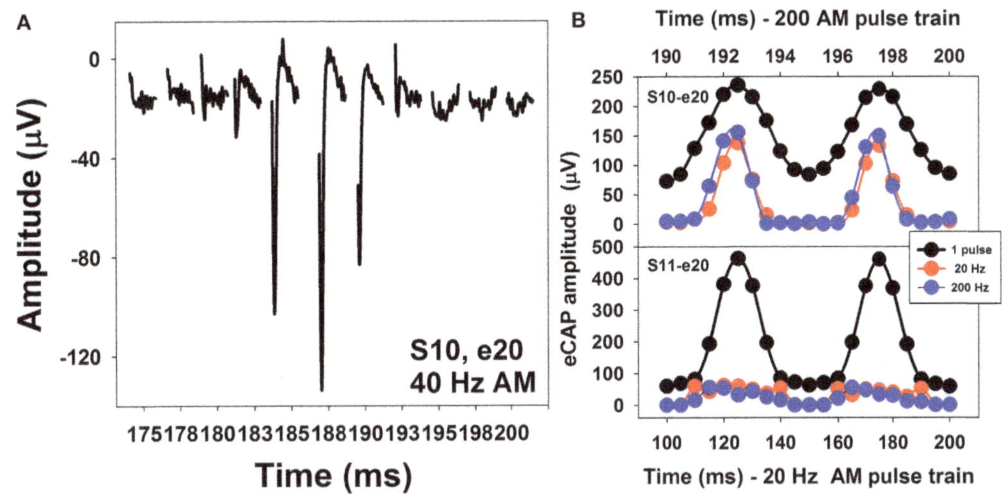

FIGURE 13 | Waveforms of eCAPs recorded at electrode 20 in S10 **(A)** and eCAP amplitude modulation functions measured at electrode 20 in S10 and S11 **(B)**.

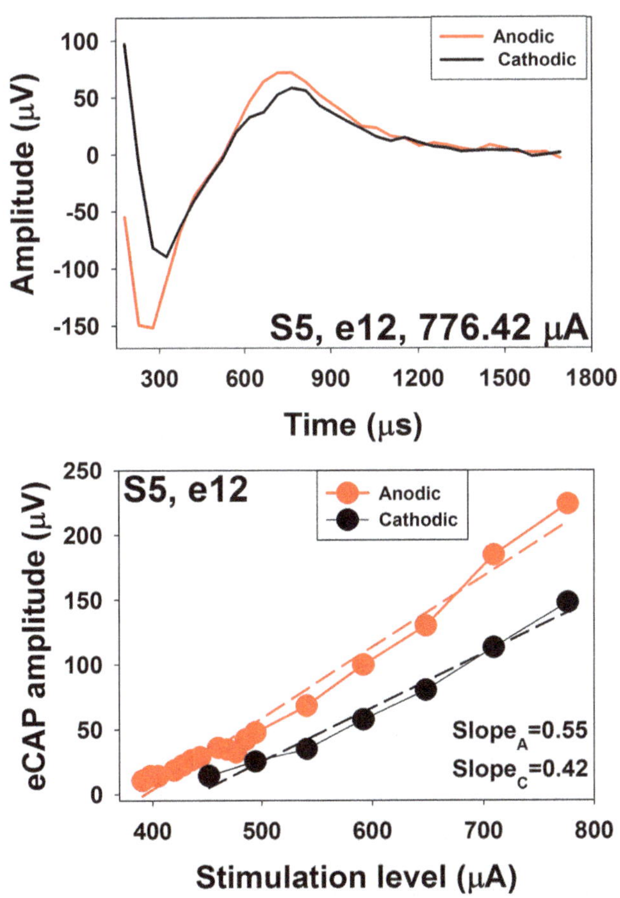

FIGURE 14 | eCAP waveforms and I/O functions measured using stimuli with reversed polarities at electrode 12 in S5.

1991; Rattay, 1999; Rattay et al., 2001; Joshi et al., 2017). In healthy auditory nerve fibers, both cathodic and anodic pulses activate peripheral processes to generate spikes at low stimulus level. At high stimulus level, the cathodic pulses still stimulate peripheral processes, whereas anodic stimuli inhibit peripheral processes and generate spikes at central axons. In cases where peripheral processes are absent or demyelinated, the only site that can be depolarized/activated by cathodic stimuli is the cell body (i.e., soma). Compared with the central axon, the soma has much higher threshold, which results in a higher cathodic threshold. In these cases, the excitability of the central axon to anodic stimuli at high stimulus levels is not affected. As a result, at an equal stimulus level, catholic-leading pulses are more effective at eliciting a neural response from intact human auditory nerve fibers, whereas anodic-leading pulses are more effective when peripheral processes are absent or demyelinated (Rattay, 1999; Rattay et al., 2001). Therefore, comparing the difference in eCAPs evoked by cathodic-leading vs anodic-leading pulses may provide useful information about neural survival of auditory nerve fibers (Undurraga et al., 2010).

Several studies have investigated polarity sensitivity of auditory nerve fibers using eCAP recordings in human CI users (Macherey et al., 2008; Undurraga et al., 2010, 2012; Glickman et al., 2016). Results of these studies suggested that auditory nerve fibers in human CI users were more sensitive to the anodic phase than the cathodic phase of the phasic pulse. Specifically, at a fixed stimulus level, eCAPs evoked by anodic-leading biphasic pulses show larger amplitudes and shorter latencies than those evoked by cathodic-leading biphasic pulses (Macherey et al., 2008; Undurraga et al., 2010; Glickman et al., 2016). In addition, eCAP I/O functions measured for anodic-leading stimuli have lower thresholds and steeper slopes than those measured for cathodic leading pulses (Undurraga et al., 2010; Glickman et al.,

2016). These results are consistent with the general belief that peripheral processes in deafened ears are demyelinated and degenerated (Fayad and Linthicum, 2006). The top panel of **Figure 14** shows an eCAP evoked by an anodic-cathodic pulse (red line) and an eCAP evoked by a cathodic-anodic pulse (black line) measured at electrode 12 in one child Cochlear 24RE CI user. It is apparent that the eCAP evoked by the anodic-leading pulse has a larger amplitude and shorter latency than that evoked by the cathodic-leading pulse. The bottom panel shows eCAP I/O functions measured for both polarities. Dashed lines show results of linear regression fits. Slopes of these functions are indicated in the low right corner. These results demonstrate that the eCAP I/O function of the anodic-leading pulse (red symbols) has lower threshold and steeper slope than that measured for the cathodic-leading pulse (black symbols). Despite these exciting and promising findings, the association between speech perception capability and polarity sensitivity has not been evaluated in human CI user.

CONCLUSIONS

This paper reviewed research efforts for investigating the utility of the eCAP in research and clinical practice, with an emphasis on new advances in knowledge and understanding that were gained within the last 10 years. Potential applications of the eCAP discussed in this paper include determining stimulus level, assessing spatial selectivity, evaluating temporal response properties and estimating neural survivals of auditory nerve fibers. It should be noted that substantial inter- and intra-subject variations across stimulating electrodes and/or pulse rates have been reported in all studies reviewed in this paper, which may reflect differences in the functional status of the neural populations that responded to electrical stimuli delivered by the CI. These variations highlight the importance of investigating to what extent differences in physioloigcal status of the auditory nerve can account for variations in auditory perception and speech perception across CI users and across stimulation sites within individual CI users. Despite these new exciting advances in our understanding of the eCAP, there are many questions that remain unknonwn. For example, it is unclear whether SOE functions measured using the eCAP can be used to determine which electrode should be used in programming MAPs for individual patients. In addition, the clinical and behavioral signfiance of different temporal response patterns of the auditory nerve remain unknown. Furthermore, whether difference in polarity sensitivity can be used to predict CI outcome for individual CI users remains unclear. These unknown questions provide exciting directions for future studies and leave room for developing new clinical applications for eCAP measures.

AUTHOR CONTRIBUTIONS

SH designed and is accountable for all aspects of this study, as well as drafted and approved the final version of this paper. HT and CB participated in study design and are accountable for all aspects of this study. They also provided critical revision and approved the final version of this paper.

FUNDING

This work was supported in parts by the R03 grant from NIH/NIDCD (1R03DC013153), and the pilot grant of Center for Perception and Communication in Children (COBRE) at Boys Town National Research Hospital from NIH/NIGMS (5P20 GM109023-03).

REFERENCES

Abbas, P. J., and Brown, C. J. (1988). Electrically evoked brainstem potentials in cochlear implant patients with multi-electrode stimulation. *Hear. Res.* 36, 153–162. doi: 10.1016/0378-5955(88)90057-3

Abbas, P. J., and Brown, C. J. (1991). Electrically evoked auditory brainstem response: refractory properties and strength-duration functions. *Hear. Res.* 51, 139–147. doi: 10.1016/0378-5955(91)90012-X

Abbas, P. J., and Brown, C. J. (2015). Assessment of responses to cochlear implant stimulation at different levels of the auditory pathway. *Hear. Res.* 322, 67–76. doi: 10.1016/j.heares.2014.10.011

Abbas, P. J., Brown, C. J., Shallop, J. K., Firszt, J. B., Hughes, M. L., Hong, S. H., et al. (1999). Summary of results using the nucleus CI24M implant to record the electrically evoked compound action potential. *Ear Hear.* 20, 45–59. doi: 10.1097/00003446-199902000-00005

Abbas, P. J., Hughes, M. L., Brown, C. J., Miller, C. A., and South, H. (2004). Channel interaction in cochlear implant users evaluated using the electrically evoked compound action potential. *Audiol. NeuroOtol.* 9, 203–213. doi: 10.1159/000078390

Abbas, P. J., Matsuoka, A. J., McDougall, V. M., Miller, C. A., and Rubinstein, J. T. (1998). "Compound action potentials in response to electrical amplitude-modulated pulse trains in the guinea pig auditory nerve," in *Paper presented at the Association for Research in Otolaryngology (ARO)*, Abstract #287.

Abbas, P. J., Miller, C. A., Rubinstein, J. T., and Hu, N. (2001). *The Neurophysiological Effects of Simulated Auditory Prosthesis Stimulation.* Eighth quarterly progress report, NIH contract N01-DC-9-2107.

Adel, Y., Hilkhuysen, G., Noreña, A., Cazals, Y., Roman, S., and Macherey, O. (2017). Forward masking in cochlear implant users: electrophysiological and psychophysical data using pulse train maskers. *J. Assoc. Res. Otolaryngol.* 18, 495–512. doi: 10.1007/s10162-016-0613-5

Avissar, M., Witting, J. H., Saunders, J. C., and Parsons, T. D. (2013). Refractoriness enhances temporal coding by auditory nerve fibers. *J. Neurosci.* 33, 7681–7690. doi: 10.1523/JNEUROSCI.3405-12.2013

Battmer, R. D., Lai, W. K., Dillier, N., Pesch, J., Killian, M. J., and Lenarz, T. (2005). "Correlation of NRT recovery function parameters and speech perception results for different stimulation rates," in *Fourth International Symposium and Workshops: Objective Measures in Cochlear Implants*, (Hannover).

Baudhuin, J. L., Hughes, M. L., and Goehring, J. L. (2016). A comparison of alternating polarity and forward masking artifact-reduction methods to resolve the electrically evoked compound action potentials. *Ear Hear.* 4, 247–255. doi: 10.1097/AUD.0000000000000288

Baudhuin, J., Cadieux, J., Firszt, J. B., Reeder, R. M., and Maxon, J. L. (2012). Optimization of programming parameters in children with the advanced bionics cochlear implant. *J. Am. Acad. Audiol.* 23, 302–312. doi: 10.3766/jaaa.23.5.2

Botros, A., and Psarros, C. (2010). Neural response telemetry reconsidered: II. The influence of neural population on the ECAP recovery function and refractoriness. *Ear Hear.* 31, 380–391. doi: 10.1097/AUD.0b013e3181cb41aa

Brill, S., Müller, J., Hagen, R., Möltner, A., Brockmeier, S. J., Startk, T., et al. (2009). Site of cochlear stimulation and its effect on electrically evoked compound action potentials using the MED-EL standard electrode array. *Biomed. Eng. Online* 16:40. doi: 10.1186/1475-925X-8-40

Brown, C. J., Abbas, P. J., and Gantz, B. (1990). Electrically evoked whole nerve action potentials: data from human cochlear implant users. *J. Acoust. Soc. Am.* 88, 1385–1391. doi: 10.1121/1.399716

Brown, C. J., Abbas, P. J., and Gantz, B. (1998). Preliminary experience with Neural Response Telemetry in the Nucleus CI24M cochlear implant. *Am. J. Otol.* 19, 320–327.

Brown, C. J., Abbas, P. J., Borland, J., and Bertschy, M. R. (1996). Electrically evoked whole number action potentials in Ineraid cochlear implant users: responses to different stimulating electrode configurations and comparison to psychophysical responses. *J. Speech Hear. Res.* 39, 453–467. doi: 10.1044/jshr.3903.453

Brown, C. J., Abbas, P. J., Etler, C. P., O'Brient, S., and Oleson, J. J. (2010). Effects of long-term use of a cochlear implant on the electrically evoked compound action potential. *J. Am. Acad. Audiol.* 21, 5–15. doi: 10.3766/jaaa.21.1.2

Brown, C. J., and Abbas, P. J. (1990). Electrically evoked whole-nerve action potentials: data from human cochlear implant users. *J. Acoust. Soc. Am.* 88, 1385–1391. doi: 10.1121/1.399716

Brown, C. J., Hughes, M. L., Luk, B., Abbas, P. J., Wolaver, A., and Gervais, J. (2000). The relationship between EAP and EABR thresholds and levels used to program the nucleus 24 speech processor: data from adults. *Ear Hear.* 21, 151–163. doi: 10.1097/00003446-200004000-00009

Cafarelli Dees, D., Dillier, N., Lai, W. K., von Wallenberg, E., van Dijk, B., Akdas, F., et al. (2005). Normative findings of electrically evoked compound action potential measurements using the neural response telemetry of the Nucleus CI24M cochlear implant system. *Audiol. Neurotol.* 10, 105–116. doi: 10.1159/000083366

Carlyon, R. P., and Deeks, J. M. (2015). Combined neural and behavioral measures of temporal pitch perception in cochlear implant users. *J. Acoust. Soc. Am.* 138, 2885–2905. doi: 10.1121/1.4934275

Cohen, L. T., Richardson, L. M., Saunders, E., and Cowan, R. S. C. (2003). Spatial spread of neural excitation in cochlear implant recipients: comparison of improved ECAP method and psychophysical forward masking. *Hear. Res.* 179, 72–87. doi: 10.1016/S0378-5955(03)00096-0

Davidson, L. S., Skinner, M. W., Holstad, B. A., Fears, B. T., Richter, M. K., Matusofsky, M., et al. (2009). The effects of instantaneous input dynamic rang setting on the speech perception of children with the Nucleus 24 implant. *Ear Hear.* 30, 340–349. doi: 10.1097/AUD.0b013e31819ec93a

Dawson, P. W., McKay, C. M., Busby, P. A., Grayden, D. B., and Clark, G. M. (2000). Electrode discrimination and speech perception in young children using cochlear implants. *Ear Hear.* 21, 597–607. doi: 10.1097/00003446-200012000-00007

Dawson, P. W., Vandali, A. E., Knight, M. R., and Heasman, J. M. (2007). Clinical evaluation of expanded input dynamic range in Nucleus cochlear implant. *Ear Hear.* 28, 163–176. doi: 10.1097/AUD.0b013e3180312651

Delgutte, B. (1980). Representation of speech-like sounds in the discharge patterns of auditory-nerve fibers. *J. Acoust. Soc. Am.* 68, 843–857. doi: 10.1121/1.384824

Delgutte, B. (1997). "Auditory neural processing of speech," in *The Handbook of Phonetic Sciences*, eds W. J. Hardcast and J. Laver (Hoboken, NJ: Blackwell Publishers), 507–538.

Delgutte, B., and Kiang, N. Y. S. (1984). Speech coding in the auditory nerve: IV. Sounds with consonant-like dynamic characteristics. *J. Acoust. Soc. Am.* 75, 897–907. doi: 10.1121/1.390599

DeVries, L., Scheperle, R., and Bierer, J. A. (2016). Assessing the electrode-neuron interface with the electrically evoked compound action potential, electrode position, and behavioral thresholds. *J. Assoc. Res. Otolaryngol.* 17, 237–252. doi: 10.1007/s10162-016-0557-9

Dhuldhoya, A. D. (2013). *Characterization of Temporal Interactions in the Auditory Nerve of Adult and Pediatric Cochlear Implant Users*. Ph.D. thesis, The University of Iowa.

Eisen, M. D., and Franck, K. H. (2004). Electrically evoked compound action potential amplitude growth functions and HiResolution programming levels in pediatric CII implant users. *Ear Hear.* 25, 528–538. doi: 10.1097/00003446-200412000-00002

Eisen, M. D., and Franck, K. H. (2005). Electrode interaction in pediatric cochlear implant subjects. *J. Assoc. Res. Otolaryngol.* 6, 160–170. doi: 10.1007/s10162-005-5057-2

Fayad, J. N., and Linthicum, F. H. Jr. (2006). Multichannel cochlear implants: relation of histopathology to performance. *Laryngoscope* 116, 1310–1320. doi: 10.1097/01.mlg.0000227176.09500.28

Finley, C. C., Holden, L. K., Holden, T. A., and Firszt, J. B. (2013). "Monopolar-coupled, ectopic stimulation in cochlear implants," in *Conference on Implantable Auditory Prostheses*, (Lake Tahoe, CA).

Finley, C. C., Wilson, B., van den Honert, C., and Lawson, D. (1997). *Speech Processors for Auditory Prostheses*. Sixth Quarterly Progress Report, NIH Project N01-DC-5-2103.

Firszt, J. B., Holden, L. K., Skinner, M. W., Tobey, E. A., Peterson, A., Gaggl, W., et al. (2004). Recognition of speech presented at soft to loud levels by adult cochlear implant recipients of three cochlear implant systems. *Ear Hear.* 25, 375–387. doi: 10.1097/01.AUD.0000134552.22205.EE

Franck, K. H., and Norton, S. J. (2001). Estimation of psychophysical levels using the electrically evoked compound action potential measured using the neural response telemetry capabilities of Cochlear Corporation's CI24M device. *Ear Hear.* 22, 289–299. doi: 10.1097/00003446-200108000-00004

Friesen, L. M., Shannon, R. V., and Cruz, R. J. (2005). Effects of stimulation rate on speech recognition with cochlear implants. *Audiol. Neurotol.* 10, 169–184. doi: 10.1159/000084027

Friesen, L. M., Shannon, R. V., Baskent, D., and Wang, X. (2001). Speech recognition in noise as a function of the number of spectral channels: comparison of acoustic hearing and cochlear implants. *J. Acoust. Soc. Am.* 110, 1150–1163. doi: 10.1121/1.1381538

Frijns, J. H., Briaire, J. J., de Laat, J. A., and Grote, J. J. (2002). Initial evaluation of the Clarion CII cochlear implant: speech perception and neural response imaging. *Ear Hear.* 23, 184–197. doi: 10.1097/00003446-200206000-00003

Fu, Q. J., and Nogaki, G. (2004). Noise susceptibility of cochlear implant users: the role of spectral resolution and smearing. *J. Assoc. Res. Otolaryngol.* 6, 19–27. doi: 10.1007/s10162-004-5024-3

Fu, Q. J., and Shannon, R. V. (2000). Effect of stimulation rate on phoneme recognition by nucleus-22 cohclear implant listeners. *J. Acoust. Soc. Am.* 107, 589–597. doi: 10.1121/1.428325

Fu, Q. J., Shannon, R. V., and Wang, X. S. (1998). Effects of noise and spectral resolution on vowel and consonant recognition: acoustic and electric hearing. *J. Acoust. Soc. Am.* 104, 3586–3596. doi: 10.1121/1.423941

Fulmer, S. L., Runge, C., Jensen, J. W., and Friedland, D. R. (2011). Rate of neural recovery in implanted children with auditory neuropathy spectrum disorder. *Otolaryngol. Head Neck Surg.* 144, 274–279. doi: 10.1177/0194599810391603

Game, C., Gibson, W., and Pauka, C. (1987). Electrically evoked brainstem auditory potential. *Ann. Otol. Rhinol. Laryngol.* 96, 94–95. doi: 10.1177/00034894870960S150

Gantz, B. J., Tyler, R. S., Woodworth, G. G., Tye-Murray, N., and Fryauf-Bertschy, H. (1994). Results of multichannel cochlear implants in congenital and acquired prelingual deafness in children: five-year follow-up. *Am. J. Otol.* 15, 1–7.

Garadat, S. N., Zwolan, T. A., and Pfingst, B. E. (2012). Across-site patterns of modulation detection: relation to speech recognition. *J. Acoust. Soc. Am.* 131, 4030–4041. doi: 10.1121/1.3701879

Garadat, S. N., Zwolan, T. A., and Pfingst, B. E. (2013). Using temporal modulation sensitivity to select stimulation sites for processor MAPs in cochlear implant listeners. *Audiol. Neurootol.* 18, 247–260. doi: 10.1159/000351302

Glickman, E. E., Hughes, M. L., Goehring, J. L., and Miller, M. (2016). "Effect of interphase gap and polarity in cochlear implant," in *American Auditory Society Scientific and Technology Meeting*, (Scottsdale, AZ).

Goldstein, M. H., and Kiang, N. Y. S. (1958). Synchrony of neural activity in electric response evoked by transient acoustic stimuli. *J. Acoust. Soc. Am.* 30, 107–114. doi: 10.1121/1.1909497

Gordon, K. A., Ebinger, K. A., Gilden, J. E., and Shapiro, W. H. (2002). Neural response telemetry in 12- and 24-month-old children. *Ann. Otol. Rhinol. Laryngol.* 189, 42–48. doi: 10.1177/00034894021110S509

Gordon, K. A., Papsin, B. C., and Harrison, R. V. (2004). Toward a battery of behavioral and objective measures to achieve optimal cochlear implant stimulation levels in children. *Ear Hear.* 25, 447–463. doi: 10.1097/01.aud.0000146178.84065.b3

Han, D. M., Chen, X. Q., Zhao, X. T., Kong, Y., Li, Y. X., Liu, S., et al. (2005). Comparison between neural response imaging thresholds, electrically evoked auditory reflex thresholds and most comfortable loudness levels in CII bionic ear users with HiResolution sound processing strategies. *Acta Otolaryngol.* 125, 732–735. doi: 10.1080/00016480510026890

Hay-McCutcheon, M., Brown, C. J., and Abbas, P. J. (2005). An analysis of the impact of auditory-nerve adaptation on behavioral measures of temporal integration in cochlear implant recipients. *J. Acoust. Soc. Am.* 118, 2444–2457. doi: 10.1121/1.2035593

He, S., Abbas, P. J., Doyle, D. V., McFayden, T. C., and Mulherin, S. (2016a). Temporal response properties of the auditory nerve in children with auditory neuropathy spectrum disorder and implanted children with sensorineural hearing loss. *Ear Hear.* 37, 397–411. doi: 10.1097/AUD.0000000000000254

He, S., McFayden, T. C., and Lopomo, P. (2016b). "Age-related changes in temporal responsiveness of the auditory nerve," in *The 39th Annual MidWinter Meeting of Association of Research in Otolaryngology*, (San Diego, CA).

He, S., Shahsavarani, B. S., McFayden, T. C., Wang, H., Gill, K. E., Xu, L., et al. (2017). Responsiveness of the electrically stimulated auditory nerve in children with cochlear nerve deficiency. *Ear Hear* (Accepted).

Henry, B. A., and Turner, C. W. (2003). The resolution of complex spectral patterns by cochlear implant and normal-hearing listeners. *J. Acoust. Soc. Am.* 113, 2861–2873. doi: 10.1121/1.1561900

Henry, B. A., McKay, C. M., McDermott, H. J., and Clark, G. M. (2000). The relationship between speech perception and electrode discrimination in cochlear implantee. *J. Acoust. Soc. Am.* 108, 1269–1280. doi: 10.1121/1.1287711

Henry, B. A., Turner, C. W., and Behrens, A. (2005). Spectral peak resoltuion and speech recognition in quiet: normal hearing, hearing impaired, and cochlear implant users. *J. Acoust. Soc. Am.* 118, 1111–1121. doi: 10.1121/1.1944567

Holden, L. K., Reeder, R. M., Firszt, J. B., and Finley, C. C. (2011). Optimizing the perception of soft speech and speech in noise with the Advanced Bionics cochlear implant system. *Int. J. Audiol.* 50, 255–269. doi: 10.3109/14992027.2010.533200

Holden, L. K., Skinner, M. W., Fourakis, M. S., and Holden, T. A. (2007). Effects of increased IIDR in the Nucleus Freedom cochlear implant system. *J. Am. Acad. Audiol.* 18, 778–791. doi: 10.3766/jaaa.18.9.6

Holstad, B. A., Sonneveldt, V. G., Fears, B. T., Davidson, L. S., Aaron, R. J., Richter, M., et al. (2009). Relation of electrically evoked compound action potential thresholds to behavioral T- and C-levels in children with cochlear implants. *Ear Hear.* 30, 115–127. doi: 10.1097/AUD.0b013e3181906c0f

Hughes, M. L. (2008). A re-evaluation of the relation between physiological channel interaction and electrode pitch ranking in cochlear implants. *J. Acoust. Soc. Am.* 124, 2711–2714. doi: 10.1121/1.2990710

Hughes, M. L., and Abbas, P. J. (2006). The relation between electrophysiologic channel interaction and electrode pitch ranking in cochlear implant recipients. *J. Acoust. Soc. Am.* 119, 1527–1537. doi: 10.1121/1.2163273

Hughes, M. L., and Goulson, A. M. (2011). Electrically evoked compound action potential measures for virtual channels versus physical electrodes. *Ear Hear.* 32, 323–330. doi: 10.1097/AUD.0b013e3182008c56

Hughes, M. L., and Stille, L. J. (2008). Psychophysical versus physiological spatial forward masking and the relation to speech perception in cochlear implants. *Ear Hear.* 29, 435–452. doi: 10.1097/AUD.0b013e31816a0d3d

Hughes, M. L., Baudhuin, J. L., and Goehring, J. L. (2014). The relation between auditory-nerve temporal responses and perceptual rate integration in cochlear implants. *Hear. Res.* 316, 44–56. doi: 10.1016/j.heares.2014.07.007

Hughes, M. L., Brown, C. J., Abbas, P. J., Wolaver, A. A., and Gervais, J. P. (2000). Comparison of ECAP thresholds with MAP levels in the nucleus 24 cochlear implant: data from children. *Ear Hear.* 21, 164–174. doi: 10.1097/00003446-200004000-00010

Hughes, M. L., Castioni, E. E., Goehring, J. L., and Baudhuin, J. L. (2012). Temporal response properties of the auditory nerve: data from human cochlear-implant recipients. *Hear. Res.* 285, 46–57. doi: 10.1016/j.heares.2012.01.010

James, C. J., Skinner, M. W., Martin, L. F., Holden, L. K., Galvin, K. L., Holden, T. A., et al. (2003). An investigation of input level range for the nucleus 24 cochlear implant system: speech perception performance, program preference, and loudness comfort ratings. *Ear Hear.* 24, 157–174. doi: 10.1097/01.AUD.0000058107.64929.D6

Jeng, F., Abbas, P. J., Hu, N., Miller, C. A., Nourski, K. V., and Robinson, B. K. (2009). Effects of temporal properties on compound action potentials in response to amplitude-modulated electric pulse trains in guinea pigs. *Hear. Res.* 247, 47–59. doi: 10.1016/j.heares.2008.10.007

Jeon, E. K., Brown, C. J., Etler, C. P., O'Brien, S., Chiou, L. K., and Abbas, P. J. (2010). Comparison of electrically evoked compound action potential thresholds and loudness estimates for the stimuli used to program the Advanced Bionics cochlear implant. *J. Am. Acad. Audiol.* 21, 16–27. doi: 10.3766/jaaa.21.1.3

Jeon, E. K., Turner, C. W., Karsten, S. A., Henry, B. A., and Gantz, B. J. (2015). Cochlear implant user's spectral ripple resolution. *J. Acoust. Soc. Am.* 138, 2350–2358. doi: 10.1121/1.4932020

Jones, G. L., Won, J. H., Drennan, W. R., and Rubinstein, J. T. (2013). Relationship between channel interaction and spectral-ripple discrimination in cochlear implant users. *J. Acoust. Soc. Am.* 133, 425–433. doi: 10.1121/1.4768881

Joshi, S. N., Dau, T., and Epp, B. (2017). A model of electrically stimulated auditory nerve fiber responses with peripheral and central site of spike generation. *J. Assoc. Res. Otolaryngol.* 18, 323–342. doi: 10.1007/s10162-016-0608-2

Kashio, A., Tejani, V. D., Scheperle, R. A., Brown, C. J., and Abbas, P. J. (2016). Exploring the source of neural response of different latencies obtained from different recording electrodes in cochlear implant users. *Audiol. Neurotol.* 21, 141–149. doi: 10.1159/000444739

Kiefer, J., Hohl, S., Stürzebecher, E., Pfennigdorff, T., and Gstöettner, W. (2001). Comparison of speech recognition with different speech coding strategies (SPEAK, CIS, and ACE) and their relationship to telemetric measure of compound action potentials in the nucleus CI 24M cochlear implant system. *Audiology* 40, 32–42. doi: 10.3109/00206090109073098

Kim, J. R., Abbas, P. J., Brown, C. J., Etler, C. P., O'Brien, S., and Kim, L. S. (2010). The relationship between electrically evoked compound action potential and speech perception: a study in cochlear implant users with short electrode array. *Otol. Neurotol.* 31, 1041–1048. doi: 10.1097/MAO.0b013e3181ec1d92

Kirby, A. E., and Middlebrooks, J. C. (2010). Auditory temporal acuity probed with cochlear implant stimulation and cortical recording. *J. Neurophysiol.* 103, 531–542. doi: 10.1152/jn.00794.2009

Kirby, A. E., and Middlebrooks, J. C. (2012). Unanesthetized auditory cortex exhibits multiple codes for gaps in cochlear implant pulse trains. *J. Assoc. Res. Otolaryngol.* 13, 67–80. doi: 10.1007/s10162-011-0293-0

Lai, W. K., and Dillier, N. (2000). A simple two-component model of the electrically evoked compound action potential in the human cochlea. *Audiol. Neurotol.* 5, 333–345. doi: 10.1159/000013899

Lee, E. R., Friedland, D. R., and Runge, C. L. (2012). Recovery from forward masking in elderly cochlear implant users. *Otol. Neurotol.* 33, 355–363. doi: 10.1097/MAO.0b013e318248ede5

Litvak, L. M., Spahr, A. J., Saoji, A. A., and Fridman, G. Y. (2007). Relationship between perception of spectral ripple and speech recognition in cochlear implant and vocoder listeners. *J. Acoust. Soc. Am.* 122, 982–991. doi: 10.1121/1.2749413

Loizou, P. C., and Poroy, O. (2001). Minimum spectral constrast needed for vowel identification by normal hearing and cochlear implant listeners. *J. Acoust. Soc. Am.* 110, 1619–1627. doi: 10.1121/1.1388004

Loizou, P. C., Poroy, O., and Dorman, M. (2000). The effect of parametric variations of cohclear implant processors on speech understanding. *J. Acoust. Soc. Am.* 108, 790–802. doi: 10.1121/1.429612

Long, C. J., Holden, T. A., McClelland, G. H., Parkinson, W. S., Shelton, C., Kelsall, D. C., et al. (2014). Examining the electro-neural interface of cochlear implant users using psychophysics, CT scans, and speech understanding. *J. Assoc. Res. Otolarynogol.* 15, 293–304. doi: 10.1007/s10162-013-0437-5

Macherey, O., Carlyon, R. P., van Wieringen, A., Deeks, J. M., and Wouters, J. (2008). Higher sensitivity of human auditory nerve fibers to positive electrical currents. *J. Assoc. Res. Otolaryngol.* 9, 241–251. doi: 10.1007/s10162-008-0112-4

Macherey, O., van Wieringen, A., Carlyon, R. P., Deeks, J. M., and Wouters, J. (2006). Asymmetric pulses in cochlear implants: effects of pulse shape, polarity and rate. *J. Assoc. Res. Otolaryngol.* 7, 253–266. doi: 10.1007/s10162-006-0040-0

Matsuoka, A. J., Abbas, P. J., Rubinstein, J. T., and Miller, C. A. (2000a). The neuronal response to electrical constant-amplitude pulse train stimulation: evoked compound action potential recordings. *Hear. Res.* 149, 115–128. doi: 10.1016/S0378-5955(00)00172-6

Matsuoka, A. J., Abbas, P. J., Rubinstein, J. T., and Miller, C. A. (2000b). The neuronal response to electrical constant-amplitude pulse train stimulation: additive Gaussian noise. *Hear. Res.* 149, 129–137. doi: 10.1016/S0378-5955(00)00173-8

McKay, C. M., and McDermott, H. J. (1998). Loudness perception with pulsatile electrical stimulation: the effect of interpulse intervals. *J. Acoust. Soc. Am.* 104, 1061–1074. doi: 10.1121/1.423316

McKay, C. M., Chandan, K., Akhoun, I., Siciliano, C., and Kluk, K. (2013). Can ECAP measures be used for totally objective programming of cochlear implants? *J. Assoc. Res. Otolaryngol.* 14, 879–890. doi: 10.1007/s10162-013-0417-9

McKay, C. M., Fewster, L., and Dawson, P. (2005). A different approach to using neural response telemetry for automated cochlear implant processor programming. *Ear Hear.* 26, 38S–44S. doi: 10.1097/00003446-200508001-00006

Miller, C. A., Abbas, P. J., and Brown, C. J. (2000). An improved method of reducing stimulus artifact in the electrically evoked whole-nerve potential. *Ear Hear.* 21, 280–290. doi: 10.1097/00003446-200008000-00003

Miller, C. A., Abbas, P. J., and Robinson, B. K. (1994). The use of long-duration current pulses to assess nerve survival. *Hear. Res.* 78, 11–26. doi: 10.1016/0378-5955(94)90039-6

Miller, C. A., Abbas, P. J., and Robinson, B. K. (2001). Response properties of the refractory auditory nerve fiber. *J. Assoc. Res. Otolaryngol.* 2, 216–232. doi: 10.1007/s101620010083

Miller, C. A., Abbas, P. J., Hay-McCutcheon, M. J., Robinson, B. K., Nourski, K. V., and Jeng, F. C. (2004). Intracochlear and extracochlear ECAPs suggest andidromic action potentials. *Hear. Res.* 198, 75–86. doi: 10.1016/j.heares.2004.07.005

Miller, C. A., Abbas, P. J., Rubinstein, J. T., Robinson, B. K., Matsuoka, A. J., and Woodworth, G. (1998). Electrically evoked compound action potentials of guinea pig and cat: responses to monopolar, monophasic stimulation. *Hear. Res.* 119, 142–154. doi: 10.1016/S0378-5955(98)00046-X

Miller, C. A., Brown, C. J., Abbas, P. J., and Chi, S. L. (2008a). The clinical application of potentials evoked from the peripheral auditory system. *Hear. Res.* 242, 184–197. doi: 10.1016/j.heares.2008.04.005

Miller, C. A., Hu, N., Zhang, F., and Abbas, P. J. (2008b). Changes across time in the temporal responses of auditory nerve fibers stimulated by electric pulse trains. *J. Assoc. Res. Otolaryngol.* 9, 122–137. doi: 10.1007/s10162-007-0108-5

Miller, C. A., Woo, J., Abbas, P. J., Hu, N., and Robinson, B. K. (2011). Neural masking by sub-threshold electric stimuli: animal and computer model results. *J. Assoc. Res. Otolaryngol.* 12, 219–232. doi: 10.1007/s10162-010-0249-9

Mino, H., and Rubinstein, J. T. (2006). Effects of neural refractoriness on spatio-temporal variability in spike initiations with electrical stimulation. *IEEE Trans. Neural Syst. Rehabil. Eng.* 14, 273–280. doi: 10.1109/TNSRE.2006.881590

Miyamoto, R., and Brown, D. (1987). Electrically evoked brainstem responses in cochlear implant recipients. *Otolaryngol. Head Neck Surg.* 96, 34–38. doi: 10.1177/019459988709600106

Morsnowski, A., Charasse, B., Collet, L., Killian, M., and Müller-Deile, J. (2006). Measuring the refractoriness of the electrically stimulated auditory nerve. *Audiol. Neurotol.* 11, 389–402. doi: 10.1159/000095966

Nelson, D. A., and Donaldson, G. S. (2002). Psychophysical recovery from pulse-train forward masking in electrical hearing. *J. Acoust. Soc. Am.* 112, 2932–2947. doi: 10.1121/1.1514935

Noble, J. H., Labadie, R. F., Gifford, R. H., and Dawant, B. M. (2013). Image-guidance enables new methods for customizing cochlear implant stimulation strategies. *IEEE Trans. Neural Syst. Rehabil. Eng.* 21, 820–829. doi: 10.1109/TNSRE.2013.2253333

Nourski, K. V., Abbas, P. J., Miller, C. A., Robinson, B. K., and Jen, F. C. (2007). Acoustic-electric interactions in the guinea pig auditory nerve: simultaneous and forward masking of the electrically evoked compound action potential. *Hear. Res.* 232, 87–103. doi: 10.1016/j.heares.2007.07.001

Pesch, J., Lai, W. K., Killian, M., Lenarz, T., and Battmer, R. D. (2005). "Characteristics of NRT^{TM} recovery functions for different stimulation parameters," in *2005 Conference on Implantable Auditory Prostheses*, (Lake Tahoe, CA).

Pfingst, B. E., Colesa, D. J., Watts, M. M., Su, G. L., Budenz, C. L., and Raphael, Y. (2014). Neurotrophin gene therapy in deafened ears with cochlear implants: long-term effects on nerve survival and functional measures. *Assoc. Res. Otolaryngol. Abs.* 37, 174.

Pfingst, B. E., Hughes, A. P., Colesa, D. J., Watts, M. M., Strahl, S. B., and Raphael, Y. (2015b). Insertion trauma and recovery of function after cochlear implantation: evidence from objective functional measures. *Hear. Res.* 330, 98–105. doi: 10.1016/j.heares.2015.07.010

Pfingst, B. E., Zhou, N., Colesa, D. J., Watts, M. M., Strahl, S. B., Garadat, S. N., et al. (2015a). Importance of cochlear health for implant function. *Hear. Res.* 322, 77–88. doi: 10.1016/j.heares.2014.09.009

Polak, M., Hodges, A. V., King, J. E., and Balkany, T. J. (2004). Further prospective findings with compound action potentials from Nucleus 24 cochlear implants. *Hear. Res.* 188, 104–116. doi: 10.1016/S0378-5955(03)00309-5

Potts, L. G., Skinner, M. W., Gotter, B. D., Strube, M. J., and Brenner, C. A. (2007). Relation between neural response telemetry thresholds, T- and C-levels, and loudness judgements in 12 adult nucleus 24 cochlear implant recipients. *Ear Hear.* 28, 495–511. doi: 10.1097/AUD.0b013e31806dc16e

Prado-Guitierrez, P., Fewster, L. M., Heasman, J. M., McKay, C. M., and Shepherd, R. K. (2006). Effect of interphase gap and pulse duration on electrically evoked potentials is correlated with auditory nerve survival. *Hear. Res.* 215, 47–55. doi: 10.1016/j.heares.2006.03.006

Ramekers, D., Versnel, H., Strahl, S. B., Smeets, E. M., Klis, S. F., and Grolman, W. (2014). Auditory-nerve responses to varied inter-phase gap and phase duration of the electric pulse stimulus as predictors for neuronal degeneration. *J. Assoc. Res. Otolaryngol.* 15, 187–202. doi: 10.1007/s10162-013-0440-x

Rattay, F. (1999). The basic mechanism for the electrical stimulation of the nervous system. *Neuroscience* 89, 335–346. doi: 10.1016/S0306-4522(98)00330-3

Rattay, F., Lutter, P., and Felix, H. (2001). A model of the electrically excited human cochlear neuron. *I.* Contribution of neural substructures to the generation and propagation of spikes. *Hear. Res.* 153, 43–63. doi: 10.1016/S0378-5955(00)00256-2

Rubinstein, J. T. (1991). Analytical theory for extracellular electrical stimulation of nerve with focal electrodes. II. Passive myelinated axon. *Bioyphys. J.* 60, 538–555. doi: 10.1016/S0006-3495(91)82084-7

Rubinstein, J. T., Wilson, B. S., Finley, C. C., and Abbas, P. J. (1999). Pseudospontaneous activity: stochastic independence of auditory nerve fibers with electrical stimulation. *Hear. Res.* 127, 108–118. doi: 10.1016/S0378-5955(98)00185-3

Scheperle, R. A., and Abbas, P. J. (2015a). Peripheral and central contributions to cortical responses in cochlear implant users. *Ear Hear.* 36, 430–440. doi: 10.1097/AUD.0000000000000143

Scheperle, R. A., and Abbas, P. J. (2015b). Relationships among peripheral and central electrophysiological measures of spatial and spectral selectivity and speech perception in cochlear implant users. *Ear Hear.* 36, 441–453. doi: 10.1097/AUD.0000000000000144

Schvartz-Leyzac, K. C., and Pfingst, B. E. (2016). Across-site patterns of electrically evoked compound action potential amplitude-growth functions in multichannel cochlear implant recipients and the effects of the interphase gap. *Hear. Res.* 341, 50–65. doi: 10.1016/j.heares.2016.08.002

Seyle, K., and Brown, C. J. (2002). Speech perception using maps based on neural response telemetry measures. *Ear Hear.* 23(Suppl.), 72S–79S. doi: 10.1097/00003446-200202001-00009

Shepherd, R. K., and Javel, E. (1999). Electrical stimulation of the auditory nerve: II. Effect of stimulus waveshape on single fibre *response properties.* Hear. Res. 130, 171–188. doi: 10.1016/S0378-5955(99)00011-8

Shepherd, R. K., Hatsushika, S., and Clark, G. M. (1993). Electrical stimulation of the auditory nerve: the effect of electrode position on neural excitation. *Hear. Res.* 66, 108–120. doi: 10.1016/0378-5955(93)90265-3

Shepherd, R. K., Roberts, L. A., and Paolini, A. G. (2004). Long-term sensorineural hearing loss induces functional changes in the rat auditory nerve. *Eur. J. Neurosci.* 20, 3131–3140. doi: 10.1111/j.1460-9568.2004.03809.x

Shpak, T. (2005). "Correlation between rate preference and NRT," in *12th NRT Research Workshop* (Hannover).

Shpak, T., Berlin, M., and Luntz, M. (2004). Objective measurements of auditory nerve recovery function in Nucleus CI24 implantees in relation to subjective preference of sitmuluation rate. *Acta Otolaryngol.* 124, 679–683. doi: 10.1080/00016480310002168

Skinner, M. W., Arndt, P. L., and Staller, S. J. (2002). Nucleus 24 advanced encoder conversion study: performance versus preference. *Ear Hear.* 23, 2S–17S. doi: 10.1097/00003446-200202001-00002

Skinner, M. W., Holden, L. K., and Holden, T. A. (1997). Speech recognition at simulated soft, conversational and raised-to-loud vocal efforts by adults with cochlear implants. *J. Acoust. Soc. Am.* 101, 3766–3782. doi: 10.1121/1.418383

Skinner, M. W., Holden, L. K., Holden, T. A., and Demorest, M. E. (1999). Comparison of two methods for selecting minimum stimulation levels used in programming the Nucleus 22 cochlear implant. *J. Speech Lang. Hear. Res.* 42, 814–828. doi: 10.1044/jslhr.4204.814

Smith, R. L. (1977). Short-term adaptation in single auditory nerve fibers: some poststimulatory effects. *Neurophysiology* 40, 1098–1112.

Smoorenburg, G. F., Willeboer, C., and van Dijk, J. E. (2002). Speech perception in Nucleus CI24M cochlear implant users with processor settings based on electrically evoked compound action potential thresholds. *Audiol. Neurotol.* 7, 335–347. doi: 10.1159/000066154

Snel-Bongers, J., Briaire, J. J., Vanpoucke, F. J., and Frijns, J. H. (2012). Spread of excitation and channel interaction in single- and dual-electrode cochlear implant stimulation. *Ear Hear.* 33, 367–376. doi: 10.1097/AUD.0b013e318234efd5

Spahr, A. J., Dorman, M. F., and Loiselle, L. H. (2007). Performance of patients using different cochlear implant systems: effects of input dynamic range. *Ear Hear.* 28, 260–275. doi: 10.1097/AUD.0b013e3180312607

Stypulkowski, P. H., and van den Honert, C. (1984). Physiological properties of the electrically stimulated auditory nerve. I. Compound action potential recordings. *Hear. Res.* 14, 205–223. doi: 10.1016/0378-5955(84)90051-0

Tejani, V. D., Abbas, P. J., and Brown, C. J. (2017). Relationship between peripheral and psychophysical measures of amplitude modulation detection in cochlear implant users. *Ear Hear.* doi: 10.1097/AUD.0000000000000417. [Epub ahead of print].

Thai-Van, H., Chanal, J. M., Coudert, C., Veuillet, E., Truy, E., and Collet, L. (2001). Relationship between NRT measurements and behavioral levels in children with the Nucleus 24 cochlear implant array over time: preliminary report. *Int. J. Pediatr. Otorhinolaryngol.* 58, 153–162. doi: 10.1016/S0165-5876(01)00426-8

Thai-Van, H., Truy, E., Charasse, B., Boutitie, F., Chanal, J. M., Cochard, N., et al. (2004). Modeling the relationship between psychophysical perception and electrically evoked compound action potential threshold in young cochlear implant recipients: clinical implications for implant fitting. *Clin. Neurophysiol.* 115, 2811–2824. doi: 10.1016/j.clinph.2004.06.024

Throckmorton, C. S., and Collins, L. M. (1999). Investigation of the effects of temporal and spatial interactions on speech-recognition skills in cochlear-implant subjects. *J. Acoust. Soc. Am.* 105, 861–873. doi: 10.1121/1.426275

Turner, C., Mehr, M., Hughes, M., Brown, C., and Abbas, P. (2002). Within-subject predictors of speech recognition in cochlear implants: a null result. *Acoust. Res. Lett. Online* 3, 95–100. doi: 10.1121/1.1477875

Undurraga, J. A., Carlyon, R. P., Macherey, O., Wouters, J., and van Wieringen, A. (2012). Spread of excitation varies for different electrical pulse shapes and stimulation modes in cochlear implants. *Hear. Res.* 290, 21–36. doi: 10.1016/j.heares.2012.05.003

Undurraga, J. A., van Wieringen, A., Carlyon, R. P., Macherey, O., and Wouters, J. (2010). Polarity effects on neural responses of the electrically stimulated auditory nerve at different cochlear sites. *Hear. Res.* 269, 146–161. doi: 10.1016/j.heares.2010.06.017

van de Heyning, P., Arauz, S. L., Atlas, M., Baumgartner, W. D., Caversaccio, M., Chester-Browne, R., et al. (2016). Electrically evoked compound action potentials are different depending on the site of cochlear stimulation. *Cochlear Implants Int.* 17, 251–262. doi: 10.1080/14670100.2016.1240427

van de Honert, C., and Stypulkowski, P. H. (1986). Characterization of the electrically evoked auditory brainstem response (EABR) in cats and humans. *Hear. Res.* 21, 109–126. doi: 10.1016/0378-5955(86)90033-X

van den Honert, C., and Stypulkowski, P. H. (1984). Physiologic properties of the electrically stimulated auditory nerve. II. Single fiber recordings. *Hear Res.* 14, 225–243. doi: 10.1016/0378-5955(84)90052-2

van der Beek, F. B., Briaire, J. J., and Frijns, J. H. (2015). Population-based prediction of fitting levels for individual cochlear implant recipients. *Audiol. Neurootol.* 20, 1–16. doi: 10.1159/000362779

van der Beek, F. B., Briaire, J. J., and Frijns, J. H. (2012). Effects of parameter manipulations on spread of excitation measured with electrically evoked compound action potentials. *Int. J. Audiol.* 51, 465–474. doi: 10.3109/14992027.2011.653446

Vandali, A. E., Whitford, L. A., Plant, K. L., and Clark, G. M. (2000). Speech perception as a function of electrical stimulation rate: using the Nucleus 24 cochlear implant system. *Ear Hear.* 21, 608–624. doi: 10.1097/00003446-200012000-00008

Viemeister, N. F., and Wakefield, G. H. (1991). Temporal integration and multiple looks. *J. Acoust. Soc. Am.* 90, 858–865. doi: 10.1121/1.401953

Weber, B. P., Lai, W. K., Dillier, N., von Wallenberg, E. L., Killian, M. J., Pesch, J., et al. (2007). Performance and preference for ACE stimulation rates obtained with nucleus RP 8 and freedom system. *Ear Hear.* 28, 46S–48S. doi: 10.1097/AUD.0b013e3180315442

Wiemes, G. R. M., Hamerschmidt, R., Moreira, A. T. R., de Fraqa, R., Tenório, S. B., and Carvalho, B. (2016). Auditory nerve recovery function in cochlear implant surgery with local anesthesia and sedation versus general anesthesia. *Audiol. Neurotol.* 21, 150–157. doi: 10.1159/000445098

Wilson, B. S., Finley, C. C., Lawson, D. T., and Zerbi, M. (1994). *Speech Processors for Auditory Prostheses.* NIH Project N01-DC-2-2401. Seventh Quarterly Progress Report.

Wilson, B. S., Finley, C. C., Lawson, D. T., and Zerbi, M. (1997). Temporal representations with cochlear implants. *Am. J. Otol.* 18, S30–S34.

Winn, M. B., and Litovsky, R. Y. (2015). Using speech sounds to test functional spectral resolution in listeners with cochlear implants. *J. Acoust. Soc. Am.* 137, 1430–1442. doi: 10.1121/1.4908308

Winn, M. B., Won, J. H., and Moon, I. J. (2016). Assessment of spectral and temporal resolution in cochlear implant users using psychoacoustic discrimination and speech cue categorization. *Ear Hear.* 37, e377–e390. doi: 10.1097/AUD.0000000000000328

Wolfe, J., and Kasulis, H. (2008). Relationships among objective measures and speech perception in adult users of the HiResolution bionic ear. *Cochlear Implant Int.* 9, 70–81. doi: 10.1179/cim.2008.9.2.70

Won, J. H., Drennan, W. R., and Rubinstein, J. T. (2007). spectral-ripple resolution correlates with speech reception in noise in cochlear implant users. *J. Assoc. Res. Otolaryngol.* 8, 384–392. doi: 10.1007/s10162-007-0085-8

Won, J. H., Humphrey, E. L., Yeager, K. R., Martinez, A. A., Robinson, C. H., Mills, K. E., et al. (2014). Relationship among the physiologic channel interactions, spectral-ripple discrimination, and vowel identification in cochlear implant users. *J. Acoust. Soc. Am.* 136, 2714–2725. doi: 10.1121/1.4895702

Zhang, F., Benson, C., Murphy, D., Boian, M., Scott, M., Keith, R., et al. (2013). Neural adaptation and behavioral measures of temporal processing and speech perception in cochlear implant recipients. *PLoS ONE* 8:e84631. doi: 10.1371/journal.pone.0084631

Zimmerling, M. J., and Hochmair, E. S. (2002). EAP recordings in ineraid patients–correlations with psychophysical measures and possible implications for patient fitting. *Ear Hear.* 23, 81–91. doi: 10.1097/00003446-200204000-00001

Zwolan, T. A., Collins, L. M., and Wakefield, G. H. (1997). Electrode discrimination and speech recognition in postlingually deafened adult cochlear implant subjects. *J. Acoust. Soc. Am.* 102, 3673–3685. doi: 10.1121/1.420401

8

Feasibility of Using Electrocochleography for Objective Estimation of Electro-Acoustic Interactions in Cochlear Implant Recipients with Residual Hearing

Kanthaiah Koka and Leonid M. Litvak*

Research and Technology, Advanced Bionics LLC, Valencia, CA, United States

***Correspondence:**
Kanthaiah Koka
kanthaiah.koka@advancedbionics.com

Although cochlear implants (CI) traditionally have been used to treat individuals with bilateral profound sensorineural hearing loss, a recent trend is to implant individuals with residual low-frequency hearing. Patients who retain some residual acoustic hearing after surgery often can benefit from electro-acoustic stimulation (EAS) technologies, which combine conventional acoustic amplification with electrical stimulation. However, interactions between acoustic and electrical stimulation may affect outcomes adversely and are time-consuming and difficult to assess behaviorally. This study demonstrated the feasibility of using the Advanced Bionics HiRes90K Advantage implant electronics and HiFocus Mid Scala/1j electrode to measure electrocochleography (ECochG) responses in the presence of electrical stimulation to provide an objective estimate of peripheral physiologic EAS interactions. In general, electrical stimulation reduced ECochG response amplitudes to acoustic stimulation. The degree of peripheral EAS interaction varied as a function of acoustic pure tone frequency and the intra-cochlear location of the electrically stimulated electrode. Further development of this technique may serve to guide and optimize clinical EAS system fittings in the future.

Keywords: residual hearing, cochlear implant, electrocochleography, ECochG, electro-acoustic stimulation, EAS and electro-acoustic interaction

INTRODUCTION

Because of advances in electrode array technology and surgical technique, patients with low-frequency residual acoustic hearing could benefit from cochlear implants (CI) (Balkany et al., 2006; Fraysse et al., 2006). Although some of these individuals lose their residual hearing completely after implant surgery, others can experience partial or full retention of their acoustic hearing (Radeloff et al., 2012; Dalbert et al., 2015). Subjects with residual hearing often can benefit from electro-acoustic stimulation (EAS) technologies, which combine conventional acoustic amplification with electrical stimulation (Von Ilberg et al., 1999; Turner et al., 2008).

One of the challenges in optimizing EAS benefit in individual patients is understanding the interactions between acoustic and electrical hearing. Psychometric studies indicate that acoustic thresholds can be increased in the presence of electrical stimulation, thereby suggesting peripheral electro-acoustic interactions (Lin et al., 2011). Systematic programming modifications such as switching off electrodes or using overlapping or non-overlapping cross-over frequencies also can characterize electro-acoustic interactions and suggest ways to improve benefit (Polak et al., 2010; Karsten et al., 2013). The drawback to these behavioral techniques is that they are subjective and require too much time, thereby making them impractical for clinical use.

Consequently, it would be valuable to take advantage of objective responses to help clinicians program EAS devices optimally. The electrically evoked compound action potential (ECAP) is a physiologic response that reflects auditory nerve activity and can serve as an objective measure of electro-acoustic interactions in the same ear (Abbas et al., 2002; Stronks et al., 2010, 2012). For example, Abbas et al. (2002) showed electro-acoustic interactions in cats with residual hearing. They observed secondary peaks in ECAP amplitudes and hypothesized that these peaks resulted from electrical stimulation of hair cells, often referred to as electrophonics. They also showed a decrease in ECAP amplitude in the presence of wide-band acoustic noise, thus indicating the presence of peripheral electro-acoustic interactions. Similarly, Stronks et al. (2012) observed a decrease in ECAP amplitude in the presence of broadband noise in guinea pigs.

Electrocochleography (ECochG) is a procedure that offers potential for assessing peripheral electro-acoustic interactions objectively. The ECochG response is comprised of electrical potentials generated by the hair cells and auditory nerve. The cochlear microphonic (CM) represents the combination of transducer currents primarily through the outer hair cell stereocilia (Dallos, 1973) and is known to follow the fine structure of the stimulus waveform. The auditory nerve neurophonic (ANN) is assumed to reflect the phase-locking activity of the auditory nerve fibers (Snyder and Schreiner, 1984; Lichtenhan et al., 2013; Fitzpatrick et al., 2014; Forgues et al., 2014). The compound action potential (CAP) is generated by the auditory nerve in response to the onset and offset of the acoustic stimulus, and the summating potential (SP) is the direct current part of the response with multiple generators.

To date, the ability to measure ECochG responses in the presence of electrical stimulation in CI recipients has been limited by CI hardware capability due to stimulus artifacts. However, the back-telemetry capability and fast-recovery amplifier in the Advanced Bionics (AB) HiRes90K® cochlear implant offers the opportunity to measure ECochG responses reliably and to explore the feasibility of using ECochG to assess peripheral electro-acoustic interactions. the AB device can record ECochG responses to low frequency pure tones. By calculating the *Difference response*, that is, the difference between responses to alternating stimulus polarities, the odd harmonics of the tone frequency are emphasized. This calculation reflects the components of the response that follow stimulus periodicity. This *Difference response* is dominated by the CM, but also includes the largest part of the ANN (Forgues et al., 2014). In contrast, by calculating the *Summation response*, that is, the sum of the responses to alternating stimulus polarities, the even harmonics of the tone frequency are emphasized. This calculation includes components of the response that do not change with stimulus phase and thus reflects asymmetric distortions in the CM and ANN. Because these distortions are greater in the ANN than the CM, the ongoing component of the *Summation response* can be dominated by the ANN, when it is present. However, this part of the ANN is only the distortions, and so is smaller than the part that appears in the difference response.

This study explored the feasibility of using ECochG to assess electro-acoustic interactions objectively in implanted subjects with residual hearing in the presence of electrical stimulation. The study focused particularly on using the fast-recovery amplifier in the AB HiRes90K® cochlear implant to measure ECochG responses. The objective of the study was to show that it is feasible to record the *Difference response* and the *Summation response* in the presence of electrical stimulus artifacts. These measurements then would provide a way to objectively estimate electro-acoustic interactions. A hypothesis that these objective electro-acoustic interactions correlate with behaviorally measured electro-acoustic interactions was tested.

METHODS

Two methods were used to explore the interaction between acoustic and electrical stimulation in CI recipients with residual hearing. Experiment 1 evaluated the feasibility of recording acoustic ECochG responses in the presence of electrical stimulation. Those responses then were used to estimate electro-acoustic interactions objectively. Experiment 2 assessed electro-acoustic interactions behaviorally by measuring changes in acoustic thresholds in presence of electrical stimulation. These behavioral interactions then were compared with the objective electro-acoustic interactions from Experiment 1.

Experiment 1

Objective

The aim of this experiment was to show the feasibility of recording acoustic ECochG responses in the presence of electrical stimulation. The *Difference response* amplitudes observed in presence of electrical stimulation were compared to baseline responses measured with no electrical stimulation to provide an objective estimation of electro-acoustic interactions.

Subjects

Twelve CI recipients with Advanced Bionics HiRes90K® cochlear implants and HiFocus MidScala® and 1J electrode arrays participated in this phase of the study. Eleven subjects were unilaterally implanted and one subject was a bilateral implant user, thereby yielding a total of 13 experimental ears. **Table 1** shows the subjects' implant devices, duration of implant use and experimental participation. **Figure 1** shows the pure-tone audiograms for these subjects, who exhibited different degrees of residual hearing. The etiology of the hearing loss is unknown for the group. All subjects provided written informed consent prior to participation. The study protocol (#20121035)

TABLE 1 | Subject demographics.

Subject ID	Implant Type	Electrode Type	Implant usage (yrs)	Exp 1	Exp 2
CI03	HiRes90K Advantage	MidScala	0.25	yes	yes
CI04L	HiRes90K Advantage	MidScala	1	yes	yes
CI04R	HiRes90K Advantage	MidScala	2	yes	yes
CI06	HiRes90K Advantage	MidScala	0.5	yes	yes
CI07	HiRes90K Advantage	MidScala	2	yes	no
CI08	HiRes90K Advantage	MidScala	1.67	yes	yes
CI09	HiRes90K Advantage	MidScala	1.5	yes	no
CI11	HiRes90K	HiFocus 1J	3	yes	no
CI12	HiRes90K Advantage	MidScala	1.5	yes	no
CI13	HiRes90K Advantage	MidScala	0.5	yes	yes
CI15	HiRes90K Advantage	MidScala	0.5	yes	yes
CI16	HiRes90K Advantage	MidScala	2	yes	no
CI19	HiRes90K Advantage	MidScala	1.5	yes	no

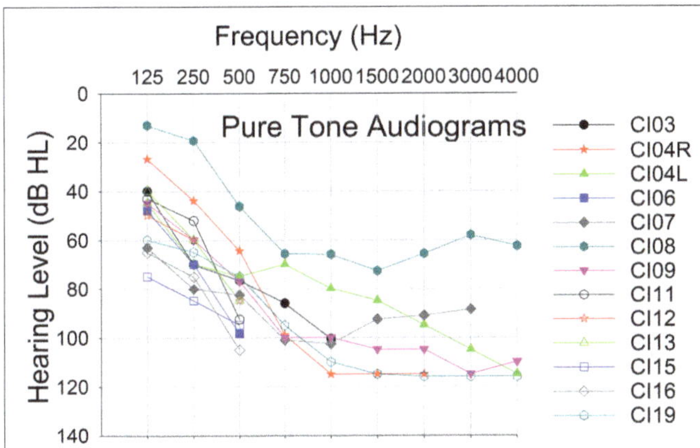

FIGURE 1 | Pure tone audiograms for 12 study participants.

was approved by the Western Institutional Review Board (WIRB).

Equipment

The stimulus delivery and measurement system for assessing ECochG responses was like that described in Koka et al. (2016). The Advanced Bionics' Bionic Ear Data Collection System (BEDCS) research software was used to control stimulus delivery and ECochG response measurement. The acoustic stimuli were generated by an NI DAQ system (NI DAQ 6216, National Instruments Corporation, Austin, TX, USA) along with an audio amplifier (Sony PHA-2, Sony Corporation, New York, NY, USA) and presented through ER-3A insert earphones (Etymotic Research, Inc. Elk Grove Village, IL, USA). An ER-7 (Etymotic Research, Inc. Elk Grove Village, IL, USA) probe MIC was used to monitor the stimulus level in the ear canal. ECochG responses were measured using an Advanced Bionics' Clinical Programming Interface (CPI-II), Platinum Series Sound Processor (PSP), and Universal Headpiece (HP). The CPI-II delivered an external trigger to synchronize acoustic stimulus generation and response measurement through the implant. Frequencies including 125, 250, 500, 750, 1,000, and 2,000 Hz were studied. The stimulus delivery system had maximum levels of 90, 100, 105, 110, 110, 110 dB HL for those audiometric frequencies.

Stimulation and Recording Parameters

The acoustic stimulus for ECochG recording consisted of 50-ms tone bursts with a ramp duration of 5 ms (Hanning window) presented at each subject's most comfortable level (MCL) or at maximum stimulus level generated by test system at test frequency. ECochG responses were recorded using 240 presentations with alternating polarity (120 rarefaction and 120 condensation). From the responses to alternating polarities, the *Difference response* (difference between responses to the two polarities) or the *Summation response* (sum of responses to the two polarities) was computed.

The electrical stimulus consisted of a 50-ms biphasic pulse train with a phase duration of 36 μS. The inter-pulse gap was varied to produce pulse rates that ranged between 400 and 1,200 pulses per second (pps). The pulse trains were delivered at each subject's MCL. Electrical stimuli were delivered to either electrode 2 or electrode 3 in a monopolar manner using the case ground as the return electrode. Electrode 1 was used as the recording electrode. In some cases, electrode 2 was used as the recording electrode, and then either electrode 1 or 3 was used for stimulation. In the AB system, electrode 1 is the most apical electrode.

For recording, the ring electrode, located on the electrode lead outside of the cochlea, served as the reference electrode for the differential recording amplifier. The amplifier on the HiRes90K® Advantage implant was configured to have a gain of 1,000. Data were sampled at a rate of 9,280 sample/s, thus supporting a fast Fourier transform (FFT) up to 4,000 Hz. The response amplitudes were estimated as the peak value at stimulus frequency in the FFT spectrum. With these settings, the AB implant offers a relatively long recording window of 54.4 ms that can record ECochG waveforms for low-frequency stimuli down to 125 Hz.

Procedures

The procedure used for electro-acoustic interaction was simultaneous presentation of electric and acoustic stimuli. The electrical pulse rates and acoustic frequencies were kept disparate so that the acoustic responses could be differentiated from electrical stimulus artifacts in the FFT spectrum. **Figure 2** illustrates the procedures used in this experiment. First, ECochG responses were recorded for the pure-tone acoustic stimulus presented alone (**Figure 2A**). Then the ECochG responses were recorded for the acoustic pure-tone stimulus and electrical pulse train presented simultaneously (**Figure 2B**). Following, ECochG responses were measured for the electrical pulse train alone (**Figure 2C**). Note that the responses in **Figures 2B,C** both show large stimulus artifacts during the electrical pulses, but the response to the acoustic stimulation still can be seen in **Figure 2B**, where the acoustic and electrical stimulation are presented together.

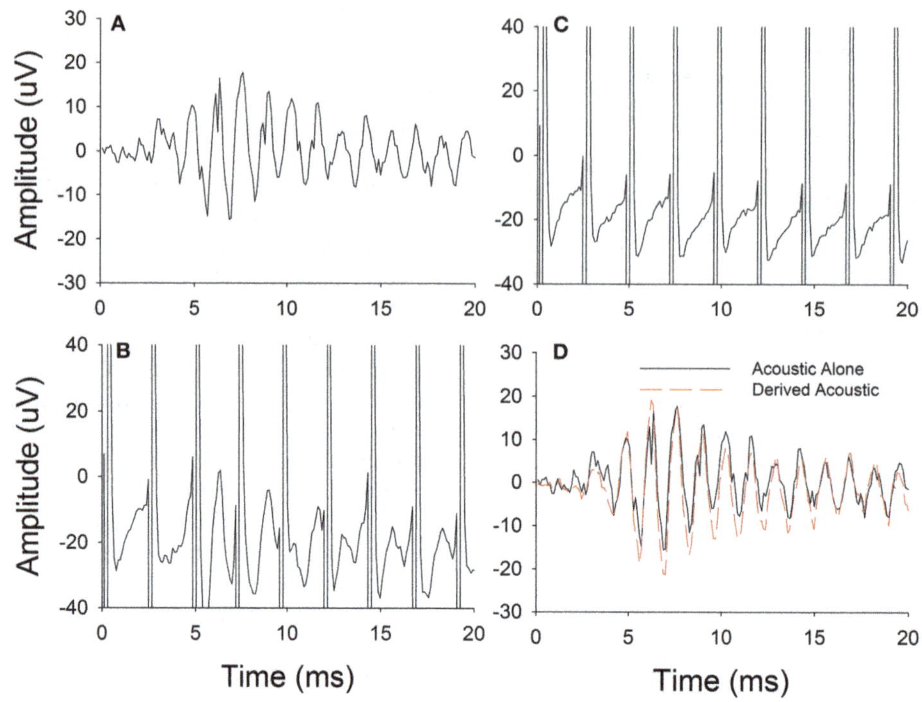

FIGURE 2 | Experimental procedure used for estimating physiological electro-acoustic interactions for simultaneous stimulations. **(A)** *Difference responses* measured for acoustic stimulus alone. **(B)** *Difference responses* measured for electric and acoustic stimulus together. **(C)** *Difference responses* measured for electric stimulus alone. **(D)** *Derived acoustic* responses estimated by subtracting electric stimulus alone responses from responses to electric and acoustic stimuli presented together.

The electric-only responses were subtracted from electro-acoustic responses. This subtracted response was defined as the *Derived acoustic* response (**Figure 2D**). Finally, the *acoustic-alone* (**Figure 2A**) and *Derived acoustic* response (**Figure 2D**) amplitudes in the frequency spectrum were compared at the stimulus frequency to determine if any electrical-acoustic interaction was present. Even though not shown in **Figure 2**, a similar computational technique was used to calculate and analyze the interactions in the ANN.

Different electrodes were used for electrical stimulation and recording of ECochG responses to minimize stimulus artifact contamination of the recordings. The fast-recovery property of the evoked potential recording amplifier designed into the HiRes90K® Advantage cochlear implant allowed the amplifier, when it encountered large saturating stimulus artifacts, to quickly return from saturation into linear operation. This capability permitted recording of responses immediately after the stimulus artifact ended. Thus, electrical pulse rates closer to clinical stimulation rates could be explored to determine the feasibility of using this ECochG technique to complement everyday clinical programming.

Experiment 2

Objective

The aim of this experiment was to estimate electro-acoustic interactions using a behavioral masking technique, i.e., the elevation of acoustic thresholds in the presence of an electrical stimulus masker. These behavioral electro-acoustic interactions were compared with the objective electro-acoustic interactions estimated in Experiment 1.

Subjects

A subset of the 6 subjects who participated in Experiment 1 took part in this phase of the study. Five were unilaterally implanted and one had two devices, resulting in a total of seven experimental ears. **Table 1** indicates the six individuals composing this subset of subjects.

Stimulation and Recording Parameters

The experiment was conducted in a quiet room. If required, a foam plug was introduced in the contralateral ear to avoid distraction. The acoustic probe stimuli consisted of tone bursts at 125, 250, 500, 750, 1,000, and 2,000 Hz. The tone duration was 200 ms with 10-ms on/off ramps.

The electrical masker consisted of 500-ms pulse train of (cathodic first) biphasic pulses with phase durations of approximately 36 μs. The pulse rate was kept constant at 421 pps. Electrical stimulation was delivered at the same MCLs used in Experiment 1. When the probe and masker were delivered simultaneously, the acoustic tone burst was centered temporally within the electrical pulse train. The experimental design was similar to Lin et al. (2011).

Procedure

Unmasked and masked acoustic thresholds were measured using a three-interval, forced-choice procedure with a three-down-one-up search rule. Initially within a run, the acoustic stimulus levels were varied in 8-dB steps. After three reversals, the step size was reduced to 2 dB. Thresholds were calculated by averaging six reversals with a step size of 2 dB. Thresholds were measured for each acoustic stimulus presented alone and with the electrical masker. The threshold track was aborted if the acoustic signal level exceeded the maximum stimulation limit. Any changes in acoustic thresholds in the presence of electrical stimulation from the unmasked condition were evidence of electro-acoustic interactions.

RESULTS

Feasibility of Recording ECochG Responses in the Presence of Electrical Stimulation (Experiment 1)

Figure 2 has shown feasibility of recording ECochG responses for an acoustic tone of 750 Hz and electrical stimulation rate of 421 pps. Then ECochG responses were also recorded for different electrical stimulation rates and *Derived acoustic responses* were estimated based on the technique described in Methods for Experiment 1. The peak amplitude of the *Difference response* to acoustic pure tones was assessed as a function of electrical pulse rate (400–1,200 pps). **Figure 3** shows an example of the effect of stimulation rate on the *Derived acoustic* response for a 750-Hz pure-tone stimulus (CI08). **Figure 3A** overlays the time domain responses to the acoustic stimulus alone with *Derived acoustic* responses for electrical stimulation delivered at 421, 843, and 1,160 pps. **Figure 3B** shows the same four responses in the frequency domain.

The time domain data show no visible residual stimulus artifacts after template subtraction. The frequency spectra show some stimulus artifacts around 1,160 Hz which appear to be harmonic or at the electrical stimulation rate. Nonetheless, these stimulus artifacts were clearly different from the *Difference response* at 750 Hz. In this example, there is no evidence of peripheral electro-acoustic interactions as indicated by no differences in the waveforms or spectra for the *Derived acoustic* responses compared to the *acoustic-alone* responses. These results demonstrate the feasibility of recording acoustic responses in the presence of electrical stimuli delivered at different stimulation rates.

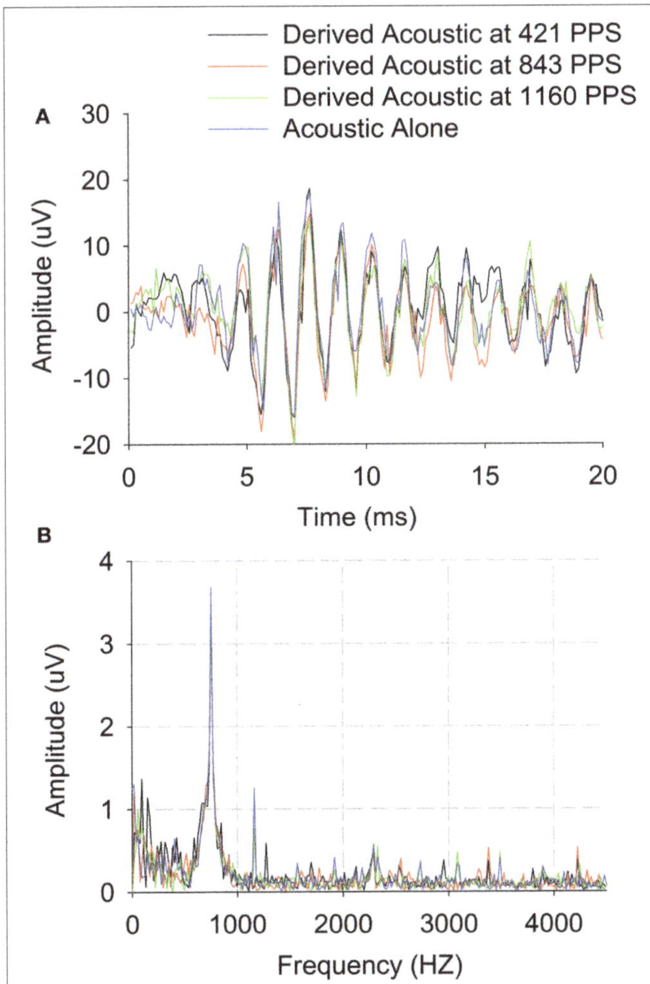

FIGURE 3 | *Derived acoustic* and *Acoustic alone responses* of *Difference responses* (difference of alternating polarities) for three three electrical stimulation rates. **(A)** Time domain. **(B)** Frequency domain.

Objective Estimation of Electro-Acoustic Interactions through ECochG Responses (Experiment 1)

Figure 4 shows an example of *Difference response* amplitude change as a function of acoustic stimulation frequency for electrical stimulation on electrode 1 vs. stimulation on electrode 2 (Subject CI04L). In this case, the pulse rate was constant at 421 pps. The *Difference response* amplitudes decreased for acoustic stimulus frequencies above 250 Hz, thereby

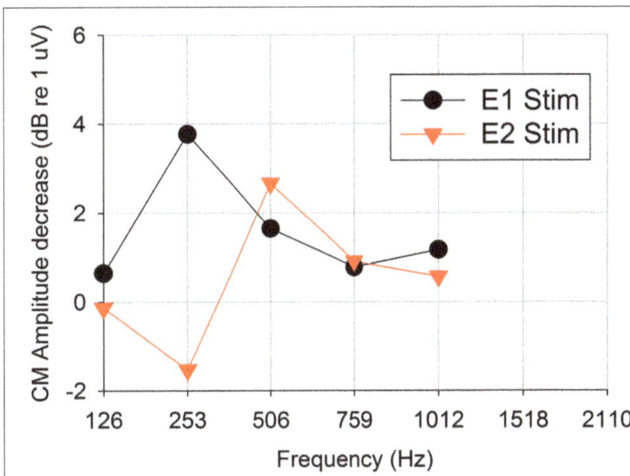

FIGURE 4 | *Difference response* amplitude changes as a function of acoustic stimulation frequency for 421-pps electrical stimulation on two two different electrodes (representative subject CI04L). Positive dB-values indicate decreases (suppression) in the acoustic response and negative dB-values indicate increases (enhancement) in the acoustic response in presence of electrical stimulation.

providing evidence of peripheral physiologic electro-acoustic interactions. The *Difference response* amplitudes decreased up to 4 dB (dB re: 1 uV) at 250 Hz and about 2 dB above 250 Hz.

Figure 5 plots *Derived acoustic* vs. *acoustic-alone* responses for *Difference responses* across all 13 experimental ears for electrical stimulation on electrodes 1–3 for all test frequencies (**Figures 5A–C**). **Figure 5** also shows the comparison of *acoustic*

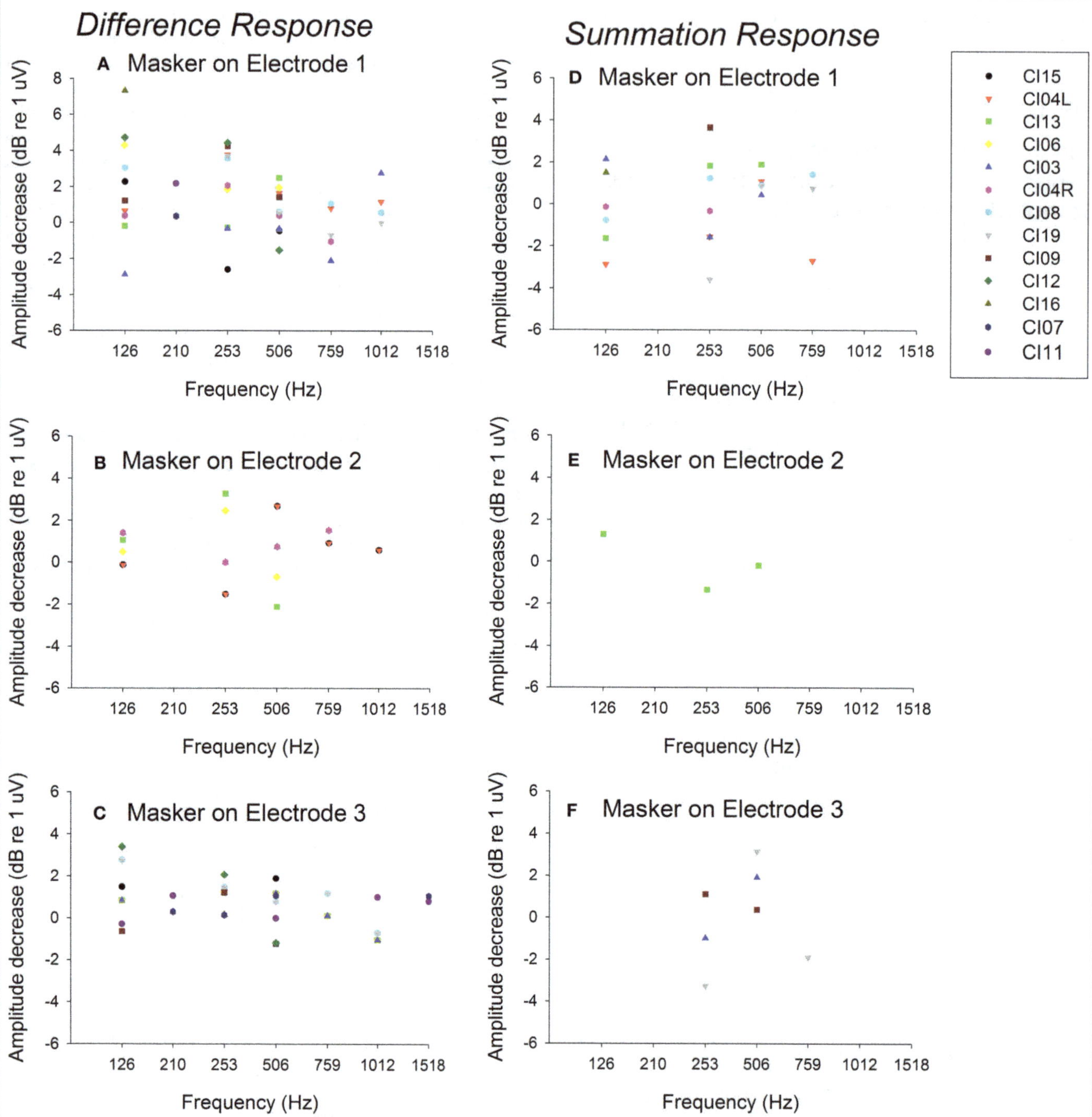

FIGURE 5 | Comparison of *Derived acoustic* vs. *acoustic alone* for *Difference responses* (difference of alternating polarities) and *Summation responses* (summation of alternating polarities) for 13 ears across multiple frequencies. **(A–C)** show the data for *Difference responses* for electrical stimulation on electrodes 1–3; **(D–F)** show the data for *Summation responses* for electrical simulation on electrodes 1–3. The points above zero indicate decrease in acoustic response in presence of electrical stimulation (suppression) and points below zero indicate increase in acoustic response in presence of electrical stimulation (enhancement).

alone and *Derived acoustic* conditions for *Summation responses* for electrical stimulation on electrodes 1–3 for all test frequencies (**Figures 5D–F**). Data points above zero indicate decrease in acoustic response due to electrical stimulation (suppression) and points below zero indicate increase in acoustic response due to electrical stimulation (enhancement). The responses show significant electro-acoustic interactions for *Difference response* and non-significant electro-acoustic interactions for *Summation responses*. The difference between *Derived acoustic responses* and *Acoustic alone responses* was significant (two tailed $p < 0.001$, paired t-test, $n = 41$ for electrical stimulation on electrode 1; two tailed $p < 0.001$, paired t-test, $n = 36$ for electrical stimulation on electrode 3, two tailed $p < 0.001$, paired t-test, $n = 20$ for electrical stimulation on electrode 2) for *Difference responses*. The difference between *Derived acoustic responses* and *Acoustic alone responses* was not significant (two tailed $p = 0.266$, paired t-test, $n = 21$ for electrical stimulation on electrode 1; two tailed $p = 0.89$, paired t-test, $n = 7$ for electrical stimulation on electrode 3, two tailed $p = 0.84$, paired t-test, $n = 3$ for electrical stimulation on electrode 2) for *Summation responses*.

Behavioral Electro-Acoustic Interaction as a Function of Acoustic Stimulus Frequency (Experiment 2)

Figure 6 shows the changes in behavioral thresholds for one ear (Subject CI04L) in the presence of the 421-pps electrical masker. The observed variance between runs was 1 dB. The behavioral thresholds increased for test frequencies 250 Hz and above, with the greatest threshold shifts observed above 500 Hz. This subject did not show frequency selectivity with respect to threshold increase for stimulation on either electrode 1 or 2.

Figure 7 shows the effect of the 421-pps electrical masker across all audiometric test frequencies for all seven ears tested in Experiment 2. The data show mean and individual threshold changes observed across subjects. Each of the panels represents electrical stimulation on a different electrode. The mean data show the threshold selectivity of ~500–750 Hz for electrode 1 stimulation and ~1,500 Hz for electrode 2.

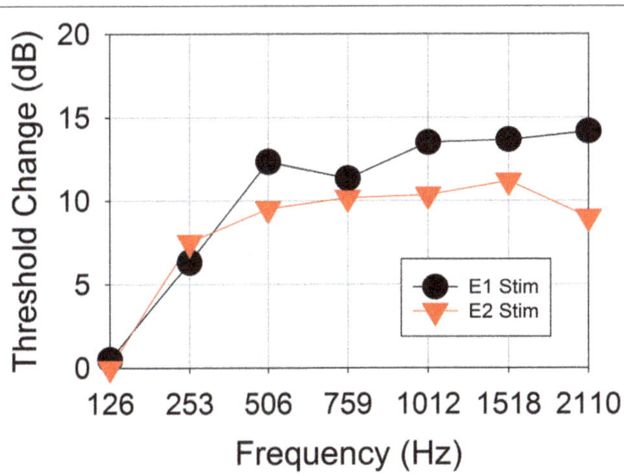

FIGURE 6 | Behavioral threshold change vs. acoustic test frequency for a representative subject CI04L. An electrical masker of 421 pps was applied to either electrode 1 or electrode 3.

Comparison of Objective and Behavioral Electro-Acoustic Interaction

Figure 5 shows *Difference response* amplitude changes across audiometric frequencies in the presence of a 421-pps electrical masker for the same seven ears assessed in Experiment 2. Again, each of the panels represents electrical stimulation on a different electrode. The behavioral threshold shifts (**Figure 7**)

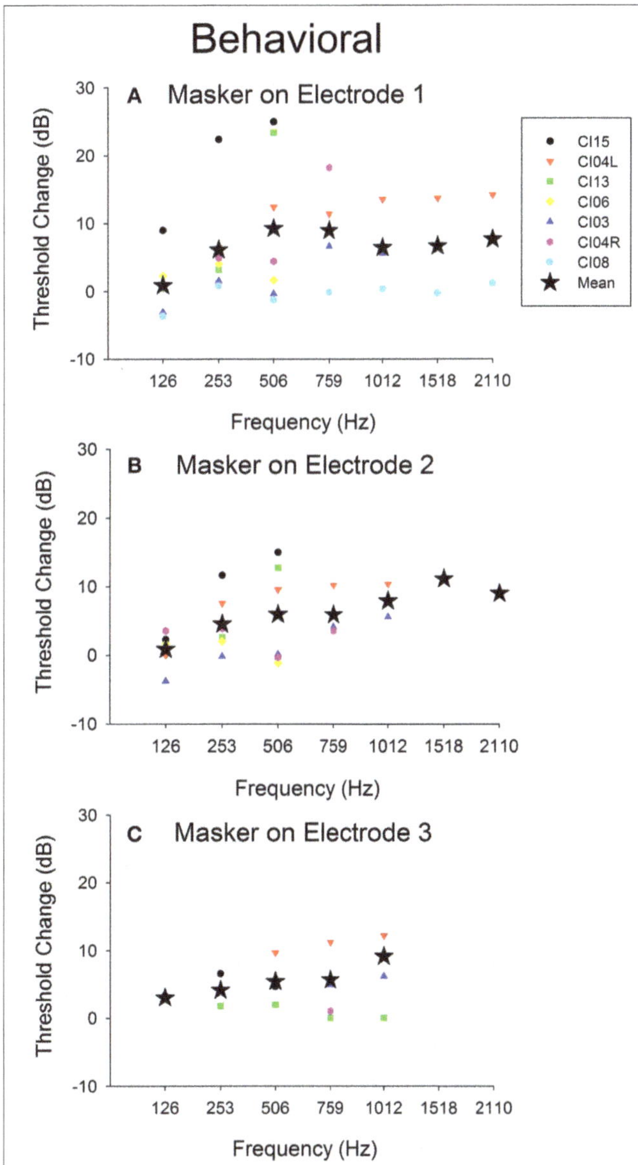

FIGURE 7 | Behavioral threshold changes and *Difference response* amplitude changes vs. acoustic test frequency vs. electrical stimulation location. **(A–C)** Behavioral threshold changes observed with electrical stimulation masker on electrodes 1–3 across frequencies and across all subjects.

varied by place of stimulation (i.e., by the electrode used for the masker) and the frequency of the acoustic probe stimulus. The behavioral thresholds show a peak around 500–750 Hz for electrical stimulation on electrode 1 and for higher frequencies for stimulation on electrodes 2 (~1,500 Hz). In contrast, the *Difference response* amplitude changes across electrodes do not show any clear peaks but do show greater shifts in amplitude for stimulation on electrode 1 than for stimulation on electrodes 2 or 3. This pattern suggests that apical stimulation results in greater physiologic electro-acoustic interactions than stimulation more basally. Notably, the objective electro-acoustic interactions estimated by *Difference response* amplitude changes (<8 dB change) were smaller than behavioral threshold changes (5–25 dB). There were no significant correlations observed between behavioral and objective electro-acoustic interactions ($p > 0.05$, $n = 48$, Pearson Correlation).

DISCUSSION

This study demonstrates the feasibility of measuring acoustic ECochG responses in the presence of electrical stimulation using the HiRes90K® Advantage cochlear implant. The fast-recovery amplifier enabled measurement of acoustic *Difference responses* and *Summation responses* for electrical pulse rates as high as 1,000 pps. Moreover, there were minimal or no residual electrical stimulation artifacts when using the technique described. Electro-acoustic interactions were observed in subset of subjects up to 4 dB of suppression in ECochG responses.

Furthermore, this is the first study to demonstrate that ECochG can be used to evaluate electro-acoustic interactions in CI recipients with residual hearing. The degree of electro-acoustic interaction was dependent on location of the stimulation and recording electrode, as well as acoustic frequency (**Figures 4, 5**). Comparison of ECochG interactions and the effect of electrical stimulation on behavioral thresholds showed a general pattern of suppression of acoustic responses with electric stimulation. Quantitatively, the physiological measures showed less suppression than those observed behaviorally. For example, in the same subject, a 0–4 dB decrease in *Difference response* (**Figure 4**) corresponded to a 0–20 dB increase in behavioral threshold (**Figure 6**). One possible explanation is that the discrepancy between the two measures may be related to the difference in the point on the psychometric function at which the measures were obtained. ECochG measures were obtained with acoustic stimulation levels near MCL or maximum stimulus level of test system, whereas acoustic levels for the behavioral experiment were near threshold. The test stimulus level varied from soft level to MCL in different subjects based on their residual hearing (see **Figure 1**). **Figure 8** shows the replot of the data from **Figure 5A** with X-axis changed to *Acoustic alone* response amplitude. This clearly shows that maximum interactions observed at smaller *acoustic alone* responses than at larger *acoustic alone* responses. The smaller *acoustic alone* response amplitudes indicate that test stimulus levels were at soft level and larger *acoustic alone* response amplitudes indicate that test stimulus levels were at MCL.

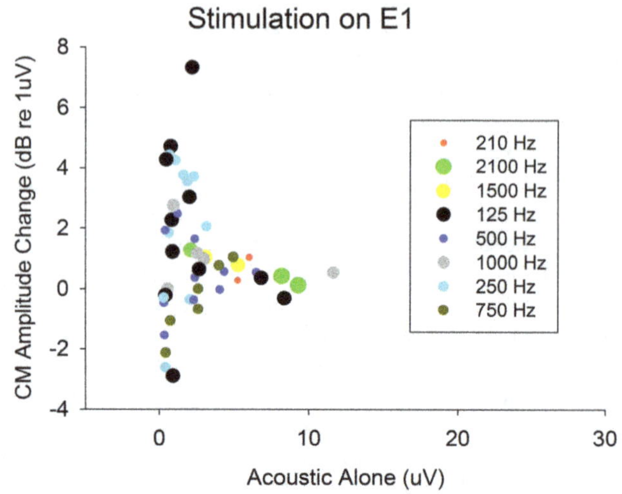

FIGURE 8 | Decrease in acoustic responses due to electrical stimulation on electrode 1. The decrease in amplitudes (indicating presence of electro-acoustic interactions) were plotted with respect actual *acoustic alone* response amplitudes. This shows amount of electro-acoustic interactions observed dependent up on *acoustic alone* response amplitude (psychometric function at which the measures were obtained). The objective measures were obtained at either MCL or maximum of stimulus level of test system. This varied from soft level to MCL based on amount of residual hearing present.

Stronks et al. (2010) reported a similar pattern where greater changes in acoustic CAPs in the presence of electric stimulation were observed near threshold compared to higher acoustic stimulus levels. Specifically, the amplitude changes observed at higher stimulation levels were around 3 dB, while amplitude changes were 10–20 dB near threshold. However, Stronks et al., study and other animal studies (Abbas et al., 2002) evaluated CAPs at higher acoustic frequencies than those used in this study. CAP techniques have limited applicability in CI recipients with low-frequency residual hearing where CAP responses cannot be measured. In contrast, *Difference responses* and *Summation responses* are measurable in these individuals at low frequencies (see **Figure 3**).

In summary, it is feasible to assess electro-acoustic interactions objectively in CI recipients with residual hearing. Further studies will explore stimulus-level-dependent electroacoustic interactions and whether these objective data can be used to guide fitting of EAS technology. Long-term, the goal is to be able to fit clinical EAS systems (1) without dependence on time-consuming psychometric methods and (2) in patients unable to undergo behavioral testing.

CONCLUSIONS

It is feasible to record ECochG responses in the presence of electrical stimulation in HiRes90® Advantage CI recipients with residual hearing, thus providing a method for objectively assessing electro-acoustic interactions.

The HiRes90K® Advantage fast-recovery recording amplifier allows electro-acoustic interactions to be measured at high electrical stimulation rates with minimal stimulus artifacts.

Future studies are required to understand the relationship between behavioral and objective electro-acoustic interactions.

AUTHOR CONTRIBUTIONS

Both authors contributed for conception and design, acquisition of data, or analysis and interpretation of data and drafting the article.

FUNDING

This study was funded by Advanced Bionics Corporation and authors are employees of Advanced Bionics.

ACKNOWLEDGMENTS

The authors would like to thank all the subjects who participated in the study and Lupe Navarro and Maria Holloway for organizing their visits.

REFERENCES

Abbas, P. J., Miller, C. A., Rubinstein, J. T., Robinson, B. K., Hu, N., Mino, H., et al. (2002). *Effects of Remaining Hair Cells on Cochlear Implant Function*. Final Report N01-DC-9-2106, NIH.

Balkany, T. J., Connell, S. S., Hodges, A. V., Payne, S. L., Telischi, F. F., Eshraghi, A. A. et al. (2006). Conservation of residual acoustic hearing after cochlear implantation. *Otol. Neurotol.* 27, 1083–1088. doi: 10.1097/01.mao.0000244355.34577.85

Dalbert, A., Sim, J. H., Gerig, R., Pfiffner, F., Roosli, C., and Huber, A. (2015). Correlation of electrophysiological properties and hearing preservation in cochlear implant patients. *Otol. Neurotol.* 36, 1172–1180. doi: 10.1097/MAO.0000000000000768

Dallos, P. (1973). *The Auditory Periphery: Biophysics and Physiology*. New York, NY: Academic Press.

Fitzpatrick, D. C., Campbell, A. T., Choudhury, B., Dillon, M. P., Forgues, M., Buchman, C. A., et al. (2014). Round window electrocochleography just before cochlear implantation: relationship to word rECochGnition outcomes in adults. *Otol. Neurotol.* 35, 64–71. doi: 10.1097/MAO.00000000000 00219

Forgues, M., Koehn, H. A., Dunnon, A. K., Pulver, S. H., Buchman, C.A., Adunka, O. F., et al. (2014). Distinguishing hair cell from neural potentials recorded at the round window. *J. Neurophysiol.* 111, 580–593. doi: 10.1152/jn.0044 6.2013

Fraysse, B., Macías, A. R., Sterkers, O., Burdo, S., Ramsden, R., Deguine, O., et al. (2006). Residual hearing conservation and electroacoustic stimulation with the nucleus 24 contour advance cochlear implant. *Otol. Neurotol.* 27, 624–633. doi: 10.1097/01.mao.0000226289.04048.0f

Karsten, S. A., Turner, C. W., Brown, C. J., Joen, E. K., Abbas, J., and Gantz, B. J. (2013). Optimising the combination of acoustic and electric hearing in the implanted ear. *Ear Hear.* 34, 142–150. doi: 10.1097/AUD.0b013e3182 69ce87

Koka, K., Saoji, A. A., and Litvak, L. M. (2016). Electrocochleography in cochlear implant recipients with residual hearing: comparison with audiometric thresholds. *Ear Hear.* 38, e161–e167. doi: 10.1097/AUD.0000000000000385

Lichtenhan, J. T., Cooper, N. P., and Guinan, J. J. Jr. (2013). A new auditory threshold estimation technique for low frequencies: proof of concept. *Ear Hear.* 34, 42–51. doi: 10.1097/AUD.0b013e31825f9bd3

Lin, P., Turner, C. W., Gantz, B. J., Djalilian, H. R., and Zeng, F.-G. (2011). Ipsilateral masking between acoustic and electric stimulations. *J. Acoust. Soc. Am.* 130, 858–865. doi: 10.1121/1.3605294

Polak, M., Lorens, A., Helbig, S., McDonald, S., and Vermeire, K. (2010). Fitting of the hearing system affects partial deafness cochlear implant performance. *Cochlear Implants Int.* 11(Suppl. 1), 117–121. doi: 10.1179/146701010X12671177544221

Radeloff, A., Shehata-Dieler, W., Scherzed, A., Rak, K., Harnisch, W., Hagen, R., et al. (2012). Intraoperative monitoring using cochlear microphonics in cochlear implant patients with residual hearing. *Otol. Neurotol.* 33, 348–354. doi: 10.1097/MAO.0b013e318248ea86

Snyder, R. L., and Schreiner, C. E. (1984). The auditory neurophonic: basic properties. *Hear. Res.* 15, 261–280.

Stronks, H. C., Prijs, V. F., Chimona, T. S., Grolman, W., and Klis, S. F. L. (2012). Spatial overlap of combined electroacoustic stimulation determines the electrically evoked response in the guinea pig cochlea. *Otol. Neurotol.* 33, 1535–1542. doi: 10.1097/MAO.0b013e318271c0b6

Stronks, H. C., Versnel, H., Prijs, V. F., and Klis, S. F. L. (2010). Suppression of the acoustically evoked auditory-nerve response by electrical stimulation in the cochlea of the guinea pig. *Hear. Res.* 259, 64–74. doi: 10.1016/j.heares.2009.10.004

Turner, C. W., Reiss, L. A. J. and Gantz, B. J. (2008). Combined acoustic and electric hearing: preserving residual acoustic hearing. *Hear. Res.* 242, 164–171. doi: 10.1016/j.heares.2007.11.008

Von Ilberg, C., Keifer, J., Tillein, J., Pfenningdorff, T., Hartmann, R., Stur-zebecher, E., et al. (1999). Electro-acoustic stimulation of the auditory system. *Otorhinolaryngol. Relat. Spec.* 61, 334–340. doi: 10.1159/000027695

9

Inner Hair Cell Loss Disrupts Hearing and Cochlear Function Leading to Sensory Deprivation and Enhanced Central Auditory Gain

Richard Salvi[1], Wei Sun[1], Dalian Ding[1], Guang-Di Chen[1], Edward Lobarinas[2], Jian Wang[3], Kelly Radziwon[1] and Benjamin D. Auerbach[1]*

[1] Center for Hearing and Deafness, University at Buffalo, Buffalo, NY, USA, [2] Callier Center, University of Texas at Dallas, Dallas, TX, USA, [3] School of Human Communication Disorders, Dalhousie University, Halifax, NS, Canada

***Correspondence:**
Richard Salvi
salvi@buffalo.edu

There are three times as many outer hair cells (OHC) as inner hair cells (IHC), yet IHC transmit virtually all acoustic information to the brain as they synapse with 90–95% of type I auditory nerve fibers. Here we review a comprehensive series of experiments aimed at determining how loss of the IHC/type I system affects hearing by selectively destroying these cells in chinchillas using the ototoxic anti-cancer agent carboplatin. Eliminating IHC/type I neurons has no effect on distortion product otoacoustic emission or the cochlear microphonic potential generated by OHC; however, it greatly reduces the summating potential produced by IHC and the compound action potential (CAP) generated by type I neurons. Remarkably, responses from remaining auditory nerve fibers maintain sharp tuning and low thresholds despite innervating regions of the cochlea with ~80% IHC loss. Moreover, chinchillas with large IHC lesions have surprisingly normal thresholds in quiet until IHC losses exceeded 80%, suggesting that only a few IHC are needed to detect sounds in quiet. However, behavioral thresholds in broadband noise are elevated significantly and tone-in-narrow band noise masking patterns exhibit greater remote masking. These results suggest the auditory system is able to compensate for considerable loss of IHC/type I neurons in quiet but not in difficult listening conditions. How does the auditory brain deal with the drastic loss of cochlear input? Recordings from the inferior colliculus found a relatively small decline in sound-evoked activity despite a large decrease in CAP amplitude after IHC lesion. Paradoxically, sound-evoked responses are generally larger than normal in the auditory cortex, indicative of increased central gain. This gain enhancement in the auditory cortex is associated with decreased GABA-mediated inhibition. These results suggest that when the neural output of the cochlea is reduced, the central auditory system compensates by turning up its gain so that weak signals once again become comfortably loud. While this gain enhancement is able to restore normal hearing under quiet conditions, it may not adequately compensate for peripheral dysfunction in more complex sound environments. In addition, excessive gain increases may convert recruitment into the debilitating condition known as hyperacusis.

Keywords: inner hair cells, carboplatin, central auditory system, auditory gain, auditory cortex, tinnitus, hyperacusis

SENSORINEURAL HEARING LOSS AND THE AUDIOGRAM

The audiogram is often considered the gold standard for assessing sensorineural hearing loss (HL). Individuals with pure tone thresholds of ≤20 dB HL would be classified as having normal hearing. However, there is growing awareness that the pure tone audiogram fails to detect certain forms of cochlear pathology and auditory processing deficits. This has led to the concept of "hidden hearing loss," i.e., the realization that significant auditory perceptual deficits can exist in listeners with normal hearing thresholds, a condition that can exist when there is considerable IHC and/or auditory nerve fiber degeneration (Schaette and McAlpine, 2011; Plack et al., 2014; Lobarinas et al., 2016). Hidden hearing loss is likely involved in some cases of auditory neuropathy and central auditory processing disorders, which are characterized by temporal processing deficits, impaired speech perception, and difficulties hearing in noisy environments (Kraus et al., 2000; Zeng et al., 2005). It may also contribute to other auditory perceptual disorders such as tinnitus and hyperacusis (Schaette and McAlpine, 2011; Hickox and Liberman, 2014). It is therefore imperative to develop ways for clinically assessing hidden hearing loss and determining the consequences of IHC/auditory nerve damage on peripheral and central auditory processing.

Electrocochleography (ECochG) can be used to interrogate the functional status of different structures in the cochlea and identify "hidden" damage to inner hair cells (IHC), outer hair cells (OHC), the IHC/type I auditory nerve fiber synapse, and spiral ganglion neurons (SGN). Sensorineural hearing loss is a complex phenomenon that not only involves the cochlea, but also numerous structures in the central auditory system capable of partially compensating for these cochlear deficits. Therefore, a more complete understanding of sensorineural hearing loss not only requires assessment with ECochG, but also examination of the neurophysiological changes occurring in the central auditory pathway. In this review, we will discuss our results from a comprehensive series of electrophysiological, neuroanatomical, behavioral, and neuropharmacological experiments in a chinchilla animal model of carboplatin-induced ototoxicity in which there is selective damage to the IHC and type I auditory nerve fibers that exclusively innervate the IHC. These studies illustrate how ECochG can be used to identify damage to the IHC and type I neurons that goes undetected (i.e., hidden) by the pure tone audiogram. Electrophysiological recordings from the inferior colliculus (IC) and auditory cortex (ACx) reveal how weak neural signals from a damaged cochlea are amplified as they ascend through the central auditory pathway. Finally, we discuss a few simple psychophysical tests we have shown can identify hearing deficits associated with damage to IHC and type I neurons.

CARBOPLATIN-INDUCED IHC AND TYPE I LESIONS

Cisplatin and other platinum based anti-cancer drugs are generally more toxic to OHC than IHC, with hair cell lesions generally progressing from the base toward the apex as the dose and duration of treatment increases (Boettcher et al., 1992; Rybak et al., 2007). Carboplatin is a second generation antineoplastic agent that is considered much less ototoxic than cisplatin (Ettinger et al., 1994), a view consistent with most studies in animal models (Saito et al., 1989; Ding et al., 1999). However, when low-to-moderate doses of carboplatin (50–75 mg/kg, i.p.) were systemically administered to chinchillas, it induced an unusual lesion that preferentially damaged IHC (**Figure 1A**), type I auditory nerve fibers (**Figure 1B**) and SGN. OHC damage was only observed at extremely high doses of carboplatin (200 mg/kg, i.p.) (Takeno et al., 1994, 1998; Hofstetter et al., 1997a; Wang et al., 1997; Ding et al., 1999). Unlike other ototoxic drugs, the IHC lesion was characterized by a relatively uniform loss of hair cells along the entire length of the cochlea (Trautwein et al., 1996; Hofstetter et al., 1997a; **Figure 1C**). Due to the systemic nature of treatment, hall cell lesions were similar in both ears (Hofstetter, 1996; Hofstetter et al., 1997a).

To gain insights into the time course of carboplatin-mediated damage, we counted the number of IHC and nerve fibers in the habenula perforata 24–72 h after treatment with a moderate dose of carboplatin (50 mg/kg, i.p.) (Wang et al., 2003). Surprisingly, 24 h after carboplatin treatment, only 50% of the nerve fibers in the habenula perforata were present whereas there was no loss of IHC (**Figure 1D**). Significant IHC loss was first observed 3 days post-carboplatin, but by this time only ~25% of the nerve fibers were still present. These results suggest that the auditory nerve fibers and their afferent synapses are especially susceptible to carboplatin ototoxicity. To explore this possibility, transmission electron microscopy was used to examine the morphological condition of the type I afferent synapse at the base of the IHC. At 24 h post-carboplatin, numerous vacuoles were present around afferent terminals at the base of the IHC (**Figure 1E**; Ding et al., 1997, 1998). Damage to the afferent nerve terminals, IHC and SGN increased considerably between 24 and 72 h whereas the morphology of the OHC remained remarkably normal. Vacuoles were also present on the proximal nerve fibers and transmission electron microscopy revealed significant loss of myelin around the nerve fibers 24–72 h post-treatment (**Figure 1F**; Ding et al., 2002; Wang et al., 2003). Taken together, these results indicate that moderate doses of carboplatin can selectively damage IHC and type I afferent neurons.

MASSIVE IHC LESIONS HAVE LITTLE EFFECT ON DISTORTION PRODUCT OTOACOUSTIC EMISSIONS

Distortion product otoacoustic emissions (DPOAE), which depend on OHC somatic electromotility (Brownell, 1990; Liberman et al., 2002), provide a noninvasive method for assessing the functional integrity of the cochlea (Brown et al., 1989; Schrott et al., 1991; Hofstetter et al., 1997a) and are widely used to screen for cochlear hearing loss in infants and adults (Stanton et al., 2005; Jakubíková et al., 2009). Subjects with normal DPOAE pass the screening test and are generally believed to have normal hearing; however, since DPOAE are specifically sensitive to OHC function, this is not always correct,

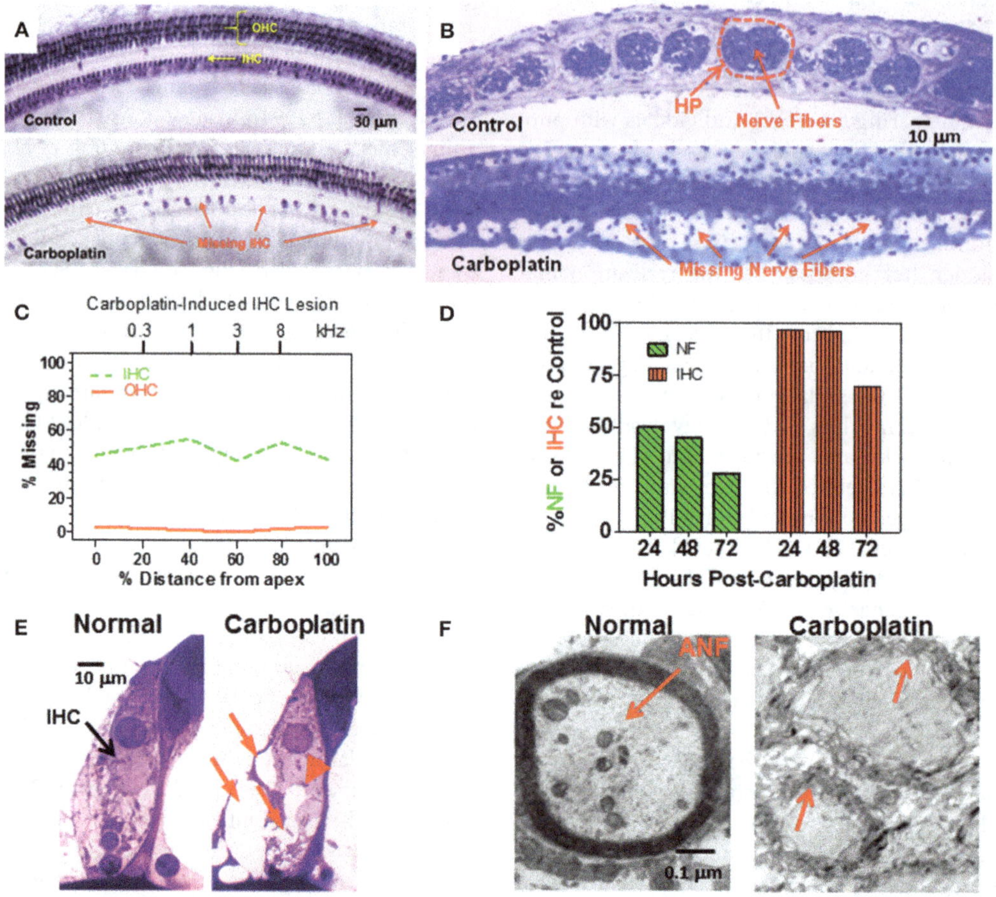

FIGURE 1 | (A) Photomicrographs of a surface preparation of the organ of Corti stained with succinate dehydrogenase, a metabolic enzyme highly expressed in OHC and IHC, but not supporting cells. Control (upper panel) shows strong staining of all OHC and IHC. One month after a moderate dose of carboplatin (50–75 mg/kg, i.p.) there are patches of stained IHC separated by large regions of missing IHC. OHC were present and appeared normal. **(B)** Photomicrographs of thin sections stained with toluidine blue taken tangential to the habenula perforata. Dashed line (upper panel) showing the darkly stained nerve fibers in the openings in the habenular perforata (HP) in the osseous spiral lamina (dashed line) of a normal control ear. Each habenular opening in control ears is filled with nerve fibers (upper panel) whereas in carboplatin-treated ears (bottom panel), many nerve fibers are missing in the habenular openings. **(C)** Schematic of a cochleogram showing the typical pattern of IHC loss induced by a moderate dose of carboplatin. In this depiction, roughly 40–50% of the IHC were missing along the length of the cochlea whereas OHC were intact. The cochleogram shows the percentage of missing IHC and OHC as a function of percent distance from the apex of the cochlea; cochlear position related to frequency on the upper x-axis. **(D)** Carboplatin induced a large and rapid loss of nerve fibers (NF) in the habenula perforata 24–72 h post-treatment. Significant nerve fiber (NF) loss occurred 24 h post-treatment; IHC occurred several days later. **(E)** Photomicrographs illustrating the condition of the synaptic region at the base of the IHC of a normal control (left) and a carboplatin-treated animal (right). At 24 h post-treatment, many large vacuoles (red arrows) were observed at the afferent terminals of the carboplatin-treated chinchilla unlike the control. Swelling distorted the basal pole of the IHC in carboplatin treated (arrowhead) animal. **(F)** Transmission electron micrograph show thick myelin sheath around a normal auditory nerve fiber (ANF). Carboplatin caused significant demyelination 24–72 h post-treatment (red arrows). Data schematized from Hofstetter et al. (1997b), Ding et al. (1999, 2001), and Wang et al. (2003).

for example in patients with auditory neuropathy (Abdala et al., 2000). Since moderate doses of carboplatin selectively damage the IHC while ostensibly leaving the OHC intact, DPOAE might be expected to be normal in ears with just IHC loss. To test this hypothesis, DPOAE input/output functions were measured in chinchillas before and after treatment with a moderate to high dose of carboplatin (Trautwein et al., 1996; Wake et al., 1996a; Hofstetter et al., 1997a). In some animals, carboplatin treatment caused near complete loss of IHC along the entire length of the cochlea, but failed to damage the OHC (**Figure 2A**). In such cases, where nearly all the IHC were missing but the OHC were intact, the DPOAE input/output functions were completely normal (**Figure 2B**; Hofstetter et al., 1997a). Thus, the presence of normal DPOAE does not mean that the cochlea is structurally intact.

MODERATE IHC LESION HAS LITTLE EFFECT ON THRESHOLD

IHC make one-to-one synaptic contact with the type I auditory nerve fibers, providing the only pathway through which acoustic information is relayed to the central auditory system (Spoendlin and Baumgartner, 1977). Therefore, massive loss of IHC would

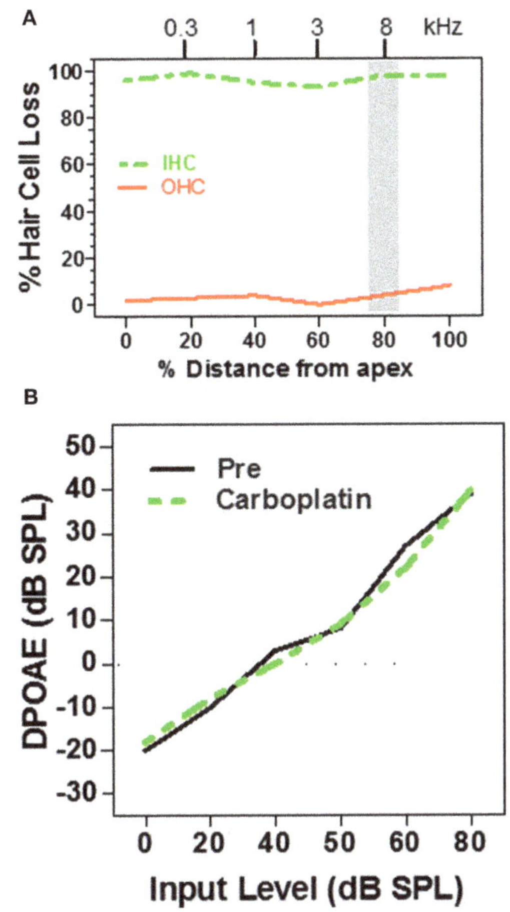

FIGURE 2 | (A) Schematic cochleogram showing a very large IHC lesion with little OHC loss induced by a high dose of carboplatin. IHC lesion extends over nearly the entire length of the cochlea. **(B)** Schematic DPOAE input/output function before and after carboplatin treatment at f1 and f2 frequencies corresponding to the shaded region in the cochleogram in **(A)**. DPOAE input/output function was normal several months post-carboplatin despite massive IHC loss, but retention of most OHC. Data schematized from Hofstetter et al. (1997a).

greatly reduce input to the central auditory system and should drastically disrupt hearing. To determine how IHC loss affects hearing thresholds, pure tone audiograms were measured in chinchillas using an avoidance conditioning paradigm before and 1–2 months after moderate to high doses of carboplatin designed to induce a range of IHC lesions (Salvi et al., 1978; Lobarinas et al., 2013). After completing the hearing tests, the cochleae were harvested to determine the magnitude and type of cochlear lesion. The schematic audiogram (**Figure 3A**) and schematic cochleogram (**Figure 3B**) illustrate the results obtained when carboplatin induced a moderate IHC lesion, but no OHC damage. In these cases, thresholds in quiet were surprisingly unaffected, increasing very little despite the fact that 40–60% of the IHC were missing (Lobarinas et al., 2013). To understand the relationship between hearing loss and IHC loss, the threshold shifts post-carboplatin were plotted as a function of percent IHC loss as schematized in **Figure 3C**. Hearing thresholds were largely unaffected by small IHC lesions (<35%). Threshold shifts gradually increased with moderate IHC lesions (40–75%), but then increased substantially once the IHC lesions exceeded 80%. One interpretation of these results is that the pure tone audiogram is very poor at detecting small to moderate sized IHC lesions and that thresholds in quiet only begin to rise after the vast majority of IHC have been destroyed. Apparently, only a few IHC and type I neurons are needed to detect a tone in a quiet environment. The important implication of the above results is that DPOAE and pure tone audiograms, two of the most commonly used techniques for assessing hearing, are insensitive to profound IHC/type I neuron damage. This suggests additional measures are likely necessary to fully assess auditory function.

IHC LESIONS HAVE LITTLE EFFECT ON THE COCHLEAR MICROPHONIC

ECochG recorded from the ear canal, round window or within the cochlea, provides researchers and clinicians with a powerful tool to assess the functional integrity of the sensory and neural structures in the cochlea. The cochlear microphonic (CM), an AC receptor potential that mirrors the waveform of the acoustic stimulus, is predominantly generated by the OHC with only a small contribution from IHC (Dallos et al., 1972). Given that carboplatin preferentially damages the IHC and does not alter DPOAE, one would predict that the CM amplitude would be largely unaffected by carboplatin treatments that primarily target the IHC. Indeed, when the CM was recorded from the round window of carboplatin treated chinchillas with large IHC lesions but near complete retention of OHC, CM input/output functions were nearly identical to control as schematized in **Figure 4A** (Trautwein et al., 1996; Wang et al., 1997). These results indicate that the IHC contribute little to the generation of the CM and that the CM cannot be used to assess IHC function.

IHC LESION SUPPRESSES THE SUMMATING POTENTIAL

The summating potential (SP), reflected as a sound-evoked DC shift near stimulus onset, is thought to be generated predominantly by the IHC receptor potential with a much smaller contribution from OHC (Russell and Sellick, 1983; Zheng et al., 1997). Given that carboplatin preferentially damages the IHC, one would predict that SP amplitude would be greatly reduced in animals with large carboplatin-induced IHC lesions. To test this hypothesis, the SP evoked by tone bursts was recorded from the round window of carboplatin treated chinchillas. In animals with large IHC lesions and complete retention of OHC, SP amplitude was greatly reduced (~60%) compared to controls as schematized by the SP input/output function in **Figure 4B** (Durrant et al., 1998). Destruction of both IHC plus OHC resulted in a further decline in SP amplitude. These results provide further confirmation that the SP is generated presynaptically primarily by IHC and this component

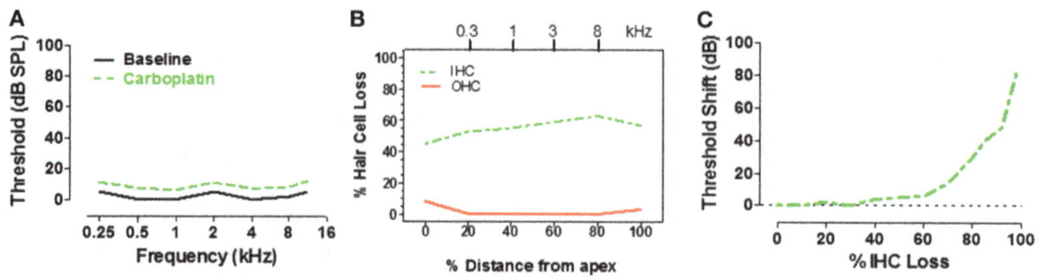

FIGURE 3 | (A) Schematic of pure tone audiogram obtained pre- and post-carboplatin in a chinchilla with ~50–60% IHC and an intact OHC population **(B)**. The post-carboplatin thresholds (green) were slightly increased from baseline (black). **(B)** Schematic of cochleogram showing 50–60% IHC and minimal OHC loss following carboplatin treatment (audiometric profile for such lesions depicted in **A**). Percent distance from the apex of cochlea shown on x-axis; position in the cochlea related to frequency on upper x-axis. **(C)** Schematic showing the approximate relationship between the threshold shift vs. the percent IHC loss induced by carboplatin. Thresholds remained nearly normal up to about 60% IHC loss, but then increased steeply once the IHC lesion exceeds 80%. Data schematized from Lobarinas et al. (2013).

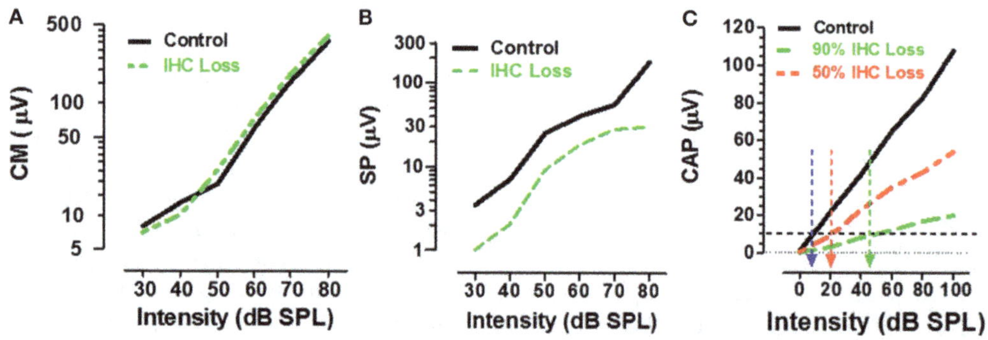

FIGURE 4 | (A) Schematic showing the CM input/output functions in control (black) vs. carboplatin-treated (green) chinchillas with large IHC loss but intact OHC. IHC loss had little effect on CM amplitude. **(B)** Schematic illustrating the SP input/output functions in control (black) vs. carboplatin-treated (green) chinchillas with large IHC lesion with retention of OHC. IHC lesion caused a large reduction (~60%) in SP amplitude. **(C)** Schematic showing the CAP input/output function in control (black) and carboplatin-treated chinchillas with a large (~90%, green) or moderate (~50%, red) IHC lesion and intact OHC. IHC loss resulted in a large decrease in CAP amplitude; the amplitude reduction was proportional to IHC loss. Black horizontal dashed line at 10 μV used to derive CAP threshold for control group (~10 dB SPL, blue arrow) vs. groups with 50% IHC loss (~20 dB SPL, red arrow) or 90% IHC loss (~45 dB SPL, green arrow). Data schematized from Trautwein et al. (1996), Wang et al. (1997), and Durrant et al. (1998).

of the ECochG can be used to assess the functional status of IHC.

IHC LOSS DEPRESSES THE COMPOUND ACTION POTENTIAL

The auditory nerve compound action potential (CAP), consisting of two negative peaks (N1 and N2), is the most widely studied component of ECochG. The CAP is most effectively elicited by acoustic stimuli with rapid rise time and is thought to reflect the synchronized onset response of type I auditory nerve fibers (Dallos, 1973; Zheng et al., 1996). Since the amplitude of the CAP is a postsynaptic response that depends on the release of excitatory neurotransmitter from the IHC, damage to the IHC would be predicted to greatly reduce the CAP. To test this hypothesis, CAP input/output functions were recorded from carboplatin-treated chinchillas with different degrees of IHC damage (Trautwein et al., 1996; Wang et al., 1997). In cases where most IHC were destroyed (80–90%) and most OHC were present, the amplitude of the CAP was greatly reduced compared to controls, whereas moderate (~50%) IHC loss resulted in a modest amplitude reduction as schematized by the CAP input/output functions in **Figure 4C**. These results indicate that the reduction in CAP amplitude is proportional to the degree of IHC loss (Wang et al., 1997; Qiu et al., 2000). CAP thresholds can be derived from the input/output functions using an amplitude criterion of 10 μV. In the schematic (**Figure 4C**), CAP threshold was ~10 dB SPL in the control group (blue arrow) and ~20 dB SPL in the carboplatin group with 50% IHC (red arrow). These results suggest that auditory nerve fiber thresholds are only slightly increased despite the moderate to severe IHC lesion. However, in cases where ~90% of the IHC were missing and very few nerve fibers would be available to generate a synchronized CAP response, the CAP threshold had increased to ~45 dB SPL (green arrow). These results suggest that the CAP amplitude and CAP threshold have the greatest utility for detecting damage to the IHC/type I auditory nerve fibers.

ACOUSTICALLY RESPONSIVE AUDITORY NERVE FIBERS HAVE LOW THRESHOLDS AND ARE SHARPLY TUNED

High impedance microelectrodes can be used to record the all or none spike discharges from single auditory nerve fibers as they leave the cochlea and enter the cochlear nucleus. Since each type I auditory nerve fiber contacts a single IHC, the neural output of a fiber reflects the activity from a discrete region of the basilar membrane. When tone bursts are used to measure the response of a single auditory nerve fiber, one can map out the frequency-intensity combinations that are just capable of evoking a response, the so-called frequency-threshold tuning curve (Salvi et al., 1982, 1983; Wang et al., 1997). Each tuning curve is characterized by a low threshold, narrowly tuned tip (**Figure 5A**). The frequency with the lowest threshold at the tip is the characteristic frequency (CF). The tuning curves of high CF and medium CF neurons are characterized by a steep high frequency slope above CF. Thresholds below CF also rise steeply, but gradually give rise to a high-threshold, broadly tuned tail. The tuning curves of low-CF neurons are more symmetrical and lack the broad low-frequency tail (Wang et al., 1997; Salvi et al., 1983, 1982).

Extensive damage to the IHC could conceivably affect the mechanical properties of the basilar membrane and alter the tuning and sensitivity of auditory nerve fibers. To evaluate this possibility, recordings were made from carboplatin-treated chinchillas with extensive IHC loss along the entire length of the cochlea as well as some OHC loss in the base of the cochlea as schematized in **Figure 5B** (Wang et al., 1997). When a microelectrode was advanced through the auditory nerve bundle, comparatively few acoustically responsive nerve fibers were encountered during the penetration, presumably due to the extensive loss of IHC and type I nerve fibers. However, when an acoustically responsive nerve fiber was encountered, CF-thresholds were low and tuning curve shapes were similar to those from normal control ears (**Figures 5C–E**; Wang et al., 1997). Thus, despite the massive IHC loss, the remaining IHC and type I neurons had low thresholds and sharp tuning which may explain why behavioral thresholds were relatively normal notwithstanding the large IHC loss. Apparently, sounds can be detected in quiet with only a weak signal from the few remaining IHC and type I neurons. Despite normal thresholds and tuning, spontaneous and suprathreshold responses from intact auditory nerve fibers were decreased in carboplatin-treated animals, indicative of subtle damage to surviving IHCs, and/or type I neurons (Wang et al., 1997).

CENTRAL GAIN COMPENSATES FOR AUDITORY DEPRIVATION

If 75% of the IHC and type I neurons were destroyed, the central auditory pathway would receive only 25% of its normal input, a condition that would lead to a severe case of auditory sensory deprivation. A shout to a carboplatin-deafferented ear would likely be perceived as muffled unless there was some form of compensation to boost the weak neural signal. To determine how the central auditory system deals with diminished neural input from a carboplatin-damaged cochlea, recordings were made from chronically implanted electrodes in the cochlea (CAP), inferior colliculus (IC), and auditory cortex (ACx) of awake chinchillas before and after carboplatin treatment (Qiu et al., 2000). The schematics in the upper half of **Figure 6** show the local field potential (LFP) input/output functions for the CAP (panel A), IC (panel C) and ACx (panel E) pre- and 5 weeks post-carboplatin treatment. The results portrayed in the upper half are representative data obtained from animals with mild IHC lesions of 20–30%. To facilitate a comparison across animals and conditions, the amplitudes are expressed as a percentage of the pre-treatment amplitude at 100 dB SPL. Consequently, all the pre-treatment values equal 100% at 100 dB SPL. In cases where 20–30% of the IHC were destroyed, the CAP amplitudes were smaller than normal. At 100 dB, the post-carboplatin CAP was reduced ~20% (80% of normal). **Figure 6B** is a schematic that shows the percent change in CAP amplitude at 80 dB as a function of percent IHC loss. CAP amplitude declines rapidly with IHC loss and the response is almost completely abolished with a loss of 90%. If the output of the auditory nerve was simply relayed up the central auditory pathway, the responses in the IC and ACx would mirror the CAP. Inspection of responses from the IC shows that the post-carboplatin input/output function is only slightly below the pre-treatment curve (**Figure 6C**; Qiu et al., 2000). The schematic in **Figure 6D** shows the percent change in IC amplitude at 80 dB vs. percent IHC loss. The slope of the IC function is roughly half that of the CAP, i.e., IC amplitude at 80 dB was only reduced ~40% compared to ~80% for the CAP. Carboplatin produced the most striking changes in the ACx where the post-exposure amplitudes were larger than pre-treatment values as schematized in **Figure 6E**. This cortical hyperactivity was dynamic, developing gradually over several days to weeks (Qiu et al., 2000). When the percent change in ACx amplitude at 80 dB is compared to percent IHC loss (**Figure 6F**), post-carboplatin amplitudes were 20–30% larger than normal (enhanced) with small to moderate IHC lesions and remarkably, only slightly below normal with near complete IHC lesions.

Taken together, these results indicate that the signal from the cochlea is progressively amplified as it is relayed to the central auditory pathway eventually leading to hyperactivity in the ACx. These findings are consistent with recent reports showing central gain enhancement with various forms of cochlear pathology; however, an unusual feature of carboplatin is that hearing thresholds are largely unaffected by the cochlea pathology (Salvi et al., 1990, 2000b; Sun et al., 2009; Stolzberg et al., 2011; Yuan et al., 2014; Brotherton et al., 2015; Chen et al., 2016). Interestingly, similar perceptual and electrophysiological changes were observed in a recent study examining ouabain treatment in mice, which selectively destroys type-1 SGN (Chambers et al., 2016). Animals with a unilateral lesion of >95% of afferent nerve fibers maintained relatively normal sound detection, likely due to a progressive recovery of sound-evoked activity along the central auditory pathway. Like the above results with carboplatin treatment (**Figure 6**), ouabain treatment greatly

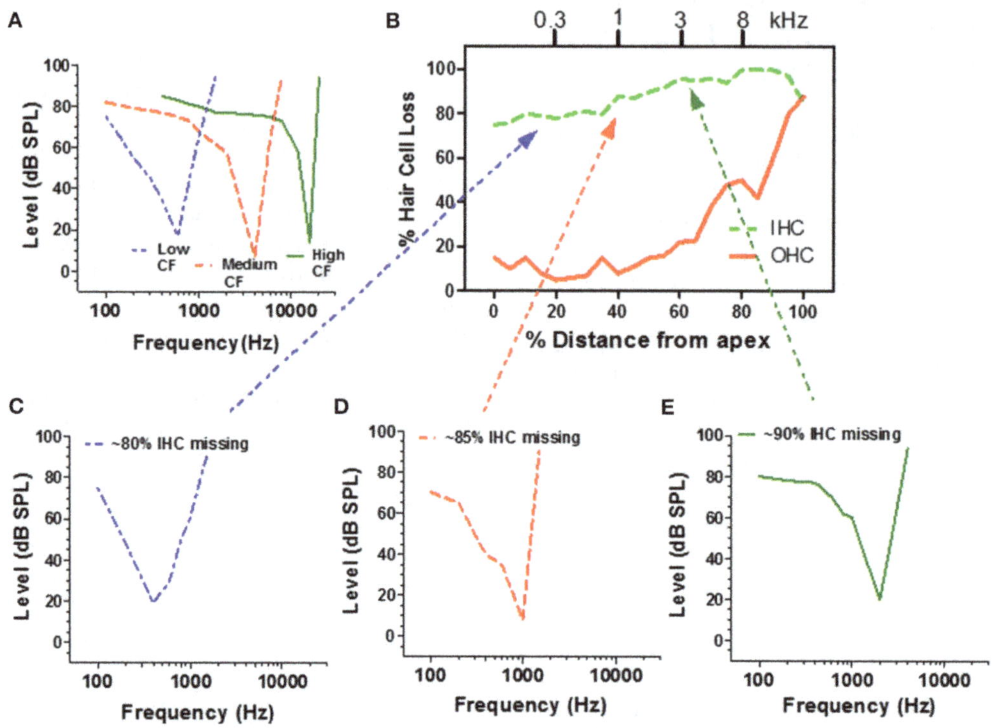

FIGURE 5 | (A) Schematic of a low, medium and high CF auditory nerve fiber frequency-threshold tuning curves. The neuron's CF maps to the tonotopic map of the cochlea (frequency-place map upper x-axis, **B**). **(B)** Schematic cochleogram showing the percentage of missing IHC and OHC in a chinchilla treated with a high dose of carboplatin that destroyed approximately 80–98% of the IHC; damage was more severe in the basal half of the cochlea. Carboplatin also damaged OHC in the base (60–100%). **(C–E)** Schematic of auditory nerve fiber tuning curves from carboplatin treated animals with CFs near 300 Hz (**C**, blue), 1000 Hz (**D**, red), and 3000 Hz (**E**, green). Dotted lines relate each neuron's CF to IHC damage on tonotopic map (upper x-axis, **B**). Data schematized from Wang et al. (1997).

diminished auditory nerve responses while neural response were partially recovered in the IC and almost completely recovered, and in some cases enhanced, at the level of the ACx. Thus, cochlear damage appears to trigger a cascade of neuroplastic changes in the central auditory pathway to compensate for the reduced neural output from a damaged cochlea. Increasing the amplitude of a weak signal would make it easier for the ACx to detect sounds; this may explain why mild to moderate IHC and/or SGN loss has so little effect on auditory thresholds.

DECREASED INHIBITION IN THE AUDITORY CORTEX

Mechanistically, the heightened level of sound-evoked activity in the ACx of carboplatin-treated chinchillas could be due to increased excitation and/or decreased inhibition (Milbrandt et al., 2000; Suneja et al., 2000; Vale and Sanes, 2002; Sanes and Kotak, 2011). Gamma aminobutyric acid (GABA), a potent and ubiquitous inhibitory neurotransmitter, is heavily expressed in the central auditory system and ACx (Hendry and Jones, 1991; Prieto et al., 1994; Ling et al., 2005; Sacco et al., 2009) Neonatal sensorineural hearing loss reduces the number of GABAa receptors in the plasma membrane of layer 2/3 neurons in ACx (Sarro et al., 2008); this would decrease GABAa-mediated inhibition and may contribute to the hyperactivity seen in the ACx with cochlear hearing loss. To determine if the sound-evoked hyperexcitability in ACx was due to reduced GABAa-mediated inhibition, we measured LFPs in the ACx of normal and carboplatin-treated chinchillas while manipulating inhibitory tone (Salvi et al., 2000a, 2014). When bicuculline, a potent GABAa antagonist was applied locally to the ACx, it increased the firing rate, broadened the tuning and lowered the threshold of many ACx neurons (Wang et al., 2000). Bicuculline applied to the surface of the ACx of normal-hearing chinchillas also dramatically increased the amplitude of the sound-evoked LFP in the ACx as schematized in **Figure 7A**; the amplitude enhancement was much greater for the negative peak than the positive peak. **Figure 7B** is a schematic that shows the time course and percent increase in the magnitude of the positive and negative peaks of the LFP response after bicuculline was applied to the ACx of a normal chinchilla. The maximum increase occurred ~5 min after bicuculline was applied to the ACx and the response gradually recovered toward baseline values over the following 30 min as bicuculline washed out. These results indicate that under normal conditions, GABA strongly inhibits sound-evoked responses in the ACx, but when GABAa receptors are blocked with bicuculline sound-evoked activity increases dramatically.

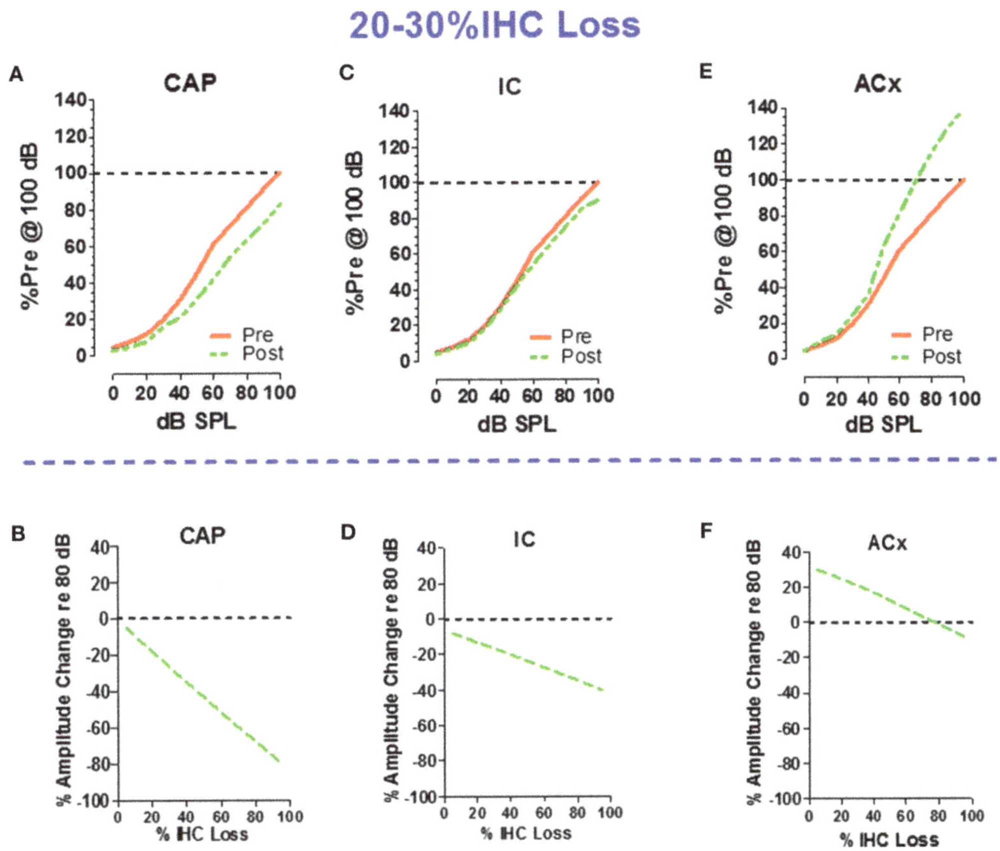

FIGURE 6 | Schematics in upper half illustrate the input/output functions recorded from the (A) round window of the cochlea (compound action potential, CAP), **(C)** inferior colliculus (IC) and **(E)** auditory cortex (ACx) before and after carboplatin treatment that induced 20–30% IHC loss. Amplitude of local field potentials (LFPs) expressed as a percentage of the pre-treatment amplitude measured at 100 dB SPL. All pre-treatment amplitudes equal 100% at 100 dB before carboplatin treatment. Schematics in lower half show the percent change in amplitude of the LFPs recorded at 80 dB SPL vs. percent IHC loss; plots show result for the cochlear CAP **(B)**, IC **(D)**, and ACx **(F)**. Values above the dashed horizontal line in panel F indicate that at 80 dB SPL LFPs in the ACx were larger than normal for small to moderate size IHC lesion, but response were smaller than normal for IHC lesions >80%. Negative slopes indicate that LFP measured at 80 dB SPL decrease as IHC lesions increase. The decrease in amplitude was greatest for the CAP and least for the ACx. Data schematized from Qiu (1998) and Qiu et al. (2000).

As noted above (**Figure 6**), sound-evoked responses in the ACx greatly increase after carboplatin treatment, potentially indicating that GABA mediated inhibition was already diminished. To investigate this possibility, bicuculline was applied to the ACx of chinchillas that had been treated with a moderate dose of carboplatin. As schematized in **Figure 7C**, bicuculline failed to increase the amplitude of the sound-evoked LFP in the ACx; instead there was a slight reduction that dissipated over time. Thus, carboplatin treatment appears to occlude the effects of bicuculline on ACx responses. Failure of bicuculline to increase sound-evoked activity could occur if there was a significant decline in GABAa receptors in the ACx, an interpretation consistent with previous findings in hearing impaired animals (Sarro et al., 2008). An alternative possibility is that less GABA is released from presynaptic neurons; however, this view is not supported by results from hearing impaired animals (Sarro et al., 2008). While altered inhibition has been observed in both cortical and subcortical auditory structures following noise-induced hearing loss (Milbrandt et al., 2000; Dong et al., 2010; Wang et al., 2011; Yang et al., 2011), it remains to be determined if changes to GABA-mediated inhibition are involved in the partial recovery of IC responses following carboplatin treatment.

CRITICAL BAND PERCEPTUAL DEFICITS WITH IHC LOSS

Taken together, the above results suggest that only a fraction of IHC and type 1 nerve fibers are required for normal hearing thresholds in quiet (**Figure 3**) because activity from the few remaining intact nerve fibers, which maintain low thresholds and sharp tuning (**Figure 5**), is progressively amplified through the central auditory system (**Figure 6**). However, listening with few IHC and type I neurons might be extremely challenging in more difficult listening environments. Each IHC is contacted by 10–20 type I nerve fibers resulting in considerable redundancy in the information relayed by each IHC to the central auditory system. Moderate IHC and type I neural loss would greatly reduce this redundancy and information transfer to the auditory brain which

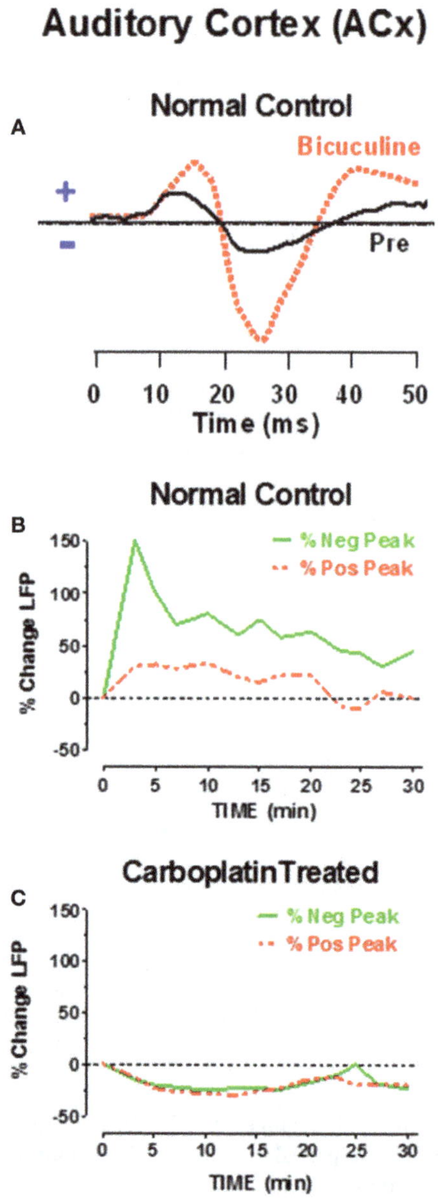

FIGURE 7 | (A) Schematic of sound-evoked local field potentials (LFPs) from the auditory cortex (ACx) before (pre, solid black line) and after applying bicuculline (dashed red line) to the surface of the ACx of a normal control. Note increase in positive and negative peaks in the ACx waveform; increase in negative peak was larger than positive peak. **(B)** Percent change in positive and negative peaks in the LFP after applying bicuculline to the ACx. Bicuculline caused a large increase in positive and negative peaks. Largest increase occurred approximately 5 min post-treatment. Amplitudes gradually recovered with bicuculline washout. **(C)** Percent change in LFP after applying bicuculline to the ACx of chinchillas that had been treated with a moderate dose of carboplatin 1–2 months earlier. Bicuculline failed to induce an increase in cortical LFP, but instead induced a small decrease in the LFP which partially recovered 30 min after applying bicuculline. Data schematized from Salvi et al. (2000a, 2014).

could result in auditory processing deficits in conditions with decreased signal to noise ratio, such as detecting sounds in noisy environments. To test this hypothesis, chinchillas were trained to detect a tone burst in broadband noise (BBN), a technique often used to investigate the internal critical band filters (Scharf, 1961, 1970). Consistent with previous results, pure tone thresholds measured in quiet were only slightly higher (3–5 dB) than baseline after administering a dose of carboplatin that destroyed ~60–70% of the IHC as schematized in **Figures 8A,B** (Lobarinas et al., 2013, 2016). Pure tone thresholds were then measured in BBN with an overall SPL of 50 dB and a spectrum level of ~7 dB as schematized in **Figure 8C**. During baseline testing, tone thresholds in BBN increased with frequency up to around 8 kHz and then plateaued similar to previous results (Seaton and Trahiotis, 1975). After carboplatin treatment, tone thresholds in BBN increased at all frequencies; the 6–11 dB increase in signal to noise ratios was statistically significant (Lobarinas et al., 2016).

According to critical band theory, detection of the signal depends on the power in the signal relative to the power passing through the width of the critical band (Scharf, 1970). The carboplatin-induced increase in critical band values could result from a widening of the critical band. However, since sharp tuning is maintained at the auditory nerve (**Figure 5**) and IC (Wake et al., 1996b), the absence of band widening would not alter the amount of noise passing through the critical band and therefore not alter the signal to noise ratios. However, it is still possible that broader neural tuning could emerge at the level of the ACx due to loss of GABA-mediated inhibition (Wang et al., 2002). Alternatively, the increase in signal to noise ratios (**Figure 8C**) could result from an increase in central gain because the total amount of noise passing through a filter is the product of the bandwidth times the gain.

NARROW BAND NOISE MASKING WITH IHC LOSS

Another approach used to assess the frequency selectivity of the auditory system is to measure tone burst thresholds at frequencies below, at and above the center frequency of a narrow band noise (NBN); a plot of threshold vs. frequency in the presence of the masker defines the NBN masking profile (Egan and Hake, 1950). The solid line in **Figure 8D** is a schematic showing a typical masking profile for a NBN (100 Hz bandwidth) centered at 4 kHz. The baseline NBN masking profile in a normal chinchilla is asymmetric. Masked thresholds are highest at the frequency of the masker, but decrease rapidly for frequencies below 4 kHz. In contrast, masked thresholds decline gradually at frequencies above the 4 kHz masker resulting in considerable upward spread of masking. To determine if the NBN masking profile was altered by the loss of IHC, chinchillas were treated with a moderate dose of carboplatin that destroyed 60–70% of the IHC (**Figure 8B**), which had little effect on thresholds in quiet (**Figure 8A**). Following carboplatin-treatment, threshold at the 4 kHz NBN masker increased approximately 10 dB, a result consistent with the BBN masking pattern. A 10–12 dB threshold increase also occurred at frequencies above the masker. Thus, the tip and high-frequency leg of the NBN masking pattern were shifted upward, but the bandwidth of the tip was essentially unchanged indicating that frequency selectivity was normal near

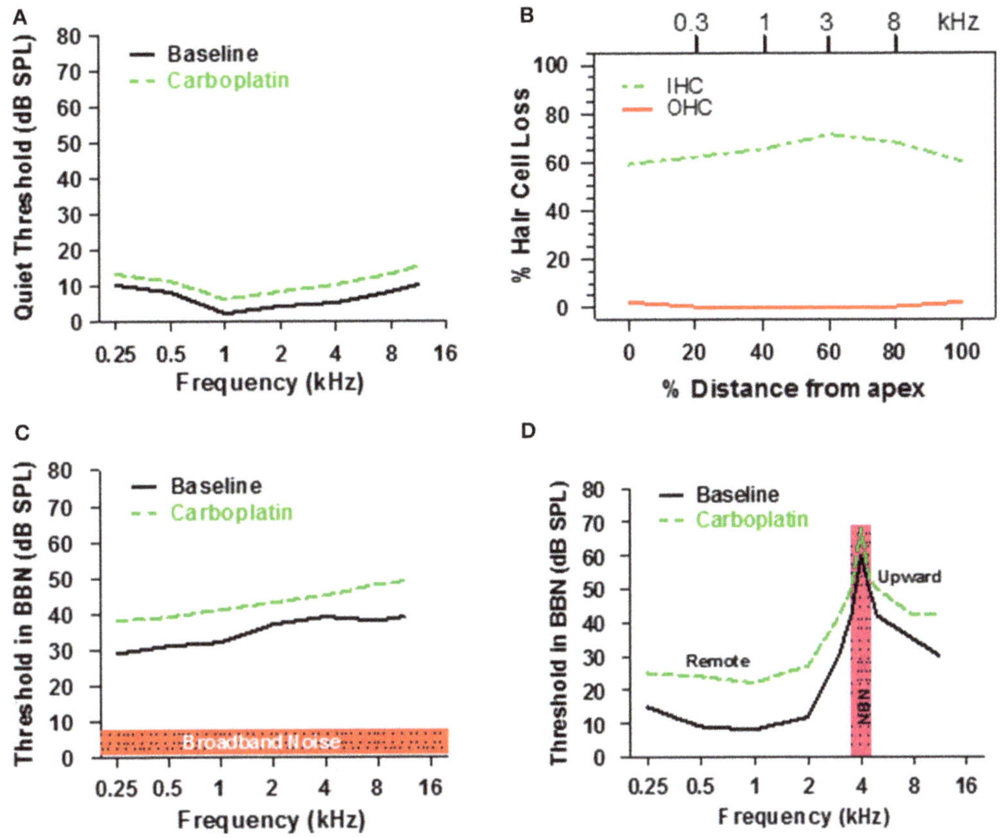

FIGURE 8 | (A) Schematic illustrating threshold in quiet before and after a moderate dose of carboplatin. **(B)** Schematic representing the IHC and OHC loss after a moderate dose of carboplatin that induces a 60–70% IHC with little or no loss of OHC. **(C)** Schematic showing the threshold in 50 dB SPL broadband noise before and after moderate dose of carboplatin. **(D)** Schematic illustrating the thresholds measured in narrowband noise (100 Hz bandwidth) centered at 4 kHz before and after a moderate dose of carboplatin. Carboplatin-induced threshold elevations above 4 kHz reflect the upward spread of masking and those below 4 kHz reflect remote masking. Data schematized from Lobarinas et al. (2016).

4 kHz. Paradoxically, masked thresholds were also elevated 10–15 dB at frequencies (0.25–2 kHz) far below the 4 kHz masker, a phenomenon known as remote masking. It has been suggested that remote masking arises from OHC electromotility and nonlinear motion of the basilar membrane because conditions that disrupt the OHC reduce remote masking (Cervellera and Quaranta, 1982; Salonna et al., 1992; Quaranta et al., 1999). Since OHC appeared functionally intact, our results suggest that IHC/type I neurons normally suppress remote masking as their loss results in greater remote masking. Thresholds in NBN were elevated over a broad range of frequencies, a pattern at odds with basilar membrane mechanics. An alternative explanation for the widespread increase in masked threshold is that it is due to the loss of GABA-mediated inhibition in the ACx since pharmacologic blockage of GABA-mediated inhibition results in broadening of ACx tuning curves both above and below CF (Wang et al., 2002).

SYNOPSIS

Much of the basic auditory research over the past century has focused on the anatomy and physiology of the cochlea. As a result, we now have noninvasive functional tests such as DPOAE to evaluate the status of the OHC in the cochlea. DPOAE are maintained at normal levels (**Figure 2**) if cochlear damage is confined to IHC, but rapidly decline if the OHC are also destroyed (Hofstetter et al., 1997a). The CM component of ECochG can also be used to evaluate the functional status of OHC as well. Selective destruction of the IHC with carboplatin had no measureable effect on the CM (**Figure 4A**), consistent with the notion that OHC are the dominant generators of this potential. In addition, the SP of ECochG provides a powerful tool for evaluating activity of IHC, since IHC loss results in a massive decline, but not complete abolition, of this potential (**Figure 4B**; Durrant et al., 1998). The CAP, the neural component of ECochG, is useful for assessing the sensitivity and global neural output of the cochlea. The decline in CAP amplitude is roughly proportional to IHC loss (**Figure 4C**) whereas changes in CAP threshold are more difficult to assess because a large decline in CAP amplitude can make it difficult to clearly identify the CAP.

One of the most remarkable psychoacoustic findings from the series of carboplatin studies reviewed here was that hearing thresholds in quiet were nearly normal despite the massive loss of IHC and type I neurons. Our auditory nerve fiber recording

(**Figure 5**) and psychoacoustic (**Figure 3**) results suggest that only a few normal functioning IHC and type I neurons are needed to hear a tone in a quiet environment. How is it that we can hear so well when only a few IHC and type I neurons are connected to the brain? The answer to this question may relate to the fact that we perceive sounds not just with the cochlea, but also with our brain. The decrease in the neural output of the cochlea likely triggers a series of homeostatic processes at multiple stages of the auditory pathway that amplify these weak signals so that by the time it reaches the IC or ACx, sound-evoked responses are normal or even supra normal (**Figure 6**; Qiu et al., 2000; Jiang et al., 2016). The increases in gain seem to be most pronounced with mild to moderate IHC lesions, where the largest increase in ACx response occurred (**Figures 6E,F**). Since carboplatin-induced damage results in relatively matched bilateral lesions, it is possible that recovery from more severe IHC loss may be observed if lesions were restricted to one ear, as was found recently for a ouabain model of auditory neuropathy (Chambers et al., 2016). However, the fact that extensive recovery of sound encoding (and even over amplification as in the ACx) is observed in carboplatin-treated animals with bilateral lesions suggests that central gain enhancement is not limited to ear- or input-specific competitive changes but can also arise from a balanced loss of input to both ears. Our results suggest that, at least for carboplatin-induced cochlear damage, enhanced central gain and neural amplification is due in part to the loss of GABA-mediated inhibition in the ACx. However, a plethora of additional mechanisms operating at multiple levels of the auditory system are likely to be involved as well (Suneja et al., 2000; Chen et al., 2007; Peppi et al., 2012; Auerbach et al., 2014).

There is currently tremendous scientific and clinical interest in a form of hidden hearing loss termed synaptopathy that affects the synaptic ribbon at the base of the IHC, glutamatergic receptors located on type I auditory nerve terminals and neurotrophin3 which provides trophic support for SGN (Liberman et al., 2011; Kujawa and Liberman, 2015; Shaheen et al., 2015; Viana et al., 2015; Shi et al., 2016a,b; Suzuki et al., 2016). Identifying the unique perceptual deficits associated with this condition will provide additional tools for identifying individuals with normal clinical audiograms that nonetheless have significant auditory processing disruptions. Although the histopathologies associated with carboplatin damage in the chinchilla are likely somewhat different than those with pure synaptopathy, our psychophysical studies suggest that a simple tone in BBN noise detection task, something that can be accomplished with a clinical audiometer, may be a sensitive method for identifying damage confined to the IHC and/or SGN. Tests of remote masking might also be useful since remote masking increased in chinchillas with selective damage to IHC and type I neurons whereas remote masking decreases with age-related hearing loss and salicylate ototoxicity, conditions likely to involve OHC pathology.

Why does loss of IHC/type I neurons result in difficulties hearing in noise? While remaining auditory nerve fibers maintain normal tuning and thresholds following carboplatin treatment (**Figure 5**), there is evidence for reduced spontaneous and maximum driven firing rates, which could lead to coding deficits in noisy conditions (Wang et al., 1997). A recent study has demonstrated that auditory nerve fibers with low spontaneous firing rates are preferentially damaged by noise exposure that causes hidden hearing loss (Furman et al., 2013). These nerve fibers are characterized by a relatively large dynamic range and wide threshold distribution and are therefore well-equipped for coding sounds in noisy backgrounds, suggesting that selective loss of these nerve fibers could lead to problems hearing in noisy environments. Interestingly, carboplatin treatment results in a decrease in the median spontaneous firing rate of auditory nerve fibers, shifting the population in favor of lower spontaneous rates rather than higher (Wang et al., 1997). This suggests that the difficulties hearing in noise experienced by carboplatin-treated chinchillas is not likely due to the loss of a specific class of auditory neurons, contrary to what is seen with noise-induced hidden hearing loss, but may be due in part to the reduced maximum driven rates seen at high sound levels (Wang et al., 1997).

Adding to the complexity of cochlear hearing loss is the fact that the central auditory system attempts to compensate for peripheral change by turning up its gain. While central gain enhancement is able to restore normal hearing under quiet conditions (**Figure 3**), it may not adequately compensate for peripheral dysfunction in more difficult sound environments (**Figure 7**) or in response to temporally complex stimuli (Lobarinas, 2006; Chambers et al., 2016). This could be because central gain enhancement is most prominent in higher auditory areas that lack the temporal precision required to follow rapid acoustic fluctuations that brainstem and peripheral auditory centers are optimized for. Alternatively, it could be a byproduct of the mechanisms by which gain enhancement is achieved. For instance, while a loss of cortical inhibition may allow for recovery of rate-intensity coding following hearing loss, it could also result in temporal coding deficits that may contribute to impaired speech perception and difficulties hearing in noisy conditions (Wehr and Zador, 2003; Scholl and Wehr, 2008).

Central adaptation to hearing loss is also likely crucial in the development of auditory perceptual disorders like tinnitus and hyperacusis. From a clinical perspective, it would be difficult to account for loudness recruitment or hyperacusis (loudness intolerance) based on the neural responses seen in the damaged cochlea (**Figures 1A,B**). The large gain enhancements seen in the ACx seem particularly relevant to loudness hyperacusis. To our knowledge, no one has tested for evidence of hyperacusis in carbolpatin-treated chinchillas to determine if loudness intolerance is related to carboplatin-induced hyperactivity. However, we have found a striking correlation between salicylate-induced hyperactivity in the central auditory system of rats with behavioral evidence of loudness hyperacusis (Chen et al., 2014, 2015). While enhanced central gain can compensate for the reduced neural output of the cochlea, too much gain at low sound levels could contribute to tinnitus whereas excess gain at high levels may give rise to loudness hyperacusis.

AUTHOR CONTRIBUTIONS

WS, DD, GC, EL, JW, KR, and BA finished the experiment. RS, WS, DD, GC, EL, and KR analyzed the results. RS, BA, and WS wrote and edited the paper.

ACKNOWLEDGMENTS

Research supported in part by the NIH National Institute on Deafness and Other Communication Disorders grants to RS (R01DC014452 and R01DC014693) and to BA (F32DC015160).

REFERENCES

Abdala, C., Sininger, Y. S., and Starr, A. (2000). Distortion product otoacoustic emission suppression in subjects with auditory neuropathy. *Ear Hear.* 21, 542–553. doi: 10.1097/00003446-200012000-00002

Auerbach, B. D., Rodrigues, P. V., and Salvi, R. J. (2014). Central gain control in tinnitus and hyperacusis. *Front. Neurol.* 5:206. doi: 10.3389/fneur.2014.00206

Boettcher, F., Gratton, M. A., Bancroft, B. R., and Spongr, V. (1992). "Interaction of noise and other agents," in *Noise Induced Hearing Loss*, eds A. Dancer, D. Henderson, R. Salvi, and R. P. Hamernik (St. Louis, MO: Mosby Year Book), 175–187.

Brotherton, H., Plack, C. J., Maslin, M., Schaette, R., and Munro, K. J. (2015). Pump up the volume: could excessive neural gain explain tinnitus and hyperacusis? *Audiol. Neurootol.* 20, 273–282. doi: 10.1159/000430459

Brown, A. M., McDowell, B., and Forge, A. (1989). Acoustic distortion products can be used to monitor the effects of chronic gentamicin treatment. *Hear. Res.* 42, 143–156. doi: 10.1016/0378-5955(89)90140-8

Brownell, W. E. (1990). Outer hair cell electromotility and otoacoustic emissions. *Ear Hear.* 11, 82–92. doi: 10.1097/00003446-199004000-00003

Cervellera, G., and Quaranta, A. (1982). Audiologic findings in presbycusis. *J. Aud. Res.* 22, 161–171.

Chambers, A. R., Resnik, J., Yuan, Y., Whitton, J. P., Edge, A. S., Liberman, M. C., et al. (2016). Central gain restores auditory processing following near-complete cochlear denervation. *Neuron* 89, 867–879. doi: 10.1016/j.neuron.2015.12.041

Chen, G. D., Radziwon, K. E., Kashanian, N., Manohar, S., and Salvi, R. (2014). Salicylate-induced auditory perceptual disorders and plastic changes in nonclassical auditory centers in rats. *Neural Plast.* 2014:658741. doi: 10.1155/2014/658741

Chen, G. D., Sheppard, A., and Salvi, R. (2016). Noise trauma induced plastic changes in brain regions outside the classical auditory pathway. *Neuroscience* 315, 228–245. doi: 10.1016/j.neuroscience.2015.12.005

Chen, Y. C., Li, X., Liu, L., Wang, J., Lu, C. Q., Yang, M., et al. (2015). Tinnitus and hyperacusis involve hyperactivity and enhanced connectivity in auditory-limbic-arousal-cerebellar network. *Elife* 4:e06576. doi: 10.7554/eLife.06576

Chen, Z., Kujawa, S. G., and Sewell, W. F. (2007). Auditory sensitivity regulation via rapid changes in expression of surface AMPA receptors. *Nat. Neurosci.* 10, 1238–1240. doi: 10.1038/nn1974

Dallos, P. (1973). *The Auditory Periphery: Biophysics and Physiology*. New York, NY: Academic Press.

Dallos, P., Billone, M. C., Durrant, J. D., Wang, C., and Raynor, S. (1972). Cochlear inner and outer hair cells: functional differences. *Science* 177, 356–358. doi: 10.1126/science.177.4046.356

Ding, D., McFadden, S. L., and Salvi, R. J. (2001). Calpain activation and morphological damage in chinchilla inner ears after carboplatin. *J. Assoc. Res. Otolaryngol.* 3, 68–79. doi: 10.1007/s101620020004

Ding, D., Wang, J., Salvi, R., Henderson, D., Hu, B. H., McFadden, S. L., et al. (1999). Selective loss of inner hair cells and type-I ganglion neurons in carboplatin-treated chinchillas. Mechanisms of damage and protection. *Ann. N.Y. Acad. Sci.* 884, 152–170. doi: 10.1111/j.1749-6632.1999.tb08640.x

Ding, D., Wang, J., and Salvi, R. J. (1997). Early damage in the chinchilla vestibular sensory epithelium from carboplatin. *Audiol. Neurootol.* 2, 155–167. doi: 10.1159/000259238

Ding, D., Wang, J., Zheng, X.-Y., and Salvi, R. J. (1998). Early damage of spiral ganglion caused by carboplatin in chinchilla. *J. Audiol. Speech Pathol.* 6, 65–67.

Ding, L., McFadden, S. L., and Salvi, R. J. (2002). Calpain immunoreactivity and morphological damage in chinchilla inner ears after carboplatin. *J. Assoc. Res. Otolaryngol.* 3, 68–79. doi: 10.1007/s101620020004

Dong, S., Rodger, J., Mulders, W. H., and Robertson, D. (2010). Tonotopic changes in GABA receptor expression in guinea pig inferior colliculus after partial unilateral hearing loss. *Brain Res.* 1342, 24–32. doi: 10.1016/j.brainres.2010.04.067

Durrant, J. D., Wang, J., Ding, D. L., and Salvi, R. J. (1998). Are inner or outer hair cells the source of summating potentials recorded from the round window? *J. Acoust. Soc. Am.* 104, 370–377. doi: 10.1121/1.423293

Egan, J. P., and Hake, H. W. (1950). On the masking pattern of simple auditory stimulus. *J. Acoust. Soc. Am.* 22, 622–630. doi: 10.1121/1.1906661

Ettinger, L. J., Gaynon, P. S., Krailo, M. D., Ru, N., Baum, E. S., Siegel, S. E., et al. (1994). A phase II study of carboplatin in children with recurrent or progressive solid tumors. A report from the Childrens Cancer Group. *Cancer* 73, 1297–1301.

Furman, A. C., Kujawa, S. G., and Liberman, M. C. (2013). Noise-induced cochlear neuropathy is selective for fibers with low spontaneous rates. *J. Neurophysiol.* 110, 577–586. doi: 10.1152/jn.00164.2013

Hendry, S. H., and Jones, E. G. (1991). GABA neuronal subpopulations in cat primary auditory cortex: co-localization with calcium binding proteins. *Brain Res.* 543, 45–55. doi: 10.1016/0006-8993(91)91046-4

Hickox, A. E., and Liberman, M. C. (2014). Is noise-induced cochlear neuropathy key to the generation of hyperacusis or tinnitus? *J. Neurophysiol.* 111, 552–564. doi: 10.1152/jn.00184.2013

Hofstetter, P. (1996). *Effects of Carboplatin on Distortion product Otoacoustic Emissions and Inner and Outer Hair Cells in the Chinchilla.* Masters, State University of New York at Buffalo, Communicative Sciences and Disorders.

Hofstetter, P., Ding, D., Powers, N., and Salvi, R. J. (1997a). Quantitative relationship of carboplatin dose to magnitude of inner and outer hair cell loss and the reduction in distortion product otoacoustic emission amplitude in chinchillas. *Hear. Res.* 112, 199–215. doi: 10.1016/S0378-5955(97)00123-8

Hofstetter, P., Ding, D., and Salvi, R. (1997b). Magnitude and pattern of inner and outer hair cell loss in chinchilla as a function of carboplatin dose. *Audiology* 36, 301–311. doi: 10.3109/00206099709071981

Jakubíková, J., Kabatová, Z., Pavlovcinová, G., and Profant, M. (2009). Newborn hearing screening and strategy for early detection of hearing loss in infants. *Int. J. Pediatr. Otorhinolaryngol.* 73, 607–612. doi: 10.1016/j.ijporl.2008.12.006

Jiang, C., Luo, B., Manohar, S., Chen, G. D., and Salvi, R. (2016). Plastic changes along auditory pathway during Salicylate-induced ototoxicity: hyperactivity and CF shifts. *Hear. Res.* doi: 10.1016/j.heares.2016.10.021. [Epub ahead of print].

Kraus, N., Bradlow, A. R., Cheatham, M. A., Cunningham, J., King, C. D., Koch, D. B., et al. (2000). Consequences of neural asynchrony: a case of auditory neuropathy. *J. Assoc. Res. Otolaryngol.* 1, 33–45. doi: 10.1007/s101620010004

Kujawa, S. G., and Liberman, M. C. (2015). Synaptopathy in the noise-exposed and aging cochlea: primary neural degeneration in acquired sensorineural hearing loss. *Hear. Res.* 330(Pt B): 191–199. doi: 10.1016/j.heares.2015.02.009

Liberman, L. D., Wang, H., and Liberman, M. C. (2011). Opposing gradients of ribbon size and AMPA receptor expression underlie sensitivity differences among cochlear-nerve/hair-cell synapses. *J. Neurosci.* 31, 801–808. doi: 10.1523/JNEUROSCI.3389-10.2011

Liberman, M. C., Gao, J., He, D. Z., Wu, X., Jia, S., and Zuo, J. (2002). Prestin is required for electromotility of the outer hair cell and for the cochlear amplifier. *Nature* 419, 300–304. doi: 10.1038/nature01059

Ling, L. L., Hughes, L. F., and Caspary, D. M. (2005). Age-related loss of the GABA synthetic enzyme glutamic acid decarboxylase in rat primary auditory cortex. *Neuroscience* 132, 1103–1113. doi: 10.1016/j.neuroscience.2004.12.043

Lobarinas, E. (2006). *Effects of Carboplatin-Induced Inner Hair Cell Loss on Auditory Perception in Chinchilla.* Ph.D. Thesis, SUNY University at Buffalo, Dept of Communicative Disorders and Sciences.

Lobarinas, E., Salvi, R., and Ding, D. (2013). Insensitivity of the audiogram to carboplatin induced inner hair cell loss in chinchillas. *Hear. Res.* 302, 113–120. doi: 10.1016/j.heares.2013.03.012

Lobarinas, E., Salvi, R., and Ding, D. (2016). Selective inner hair cell dysfunction in chinchillas impairs hearing-in-noise in the absence of outer hair cell loss. *J. Assoc. Res. Otolaryngol.* 17, 89–101. doi: 10.1007/s10162-015-0550-8

Milbrandt, J. C., Holder, T. M., Wilson, M. C., Salvi, R. J., and Caspary, D. M. (2000). GAD levels and muscimol binding in rat inferior colliculus following acoustic trauma. *Hear. Res.* 147, 251–260. doi: 10.1016/S0378-5955(00)00135-0

Peppi, M., Landa, M., and Sewell, W. F. (2012). Cochlear kainate receptors. *J. Assoc. Res. Otolaryngol.* 13, 199–208. doi: 10.1007/s10162-011-0309-9

Plack, C. J., Barker, D., and Prendergast, G. (2014). Perceptual consequences of "hidden" hearing loss. *Trends Hear* 18, 1–11. doi: 10.1177/2331216514550621

Prieto, J. J., Peterson, B. A., and Winer, J. A. (1994). Morphology and spatial distribution of GABAergic neurons in cat primary auditory cortex (AI). *J. Comp. Neurol.* 344, 349–382. doi: 10.1002/cne.903440304

Qiu, C. X. (1998). *The Effects of Selective Inner Hair Cell Loss on the Amplitude of the Evoked Responses from the Auditory Nerve, Inferior Colliculus and Auditory Cortex.* Ph.D. Thesis: SUNY University at Buffalo, Communicative Disorders and Sciences.

Qiu, C., Salvi, R., Ding, D., and Burkard, R. (2000). Inner hair cell loss leads to enhanced response amplitudes in auditory cortex of unanesthetized chinchillas: evidence for increased system gain. *Hear. Res.* 139, 153–171. doi: 10.1016/S0378-5955(99)00171-9

Quaranta, A., Portalatini, P., Camporeale, M., and Sallustio, V. (1999). Effects of salicylates on evoked otoacoustic emissions and remote masking in humans. *Audiology* 38, 174–179. doi: 10.3109/00206099909073019

Russell, I. J., and Sellick, P. M. (1983). Intracellular studies of hair cells in the mammalian cochlea. *J. Physiol. (Lond)* 284, 261–290. doi: 10.1113/jphysiol.1978.sp012540

Rybak, L. P., Whitworth, C. A., Mukherjea, D., and Ramkumar, V. (2007). Mechanisms of cisplatin-induced ototoxicity and prevention. *Hear. Res.* 226, 157–167. doi: 10.1016/j.heares.2006.09.015

Sacco, C. B., Tardif, E., Genoud, C., Probst, A., Tolnay, M., Janzer, R. C., et al. (2009). GABA receptor subunits in human auditory cortex in normal and stroke cases. *Acta Neurobiol. Exp. (Wars).* 69, 469–493.

Saito, T., Saito, H., Saito, K., Wakui, S., Manabe, Y., and Tsuda, G. (1989). Ototoxicity of carboplatin in guinea pigs. *Auris Nasus Larynx* 16, 13–21. doi: 10.1016/S0385-8146(89)80003-3

Salonna, I., Bartoli, R., Berardi, P., and Quaranta, A. (1992). Psychoacoustic tests: effects of atropine. *Boll. Soc. Ital. Biol. Sper.* 68, 633–639.

Salvi, R., Ding, D., Sun, W., Lobarinas, S., and Wang, J. (2014). "Animal model with auditory neuropathy-like characteristics," in *The Hearing Aid Technician's Handbook,* eds U. Ambrosetti, F. di Berardino, and L. del Bo (Torino: Edizioni Minerva Medica), 247–263.

Salvi, R. J., Hamernik, R. P., and Henderson, D. (1978). Discharge patterns in the cochlear nucleus of the chinchilla following noise induced asymptotic threshold shift. *Exp. Brain Res.* 32, 301–320. doi: 10.1007/BF00238704

Salvi, R. J., Henderson, D., Hamernik, R., and Ahroon, W. A. (1983). Neural correlates of sensorineural hearing loss. *Ear Hear.* 4, 115–129. doi: 10.1097/00003446-198305000-00001

Salvi, R. J., Perry, J., Hamernik, R. P., and Henderson, D. (1982). "Relationship between cochlear pathologies and auditory nerve and behavioral responses following acoustic trauma," in *New Perspectives on Noise-Induced Hearing Loss,* eds R. P. Hamernik, D. Henderson, and R. J. Salvi (New York, NY: Raven Press), 165–188.

Salvi, R. J., Saunders, S. S., Gratton, M. A., Arehole, S., and Powers, N. (1990). Enhanced evoked response amplitudes in the inferior colliculus of the chinchilla following acoustic trauma. *Hear. Res.* 50, 245–257. doi: 10.1016/0378-5955(90)90049-U

Salvi, R. J., Sun, W., Wang, J., Guo, Y. Q., Ding, D. L., and Burkard, R. (2000a). "Diminished GABA-A mediated inhibition in auditory cortex following carboplatin-induced inner hair cell loss," in *Abstracts of the Association for Research in Otolaryngology* (Mt Royal, NJ).

Salvi, R. J., Wang, J., and Ding, D. (2000b). Auditory plasticity and hyperactivity following cochlear damage. *Hear. Res.* 147, 261–274. doi: 10.1016/S0378-5955(00)00136-2

Sanes, D. H., and Kotak, V. C. (2011). Developmental plasticity of auditory cortical inhibitory synapses. *Hear. Res.* 279, 140–148. doi: 10.1016/j.heares.2011.03.015

Sarro, E. C., Kotak, V. C., Sanes, D. H., and Aoki, C. (2008). Hearing Loss alters the subcellular distribution of presynaptic GAD and postsynaptic GABAA receptors in the auditory cortex. *Cereb. Cortex* 18, 2855–2867. doi: 10.1093/cercor/bhn044

Schaette, R., and McAlpine, D. (2011). Tinnitus with a normal audiogram: physiological evidence for hidden hearing loss and computational model. *J. Neurosci.* 31, 13452–13457. doi: 10.1523/JNEUROSCI.2156-11.2011

Scharf, B. (1961). Complex sounds and critical bands. *Psychol. Bull.* 58, 205–217. doi: 10.1037/h0049235

Scharf, B. (1970). "Critical bands," in *Foundations of Modern Auditory, I.* ed J. Tobias (New York, NY: Academic Press), 157–202.

Scholl, B., and Wehr, M. (2008). Disruption of balanced cortical excitation and inhibition by acoustic trauma. *J. Neurophysiol.* 100, 646–656. doi: 10.1152/jn.90406.2008

Schrott, A., Puel, J. L., and Rebillard, G. (1991). Cochlear origin of 2f1-f2 distortion products assessed by using 2 types of mutant mice. *Hear. Res.* 52, 245–253. doi: 10.1016/0378-5955(91)90204-M

Seaton, W. H., and Trahiotis, C. (1975). Comparison of critical ratios and critical bands in the monaural chinchilla. *J. Acoust. Soc. Am.* 57, 193–199. doi: 10.1121/1.380414

Shaheen, L. A., Valero, M. D., and Liberman, M. C. (2015). Towards a diagnosis of cochlear neuropathy with envelope following responses. *J. Assoc. Res. Otolaryngol.* 16, 727–745. doi: 10.1007/s10162-015-0539-3

Shi, L., Chang, Y., Li, X., Aiken, S. J., Liu, L., and Wang, J. (2016a). Coding deficits in noise-induced hidden hearing loss may stem from incomplete repair of ribbon synapses in the cochlea. *Front. Neurosci.* 10:231. doi: 10.3389/fnins.2016.00231

Shi, L., Chang, Y., Li, X., Aiken, S., Liu, L., and Wang, J. (2016b). Cochlear synaptopathy and noise-induced hidden hearing loss. *Neural Plast.* 2016:6143164. doi: 10.1155/2016/6143164

Spoendlin, H., and Baumgartner, H. (1977). Electrocochleography and cochlear pathology. *Acta Otolaryngol.* 83, 130–135. doi: 10.3109/00016487709128822

Stanton, S. G., Ryerson, E., Moore, S. L., Sullivan-Mahoney, M., and Couch, S. C. (2005). Hearing screening outcomes in infants of pregestational diabetic mothers. *Am. J. Audiol.* 14, 86–93. doi: 10.1044/1059-0889(2005/008)

Stolzberg, D., Chen, G. D., Allman, B. L., and Salvi, R. J. (2011). Salicylate-induced peripheral auditory changes and tonotopic reorganization of auditory cortex. *Neuroscience* 180, 157–164. doi: 10.1016/j.neuroscience.2011.02.005

Sun, W., Lu, J., Stolzberg, D., Gray, L., Deng, A., Lobarinas, E., et al. (2009). Salicylate increases the gain of the central auditory system. *Neuroscience* 159, 325–334. doi: 10.1016/j.neuroscience.2008.12.024

Suneja, S. K., Potashner, S. J., and Benson, C. G. (2000). AMPA receptor binding in adult guinea pig brain stem auditory nuclei after unilateral cochlear ablation. *Exp. Neurol.* 165, 355–369. doi: 10.1006/exnr.2000.7471

Suzuki, J., Corfas, G., and Liberman, M. C. (2016). Round-window delivery of neurotrophin 3 regenerates cochlear synapses after acoustic overexposure. *Sci. Rep.* 6:24907. doi: 10.1038/srep24907

Takeno, S., Harrison, R. V., Mount, R. J., Wake, M., and Harada, Y. (1994). Induction of selective inner hair cell damage by carboplatin. *Scanning Microsc.* 8, 97–106.

Takeno, S., Wake, M., Mount, R. J., and Harrison, R. V. (1998). Degeneration of spiral ganglion cells in the chinchilla after inner hair cell loss induced by carboplatin. *Audiol. Neurootol.* 3, 281–290. doi: 10.1159/000013800

Trautwein, P., Hofstetter, P., Wang, J., Salvi, R., and Nostrant, A. (1996). Selective inner hair cell loss does not alter distortion product otoacoustic emissions. *Hear. Res.* 96, 71–82. doi: 10.1016/0378-5955(96)00040-8

Vale, C., and Sanes, D. H. (2002). The effect of bilateral deafness on excitatory and inhibitory synaptic strength in the inferior colliculus. *Eur. J. Neurosci.* 16, 2394–2404. doi: 10.1046/j.1460-9568.2002.02302.x

Viana, L. M., O'Malley, J. T., Burgess, B. J., Jones, D. D., Oliveira, C. A., Santos, F., et al. (2015). Cochlear neuropathy in human presbycusis: confocal analysis of hidden hearing loss in post-mortem tissue. *Hear. Res.* 327, 78–88. doi: 10.1016/j.heares.2015.04.014

Wake, M., Anderson, J., Takeno, S., Mount, R. J., and Harrison, R. V. (1996a). Otoacoustic emission amplification after inner hair cell damage. *Acta Otolaryngol.* 116, 374–381. doi: 10.3109/00016489609137860

Wake, M., Takeno, S., Mount, R. J., and Harrison, R. V. (1996b). Recording from the inferior colliculus following cochlear inner hair cell damage. *Acta Otolaryngol.* 116, 714–720. doi: 10.3109/00016489609137912

Wang, H., Brozoski, T. J., and Caspary, D. M. (2011). Inhibitory neurotransmission in animal models of tinnitus: maladaptive plasticity. *Hear. Res.* 279, 111–117. doi: 10.1016/j.heares.2011.04.004

Wang, J., Caspary, D., and Salvi, R. J. (2000). GABA-A antagonist causes dramatic expansion of tuning in primary auditory cortex. *Neuroreport* 11, 1137–1140. doi: 10.1097/00001756-200004070-00045

Wang, J., Ding, D., and Salvi, R. J. (2003). Carboplatin-induced early cochlear lesion in chinchillas. *Hear. Res.* 181, 65–72. doi: 10.1016/S0378-5955(03)00176-X

Wang, J., McFadden, S. L., Caspary, D., and Salvi, R. (2002). Gamma-aminobutyric acid circuits shape response properties of auditory cortex neurons. *Brain Res.* 944, 219–231. doi: 10.1016/S0006-8993(02)02926-8

Wang, J., Powers, N. L., Hofstetter, P., Trautwein, P., Ding, D., and Salvi, R. (1997). Effects of selective inner hair cell loss on auditory nerve fiber threshold, tuning and spontaneous and driven discharge rate. *Hear. Res.* 107, 67–82. doi: 10.1016/S0378-5955(97)00020-8

Wehr, M., and Zador, A. M. (2003). Balanced inhibition underlies tuning and sharpens spike timing in auditory cortex. *Nature* 426, 442–446. doi: 10.1038/nature02116

Yang, S., Weiner, B. D., Zhang, L. S., Cho, S. J., and Bao, S. (2011). Homeostatic plasticity drives tinnitus perception in an animal model. *Proc. Natl. Acad. Sci. U.S.A.* 108, 14974–14979. doi: 10.1073/pnas.1107998108

Yuan, Y., Shi, F., Yin, Y., Tong, M., Lang, H., Polley, D. B., et al. (2014). Ouabain-induced cochlear nerve degeneration: synaptic loss and plasticity in a mouse model of auditory neuropathy. *J. Assoc. Res. Otolaryngol.* 15, 31–43. doi: 10.1007/s10162-013-0419-7

Zeng, F. G., Kong, Y. Y., Michalewski, H. J., and Starr, A. (2005). Perceptual consequences of disrupted auditory nerve activity. *J. Neurophysiol.* 93, 3050–3063. doi: 10.1152/jn.00985.2004

Zheng, X. Y., Ding, D. L., McFadden, S. L., and Henderson, D. (1997). Evidence that inner hair cells are the major source of cochlear summating potentials. *Hear. Res.* 113, 76–88. doi: 10.1016/S0378-5955(97)00127-5

Zheng, X. Y., Wang, J., Salvi, R. J., and Henderson, D. (1996). Effects of kainic acid on the cochlear potentials and distortion product otoacoustic emissions in chinchilla. *Hear. Res.* 95, 161–167. doi: 10.1016/0378-5955(96)00047-0

10

Characterizing Electrocochleography in Cochlear Implant Recipients with Residual Low-Frequency Hearing

Christofer W. Bester[1,2], Luke Campbell[1], Adrian Dragovic[1], Aaron Collins[1] and Stephen J. O'Leary[1,2]*

[1] *Department of Otolaryngology, University of Melbourne, Melbourne, VIC, Australia,* [2] *Royal Victorian Eye and Ear Hospital, Melbourne, VIC, Australia*

Correspondence:
Christofer W. Bester
christofer.bester@unimelb.edu.au

Objective: Lay the groundwork for using electrocochleography (ECochG) as a measure of cochlear health, by characterizing typical patterns of the ECochG response observed across the electrode array in cochlear implant recipients with residual hearing.

Methods: ECochG was measured immediately after electrode insertion in 45 cochlear implant recipients with residual hearing. The Cochlear Response Telemetry system was used to record ECochG across the electrode array, in response to 100- or 110-dB SPL pure tones at 0.5-kHz, presented at 14 per second and with alternating polarities. Hair cell activity, as the cochlear microphonic (CM), was estimated by taking the difference (DIF) of the two polarities. Neural activity, as the auditory nerve neurophonic (ANN), was estimated by taking the sum (SUM) of the two polarities. Prior work in humans and animal studies suggested that the expected ECochG pattern in response to a 0.5-kHz pure tone is an apical-peak in CM amplitude and latency.

Results: The most prevalent pattern was a peak in the DIF amplitude near the most apical electrode, with a prolongation of latency toward the electrode tip; this was found in 21/39 individuals with successful ECochG recordings. The 21 apical-peak recipients had the best low-frequency hearing. A low amplitude, long-latency DIF response that remained relatively constant across the electrode array was found in 10/39 individuals, in a group with the poorest low- and high-frequency hearing. A third, previously undescribed, pattern occurred in 8/39 participants, with mid-electrode peaks in DIF amplitude. These recipients had the best high-frequency hearing and a progressive prolongation of DIF latency around the mid-electrode peaks consistent with the presence of discrete populations of hair cells.

Conclusions: The presence of distinct patterns of the ECochG response with relationships to pre-operative hearing levels supports the notion that ECochG across the electrode array functions as a measure of cochlear health.

Keywords: cochlea, cochlear implant, cochlear microphonic, electrocochleography, hearing loss

INTRODUCTION

Cochlear implants (CIs) are no longer restricted to individuals with severe-to-profound hearing loss. Instead, many implant recipients have substantial levels of low-frequency residual hearing, and a goal of modern implant designs and surgical techniques is to preserve this hearing for electro-acoustic stimulation (EAS; Gantz et al., 2005). Efforts to combine residual hearing and EAS have been hampered by the absence of methods to map the function of neurosensory elements along the cochlea. Such a map would identify frequencies that are appropriate for acoustic stimulation and those that require electrical stimulation, identified as an important factor in the success of this combined delivery method (Gantz and Turner, 2004). Here we demonstrate that this can be achieved with the direct recording of electrocochleography (ECochG) along the length of a cochlear implant electrode.

ECochG has recently become available using intra-cochlear electrodes in CI recipients (Calloway et al., 2014; Campbell et al., 2015; Dalbert et al., 2015). It is a cochlear potential derived from neural and sensory sources in response to transient acoustic stimuli presented with alternating polarity. A frequency-following hair cell response known as the cochlear microphonic (CM) is derived by taking the difference of the two alternating responses (DIF) (Ruben et al., 1961; Dallos, 1973; Patuzzi et al., 1989). ECochG also contains the phase-locked neural response of the auditory nerve as the auditory nerve neurophonic (ANN). As phase-locking occurs preferentially as inner hair cells depolarize (Palmer and Russell, 1986), it results in distortions in the ECochG trace that occur at even harmonics of the acoustic input. Therefore, the ANN is derived by summing the alternating phase responses (SUM), and isolating the 2nd harmonic of the stimulus frequency (Weinberger et al., 1970). It is important to note that the DIF trace, while dominated by the CM, will contain some neural response as demonstrated by Forgues et al. (2014). Similarly, while the SUM trace is dominated by the ANN, at the high sound intensities required for ECochG in CI recipients this response may include some hair cell activity due to asymmetric saturation in the input-output function of the hair cell response (Teich et al., 1989).

ECochG has been recorded from intracochlear electrodes in hearing animals responding to pure acoustic tones. As the site of recording progresses from the base of the cochlea toward the location where the cochlea is most sensitive to the stimulus, there is an exponential increase in CM amplitude and prolongation of its latency. The CM amplitude decreases rapidly at cochlear sites apical to this "characteristic" frequency (Honrubia and Ward, 1968). There have been three previous reports of ECochG recorded from multiple locations along the human cochlea (Calloway et al., 2014; Dalbert et al., 2015; Campbell et al., 2016). Dalbert et al. (2015) recorded ECochG from multiple electrodes along a mid-scalar electrode array (HiFocus Mid-Scala electrode, Advanced Bionics, USA), 12 or more weeks after implantation. Contrary to Calloway et al. (2014), all eight participants exhibited ECochG responses with relatively constant amplitude across the array, or showed a peak in the CM response on basal electrodes in response to 0.5- or 1-kHz tones. It was suggested that the unexpectedly flat responses and basal-peak responses arose from the proximity of the electrode to the auditory nerve, or the influence of intra-scalar fibrosis on the current path in the vicinity of the electrode (also suggested by Campbell et al., 2015). In contrast, Formeister et al. (2015) made recordings at multiple insertion depths from a single recording electrode on a flexible carrier that was inserted into the cochlea during surgery, just prior to implantation of the commercial CI. These investigators found the relationship seen in the previous animal experiments of Honrubia and Ward (1968), with five of eight patients exhibiting a rise in CM amplitude as depth increased, in response to a 0.5-kHz tone. We have made similar observations when recording ECochG from the apical-most electrode of an implant manufactured by Cochlear Ltd during its insertion into the cochlea (Campbell et al., 2016). Whether the difference in response patterns observed between these studies reflects differences in the time between implantation and recording, differences in residual hearing between CI recipients, or the intracochlear position of the recording electrode between devices remains unclear.

In the present work intracochlear ECochG was recorded across the electrode array during surgery, immediately after insertion of the electrode array, in 45 CI recipients who received Cochlear's CI422 or 522 implants. These devices have a thin, flexible electrode that traverses the lateral wall of the cochlea. The aim of the present work was to characterize patterns of ECochG across the electrode array and relate these patterns of response to pre-operative hearing levels. We predicted that there would be a restricted number of patterns of ECochG response, and that these would be associated with the shape of the pre-operative audiogram.

METHODS

Clinical Information

Forty-five adults who received a CI422 or CI522 cochlear implant (Cochlear Ltd, Sydney, Australia) with the "Slim Straight" electrode array had ECochG recordings made from the electrode array immediately after its insertion. All participants had pre-operative hearing thresholds lower than 100-dB HL at 0.5-kHz and a post-lingual hearing loss.

The CI422 and CI522 implants have Cochlear's Slim Straight electrode, an array with 22 half-band intra-cochlear electrodes. The cochlea was approached via a posterior tympanotomy, and the electrode inserted through an incision made in the round window to a depth of between 20- and 25-mm, at the surgeon's discretion. All participants had a full insertion of at least 20-mm, confirmed at the time of surgery and with a post-operative cone-beam CT scan.

This research was conducted under the auspices of the Human Research and Ethics Committee of the Royal Victorian Eye and Ear Hospital HREC (#14/1171H). All patients provided informed, written consent for their participation in the study, and for its dissemination through publication.

Equipment and Information Processing

Electrocochleography was recorded using the Cochlear Response Telemetry (CRT) system previously described by the investigators (Campbell et al., 2015, 2016). Acoustic stimuli were generated digitally using a USB data acquisition card (DT9847, Data Translation, USA), and presented using an ER3A insert earphone (Etymotics, USA). The acoustic stimuli were 12-ms in length with 1-ms linear onset and offset ramps and a 50-ms inter-stimulus interval. Alternating rarefaction and condensation phases were presented, and stored separately. The intensity of the acoustic stimuli was calibrated with peak-to-peak amplitudes equal to the dB HL scale for insert earphones (ISO 389-2:1994).

The CRT system uses the implant's Neural Response Telemetry™ (NRT) amplifier to record from the intra-cochlear CI electrodes. These recordings are made between any one of the intra-cochlear electrodes and the extra-cochlear plate electrode located on the body of the implant. Recording windows were 20-ms in duration, digitized at 20-kHz and streamed to a Dell laptop (Dell, USA), via a Cochlear Freedom™ programming POD. Each ECochG waveform is an average of 100 presentations. The stimuli and recording were coordinated by in-house custom-written software, which interfaced with the Freedom™ sound processor using the Cochlear Device Interface (CDI) libraries (4.15.02). ECochG was recorded from the most apical electrode (22) and then every second electrode until the second most basal electrode. In this study, ECochG was characterized across the electrode array in response to a 0.5-kHz tone pip, delivered at either 100- for patients with ≤70 dB HL at 0.5-kHz or 110-dB for those with >70 dB HL. The 0.5-kHz stimulus frequency was chosen as the closest frequency apical to the average angular insertion depth in a CI422/CI522 patient (410°, or ~0.75-kHz, O'Connell et al., 2016) for which audiometric thresholds are routinely measured. The 1-ms linear onset and offset ramps will result in a loss of frequency specificity (Skinner and Jones, 1968), calculated by FFT to be a broadening of the stimulus by 0.075-kHz either side of 0.5-kHz starting at −20 dB to the peak at 0.5-kHz. Frequency specificity is already decreased due to the high sound pressure level used (Russell and Nilsen, 1997), and considerable sensorineural hearing loss present in the cohort (Gummer and Johnstone, 1984).

To estimate the CM and ANN components of the ECochG waveform, the recordings were processed by either adding the alternating phases responses (SUM) to estimate the ANN or by subtracting them (DIF) to estimate the CM (Adunka et al., 2006; Choudhury et al., 2012; Campbell et al., 2015). To isolate the magnitude of the stimulus frequency-matching CM in the DIF trace, the magnitude at the stimulus frequency was calculated by Fast Fourier Transform (FFT). For the ANN, the asymmetric neural saturating response in the SUM trace was isolated using the FFT magnitude at the 2nd harmonic. The latency of these responses was measured by calculating the FFT phase difference from the response at the most basal electrode to each successive electrode, which used the 2nd harmonic of the SUM trace or the 1st harmonic of the DIF trace. A noise floor for each trace was calculated from FFT bins ± 2 from the frequency of interest, where each FFT bin was 62.5 Hz wide, and ECochG responses were considered robust if the amplitude exceeded the calculated noise floor plus 3 standard deviations.

The absolute latency of the DIF response was measured as the first deflection from baseline after the first pressure change in the ear canal (calibrated using a Bruel and Kjaer ½ inch microphone, oscilloscope, and 2cc coupler) from either the most basal or most apical electrode.

An electrode was considered to have a CM peak if its magnitude was >30% above the mean magnitude across the electrode array. If more than one electrode satisfied this condition, then the electrode with the largest CM was considered the peak. Multiple peaks were recorded if there was an electrode with a greater than 30% drop between one peak and the next more apical electrode.

RESULTS

Electrocochleography could be recorded across the electrode array in response to 0.5-kHz tone in all but six participants, in whom there was no detectable ECochG response on any electrode. **Figure 1** shows example DIF and SUM traces, with power spectral density functions from a single CI recipient with <60 dB HL at 0.5-kHz. **Figure 1** demonstrates that the bulk of response power in the DIF trace is located at the stimulus frequency, consistent with a primary contribution by the CM, whereas the power in the SUM trace is concentrated at the secondary harmonic, consistent with asymmetric saturation in the neural response.

Median hearing level for all participants who showed a detectable ECochG was 60-, 65-, 85-, 100-, and 110-dB HL at 0.25-, 0.5-, 1-, 2-, and 4-kHz.

Apical Peak

The acoustic stimulus was a 0.5-kHz tone, and ECochG was recorded from 11 electrodes across the array. The most prevalent response pattern (21 participants) was a growth of the DIF amplitude to a peak near the apical tip of the electrode, defined as a single CM peak on the most apical 6 electrodes located proximal to the 0.5-kHz characteristic frequency region in the cochlea. The major acoustic generator contributing to this response is the CM (Dallos, 1973; Patuzzi et al., 1989). The DIF and SUM amplitudes, and DIF latencies are shown relative to the electrode with the peak DIF amplitude in **Figure 2**. In this figure, the amplitude of the responses has been normalized relative to the peak amplitude in the respective individual. The mean absolute DIF amplitude on electrodes basal to the peak DIF responses was 3.4 μV ± 0.3 SEM. The mean maximum absolute DIF amplitude on apical peaks was 22.1 μV ± 5.6 SEM. In these participants, the peak DIF amplitude was located at one of the more apical electrodes, specifically on electrodes 22 (i.e., at the tip, n = 9), 20 (n = 6), 18 (n = 4), or 16 (n = 2). A rapid increase in DIF amplitude was found up to the electrode exhibiting the peak, with a comparably rapid drop off in amplitude once that at more apical electrodes. The SUM response showed a similar pattern with gradual increase in amplitude that reached its maximum at, or slightly above, the peak electrode. The SUM response is largely derived from the frequency-following potential of the auditory nerve, the ANN (Weinberger et al., 1970). Across the group, there was a moderate to strong positive correlation between DIF and SUM amplitudes (Pearson product-moment correlation coefficient, mean r = 0.68, ranging from 0.18 to 0.94). While this correlation was strong, the peak SUM response was on a more apical electrode than the peak DIF response in the majority of patients (n = 12), and less frequently on the same (n = 7), or a more basal electrode (n = 2). In this group, absolute latency increased across the electrode array from 1.22-ms ± 0.67 until the peak was reached (2.40-ms ± 0.66) and there was a strong, positive correlation between the DIF

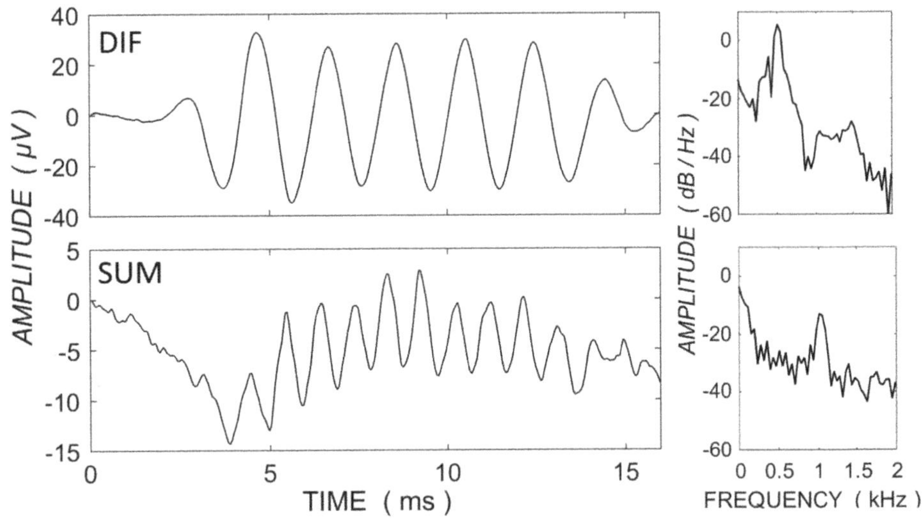

FIGURE 1 | ECochG traces for the difference (DIF - upper panels) and sum (SUM - lower panels) responses in a single CI recipient with <70 dB HL at 0.5-kHz and in response to a 0.5-kHz tone burst at 100 dB HL. Power spectral density functions are shown to the right of the traces (expressed as dB relative to 1 μV). The primary power for the DIF trace is concentrated at the fundamental frequency, consistent with a contribution primarily by the frequency-matching hair cell response, whereas the power in the SUM trace is concentrated at the secondary harmonic, consistent with the neural saturating response.

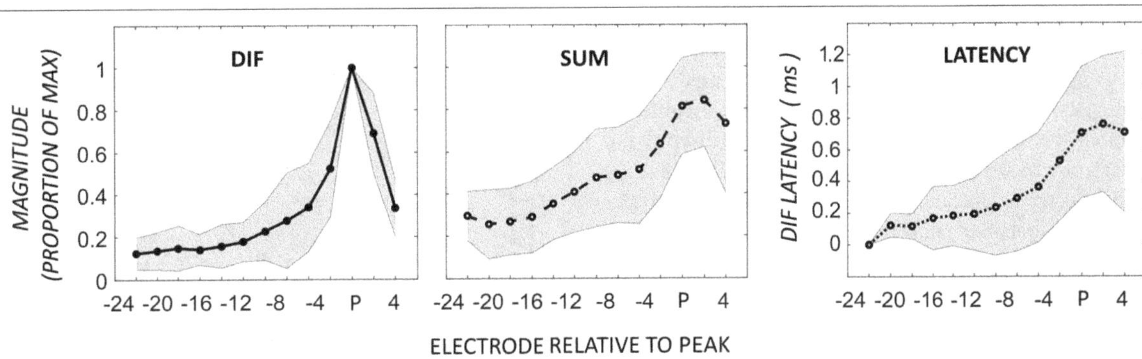

FIGURE 2 | ECochG responses in 21 patients with the maximum DIF amplitude at apical electrodes. Responses here have been normalized to the maximum response in each individual, as well as to the electrode with the peak DIF response (P). The amplitudes of the SUM response are reported normalized to the electrode with the peak DIF response. The DIF latency is reported relative to the response on the most basal electrode in each individual. Shaded area represents ± 1 *SD*.

amplitudes and latencies (Pearson product-moment correlation coefficient mean $r = 0.76$, ranging from 0.45 to 0.96).

Flat-Response

In addition to the pattern of ECochG with an apical peak in DIF amplitude, we observed a pattern of flat DIF amplitudes across the electrode array in 10 participants, defined as individuals with no detected CM peaks. The DIF and SUM amplitudes, and DIF latencies are shown across the electrode array in this group in **Figure 3**.

In this group, there was no apical rise in DIF amplitudes proximal to the 0.5-kHz region in the cochlea. However, absolute DIF amplitues across the whole electrode array in the flat-responders were not significantly different to the responses across the basal electrodes in the apical-peak group (means of 3.4 ± 6.5 and 1.3 ± 0.4 μV for the apical-peak and flat-response groups respectively, all responses passed 1-sample Kolmogorov–Smirnov tests for normality). The flat-responders showed a gradual increase in SUM amplitude with increasing electrode depth, and there was a weak relationship between DIF and SUM amplitudes (Pearson product-moment correlation coefficient mean $r = 0.36$, with a range from -0.63 to 0.92). The latency of the DIF response rose from 2.31-ms ± 1.1 on the most basal electrode to 2.6-ms ± 1.2 at the most apical. The latency on the most basal electrode in this group was comparable to that recorded from the tip electrodes in the apical-peak group.

Mid-Electrode Peaks

A third, previously undescribed, pattern showed a mid-electrode peak of DIF amplitude with or without a second apical peak ($n = 8$). The mid-electrode peaks occurred most frequently on electrode 12 ($n = 5$), and less frequently on electrodes 14 ($n =$

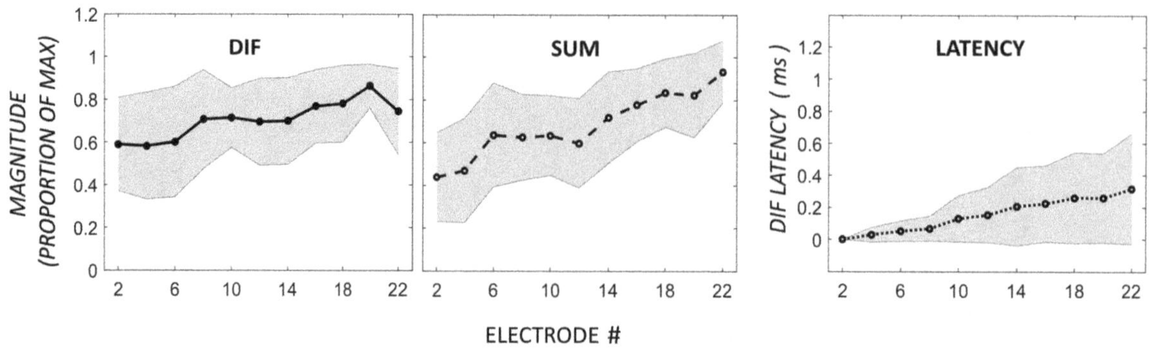

FIGURE 3 | Comparison of DIF, SUM, and DIF latency responses in 10 participants with a flat response across electrodes 2–22. Note that the horizontal axis in this figure is not normalized to the maximum DIF response as in **Figure 2**, as these subjects showed a flat response pattern without a distinct maximum.

2), and 8 ($n = 1$). Apical to the mid-electrode peaks, the DIF amplitude increased to a second peak on apical electrodes in half of the participants in this group ($n = 4$), and decrease to a flat response in half ($n = 4$). Examples of these patterns are shown in **Figure 4**, demonstrating a second apical peak (**Figure 4A**) or a single mid-electrode peak (**Figure 4B**).

Figure 5 demonstrates the normalized DIF and SUM magnitudes, and the DIF latencies, that have been averaged across the patients for each of the electrodes in the mid-electrode peak group. The DIF amplitudes at these mid-electrode peaks (27.7 μV ± 10.4 SEM) were comparable to the maximal amplitudes seen in the apical-peak group. The latency increased from the most basal electrode (1.0-ms ±.52) to a mean of 2.55-ms ±.70 at the tip of the electrode. Because the electrode upon which the peak occurred varied between subjects, these data were replotted, but now referenced to the mid-electrode peak for each individual (**Figure 6**). By aligning these peaks, it is apparent that the SUM amplitude peaks on the same electrode as the DIF amplitude. In addition, latency grew progressively across the peak.

As the ECochG signal is comprised of potentials derived from both neural and sensory elements, one possible explanation for the mid-electrode peaks was that these were generated by constructive or destructive interference between the phases of these potentials. If this were the case, it would be expected that the phase of the DIF and SUM components would be constructive at the peak electrode. In contrast to this expectation, there was no consistent relationship between the phase of the DIF and SUM components at the peak, or the surrounding electrodes. The difference in phase between peak electrode and the next most basal electrode averaged $-1.7^\circ \pm 16$, and between peak electrode and next most apical the phase difference was $-15.7^\circ \pm 41$, which is not consistent with an advancement from destructive to constructive interference between the CM and ANN on the mid-electrode peaks.

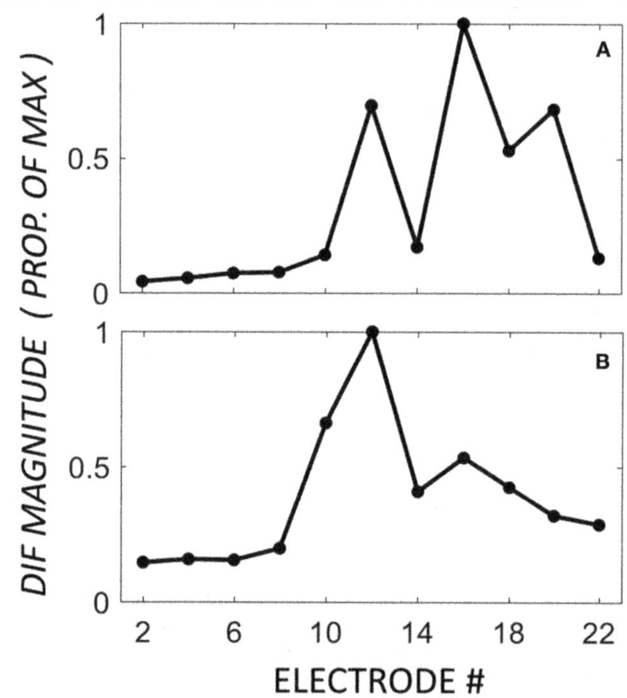

FIGURE 4 | DIF amplitude across the electrode array in two individuals from the mid-electrode peak group. In these individuals, the mid-electrode peaks were on electrode 12. For **(A)**, the DIF amplitude increased to a second peak on an apical electrode (16). For **(B)**, the DIF amplitude decreases across the final 5 recording electrodes.

Patterns Relationship to Hearing Level

Figure 7 summarizes the audiometric results for each of the three response patterns. Audiometric thresholds at 0.5-kHz were significantly lower in the apical peak group than the other two groups [Kruskal–Wallis test, $H(2) = 7.43$, $p = 0.024$]. The flat-response group showed the highest level of low-frequency hearing loss. The mid-electrode peak group showed the lowest level of high-frequency hearing loss and peaks in DIF amplitude that were at cochlear locations proximal to these high-frequency regions in the cochlea.

DISCUSSION

Here we describe three different response patterns, characterized as the response to a high intensity 0.5-kHz acoustic stimulus,

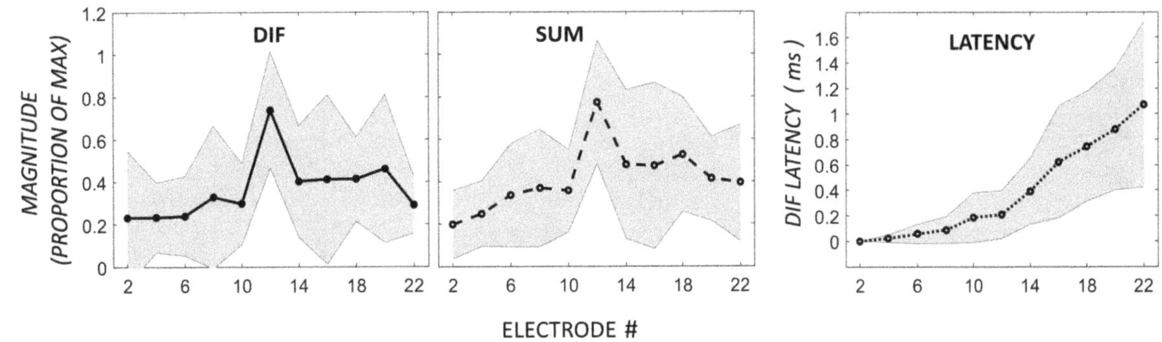

FIGURE 5 | DIF, SUM, and DIF latency responses in 8 participants with a mid-electrode peak, for electrodes 2–22.

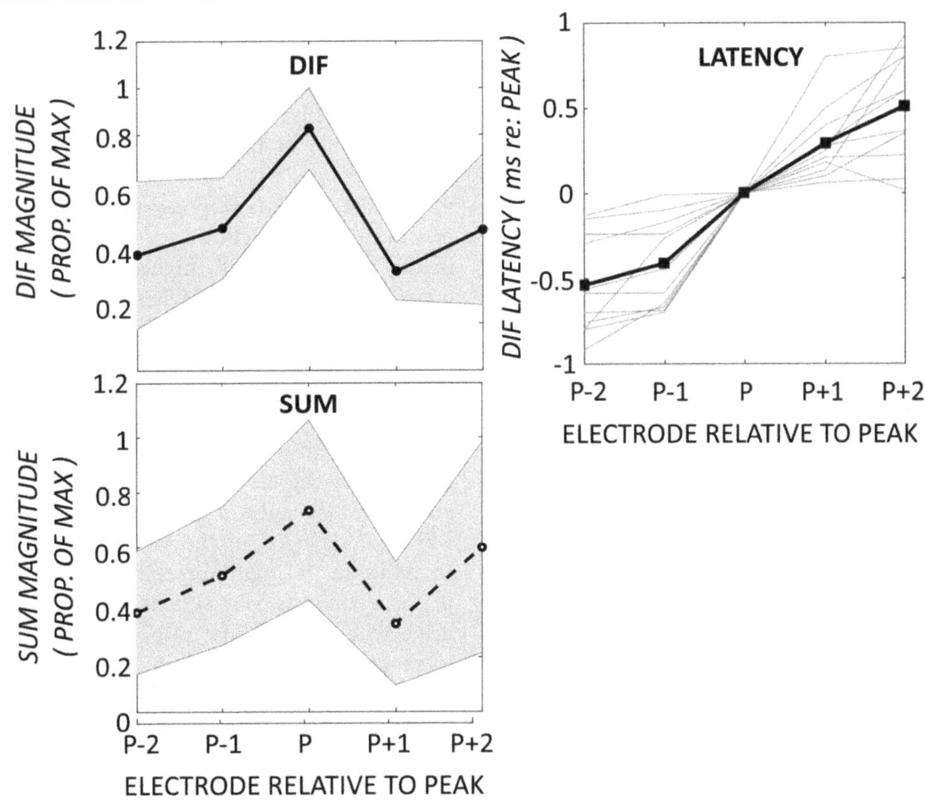

FIGURE 6 | Changes in DIF and SUM amplitudes and DIF latencies have been aligned to the electrode exhibiting the mid-electrode peak (P). The DIF and SUM responses show peaks on the same electrodes. The DIF latency increased progressively across the peak. Shaded area represents ± 1 *SD*.

when ECochG was recorded along the length of a cochlear electrode immediately after surgical implantation of the array. All patients had residual hearing recorded on their pre-operative audiograms.

For ease of communication the term CM will be used to refer to the first harmonic of the DIF response, and the ANN to the second harmonic of the SUM response. It is acknowledged that other cochlear generators may have contributed to these responses, such as a neural response to the first harmonic of the DIF response (Forgues et al., 2014), and hair cell distortion products to the second harmonic of the SUM (Teich et al., 1989), but these are of smaller magnitude and do not impact significantly upon the response characterization proposed here.

The apical response pattern that was expected from cochleae with functioning hair cells in the more apical cochlear regions. This is supported by the growth of CM amplitude along the length of the cochlea, and by the relatively low audiometric thresholds at 0.25 and 0.5-kHz. In these patients hearing dropped to a median of 85-dB at 1-kHz, and to profound levels above this. The latency of the CM is also consistent with this interpretation,

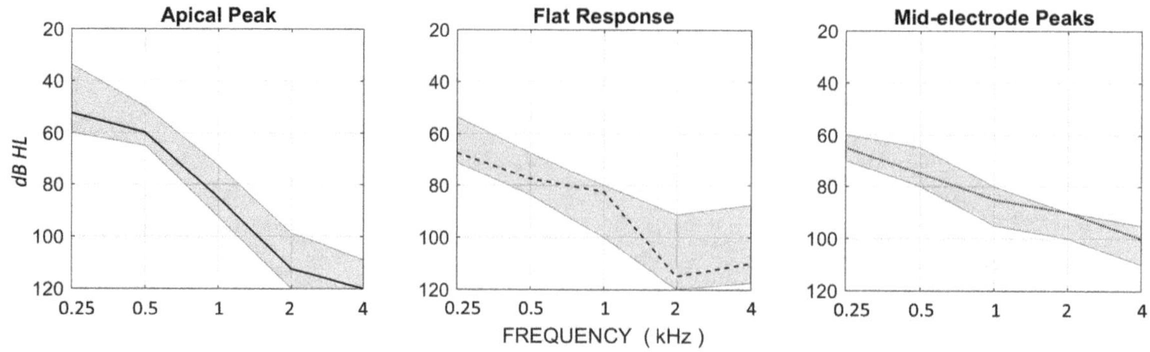

FIGURE 7 | Median HL for the Apical Peak, Flat Response, and Mid-electrode Peak groups, with upper and lower quartile ranges. The Apical Peak group has the best low-frequency thresholds, and the Mid-electrode Peak group has the best high-frequency thresholds. The Flat Response group has poor thresholds across the audiometric range.

as it became more prolonged toward the tip of the electrode, especially in responses recorded from electrodes in the apical half of the array where the response amplitude was growing more rapidly. This is what might be expected if the ECochG recorded from each electrode reflected the response of local populations of hair cells, in response to a cochlear traveling wave generated by a 0.5-kHz tone. Further support for this notion comes from the latency growth observed along the electrode, which was similar—but slightly shorter than—that seen in human psychophysical experiments for a traveling wave traversing this region of the cochlea (Eggermont, 1979; Schoonhoven et al., 2001). The shorter latency may reflect a basal-ward shift in the cochlear site of excitation arising from the high intensity of the acoustic stimulus (Honrubia and Ward, 1968; Russell and Nilsen, 1997). The peak CM amplitude occurred a few electrodes away from the tip in some patients, and dropped dramatically in magnitude on the more apical electrodes. This we suspect is a result of the tip of the electrode passing the 0.5-kHz place on the basilar membrane. Alternatively, this response characteristic might have been caused by the most apical implant electrodes contacting the basilar membrane, as this would prevent motion of the basilar membrane and dampen hearing at the point(s) of contact. The ANN response amplitude correlated well with the CM in this group of patients, presumably reflecting good innervation of the residual hair cells. However, the electrode upon which the CM and ANN peaks occurred differed in more than half the patients, usually with the CM peak on a more basal electrode. The reason(s) for this discrepancy are not apparent.

The CM latency for the mid-electrode peak group resembled that of the apical peak responders, as is apparent in **Figures 4, 5**. This suggests that the mid-electrode peak may arise from surviving populations of hair cells in more basal regions of the cochlea, as this electrode is typically located around 10-mm into the cochlea, near the 2-kHz region, and this group had the best audiometric thresholds at 2-kHz (90 dB HL in the mid-electrode peak group, compared with 112.5 or 115 in the Apical Peak or Flat Response groups, respectively). An alternative explanation for a mid-electrode peak might be the constructive interference of the phases of CM and ANN, but there was no evidence to support this in the data presented. Our results suggest that those hair cells which are present are likely to be innervated, as the profile of the ANN response mirrors that of the CM response.

The flat ECochG response pattern was also found in Dalbert et al. (2015) and Calloway et al. (2014). This pattern occurred in the individuals with higher levels of hearing loss than the other two groups, with median audiometric thresholds that were 15-dB worse at 0.25-kHz and 17.5-dB at 0.5-kHz than those in the apical peak group. Thresholds in response to higher frequencies were similar to those seen in patients exhibiting an apical response. The very slow CM amplitude growth across the electrode, with a long latency response (>2 ms) that changed little across the electrode suggests that the response detected arose from the apex of the cochlea, and that hair cell responses were not detected in the vicinity of the implant's electrodes. In addition, it might be that with the poorer hearing seen in these subjects, our system did not have sufficient acoustic drive to elicit a robust response. Based on these findings, it is suggested that flat responders reflect cochleae with "dead regions," namely cochlear places without significant numbers of functioning hair cells. The identification of dead regions is of clinical significance, as they will limit any benefit of EAS.

The present work identified discrete patterns of ECochG profile across the electrode that related to the patient's residual hearing. By recording ECochG across the electrode array, it was possible to map out the location of functioning hair cells and infer whether these were innervated. These data may improve the fitting of electro-acoustic hearing aids in the future, as specific regions with hair cell survival can be targeted with the acoustic component. The approach provides a detailed assessment of cochlear health at the time of cochlear implantation that provides a baseline for longitudinal monitoring of residual hearing. It is hoped that this will provide unique insights into the nature of hearing loss in the months after implant surgery. Furthermore, as these responses are better characterized, it will be possible to correlate the ECochG profile with speech perception and determine whether particular cochlear pathologies predict the outcome of cochlear implantation.

AUTHOR CONTRIBUTIONS

CB and SO: Design of study, data collection and analysis, writing and proofreading of manuscript. LC: Design of study, data collection and analysis, and proofreading of manuscript. AD: Data collection and analysis, and proofreading of manuscript. AC: Data analysis and proofreading of manuscript.

FUNDING

SO was funded by the National Health and Medical Research Council (Australia), GNT0628679 and GNT1078673.

REFERENCES

Adunka, O., Roush, P., Grose, J., Macpherson, C., and Buchman, C. A. (2006). Monitoring of cochlear function during cochlear implantation. *Laryngoscope* 116, 1017–1020. doi: 10.1097/01.mlg.0000217224.94804.bb

Calloway, N., Fitzpatrick, D. C., Campbell, A. P., Iseli, C., Pulver, S. H., Buchman, C. A., et al. (2014). Intracochlear electrocochleography during cochlear implantation. *Otol. Neurotol.* 35, 1451–1457. doi: 10.1097/MAO.0000000000000451

Campbell, L., Kaicer, A., Briggs, R., and O'Leary, S. (2015). Cochlear response telemetry: intracochlear electrocochleography via cochlear implant neural response telemetry pilot study results. *Otol. Neurotol.* 36, 399–405. doi: 10.1097/MAO.0000000000000678

Campbell, L., Kaicer, A., Sly, D., Iseli, C., Wei, B., Briggs, R., et al. (2016). Intraoperative real-time cochlear response telemetry predicts hearing preservation in cochlear implantation. *Otol. Neurotol.* 37, 332–338. doi: 10.1097/mao.0000000000000972

Choudhury, B., Fitzpatrick, D. C., Buchman, C. A., Wei, B. P., Dillon, M. T., He, S., et al. (2012). Intraoperative round window recordings to acoustic stimuli from cochlear implant patients. *Otol. Neurotol.* 33, 1507–1515. doi: 10.1097/MAO.0b013e31826dbc80

Dalbert, A., Pfiffner, F., Röösli, C., Thoele, K., Sim, J. H., Gerig R., et al. (2015). Extra- and intracochlear electrocochleography in cochlear implant recipients. *Audiol. Neurotol.* 20, 339–348. doi: 10.1159/000438742

Dallos, P. (1973). "Cochlear potentials and cochlear mechanics," in *Basic Mechanisms in Hearing*, ed A. Moller (New York, NY; London, UK: Acadamic Press, Inc.), 335–372. doi: 10.1016/B978-0-12-504250-5.50017-5

Eggermont, J. (1979). Narrow-band AP latencies in normal and recruiting human ears. *J. Acoust. Soc. Am.* 65, 463–470. doi: 10.1121/1.382345

Forgues, M., Koehn, H. A., Dunnon, A. K., Pulver, S. H., Buchman, C. A., Adunka, O. F., et al. (2014). Distinguishing hair cell from neural potentials recorded at the round window. *J. Neurophysiol.* 111, 580–593. doi: 10.1152/jn.00446.2013

Formeister, E. J., McClellan, J. H., Merwin, W. H. III, Iseli, C. E., Calloway, N. H., Teagle, H. F., et al. (2015). Intraoperative round window electrocochleography and speech perception outcomes in pediatric cochlear implant recipients. *Ear Hear.* 36, 249–260. doi: 10.1097/AUD.0000000000000106

Gantz, B. J., and Turner, C. (2004). Combining acoustic and electrical speech processing: Iowa/Nucleus hybrid implant. *Acta Otolaryngol.* 124, 344–347. doi: 10.1080/00016480410016423

Gantz, B. J., Turner, C., Gfeller, K. E., and Lowder, M. W. (2005). Preservation of hearing in cochlear implant surgery: advantages of combined electrical and acoustical speech processing. *Laryngoscope* 115, 796–802. doi: 10.1097/01.MLG.0000157695.07536.D2

Gummer, A. W., and Johnstone, B. M. (1984). Group delay measurement from spiral ganglion cells in the basal turn of the guinea pig cochlea. *J. Acoust. Soc. Am.* 76, 1388–1400. doi: 10.1121/1.391456

Honrubia, V., and Ward, P. H. (1968). Longitudinal distribution of the cochlear microphonics inside the cochlear duct (guinea pig). *J. Acoust. Soc. Am.* 44, 951–958. doi: 10.1121/1.1911234

O'Connell, B. P., Hunter, J. B., Gifford, R. H., Rivas, A., Haynes, D. S., Noble, J. H., et al. (2016). Electrode location and audiologic performance after cochlear implantation: a comparative study between Nucleus CI422 and CI512 electrode arrays. *Otol. Neurotol.* 37, 1032–1035. doi: 10.1097/MAO.0000000000001140

Palmer, A. R., and Russell, I. J. (1986). Phase-locking in the cochlear nerve of the guinea-pig and its relation to the receptor potential of inner hair-cells. *Hear. Res.* 24, 1–15. doi: 10.1016/0378-5955(86)90002-X

Patuzzi, R. B., Yates, G. K., and Johnstone, B. M. (1989). Changes in cochlear microphonic and neural sensitivity produced by acoustic trauma. *Hear. Res.* 39, 189–202. doi: 10.1016/0378-5955(89)90090-7

Ruben, R. J., Bordley, J., and Lieberman, A. (1961). Cochlear potentials in man. *Laryngoscope* 71, 1141–1164. doi: 10.1288/00005537-196110000-00001

Russell, I. J., and Nilsen, K. E. (1997). The location of the cochlear amplifier: spatial representation of a single tone on the guinea pig basilar membrane. *Proc. Natl. Acad. Sci. U.S.A.* 94, 2660–2664. doi: 10.1073/pnas.94.6.2660

Schoonhoven, R., Prijs, V. F., and Schneider, S. (2001). DPOAE group delays versus electrophysiological measures of cochlear delay in normal human ears. *J. Acoust. Soc. Am.* 109, 1503–1512. doi: 10.1121/1.1354987

Skinner, P. H., and Jones, H. C. (1968). Effects of signal duration and rise time on the auditory evoked potential. *J. Speech Hear. Res.* 11:301. doi: 10.1044/jshr.1102.301

Teich, M. C., Khanna, S. M., and Keilson, S. E. (1989). Nonlinear dynamics of cellular vibrations in the organ of Corti. *Acta Otolaryngol.* 108, 265–279. doi: 10.3109/00016488909138347

Weinberger, N., Kitzes, L., and Goodman, D. (1970). Some characteristics of the 'auditory neurophonic'. *Experientia* 26, 46–48. doi: 10.1007/BF01900383

11

Intra- and Postoperative Electrocochleography may be Predictive of Final Electrode Position and Postoperative Hearing Preservation

Brendan P. O'Connell[1], Jourdan T. Holder[2], Robert T. Dwyer[2], René H. Gifford[1, 2], Jack H. Noble[1, 3], Marc L. Bennett[1], Alejandro Rivas[1], George B. Wanna[1], David S. Haynes[1] and Robert F. Labadie[1, 3]*

[1] Department of Otolaryngology, Vanderbilt University Medical Center, Nashville, TN, United States, [2] Department of Hearing and Speech Sciences, Vanderbilt University Medical Center, Nashville, TN, United States, [3] Department of Computer Science and Electrical Engineering, Vanderbilt University, Nashville, TN, United States

***Correspondence:**
Jourdan T. Holder
jourdan.t.holder@vanderbilt.edu

Introduction: The objectives of the current study were to (1) determine the relationship between electrocochleography (ECochG), measured from the cochlear implant (CI) electrode array during and after implantation, and postoperative audiometric thresholds, (2) determine the relationship between ECochG amplitude and electrode scalar location determined by computerized tomography (CT); and (3) determine whether changes in cochlear microphonic (CM) amplitude during electrode insertion were associated with postoperative hearing.

Materials and Methods: Eighteen subjects undergoing CI with an Advanced Bionics Mid-Scala device were prospectively studied. ECochG responses were recorded using the implant coupled to a custom signal recording unit. ECochG amplitude collected intraoperatively concurrent with CI insertion and at activation was compared with audiometric thresholds postoperatively. Sixteen patients also underwent postoperative CT to determine scalar location and the relationship to ECochG measures and residual hearing.

Results: Mean low-frequency pure tone average (LFPTA) increased following surgery by an average of 28 dB (range 8–50). Threshold elevation was significantly greater for electrodes with scalar dislocation. No correlation was found between intraoperative ECochG and postoperative behavioral thresholds collapsed across frequency; however, mean differences in thresholds measured by intraoperative ECochG and postoperative audiometry were significantly smaller for electrodes inserted completely within scala tympani (ST) vs. those translocating from ST to scala vestibuli. A significant correlation was observed between postoperative ECochG thresholds and behavioral thresholds obtained at activation.

Discussion: Postoperative audiometry currently serves as a marker for intracochlear trauma though thresholds are not obtained until device activation or later. When measured at the same time-point postoperatively, low-frequency ECochG thresholds correlated with behavioral thresholds. Intraoperative ECochG thresholds, however, did not correlate significantly with postoperative behavioral thresholds suggesting that changes in cochlear physiology occur between electrode insertion and activation. ECochG may hold clinical utility providing surgeons with feedback regarding insertion trauma due to scalar translocation, which may be predictive of postoperative hearing preservation.

Conclusion: CI insertion trauma is generally not evident until postoperative audiometry when loss of residual hearing is confirmed. ECochG has potential to provide estimates of trauma during insertion as well as reliable information regarding degree of hearing preservation.

Keywords: cochlear implant, electrocochleography, residual hearing, audiometry, cochlear microphonic, hearing loss, hearing preservation

INTRODUCTION

Cochlear implants (CI) are surgically-implanted medical devices capable of restoring audibility and speech understanding to individuals with sensorineural hearing loss (SNHL) who do not receive benefit from appropriately fit amplification. Traditionally, CIs have been used to treat individuals with severe-to-profound hearing loss; however, indications for implantation have expanded to include individuals with significant low-frequency hearing and poor-to-fair speech understanding. Furthermore, advances in electrode design (e.g., increased flexibility and smaller dimensions) and surgical techniques (e.g., surgical approach, insertion angle, insertion speed, etc.) have introduced a new generation of implant recipients with preserved low-frequency hearing in the implanted ear.

The importance of low-frequency hearing in the implanted ear has been well-documented. Preservation of acoustic hearing allows individuals with CIs to take advantage of periodicity, commonly referred to as voice pitch, and temporal fine structure (e.g., Rosen, 1992), offering improved spectral resolution. Periodicity and fine structure provided via residual low-frequency hearing in the implanted ear afford significant improvement for speech understanding in complex listening environments over electric only listening and traditional bimodal hearing combining the CI with acoustic hearing originating from the non-implanted ear (e.g., Dorman and Gifford, 2010; Dunn et al., 2010; Gifford et al., 2013, 2015, 2017; Rader et al., 2013; Loiselle et al., 2016), as well as, significant improvements in sound localization (Dunn et al., 2010; Gifford et al., 2014; Loiselle et al., 2016; Plant and Babic, 2016). The degree of mean hearing preservation benefit ranges from 10- to 20-percentage points for fixed signal-to-noise ratio (SNR) conditions (e.g., Gifford et al., 2013, 2017; Loiselle et al., 2015) and 2–3-dB for adaptive SNR testing (e.g., Dunn et al., 2010; Gifford et al., 2013, 2015). Despite the success of hearing preservation surgery and associated functional benefit, there is still considerable variability in benefit across listeners, and rates of hearing preservation are highly variable across patients, electrode types (perimodiolar and straight), and insertion depths.

Previous studies have demonstrated the benefits associated with low frequency acoustic hearing, but given current resources, surgeons are able to achieve hearing preservation—defined as postoperative audiometric thresholds within 10 dB of preoperative levels—in, at most, 50% of cases (Jurawitz et al., 2014; Santa Maria et al., 2014; Van Abel et al., 2015; Dedhia et al., 2016; Eshraghi et al., 2016; Skarzynski et al., 2016). The pathophysiology of hearing loss during and following surgery is still largely unknown, but it is believed to be a result of (1) intraoperative physical trauma including fracture of the osseous spiral lamina, trans-scalar dislocation, and/or insult to spiral ligament or stria vascularis and/or (2) postoperative inflammatory responses and subsequent fibrosis, neo-osteogenesis and/or cellular apoptosis (e.g., Eshraghi and Van de Water, 2006; Eshraghi et al., 2013; Kamakura and Nadol, 2016).

At present, surgeons and audiologists have no way of knowing whether residual hearing was preserved until the patient returns for audiometric evaluation approximately 2 weeks after surgery. More often than not, there are no indications of physical trauma associated with insertion given the lack of visualization beyond the basal turn. Even experienced surgeons cannot reliably detect the subtle intraoperative forces, which can impart damage to delicate intracochlear structures. Previous retrospective research has shown that the frequent occurrence of translocation from scala tympani (ST) to scala vestibuli (SV) during insertion—occurring in approximately 42% of perimodiolar electrode insertions—has detrimental effects on CI outcomes (Adunka et al., 2004; Finley et al., 2008; Choudhury et al., 2012; Holden et al., 2013; Wanna et al., 2014; Dalbert et al., 2016).

If an intraoperative metric existed that could alert surgeons to physiological damage, such information would potentially allow him/her to modify the surgical procedure and potentially improve outcomes. One emerging solution is the use of intraoperative, intracochlear electrocochleography (ECochG) in providing continuous real-time recordings of physiological activity of intracochlear tissue during and after electrode insertion. ECochG can be recorded for patients with profound hearing loss and even in some individuals with no measurable audiometric thresholds (Choudhury et al., 2012).

ECochG is a technique used to record acoustically evoked electrical potentials generated by the inner ear and auditory nerve. Acoustic stimulation (i.e., a tone burst) is presented to the external ear, and the resulting electrical potentials are measured from the cochlea. The ECochG response is comprised of the cochlear microphonic (CM), summating potential (SP), compound action potential (CAP), and auditory nerve neurophonic (ANN). Each of these responses comes from different parts of the intricate inner auditory system. The CM is thought to represent the electrical potential generated by the stereocilia of the outer hair cells (Sohmer et al., 1980; Patuzzi et al., 1989; Verpy et al., 2008); the SP from the direct current shift of the receptor potential of the inner hair cells and some outer hair cells (Palmer and Russell, 1986; Durrant et al., 1998); the CAP from VIIIth nerve activity (ABR wave I) (Durrant et al., 1998); and the ANN from the inner hair cells (first order generator) and the phase-locked responses of VIIIth nerve fibers, which are used for hearing speech in background noise, localizing sounds, and perceiving/differentiating pitch (Palmer and Russell, 1986; Forgues et al., 2014).

ECochG responses were first recorded using surface electrodes (Poch-Broto et al., 2009), trans-tympanic electrodes (Yoshie et al., 1967; Prijs, 1991; Schoonhoven et al., 1996), or extra-tympanic electrodes (Cullen et al., 1972; Yoshie, 1973; Ferraro, 2010; Zhang, 2012). More recently, potentials have been recorded directly from the cochlea using a needle electrode placed at the round window (Mandala et al., 2012; Radeloff et al., 2012; Dalbert et al., 2015b; Adunka et al., 2016), a needle electrode placed inside the round window (Calloway et al., 2014), or an electrode on the cochlear implant array being implanted (Campbell et al., 2015; Dalbert et al., 2015a).

Relationship between Intraoperative ECochG and Postoperative Word Recognition

Fitzpatrick et al. (2014) recorded ECochG responses at the round window intraoperatively prior to CI insertion in 21 adults and subsequently correlated ECochG magnitude with postoperative CNC word recognition scores. In this study, the metric for ECochG magnitude was termed total response (TR) and defined as the sum of all significant first and second harmonic responses across all frequencies at the highest sound level (90 dB nHL). They reported that TR accounted for 47% of variability in outcomes on the CNC word recognition task making it, at the time, the highest known predictor of CI outcomes even over other predictors such as duration of deafness (<25%; e.g., Rubinstein et al., 1999; Friedland et al., 2003; Plant et al., 2016) and degree of residual hearing (e.g., Plant et al., 2016). Scott et al. (2016) completed intraoperative ECochG with a needle electrode at the round window prior to electrode insertion for 238 CI recipients with postoperative CNC word recognition obtained for 51 adult CI recipients. Similar to Fitzpatrick et al. (2014), they found a significant correlation between TR and CNC word recognition at 6 months post activation ($r = 0.43$); however, the ECochG CAP only weakly correlated postoperative word recognition ($r = 0.20, p < 0.001$). Thus, while ECochG appears to be a promising measure for helping explain postoperative outcomes, much additional research is needed to carefully investigate this relationship.

Relationship between Intraoperative ECochG and Acoustic Hearing Preservation

Researchers have also investigated the relationship between intraoperative ECochG and acoustic hearing preservation in the implanted ear. Adunka et al. (2016) recorded ECochG at the round window before and after CI insertion and found no correlation between the ECochG response and postoperative residual hearing as measured by audiometric thresholds—though the results may have been limited by the extracochlear nature of the recording electrode.

ECochG can also be recorded using the CI electrode array which offers advantages given its proximity to the organ of Corti. Koka et al. (2016) measured difference and summation responses from ECochG waveforms postoperatively from patients with residual hearing and compared with behavioral audiometric thresholds. The group found that 87% percent of the variability in postoperative behavioral audiometric thresholds across all frequencies tested could be predicted by difference response thresholds and 82% predicted by summation response thresholds; concluding that ECochG thresholds may be useful to estimate postoperative preserved acoustic hearing in CI patients who cannot participate in behavioral audiometry.

Campbell et al. (2016) recorded ECochG measurements intraoperatively from the CI array in 18 recipients with residual acoustic hearing and (1) explored providing real-time surgical feedback as well as (2) investigated the correlation between ECochG recordings and postoperative acoustic hearing. They found this method to be potentially useful for providing feedback regarding surgical trauma and that patients who had a preserved ECochG at the end of surgery were more likely to have preserved hearing. In fact, postoperative audiometric thresholds for patients with preserved CM were, on average, 15 dB better than individuals without a preserved ECochG. Similar findings were reported by Acharya et al. (2016) for two pediatric patients.

Building on this previous work, in the present study intracochlear ECochG responses were measured for 18 ($n = 18$) adult Advanced Bionics (AB) CI recipients with preoperative acoustic hearing in the ear to be implanted. ECochG measurements were made both during and after CI insertion, and these measures were compared with pre- and postoperative audiometric thresholds. Sixteen ($n = 16$) participants also underwent postoperative computerized tomography (CT) scanning to verify scalar placement. The objectives of the current study were (1) to determine the relationship between ECochG, measured from the CI array either during cochlear implantation or after surgery, and postoperative audiometric thresholds, (2) to determine if the CM amplitudes correlated with electrode scalar location/translocation as determined by CT scanning, and

(3) to determine if change in CM during electrode insertion is associated with postoperative residual hearing.

METHODS

Subjects

Adult patients with residual acoustic hearing (≤80 dB HL at 250 Hz) who were seeking cochlear implantation with an Advanced Bionics (AB) Mid-Scala device between April and December 2016 were prospectively recruited for participation. Exclusion criteria included previous history of middle ear surgery, sudden sensorineural hearing loss, auditory neuropathy spectrum disorder (ANSD), single-sided deafness, and/or abnormal anatomy as detected by CT or MRI scanning. Eighteen ($n = 18$) subjects met inclusion criteria and were implanted by one of five cochlear implant surgeons using a round window ($n = 14$) or extended round window approach ($n = 4$). Patient demographics are shown in **Table 1**. The methods used in this study were in accordance with the ethical standards of the institutional review board at Vanderbilt University (IRB approval: 151808), and all subjects provided written informed consent before participation.

TABLE 1 | Subject demographics, RW, round window; ERW, extended round window; LFPTA, low frequency pure tone average (average threshold for 125, 250, and 500 Hz, in dB HL); ST, scala tympani; SV, scala vestibuli; Preop, preoperative; Postop, postoperative.

Subject	Surgical approach	Preop LFPTA	Postop LFPTA	LFPTA shift	Scalar location
1	ERW	50.0	61.7	11.7	ST
2	ERW	51.7	85.0	33.3	ST-SV
3	RW	60.0	105.0*	45.0	ST-SV
4	RW	68.3	88.3	20.0	ST
5	RW	63.3	105.0*	41.7	ST-SV
6	RW	41.7	76.7	35.0	ST-SV
7	RW	31.7	81.7	50.0	–
8	ERW	31.7	56.7	25.0	ST
9	RW	56.7	105.0*	48.3	ST-SV
10	RW	66.7	105.0*	38.3	ST (* BM)
11	RW	66.7	76.7	10.0	ST-SV
12	RW	26.7	45.0	18.3	ST
13	RW	45.0	70.0	25.0	ST
14	ERW	53.3	66.7	13.3	ST
15	RW	58.3	105.0*	46.7	–
16	RW	75.3	83.3	8.0	ST
17	RW	66.7	75.0	8.3	ST
18	RW	60.0	80.0	20.0	ST
MEAN	**-**	**54.1**	**81.8**	**27.7**	**-**

Thresholds with asterisk represent no behavioral response at the limits of the audiometer.
**BM indicates the electrode pushing against the basilar membrane.*

Equipment

The equipment used for data collection was previously described by Koka et al. (2016). The Bionic Ear Data Collection System (BEDCS) was used to measure ECochG responses. A NI DAQ system (NI DAQ 6216, National Instruments Corporation, 11500 Mopac Expwy, Austin, TX) and an audio amplifier (Sony PHA-2, Sony Corporation, New York, NY) were used to generate the acoustic stimuli, which was presented through an ER-3A (Etymotic Research, Inc. 61 Martin Lane, Elk Grove Village, IL) insert earphone. An ER-7 (Etymotic Research, Inc. 61 Martin Lane, Elk Grove Village, IL) probe microphone was used to calibrate and monitor the stimulus level in the ear canal. The ECochG response was measured using an AB Clinical Programming Interface Platinum Series Sound Processor (PSP) and Universal Headpiece (UHP) with additional magnets for retention and secure connection.

Pure-Tone Audiometry (PTA)

Pure-tone audiometry was assessed prior to implantation and at activation approximately 2–3 weeks after surgery. Audiometric thresholds were completed in a double-walled sound treated booth. Air-conduction thresholds were obtained for all octaves and inter-octave frequencies from 125 to 8,000 Hz using an insert earphone. Bone-conduction thresholds were obtained for octave frequencies from 500 to 4,000 Hz using a bone oscillator placed on the mastoid. Contralateral masking was implemented when appropriate. Low-frequency PTA was calculated using the average of unaided air-conduction thresholds at 125, 250, and 500 Hz.

ECochG Recording

ECochG potentials were measured from the most apical electrode of the implant array intraoperatively as the surgeon was inserting the CI and postoperatively at each subject's CI activation. Intraoperatively, after the patient was intubated, an ER-3A (Etymotic Research, Inc. 61 Martin Lane, Elk Grove Village, IL) insert earphone and an ER-7 (Etymotic Research, Inc. 61 Martin Lane, Elk Grove Village, IL) probe microphone were placed in the external auditory canal of the surgical ear (See Koka et al., 2016, **Figure 1**). Since the insert earphone and probe microphone were not sterilized, these pieces were kept out of the sterile field by folding the pinna anteriorly and securing it with a large Tegaderm® transparent adhesive film dressing (3M, 2501 Hudson Rd., Maplewood, MN) taking caution to not compromise the tube delivering sound to the ear. At this point, calibration was completed to ensure that the tube was not crimped or that the insert placement was faulty. The cables/tubes connecting the insert earphone and probe microphone to the measurement equipment were then disconnected, wrapped in a cloth, and placed underneath the surgical table so as to minimize interference with the surgical procedure. The surgical preparation (i.e., sterilization and draping) and surgical procedure (cortical mastoidectomy, facial recess, and round window exposure) then progressed according to normal protocols until just before insertion of the electrode array at which point the cables/tubes were reconnected to the recording equipment and the Universal Headpiece and cable were covered with a sterile ultrasound bag and magnetically coupled to the patient's newly implanted receiver/stimulator. Calibration was repeated, and the ECochG

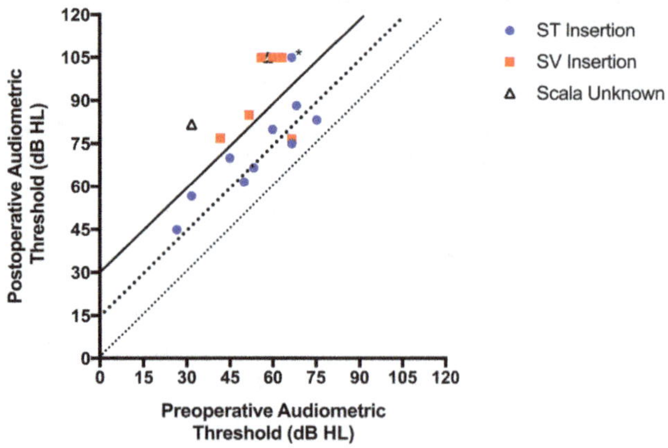

FIGURE 1 | Pre- and postoperative pure-tone thresholds; each symbol represents an individual patient. Scalar location of electrode, when available, has been denoted (the * represents the electrode abutting the basilar membrane). Diagonal lines are used to depict hearing preservation in relation to pure-tone average (PTA) shift bins as follows: PTA shift <15 dB, PTA shift between 15–30 dB, and PTA shift >30 dB.

recording was started. The CI electrode was introduced via the round window or extended round window and inserted according to the manufacturer's recommendations (i.e., insertion with the stylet to the first blue marker at which point the pre-curved electrode was advanced off the stylet until the second blue marker was located at the round window). The surgeon reported a full insertion in all cases. While the surgeon was inserting the electrode, the audiologist used markers to identify different key points during the surgery (i.e., round window, first blue marker, second blue marker, complete insertion). For the duration of electrode insertion and ECochG insertion, an acoustic tone burst was delivered via the insert earphone (500-Hz, toneburst, 110 dB SPL or 97 dB HL, alternating polarity, 50-ms duration with 5-ms onset/offset ramp time) while the ECochG response was recorded from the most apical electrode. The neural response imaging (NRI) amplifier in the implant was used for amplification of the response (gain of 1,000). The recordings were done with alternating polarities (2 rarefaction and 2 condensation traces) and averaged in the implant amplifier, then transferred to the processor. Data plotting for the insertion tracks depends on SNR of the signal, which usually averages and plots at a single point until SNR reaches 18 dB, or 8 averages have been performed (internally 16 averages). The SNR benefit can be achieved by 55 ms recordings that can be seen in frequency spectrum with larger acquisition times; the acquisitions were done at 4–6 stimuli per second. In presenting this data, the CM amplitude during the insertion track is normalized with respect to the amplitude obtained at the round window, therefore values are presented as dB. After insertion was complete, the recording electrode was changed to 1, 5, 9, and then 13; additional ECochG measurements were obtained from these electrodes to try and understand electrode location with respect to the 500-Hz stimulus. Subsequently, the stimulus frequency was changed from 125 to 2,000 Hz in octave steps using electrode 1 as the recording electrode to estimate each subject's CM threshold in dB HL at each frequency. Surgery concluded per standard. It is estimated that intraoperative ECochG testing added approximately 5 min of time to each case. It should be noted that for this study, the surgeon was not informed of the ECochG results during the insertion of the electrode.

Postoperative ECochG measurement occurred in the audiology clinic on the same day as the patient's CI activation appointment, typically 2 weeks after surgery. An ER-3A (Etymotic Research, Inc. 61 Martin Lane, Elk Grove Village, IL) insert earphone and an ER-7 (Etymotic Research, Inc. 61 Martin Lane, Elk Grove Village, IL) probe microphone were placed in the external auditory canal of the implanted ear, and the Universal Headpiece was coupled with the patient's receiver stimulator. Calibration was completed to ensure that the tube was not crimped or that the insert placement was faulty. Tone bursts were presented sequentially at 125, 250, 500, 1,000, and 2,000 Hz. The patient's ECochG response was measured from the apical electrode and recorded for each frequency. These frequency scan responses were used to estimate subjects' CM thresholds.

Stimuli and Recording Parameters

The amplitude of the ECochG response was calculated using fast Fourier transformation (FFT) analysis within the Bionic Ear Data Collection System. A sample rate of 9,280 and a low pass filter of 5 kHz in the NRI amplifier were used to acquire the responses over a 54.5 ms recording duration through back-telemetry.

Computerized Tomography (CT) Scanning

A subset ($n = 16$) of patients received postoperative CT scans using a low-dose, flat-panel, volumetric computerized tomography machine (Xoran XCAT, Xoran Technologies; Ann Arbor, MI). Using previously described and validated image-processing algorithms (Noble et al., 2011) scans were analyzed for scalar location of the electrode array (Noble et al., 2011). ST insertions were defined as insertions in which all electrode contacts were located entirely within the ST. Conversely, SV insertions were characterized by electrode arrays that translocated from the ST into the SV, such that at least one electrode contact was located within the SV.

Statistical Methods

Data were plotted and analyzed using GraphPad Prism 7.0 software (GraphPad Software Inc, 2012). Continuous variables were tested for normal distribution with D'Agostino and Pearson omnibus normality test.

Correlations were performed to examine the relationships between ECochG thresholds and behavioral thresholds at individual frequencies (125, 250, and 500 Hz). Parametric and nonparametric data were examined using a Pearson or Spearman correlation analysis, respectively. Spearman correlation was also used if the sample size of a group was too small to determine distribution of data. Given that correlations were performed at multiple frequencies, the Bonferroni correction was used adjusting the critical p-value. Patients were then categorized by the scalar location of their electrode array (ST and SV), and correlations between ECochG and behavioral thresholds within both these groups were assessed.

The following dependent variables were also assessed: (1) the absolute difference between ECochG thresholds and behavioral thresholds at individual frequencies (125, 250, and 500 Hz), (2) low-frequency PTA shift, (3) rise in CM amplitude from start of insertion to the peak value during insertion, and (4) the drop in CM amplitude from the peak value during insertion to completion of insertion. Patients were again characterized into groups according to scalar location and comparisons of the aforementioned variables were made between ST vs. SV insertions with an independent *t*-test (normal distribution) or a Mann-Whitney *U*-test (non-normal distribution). A $p < 0.05$ was considered indicative of statistical significance, with the exception of data pertaining to absolute differences between ECochG thresholds and behavioral thresholds, as multiple frequencies were analyzed; the Bonferroni correction was used in these analyses.

RESULTS

Demographics and Operative Characteristics

Eighteen patients met inclusion criteria and were prospectively enrolled (**Table 1**). The median age at the time of surgery was 67 years (range 23–80); 61% of the patients were male. Round window insertions were performed in the 78% of cases ($n = 14$), with extended round window insertions used in the remaining 22% ($n = 4$). Surgeons reported full insertion in all cases. Resistance during insertion was subjectively noted in one case; with electrode repositioning resistance subsided and a full insertion was achieved.

Electrode Location

Sixteen patients consented to undergo postoperative CT imaging such that scalar electrode location could be determined. Two patients electively chose not to participate in the postoperative imaging portion of the study, therefore scalar location of these electrode arrays could not be determined. Because all insertions were performed through either round window or extended round window approaches, all electrodes were initially inserted into the ST within the basal turn. In six patients (38%), electrode translocation from the ST into the SV was observed. In one patient, after analysis, the electrode array was pushing against the basilar membrane but did not clearly translocate into the SV; interestingly, this was the case in which resistance was subjectively felt during insertion. Because of the limits of our image processing algorithms, this patient was excluded from subsequent statistical analyses that examined the impact of scalar location on audiologic outcomes.

Hearing Preservation

Preoperatively, all patients had functional residual hearing (≤80 dB HL at 250 Hz) prior to surgery. The mean preoperative low-frequency PTA was 54 dB HL (range 27–75). At activation, the majority of patients ($n = 12$, 66%) demonstrated measurable unaided air-conduction thresholds at 125, 250, and 500 Hz. One patient had measurable thresholds at 125, and 250 Hz but did not respond to unaided pure-tones at 500 Hz; the remaining 5 patients demonstrated no responses at 125, 250, and 500 Hz.

Eleven patients (61%) maintained thresholds ≤80 dB HL at 250 Hz. Mean low-frequency PTA at activation was 82 dB HL (range 45–105), yielding an average low-frequency PTA shift of 28 dB (range 8–50). As depicted in **Figure 1**, 5 patients (28%) demonstrated low-frequency PTA shift <15 dB, 5 patients (28%) demonstrated low-frequency PTA shift between 15 and 30 dB, and the remaining 8 patients demonstrated low-frequency PTA shift >30 dB (44%).

The impact of demographic and surgical variables on low-frequency PTA shift was then assessed. No relation between age at surgery and postoperative PTA shift was noted ($r = 0.13$, $p = 0.60$). Further, no difference in median PTA shift was observed when round window insertions (23 dB, range 8–50) were compared to extended round window insertions (22 dB, range 12–47, $p = 0.81$). The median low-frequency PTA shift was significantly lower for electrodes entirely inserted into the ST (16 dB, range 8–25) as compared to electrodes that translocated into the SV (38 dB, range 10–48, $p = 0.02$; **Figure 2**).

Intraoperative ECochG Thresholds vs. Postoperative Behavioral Thresholds

The relationship between intraoperative ECochG thresholds and postoperative behavioral audiometric thresholds was analyzed. Intraoperative ECochG thresholds were successfully measured in 17 patients (94.4%); connection between the receiver stimulator and external monitoring equipment was lost in one patient. The absolute mean difference between intraoperative ECochG thresholds and postoperative behavioral thresholds for 125,

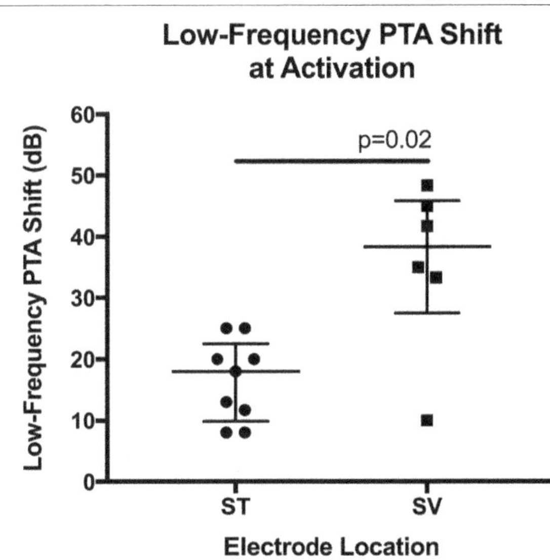

FIGURE 2 | Scatter plot of low-frequency pure-tone average (PTA) shift depicted according to scalar electrode location. Lower median shift (i.e., better hearing preservation) was noted when comparing electrodes inserted entirely into the scala tympani (ST) to electrodes that translocated into scala vestibuli (SV). Shown are the median and the range of the 25–75th percentile.

250, and 500 Hz is shown in **Table 2**. The absolute difference between intraoperative ECochG thresholds and postoperative audiometric thresholds was significantly lower (i.e., better) for ST insertions compared to SV insertions at 125 and 250 Hz frequencies ($p = 0.001$ for both analyses). In the overall cohort, no significant correlations between intraoperative ECochG thresholds and postoperative behavioral thresholds were noted at 125 Hz ($r = 0.12$, $p = 0.64$), 250 Hz ($r = 0.08$, $p = 0.77$), or 500 Hz ($rs = 0.46$, $p = 0.07$; **Figure 3**). The relationship between ECochG and behavioral thresholds at activation is also plotted as a function of scalar location.

Postoperative ECochG Thresholds vs. Postoperative Behavioral Thresholds

Postoperative ECochG thresholds were successfully measured in 17 patients (94%) at activation; testing in one patient was limited by time constraints and patient preference. The mean difference between ECochG thresholds and behavioral thresholds at activation is shown in **Table 3**. At 125 Hz, the difference between postoperative ECochG threshold and pure tone thresholds was significantly lower (i.e., better) for ST insertions compared to SV insertions ($p = 0.0007$). A significant correlation between ECochG thresholds and behavioral thresholds at activation was observed at 125 Hz ($r = 0.83$, $p < 0.0001$), 250 Hz ($r = 0.88$, $p < 0.0001$), and 500 Hz ($r = 0.88$, $p < 0.0001$; **Figure 4**). These relationships are also shown according to scalar location. Bland-Altman plots assessing agreement between methods at activation for low-frequencies are shown in **Figure 5**.

ECochG Insertion Monitoring

Changes in CM amplitude during electrode insertion were then analyzed. As mentioned previously, intraoperative ECochG could not be performed in one patient; in addition, the insertion scans from four other patients were invalid secondary to monitoring issues. Insertion scans from the remaining 13 patients are depicted in **Figure 6** according to scalar electrode location. The mean rise in CM amplitude from start of insertion at the round window to the peak value during insertion, was 22 dB (range 5–40). On average, the CM amplitude dropped 3 dB (range 0–8) from the peak value during insertion to completion of insertion. These objective measures of CM amplitude change were compared between ST and SV insertions; no significant differences were noted ($p = 0.35$ and $p = 0.61$; **Table 4**). Further, low-frequency PTA shift did not correlate significantly with round window to peak amplitude ($r = -0.40$, $p = 0.17$) nor drop from peak to completion of insertion ($r = 0.26$, $p = 0.38$).

DISCUSSION

In the current study, we completed ECochG obtaining CM amplitude at various stages in the electrode insertion as well as an estimate obtained at the activation appointment. We did not observe a significant relationship between CM amplitude obtained during electrode insertion and scalar electrode location for our group of 16 patients with postoperative CT scans. Intraoperative ECochG thresholds, via frequency scan, did not

TABLE 2 | The mean absolute difference between intraoperative electrocochleography (ECochG) thresholds and postoperative behavioral thresholds at 125, 250, and 500 Hz frequencies are shown in the overall cohort.

Frequency (Hz)	Δ Intraop ECochG and postop behavioral thresholds, overall mean in dB HL (range)	Δ Intraop ECochG and postop behavioral thresholds, ST Insertion mean in dB HL (range)	Δ Intraop ECochG and postop behavioral thresholds, SV insertion mean in dB HL (range)	*p*-value
125	29 (1–69)	16 (1–28)	46 (33–69)	0.001
250	24 (2–55)	13 (2–29)	41 (30–55)	0.001
500	19 (2–40)	12 (2–38)	22 (6–35)	0.310

Differences are also depicted according to scalar location of the electrode array; the P value represents the comparison between scala tympani (ST) insertions and scala vestibuli (SV) insertions. Means and ranges are reported. Bonferroni correction is applied for multiple comparisons, with p < 0.017 indicative of statistical significance.

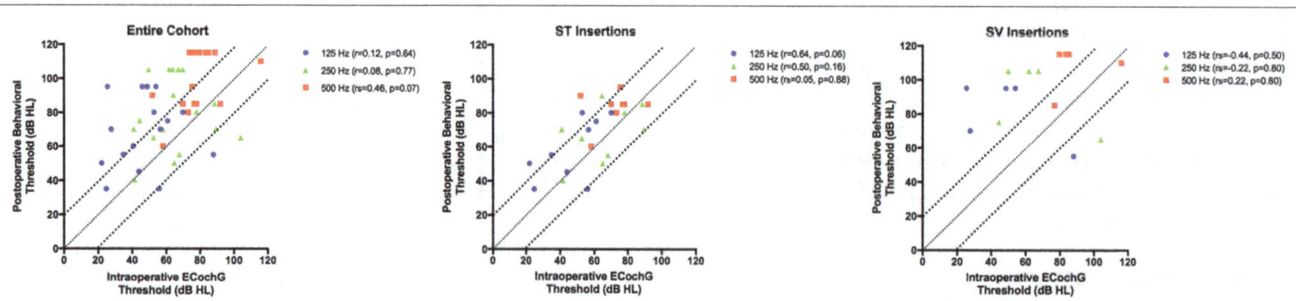

FIGURE 3 | The relationship between intraoperative ECochG thresholds, in dB HL, and postoperative behavioral thresholds, also in dB HL, for 125, 250, and 500 Hz are depicted in the entire cohort, and for those cases in which scalar location is known. Bonferroni correction is applied for multiple comparisons, with $p < 0.017$ indicative of statistical significance. The diagonal and dotted lines represent the ±20 dB difference between ECochG thresholds and behavioral thresholds.

TABLE 3 | The mean absolute difference between postoperative electrocochleography (ECochG) thresholds and postoperative behavioral thresholds at 125, 250, and 500 Hz frequencies are shown in the overall cohort.

Frequency (Hz)	Δ Postop ECochG and postop behavioral thresholds, overall mean in dB HL (range)	Δ Postop ECochG and postop behavioral thresholds, ST insertion mean in dB HL (range)	Δ Postop ECochG and postop behavioral thresholds, SV insertion mean in dB HL (range)	*p*-value
125	15 (0–37)	7 (0–14)	22 (15–37)	0.0007
250	9 (0–23)	8 (4–14)	11 (0–23)	0.42
500	6 (0–29)	4 (1–11)	6 (0–13)	0.99

Differences are also depicted according to scalar location of the electrode array; the P-value represents the comparison between scala tympani (ST) insertions and scala vestibuli (SV) insertions. Means and ranges are reported. Bonferroni correction is applied for multiple comparisons, with $p < 0.017$ indicative of statistical significance.

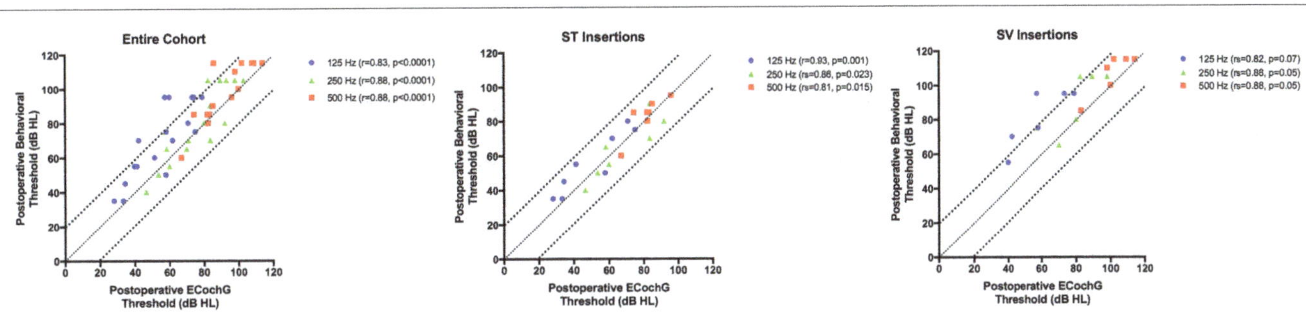

FIGURE 4 | The relationship between postoperative ECochG thresholds and postoperative behavioral thresholds for 125, 250, and 500 Hz frequencies are depicted in the entire cohort, and for those cases in which scalar location is known. Bonferroni correction is applied for multiple comparisons, with $p < 0.017$ indicative of statistical significance.

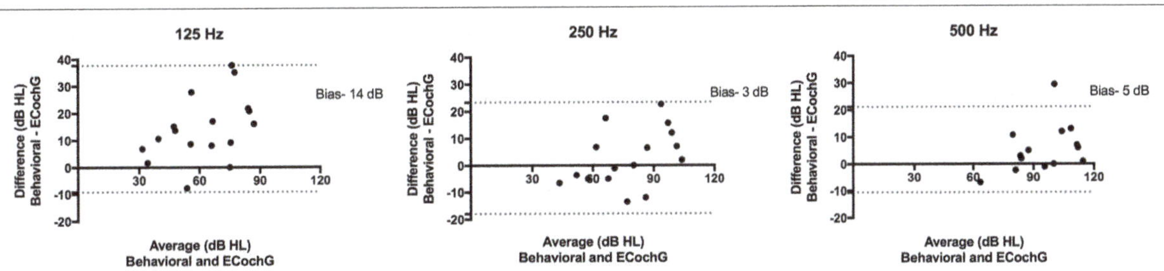

FIGURE 5 | Bland-Altman plots depict the average and difference between postoperative behavioral and ECochG thresholds at 125, 250, and 500 Hz. The 95% limits of agreement are shown as two dotted lines. The biases, or average of the differences at each frequency, are reported.

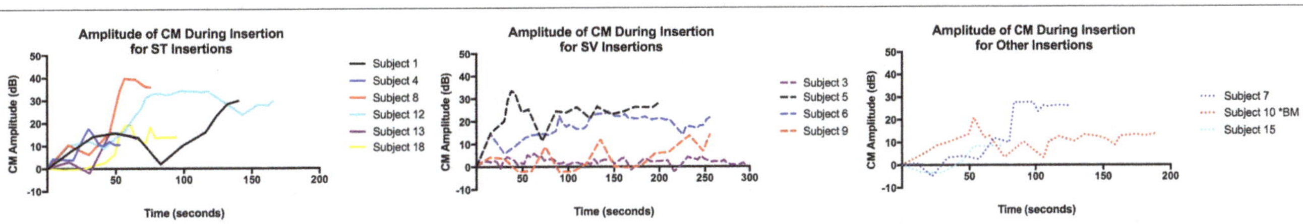

FIGURE 6 | Change in cochlear microphonic (CM) amplitude, in dB re: microVolts, during insertion is shown according to scalar location of the electrode array.

correlate significantly with postoperative audiometric thresholds; however, a trend was noted between ECochG thresholds and behavioral thresholds for electrodes inserted entirely into the ST at 125 Hz (p = 0.06). Further, the mean difference between intraoperative ECochG thresholds and postoperative audiometric thresholds was significantly smaller for electrodes in ST as compared to those which translocated into SV at 125 and 250 Hz.

TABLE 4 | Various objective measures of change in cochlear microphonic (CM) amplitude during insertion are compared between scala tympani (ST) and scala vestibuli (SV) insertions.

Δ CM Amplitude during insertion	ST Insertion median in dB (range)	SV Insertion median in dB (range)	*p*-value
Round window to peak amplitude	25 (16–40)	19 (5–33)	0.35
Peak amplitude to complete insertion	5 (0–8)	3 (0–5)	0.61

At present, postoperative audiometric thresholds represent a marker for intracochlear insertion trauma. We hypothesize that intraoperative ECochG may provide us with valuable information at the time of surgery that may be significantly correlated with behavioral audiometric thresholds obtained at activation *if electrodes remain within ST*. Though we did not observe a significant correlation between ECochG thresholds obtained intraoperatively (measured via frequency scan immediately after insertion) and postoperative audiometric thresholds at activation, the difference between intraoperative ECochG thresholds and postoperative audiometric thresholds was *significantly lower* (i.e., better) for electrodes completely located in ST. These data support the notion that changes in cochlear physiology occur in the time period between electrode insertion and activation, and are more pronounced for electrodes that translocate into the SV. Further, these data suggest that ECochG may hold clinical utility providing surgeons with feedback regarding insertion trauma as well as information regarding expected hearing preservation. Additional data are needed with larger sample sizes and broader distributions of preoperative audiometric thresholds in the low-frequency region to thoroughly investigate this relationship.

We also sought to examine whether various objective measures of CM amplitude during electrode insertion (measured via insertion scan) were related to either scalar location or hearing preservation outcomes. In order to objectively assess this relationship, we chose to record the following: (1) rise in CM amplitude from start of insertion at the round window to the peak value during insertion, and (2) drop in CM from the peak value during insertion to completion of insertion. Neither of these measures was found to be associated with scalar location or hearing preservation. It is possible that the small sample size of adequate insertion scans ($n = 13$) limited our analysis in this regard. Alternatively, we may have chosen outcomes measures that lack sensitivity to pick up differences between groups. Further studies assessing amplitude and phase characteristics of the ECochG waveform are warranted. It should be emphasized that no feedback was provided to the surgeon in the current study; we do however, plan to commence a thorough study of the utility of intraoperative ECochG in helping to guide surgical insertion. Should ECochG data obtained during insertion serve as a tool guiding surgical insertion, such feedback may allow for surgical modifications (e.g., redirecting insertion vector) resulting in less traumatic insertions, preservation of intracochlear structures, and potentially, higher rates of hearing preservation.

Current clinical practice uses audiometric thresholds (e.g., Carlson et al., 2011; Cosetti et al., 2013; Sweeney et al., 2016) and retained unaided word recognition in the postoperative period as markers of surgical trauma (inflammation, fibrosis, and/or bone growth). Postoperative audiograms, however, provide only a gross estimate of peripheral auditory function. Furthermore, in standard clinical practice, postoperative acoustic word recognition is rarely obtained for the implanted ear. In some cases, preoperative acoustic word recognition is near zero, rendering retention of word recognition potentially an irrelevant measure. Despite these challenges, the biggest restriction in our current clinical practice is that we are currently unable to assess the effects of implantation trauma until the damage has occurred which is likely irreversible. Thus, we need a measure capable of providing real-time estimates of insertion trauma providing feedback to surgeons during electrode insertion. Theoretically speaking, reducing insertion trauma will potentially result in less fibrosis, bony growth, and cellular apoptosis—though the patient-specific inflammatory response remains an unknown variable. Additional value from such a measure of insertion trauma may help guide clinical decision making regarding administration of postoperative steroids in cases where concerns may arise regarding acoustic hearing preservation.

In addition to investigating the effect of cochlear implantation on ECochG responses measured during surgical insertion, ECochG responses at postoperative activation were also assessed. Significant correlations between postoperative ECochG thresholds and pure-tone behavioral thresholds were noted across low frequencies. Our findings corroborate data recently published by Koka et al. (2016), in which strong agreement between postoperative ECochG thresholds and behavioral thresholds was also demonstrated. As physiologic estimates of hearing thresholds (via ECochG frequency scan) and behavioral measurements of hearing (pure-tone audiometry) correlate well when measured at the same time-point, the fact that intraoperative ECochG thresholds did not correlate with postoperative behavioral hearing herein further supports that cochlear physiology changes in the time between electrode insertion and activation. Future studies examining the differential changes that result directly from electrode insertion vs. those that occur in the acute post-insertion period are needed; controlling for scalar location in such reports appears to be very important. Taken together, ECochG thresholds may be capable of quantifying the degree on insertion trauma and resultant intracochlear physiological changes impacting behavioral hearing thresholds. Lastly, our data may also hold significant clinical value for patients unable to provide reliable behavioral data at the activation appointment and even possibly at subsequent postoperative audiology appointments.

Limitations

The primary limitation of the current study was the sample size ($n = 18$) and as a result, generalizations cannot be made at this time. Further, though ECochG including CM peak amplitude with electrode insertion may hold future surgical value regarding insertion trauma, no feedback was provided to the surgeons during the insertions on any of the cases included here. In order to thoroughly investigate the utility of this measure—particularly in helping to avoid scalar dislocation—real-time feedback is likely a necessary component. Finally, all participants in the current study were recipients of a conventional, pre-curved electrode, the AB mid-scala electrode. That is, none of the subjects were implanted with a lateral-wall electrode *specifically designed* for hearing preservation. Thus, it is possible that ECochG thresholds may not generalize to recipients of a shorter, lateral-wall electrode who may have lower, and potentially better, audiometric thresholds across a broader range of frequencies. Our research team is actively involved in ongoing efforts to investigate the clinical utility of ECochG as both a measure of intracochlear insertion trauma and postoperative audiometric thresholds in larger sample sizes with patients of varying residual hearing in the low-frequency and both pre-curved and lateral-wall electrodes.

Summary

More patients are presenting for CI who have measureable and clinically significant preoperative hearing thresholds. However, we are unable to appreciate the effects of CI insertion trauma and resultant postoperative audiometric thresholds until the point of device activation or even later when behavioral hearing thresholds are measured. The current study investigated the relationship between intraoperative and postoperative ECochG measurements and postoperative audiometry in a group of 18 patients with preoperative 250-Hz thresholds up to 80 dB HL who were implanted with an AB mid-scala electrode. Sixteen of the 18 patient consented to postoperative CT imaging allowing for determination of electrode scalar location. From the current dataset, the primary conclusions were as follows:

- Scalar translocation from ST to SV was associated with significantly higher shifts in low-frequency PTA when compared to electrodes inserted entirely within ST.
- There was no statistically significant relationship between intraoperative ECochG thresholds and postoperative audiometric thresholds at the group level.
    - However, a trend was noted between intraoperative ECochG thresholds and postoperative audiometric thresholds when excluding patients for whom electrode crossed from ST to SV.
    - Further, the difference between intraoperative ECochG thresholds and postoperative audiometric thresholds was *significantly lower* (i.e., better) for electrodes completely located in ST.
    - This leads us to conclude that ECochG may hold clinical utility providing surgeons with intraoperative feedback regarding insertion trauma as well as information regarding expected hearing preservation.
- There was a significant relationship between postoperative ECochG thresholds and postoperative audiometric thresholds.
    - This measure may hold significant clinical value for patients unable to provide reliable behavioral data at the activation appointment (e.g., young children) and potentially for appointments when time does not allow for comprehensive device programming and behavioral audiometry.
    - Further this suggests that changes in cochlear physiology following cochlear implantation may be evidenced by changes noted in ECochG data obtained intraoperatively and at various postoperative time points.

AUTHOR CONTRIBUTIONS

JH, BO, RD, RG, JN, and RL all collaborated on experimental design, data analysis, and manuscript preparation. JH, RD, BO, RL, and RG recruited participants and collected data. BO and RL organized the results and conducted statistical analyses. RL was responsible for the supervision of the operating room methods and CT imaging. JN completed analyses of pre- and post-implant CT imaging. MB, AR, RL, DH, and GW inserted electrode arrays used for data collection. RL and RG supervised the project, secured funding, and provided guidance for methodology and interpretation of findings.

ACKNOWLEDGMENTS

This research was supported by the Vanderbilt University School of Medicine and the National Institute of Health (NIH, R01DC008408, R01DC009404, and R01DC014037). The methods of this study were approved by the Vanderbilt Institutional Review Board (IRB# 151808). The authors would like to express sincere gratitude to the following individuals: Dr. Kanthaiah Koka for his counsel regarding software and comments on a previous version of this manuscript, Dr. Mary Dietrich for her statistical guidance, Dr. Linsey Sunderhaus for her assistance with managing the CT images, Ashudee Kirk, M.S. for her assistance with obtaining the CT images, and Dr. Ally Sisler-Dinwiddie, Dr. Adrian Taylor, and Alex Chern for their assistance with data collection. Portions of this dataset will be presented at the Combined Otolaryngology Spring Meetings (COSM) in San Diego, CA, April 26–30, 2017 and at the 15th Symposium on Cochlear Implants in Children in San Francisco, CA, July 26–29, 2017.

REFERENCES

Acharya, A. N., Tavora-Vieira, D., and Rajan, G. P. (2016). Using the implant electrode array to conduct real-time intraoperative hearing monitoring during pediatric cochlear implantation: preliminary experiences. *Otol. Neurotol.* 37, e148–e153. doi: 10.1097/mao.0000000000000950

Adunka, O. F., Giardina, C. K., Formeister, E. J., Choudhury, B., Buchman, C. A., and Fitzpatrick, D. C. (2016). Round window electrocochleography before and after cochlear implant electrode insertion. *Laryngoscope* 126, 1193–1200. doi: 10.1002/lary.25602

Adunka, O., Gstoettner, W., Hambek, M., Unkelbach, M. H., Radeloff, A., and Kiefer, J. (2004). Preservation of basal inner ear structures in cochlear implantation. *ORL* 66, 306–312. doi: 10.1159/000081887

Calloway, N. H., Fitzpatrick, D. C., Campbell, A. P., Iseli, C., Pulver, S., Buchman, C. A., et al. (2014). Intracochlear electrocochleography during cochlear implantation. *Otol. Neurotol.* 35, 1451–1457. doi: 10.1097/MAO.0000000000000451

Campbell, L., Kaicer, A., Briggs, R., and O'Leary, S. (2015). Cochlear response telemetry: intracochlear electrocochleography via cochlear implant neural response telemetry pilot study results. *Otol. Neurotol.* 36, 399–405. doi: 10.1097/MAO.0000000000000678

Campbell, L., Kaicer, A., Sly, D., Iseli, C., Wei, B., Briggs, R., et al. (2016). Intraoperative real-time cochlear response telemetry predicts hearing preservation in cochlear implantation. *Otol. Neurotol.* 37, 332–338. doi: 10.1097/mao.0000000000000972

Carlson, M. L., Driscoll, C. L. W., Gifford, R. H., Service, G. J., Tombers, N. M., Hughes-Borst, B. J., et al. (2011). Implications of minimizing trauma during conventional cochlear implantation. *Otol. Neurotol.* 32, 962–968. doi: 10.1097/MAO.0b013e3182204526

Choudhury, B., Fitzpatrick, D. C., Buchman, C. A., Wei, B. P., Dillon, M. T., He, S., et al. (2012). Intraoperative round window recordings to acoustic stimuli from cochlear implant patients. *Otol. Neurotol.* 33, 1507–1515. doi: 10.1097/MAO.0b013e31826dbc80

Cosetti, M. K., Friedmann, D. R., Zhu, B. Z., Heman-Ackah, S. E., Fang, Y., Keller, R. G., et al. (2013). The effects of residual hearing in traditional cochlear implant candidates after implantation with a conventional electrode. *Otol. Neurotol.* 34, 516–521. doi: 10.1097/MAO.0b013e3182785210

Cullen, J. K., Ellis, M. S., Berlin, C. I., and Lousteau, R. J. (1972). Human acoustic nerve action potential recordings from the tympanic membrane without anesthesia. *Acta Otolaryngol.* 74, 15–22. doi: 10.3109/00016487209128417

Dalbert, A., Huber, A., Veraguth, D., Roosli, C., and Pfiffner, F. (2016). Assessment of cochlear trauma during cochlear implantation using electrocochleography and cone beam computed tomography. *Otol. Neurotol.* 37, 446–453. doi: 10.1097/MAO.0000000000000998

Dalbert, A., Pfiffner, F., Röösli, C., Thoele, K., Sim, J. H., Gerig, R., et al. (2015a). Extra- and intracochlear electrocochleography in cochlear implant recipients. *Audiol. Neurootol.* 20, 339–348. doi: 10.1159/000438742

Dalbert, A., Sim, J. H., Gerig, R., Pfiffner, F., Roosli, C., and Huber, A. (2015b). Correlation of electrophysiological properties and hearing preservation in cochlear implant patients. *Otol. Neurotol.* 36, 1172–1180. doi: 10.1097/mao.0000000000000768

Dedhia, K., Worman, T., Meredith, M. A., and Rubinstein, J. T. (2016). Patterns of long-term hearing loss in hearing preservation cochlear implant surgery. *Otol. Neurotol.* 37, 478–486. doi: 10.1097/MAO.0000000000001011

Dorman, M. F., and Gifford, R. H. (2010). Combining acoustic and electric stimulation in the service of speech recognition. *Int. J. Audiol.* 49, 912–919. doi: 10.3109/14992027.2010.509113

Dunn, C. C., Perreau, A., Gantz, B., and Tyler, R. S. (2010). Benefits of localization and speech perception with multiple noise sources in listeners with a short-electrode cochlear implant. *J. Am. Acad. Audiol.* 21, 44–51. doi: 10.3766/jaaa.21.1.6

Durrant, J. D., Wang, J., Ding, D. L., and Salvi, R. J. (1998). Are inner or outer hair cells the source of summating potentials recorded from the round window? *J. Acoust. Soc. Am.* 104, 370–377.

Eshraghi, A. A., Ahmed, J., Krysiak, E., Ila, K., Ashman, P., Telischi, F. F., et al. (2016). Clinical, surgical, and electrical factors impacting residual hearing in cochlear implant surgery. *Acta Otolaryngol.* 137, 384–388. doi: 10.1080/00016489.2016.1256499

Eshraghi, A. A., Gupta, C., Van De Water, T. R., Bohorquez, J. E., Garnham, C., Bas, E., et al. (2013). Molecular mechanisms involved in cochlear implantation trauma and the protection of hearing and auditory sensory cells by inhibition of c-Jun-N-terminal kinase signaling. *Laryngoscope* 123(Suppl.), S1–S14. doi: 10.1002/lary.23902

Eshraghi, A. A., and Van de Water, T. R. (2006). Cochlear implantation trauma and noise-induced hearing loss: apoptosis and therapeutic strategies. *Anat. Rec. A Discov. Mol. Cell. Evol. Biol.* 288, 473–481. doi: 10.1002/ar.a.20305

Ferraro, J. (2010). Electrocochleography: a review of recording approaches, clinical applications, and new findings in adults and children. *J. Am. Acad. Audiol.* 21, 145–152. doi: 10.3766/jaaa.21.3.2

Finley, C. C., Holden, T. A., Holden, L. K., Whiting, B. R., Chole, R. A., Neely, G. J., et al. (2008). Role of electrode placement as a contributor to variability in cochlear implant outcomes. *Otol. Neurotol.* 29, 920–928. doi: 10.1097/MAO.0b013e318184f492

Fitzpatrick, D. C., Campbell, A., Choudhury, B., Dillon, M., Forgues, M., Buchman, C. A., et al. (2014). Round window electrocochleography just prior to cochlear implantation: relationship to word recognition outcomes in adults HHS public access. *Otol. Neurotol.* 35, 64–71. doi: 10.1097/MAO.0000000000000219

Forgues, M., Koehn, H. A., Dunnon, A. K., Pulver, S. H., Buchman, C. A., Adunka, O. F., et al. (2014). Distinguishing hair cell from neural potentials recorded at the round window. *J. Neurophysiol.* 111, 580–593. doi: 10.1152/jn.00446.2013

Friedland, D. R., Venick, H. S., and Niparko, J. K. (2003). Choice of ear for cochlear implantation: the effect of history and residual hearing on predicted postoperative performance. *Otol. Neurotol.* 24, 582–589. doi: 10.1097/00129492-200307000-00009

Gifford, R. H., Davis, T. J., Sunderhaus, L. W., Menapace, C., Buck, B., Crosson, J., et al. (2017). Combined electric and acoustic stimulation (EAS) with hearing preservation: effect of cochlear implant low-frequency cutoff on speech understanding and perceived listening difficulty. *Ear Hear.* doi: 10.1097/AUD.0000000000000418. [Epub ahead of print].

Gifford, R. H., Dorman, M. F., Skarzynski, H., Lorens, A., Polak, M., Driscoll, C. L. W., et al. (2013). Cochlear implantation with hearing preservation yields significant benefit for speech recognition in complex listening environments. *Ear Hear.* 34, 413–425. doi: 10.1097/AUD.0b013e31827e8163

Gifford, R. H., Driscoll, C. L. W., Davis, T. J., Fiebig, P., Micco, A., and Dorman, M. F. (2015). A within-subject comparison of bimodal hearing, bilateral cochlear implantation, and bilateral cochlear implantation with bilateral hearing preservation: high-performing patients. *Otol. Neurotol.* 36, 1331–1337. doi: 10.1097/MAO.0000000000000804

Gifford, R. H., Grantham, D. W., Sheffield, S. W., Davis, T. J., Dwyer, R., and Dorman, M. F. (2014). Localization and interaural time difference (ITD) thresholds for cochlear implant recipients with preserved acoustic hearing in the implanted ear. *Hear. Res.* 312, 28–37. doi: 10.1016/j.heares.2014.02.007

Holden, L. K., Finley, C. C., Firszt, J. B., Holden, T. A., Brenner, C., Potts, L. G., et al. (2013). Factors affecting open-set word recognition in adults with cochlear implants. *Ear Hear.* 34, 342–360. doi: 10.1097/AUD.0b013e3182741aa7

Jurawitz, M.-C., Büchner, A., Harpel, T., Schüssler, M., Majdani, O., Lesinski-Schiedat, A., et al. (2014). Hearing preservation outcomes with different cochlear implant electrodes: nucleus® HYBRID™-L24 and nucleus freedom™ CI422. *Audiol. Neurootol.* 19, 293–309. doi: 10.1159/000360601

Kamakura, T., and Nadol, J. B. (2016). Correlation between word recognition score and intracochlear new bone and fibrous tissue after cochlear implantation in the human. *Hear. Res.* 339, 132–141. doi: 10.1016/j.heares.2016.06.015

Koka, K., Saoji, A. A., and Litvak, L. M. (2016). Electrocochleography in cochlear implant recipients with residual hearing: comparison with audiometric thresholds Ear Hear. 38, e161–e167. doi: 10.1097/AUD.0000000000000385

Loiselle, L. H., Dorman, M. F., Yost, W. A., Cook, S. J., and Gifford, R. H. (2016). Using ILD or ITD cues for sound source localization and speech understanding in a complex listening environment by listeners with bilateral and with hearing-preservation cochlear implants. *J. Speech Lang. Hear. Res.* 59, 810. doi: 10.1044/2015_JSLHR-H-14-0355

Loiselle, L. H., Dorman, M. F., Yost, W. A., and Gifford, R. H. (2015). Sound source localization by hearing preservation patients with and without symmetrical low-frequency acoustic hearing. *Audiol. Neurootol.* 20, 166–171. doi: 10.1159/000367883

Mandala, M., Colletti, L., Tonoli, G., and Colletti, V. (2012). Electrocochleography during cochlear implantation for hearing preservation. *Otolaryngol. Head Neck Surg.* 146, 774–781. doi: 10.1177/0194599811435895

Noble, J. H., Schuman, T. A., Wright, C. G., Labadie, R. F., and Dawant, B. M. (2011). Automatic identification of cochlear implant electrode arrays for post-operative assessment. *Proc. SPIE Int. Soc. Opt. Eng.* 7962. doi: 10.1117/12.878490

Palmer, A. R., and Russell, I. J. (1986). Phase-locking in the cochlear nerve of the guinea-pig and its relation to the receptor potential of inner hair-cells. *Hear. Res.* 24, 1–15.

Patuzzi, R. B., Yates, G. K., and Johnstone, B. M. (1989). Outer hair cell receptor current and sensorineural hearing loss. *Hear. Res.* 42, 47–72. doi: 10.1016/0378-5955(89)90117-2

Plant, K., and Babic, L. (2016). Utility of bilateral acoustic hearing in combination with electrical stimulation provided by the cochlear implant. *Int. J. Audiol.* 55(Suppl. 2), S31–S38. doi: 10.3109/14992027.2016.1150609

Plant, K., McDermott, H., van Hoesel, R., Dawson, P., and Cowan, R. (2016). Factors predicting postoperative unilateral and bilateral speech recognition in adult cochlear implant recipients with acoustic hearing. *Ear Hear.* 37, 153–163. doi: 10.1097/AUD.0000000000000233

Poch-Broto, J., Carricondo, F., Bhathal, B., Iglesias, M.-C., López-Moya, J., Rodríguez, F., et al. (2009). Cochlear microphonic audiometry: a new hearing test for objective diagnosis of deafness. *Acta Otolaryngol.* 129, 749–754. doi: 10.1080/00016480802398962

Prijs, V. F. (1991). Evaluation of electrocochleographic audiogram determination in infants. *Acta Otolaryngol. Suppl.* 482, 27–33. doi: 10.3109/00016489109128025

Radeloff, A., Shehata-Dieler, W., Scherzed, A., Rak, K., Harnisch, W., Hagen, R., et al. (2012). Intraoperative monitoring using cochlear microphonics in cochlear implant patients with residual hearing. *Otol. Neurotol.* 33, 348–354. doi: 10.1097/MAO.0b013e318248ea86

Rader, T., Fastl, H., and Baumann, U. (2013). Speech perception with combined electric-acoustic stimulation and bilateral cochlear implants in a multisource noise field. *Ear Hear.* 34, 324–332. doi: 10.1097/AUD.0b013e318272f189

Rosen, S. (1992). Temporal information in speech: acoustic, auditory and linguistic aspects. *Philos. Trans. R. Soc. Lond.* 336, 367–373. doi: 10.1098/rstb.1992.0070

Rubinstein, J. T., Parkinson, W. S., Tyler, R. S., and Gantz, B. J. (1999). Residual speech recognition and cochlear implant performance: effects of implantation criteria. *Am. J. Otol.* 20, 445–452.

Santa Maria, P. L., Gluth, M. B., Yuan, Y., Atlas, M. D., and Blevins, N. H. (2014). Hearing preservation surgery for cochlear implantation: a meta-analysis. *Otol. Neurotol.* 35, e256–e269. doi: 10.1097/MAO.0000000000000561

Schoonhoven, R., Prijs, V. F., and Grote, J. J. (1996). Response thresholds in electrocochleography and their relation to the pure tone audiogram. *Ear Hear.* 17, 266–275. doi: 10.1097/00003446-199606000-00009

Scott, W. C., Giardina, C. K., Pappa, A. K., Fontenot, T. E., Anderson, M. L., Dillon, M. T., et al. (2016). The compound action potential in subjects receiving a cochlear implant. *Otol. Neurotol.* 37, 1654–1661. doi: 10.1097/MAO.0000000000001224

Skarzynski, H., Matusiak, M., Lorens, A., Furmanek, M., Pilka, A., and Skarzynski, P. H. (2016). Preservation of cochlear structures and hearing when using the Nucleus Slim Straight (CI422) electrode in children. *J. Laryngol. Otol.* 130, 332–339. doi: 10.1017/S0022215115003436

GraphPad Software Inc. (2012). *GraphPad Prism*. GraphPad.

Sohmer, H., Kinarti, R., and Gafni, M. (1980). The source along the basilar membrane of the cochlear microphonic potential recorded by surface electrodes in man. *Electroencephalogr. Clin. Neurophysiol.* 49, 506–514. doi: 10.1016/0013-4694(80)90393-4

Sweeney, A. D., Hunter, J. B., Carlson, M. L., Rivas, A., Bennett, M. L., Gifford, R. H., et al. (2016). Durability of hearing preservation after cochlear implantation with conventional-length electrodes and scala tympani insertion. *Otolaryngol. Head Neck Surg.* 154, 907–913. doi: 10.1177/0194599816630545

Van Abel, K. M., Dunn, C. C., Sladen, D. P., Oleson, J. J., Beatty, C. W., Neff, B. A., et al. (2015). Hearing preservation among patients undergoing cochlear implantation. *Otol. Neurotol.* 36, 416–421. doi: 10.1097/MAO.0000000000000703

Verpy, E., Weil, D., Leibovici, M., Goodyear, R. J., Hamard, G., Houdon, C., et al. (2008). Stereocilin-deficient mice reveal the origin of cochlear waveform distortions. *Nature* 456, 255–258. doi: 10.1038/nature07380

Wanna, G. B., Noble, J. H., Carlson, M. L., Gifford, R. H., Dietrich, M. S., Haynes, D. S., et al. (2014). Impact of electrode design and surgical approach on scalar location and cochlear implant outcomes. *Laryngoscope* 124, S1–S7. doi: 10.1002/lary.24728

Yoshie, N. (1973). Diagnostic significance of the electrocochleogram in clinical audiometry. *Audiology* 12, 504–539. doi: 10.3109/00206097309071666

Yoshie, N., Ohashi, T., and Suzuki, T. (1967). Non-surgical recording of auditory nerve action potentials in man. *Laryngoscope* 77, 76–85. doi: 10.1288/00005537-196701000-00006

Zhang, M. (2012). High-frequency hearing impairment assessed with cochlear microphonics. *Acta Otolaryngol.* 132, 967–973. doi: 10.3109/00016489.2012.679688

12

Putative Auditory-Evoked Neurophonic Measurements Using a Novel Signal Processing Technique

Alison M. Cook[1,2], *Ashleigh J. Allsop*[1] *and Greg A. O'Beirne*[1,2*]

[1] *New Zealand Institute of Language Brain and Behaviour, University of Canterbury, Christchurch, New Zealand,* [2] *Eisdell Moore Centre, Auckland, New Zealand*

Correspondence:
Greg A. O'Beirne
gregory.obeirne@canterbury.ac.nz

With changes to cochlear implant candidacy and improvements in surgical technique, there is a need for accurate intraoperative assessment of low-frequency hearing thresholds during cochlear implantation. In electrocochleography, onset compound action potentials (CAPs) typically allow estimation of auditory threshold for frequencies above 1 kHz, but they are less accurate at lower frequencies. Auditory nerve neurophonic (ANN) waveforms, on the other hand, may overcome this limitation by allowing phase-locked neural activity to be tracked during a prolonged low-frequency stimulus rather than just at its onset (Henry, 1995). Lichtenhan et al. (2013) have used their auditory nerve overlapped waveform (ANOW) technique to measure these potentials from the round windows of cats and guinea pigs, and reported that in guinea pigs these potentials originate in the cochlear apex for stimuli below 70 dB SPL (Lichtenhan et al., 2014). Human intraoperative round window neurophonic measurements have been reported by Choudhury et al. (2012). We have done the same in hearing impaired awake participants, and present here the results of a pilot study in which we recorded responses evoked by 360, 525, and 725 Hz tone bursts from the cochlear promontory of one participant. We also present a modification to the existing measurement technique which halves recording time, extracting the auditory neurophonic by recording a single averaged waveform, and then subtracting from it a 180° group-delayed version of itself, rather than using alternating condensation and rarefaction sound stimuli. We cannot conclude that the waveforms we measured were purely neural responses originating from the apex of the cochlea: as with all neurophonic measurement procedures, the neural responses of interest cannot be separated from higher harmonics of the cochlear microphonic without forward masking, regardless of electrode location, stimuli or post-processing algorithm. In conclusion, the extraction of putative neurophonic waveforms can easily be incorporated into existing electrocochleographic measurement paradigms, but at this stage such measurements should be interpreted with caution.

Keywords: cochlea, electrocochleography, cochlear microphonic, auditory neurophonic, hearing impairment

INTRODUCTION

Over time, changes in the criteria for cochlear implant (CI) candidacy have led to growing numbers of CI candidates presenting with useable low-frequency (LF) hearing thresholds (i.e., <1 kHz). Improvements in minimally traumatic surgical techniques and the availability of "atraumatic" electrodes have improved the chances that this residual hearing may be preserved, enabling improved speech perception and appreciation of music (Gantz et al., 2005; Dorman and Gifford, 2010; Adunka et al., 2013). Intraoperative monitoring of LF hearing has the potential to help preserve this residual hearing (Mandalà et al., 2012). One approach has been to use cochlear response telemetry, using the CI electrodes themselves to monitor cochlear responses (Radeloff et al., 2012; Campbell et al., 2016). Of the cochlear potentials measurable using this technique, Campbell et al. have found that the onset compound action potential (CAP) and summating potential (SP) had poorer signal-to-noise ratios than the cochlear microphonic potential (CM), leading them to rely on the CM for intraoperative monitoring. While CM changes may indicate damage to the organ of Corti, the low-frequency CM amplitude recorded in the basal turn is not frequency specific (Patuzzi et al., 1989). It also does not provide information about the function of residual inner hair cells (IHCs) or neurons, and cannot be used for participants with non-functional outer hair cells (OHCs). Similarly, practitioners of electrocochleography (ECochG) have reported that while tone-burst stimuli allow estimation of auditory threshold for frequencies above 1 kHz, tone burst CAPs below 1 kHz are often smaller, because the slow onset/offset ramps required to avoid spectral splatter are less effective at eliciting synchronized neural firing at the onset of the tone burst, thereby underestimating LF sensitivity. Therefore, there is a need for a reliable intraoperative assay of very low frequency (<1 kHz) IHC/neural function in CI recipients.

One such assay may be the synchronized neural firing evoked *during* longer-duration LF tones. The cochlear response to ongoing tones has been measured since the earliest studies of cochlear potentials (Wever and Bray, 1930). Then, as now, a major issue was determining the source of the measured potential (i.e., cochlear or brain stem, OHC or neural). Because assumptions about generator sites are closely linked to the names given to such responses, nomenclature must be carefully considered. Over the decades, the response to ongoing tones has been given various names. In the earliest studies of cochlear potentials, the response termed the "Wever and Bray phenomenon" (Wever and Bray, 1930) in due course came to be understood as having both hair cell (cochlear microphonic) and neural contributions (Adrian, 1930; Adrian et al., 1931; Derbyshire and Davis, 1935). Similar responses measured with intra-cranial electrodes within various parts of the auditory brainstem were called "frequency following responses" (Boudreau and Tsuchitani, 1964; Worden and Marsh, 1968) but were later dubbed "auditory neurophonic" by Weinberger et al. (1970) to reflect their neural origin, and their similarity with the cochlear microphonic potential. Snyder and Schreiner (1984) reused this terminology but re-defined the "auditory neurophonic" as the response of individual auditory brainstem nuclei, and used the more specific term of "auditory nerve neurophonic" (ANN) to refer to the neurophonic measured differentially along the auditory nerve. Moreover, they reserved the (previously used) term "frequency-following response" to refer to activity measured from the scalp, which included auditory neurophonics from the auditory nerve, as well as higher auditory brainstem structures (Snyder and Schreiner, 1984, 1985). Henry (1995, 1997) and Choudhury et al. (2012) also used the term ANN, but this time referring to the neural component of the response measured from the round window (RW) of gerbils and humans, respectively. These authors used alternating condensation and rarefaction sound stimuli to cancel the first harmonic of the contributions to the averaged waveforms (assuming this to be dominated by the CM). This processing strategy cancels out the fundamental frequency of all response components, including the CM, leaving a smaller amplitude, frequency-doubled residual waveform containing the higher harmonics and baseline shifts of the hair cell and neural responses (Sellick et al., 2003). It is worth emphasizing that this frequency-doubling is a consequence of the summing of responses to alternating stimuli, and that any neural response in the *unprocessed* waveform will repeat at the stimulation frequency f, rather than at $2f$. Lichtenhan et al. (2013) subsequently used the term the "auditory nerve overlapped waveform" (ANOW) to describe this same residual waveform recorded from the RW or nearby bone in cats and guinea pigs, albeit with the baseline shift removed to facilitate measurement of the AC component. Using a name other than "ANN" avoids the insinuation that the residual waveform is purely neural. However, the inclusion of "auditory nerve" in the "ANOW" name may also be problematic: any such waveform will inevitably contain both neural (ANN) and residual hair cell (CM) contributions, and it is not possible to determine the source of these higher harmonics by this processing strategy alone (see Section Discussion). In addition to "ANOW", Lichtenhan et al. (2014) also used the term $CR_{ave,mid}$ (i.e., the averaged cochlear response from the middle of the alternating tone burst) to acknowledge that multiple cochlear generators contribute to this response over a range of sound levels. In light of this ambiguity, here we will also refer to the response as $CR_{ave,mid}$, or as the "putative neurophonic".

We present here examples of the waveform recorded from the cochlear promontory in one participant (one ear). The invasive nature of the measurements limited our participant pool to subjects with suspected cochlear pathologies already undergoing transtympanic ECochG. We present in-depth results from one participant chosen for their clear tone-burst CAP responses and cochlear microphonic waveforms as seen in standard ECochG recordings, and use these (i) to demonstrate a novel technique that halves the averaging time for extracting steady-state tone responses and obviates the need for alternating condensation and rarefaction stimuli; (ii) to demonstrate that these measurements can be made as a relatively quick addition to any standard ECochG protocol; and (iii) to highlight the inherent ambiguity in any such waveform regarding contributions from the non-linear OHC receptor current (CM), and non-linear neural responses. This ambiguity is not an artifact of any particular processing algorithm, stimuli or electrode placement, but is intrinsic to the physiological mechanisms generating the CM and neurophonic. This point is critical, given the renewed clinical interest in the use of ECochG for intraoperative monitoring, and must be addressed before the relationship between neurophonic and audiometric thresholds can be established. It is not possible to confirm the neural origin of such a response without, for example, showing it is susceptible to forward masking (unlike hair cell responses), or by using neurotoxins such as tetrodotoxin or kainate, as is possible in experimental animals.

METHODS

Patient Selection and Pre-testing

This study was carried out in accordance with the recommendations of the National Ethics Advisory Committee's "Ethical Guidelines for Intervention Studies". The participant gave written informed consent in accordance with the Declaration of Helsinki. The protocol was approved by the Southern Health and Disability Ethics Committee (Ethics Ref: 14/STH/92). Following air- and bone-conduction audiometry and tympanometry, the participant underwent routine transtympanic ECochG in one ear only, as part of diagnosis for suspected Menière's syndrome (Allsop, 2016). In the end, for this participant the SP/CAP ratios in response to both clicks and tone bursts were not consistent with hydrops in the ear tested, according to Gibson's criteria (see Hornibrook et al., 2012). Audiometry revealed that the participant had a mild-to-moderate sensorineural hearing impairment in that ear: air conduction thresholds in dB HL (dB SPL in brackets) were 30 (55) at 250 Hz, 25 (35) at 500 Hz, 40 (45) at 1 kHz, 40 (50) at 2 kHz, 25 (35) at 4 kHz, 55 (70) at 6 kHz, and 60 (75) at 8 kHz, with bone conduction thresholds within 5 dB of air-conduction at the four frequencies tested (0.5, 1, 2, and 4 kHz). The contralateral ear showed a profound hearing loss, with responses unable to be measured at the limits of the audiometer.

ECochG Procedure

ECochG procedures used were the same as described in Hornibrook et al. (2012). The combined reference/ground electrode was placed on the forehead. Both electrodes were Ag/AgCl ECG electrodes (Blue Sensor; Ambu, Denmark). The tympanic membrane and ear canal were numbed with phenol before placing the monopolar transtympanic needle electrode (TECA; CareFusion, USA) onto the cochlear promontory. The electrode was held in place by a custom-made headphone holder, over which the magnetically shielded supra-aural headphone was placed.

Custom-written software was used to generate the stimuli, and record and process the responses. Tone burst stimuli at 360, 525, and 725 Hz (30 ms duration, 2 cycle rise-fall time) were presented at 18 stimuli/second at calibrated levels through the supra-aural headphone via a digital-to-analog converter (NI9269; National Instruments, TX, USA), and a battery-powered amplifier (MX28 MiniMix VI, Rolls Corporation). Sound stimuli frequencies were chosen to avoid harmonics of the 50 Hz mains power frequency. Where time constraints allowed (i.e., for 525 and 725 Hz), presentation levels were incremented in 5 dB steps, to obtain at least two responses above and below onset-CAP threshold. Sound levels are presented here as dB peSPL, which should allow the reader to reconstruct the stimuli used in this study. While we did not measure psychophysical detection thresholds to these stimuli, we assume they would lie between those recorded by Poulsen and Legarth (2008) for 5 ms tone bursts, and the long-duration tones used in audiometry (ANSI, 2004).

The ECochG response was amplified with an electrically isolated bioamplifier (MK15; Amplaid, Milan, Italy), band-pass filtered at 0.5 Hz and 3 kHz (1st order high-pass, 2nd order low-pass), and sampled at 44.1 kHz (NI9222; National Instruments, TX, USA). Averaging and processing of the responses was performed by our software. Whole averaged ECochG waveforms (n = 300–310) were recorded, and the plateau region of the response was used for post-processing.

The analysis window was chosen to be during the plateau (*after* the tone burst onset CAP), where the amplitude of the response has largely adapted. The exact analysis window varied with frequency, commencing 1.5 stimulus cycles after the onset CAP at response threshold, and included an integer number of stimulus cycles (4 cycles for 360 Hz, 8 for 525 Hz, and 13 for 725 Hz) before the start of the stimulus offset ramp. The noise floor and pre-stimulus DC offset were calculated from the 5 ms pre-stimulus window. The entire averaging process lasted ~10 min per ear when presenting alternating stimuli at three frequencies and six sound levels.

Responses from condensation ("CON") and rarefaction ("RAR") tone bursts were averaged separately. After removing any DC offset, the CON and RAR waveforms were summed and divided by 2 to produce the "SUM" waveform (see **Figure 1**) with the aim of canceling, or at least minimizing, any contributions that are of opposite polarities in the CON and RAR responses (assumed to be dominated by CM). The RAR waveform was subtracted from the CON waveform, and the result divided by 2 to produce the "DIFF" waveform, which allowed examination of the putative CM contribution.

The SUM waveform contained a slow baseline shift, which could be removed by subtracting a bandpass filtered version of the SUM response (high-pass at 0.01 Hz, low-pass at stimulus frequency, both with 35 dB/octave roll-off) from the unfiltered SUM waveform, leaving the $CR_{ave,mid}$ waveform that is the focus of this study.

Averaging Within the Tone Burst

As in Lichtenhan et al. (2013), the signal-to-noise ratio of the waveform could be further improved by dividing the analysis region of the $CR_{ave,mid}$ waveform into epochs the length of one cycle of the stimulus frequency f (or two cycles of the $2f$ $CR_{ave,mid}$). These epochs were then averaged together (**Figure 1**). For the 360 Hz tone burst, 4 stimulus cycles were averaged, increasing the SNR by 6 dB ($\sqrt{4}$) or reducing the time taken to reach a given SNR by 4-fold. Similarly, averaging time was reduced at 525 Hz and 725 Hz by 8-fold and 13-fold, respectively, with increases in SNR of 9 dB and 11 dB, respectively.

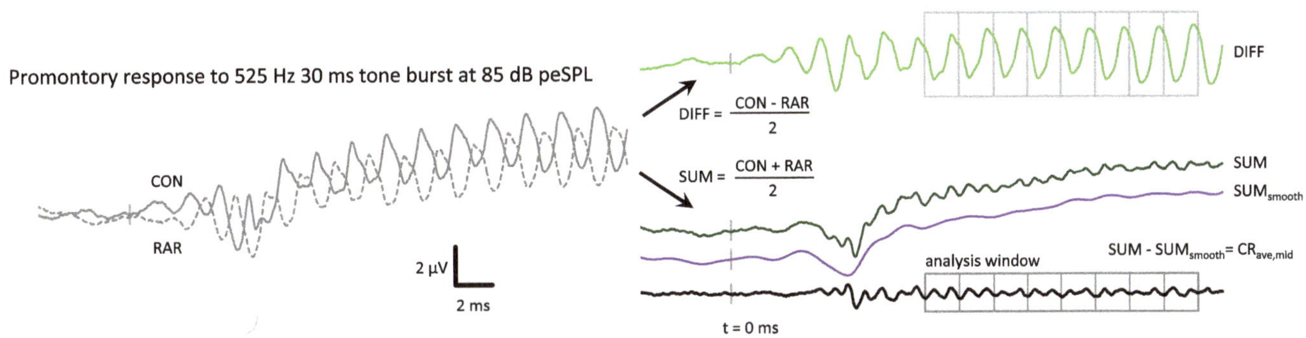

FIGURE 1 | The post-processing steps to produce the $CR_{ave,mid}$ from the ECochG response, in this case a 525 Hz 85 dB peSPL tone burst. CON and RAR are the averaged ECochG responses to condensation and rarefaction tone bursts, respectively. The $CR_{ave,mid}$ is the sum of the CON and RAR responses, with the baseline shift removed. The SUM_{smooth} waveform was produced by low-pass filtering the SUM waveform at *f*. The analysis window was further divided into epochs with a duration of one cycle of the stimulus in length for further averaging of the $CR_{ave,mid}$. The averaged $CR_{ave,mid}$ waveform therefore contains 2 cycles of $CR_{ave,mid}$ at 2*f*.

Sham Control Responses

As in any electrophysiological response that follows the sound stimulus, it is essential to confirm that the recorded responses are not the result of electromagnetic feed through between the headphone and the recording electrode. If using insert earphones, control responses could be obtained simply by clamping off the sound delivery tube or blocking the ear canal, but this was not possible with the supra-aural headphones used in this study, with an electrode placed through the tympanic membrane. This is a limitation of this study. However, as shown in **Figure 2**, the $CR_{ave,mid}$ and DIFF responses did not grow with sound level by 1dB/dB (gray lines in Panels G and H), as would be expected from electrical capacitive feedthrough from the headphone transducer. Moreover, our focus on the higher harmonics of the averaged responses makes any residual linear feed-through of little concern.

RESULTS

Figure 1 shows an example of the sequence of post-processing steps to produce a $CR_{ave,mid}$ waveform. The $CR_{ave,mid}$ waveform is essentially the sum of the condensation and rarefaction tone burst responses, with the baseline shift removed to facilitate processing (i.e., further averaging within the plateau region analysis window). Note that the $CR_{ave,mid}$ appears as a frequency-doubled waveform (i.e., at 2*f*) as a result of the summing of condensation and rarefaction stimuli. The putative neurophonic appears in the CON and RAR waveforms at *f*, where it contributes to their distorted wave shapes (**Figure 1**).

In **Figure 2** panels A, C, and E are plots of the entire 30 ms- long SUM and DIFF waveforms over a range of stimulus sound levels. The CAP at the tone-burst onset is visible in the SUM waveform (indicated by an asterisk in Panels A, C, and E). The SUM waveform is equivalent to the averaged response from alternating stimuli commonly used in ECochG. The decrease in CAP latency with increasing stimulus sound level can also be clearly seen for 525 and 725 Hz. Unfortunately, due to time constraints, not all sound stimulus levels were tested at 360 Hz. Panels B, D, and F of **Figure 2** show the corresponding $CR_{ave,mid}$ waveforms for each sound level, obtained as shown in **Figure 1**. The gray traces above and below these averaged $CR_{ave,mid}$ waveforms (shown in black) represent $\pm$ 1 standard deviation (calculated across the number of averaged stimulus cycles in the analysis window; i.e., $n = 4$, 8, and 13 for 360, 525, and 725 Hz, respectively).

Panels G and H of **Figure 2** show input-output functions for the $CR_{ave,mid}$ and DIFF. The amplitude values of $CR_{ave,mid}$ and DIFF were obtained from the spectrum at 2*f* and *f*, respectively. Responses below the noise floor are shown with open symbols. The noise floor for visual detection for each input/output function was calculated as the mean RMS amplitude of the averaged trace in the pre-stimulus window (5 ms before tone-burst onset).

The growth of the $CR_{ave,mid}$ and DIFF responses out of the noise floor shown in the input-output functions can be seen in the averaged traces (**Figures 2A,C,E**). The diagonal lines in panels G and H of **Figure 2** represent the 1 dB/dB growth expected for a capacitive feed-through electrical artifact.

An Alternative Processing Strategy

Because the analysis time window covered a relatively stable region of the LF-evoked promontory response waveform and excluded any onset components, we were able to employ a novel variation of the technique described above that halved the time taken to obtain an averaged response. This was achieved by presenting only CON tone bursts, and using a 180° group-delayed version of the CON response to replace the RAR responses during the processing described above, producing the trace shown as the $CR_{ave,mid,180°CON}$ waveform in **Figure 3**. Similarly, if only rarefaction tone bursts were presented then group-delayed RAR responses could be used instead of CON responses ($CR_{ave,mid,180°RAR}$ in **Figure 3**). In both cases, the exact delay applied corresponded to half of one cycle of the stimulus frequency. These three processing methods are compared in **Figure 3**, both in the time and frequency domains.

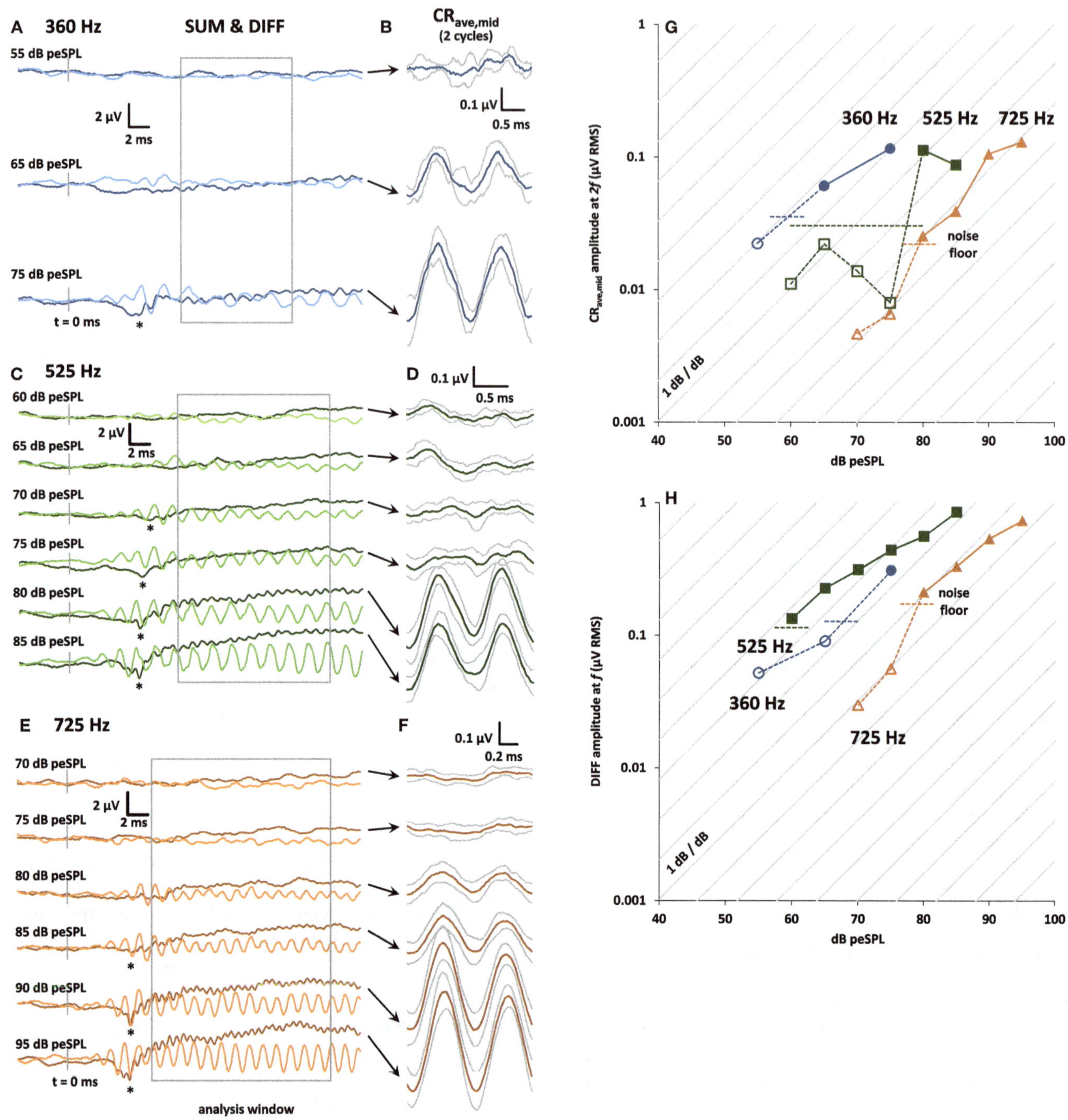

FIGURE 2 | (A) Plots of averaged SUM (dark trace) and DIFF (light trace) responses to 30 ms condensation and rarefaction tone bursts at 360 Hz. The SUM trace is equivalent to averaged ECochG responses to alternating stimuli. The onset CAP can be seen in the SUM trace at the highest level presented (asterisk). The analysis window is shown in gray. **(B)** $CR_{ave,mid}$ waveforms (±1 s.d.) obtained by further averaging of the baseline-shifted SUM waveforms shown in **(A)**. The analysis window was divided into integer multiples of the stimulus cycle at *f*, and so contains 2 cycles of the $CR_{ave,mid}$ at *2f*. **(C)** and **(E)**: As for **(A)**, with tone bursts at 525 and 725 Hz, respectively. **(D)** and **(F)**: As for **(B)**, with tone bursts at 525 and 725 Hz, respectively. **(G)** Input-output curves for the $CR_{ave,mid}$ response amplitude, calculated from the amplitude of the *2f* spectral peak of the baseline shifted SUM waveforms at 360 Hz (blue circles), 525 Hz (green squares), and 725 Hz (orange triangles). The noise floor (horizontal dashed lines) was calculated from the RMS amplitude of the waveforms in the 5 ms pre-stimulus window for each frequency and stimulus presentation level, and then averaged to produce the average noise floor value shown for each frequency. $CR_{ave,mid}$ amplitudes that are below the noise floor are shown with open symbols and dotted lines. **(H)** Input-output curves for the DIFF response amplitude, calculated from the amplitude of its spectral peak at *f*.

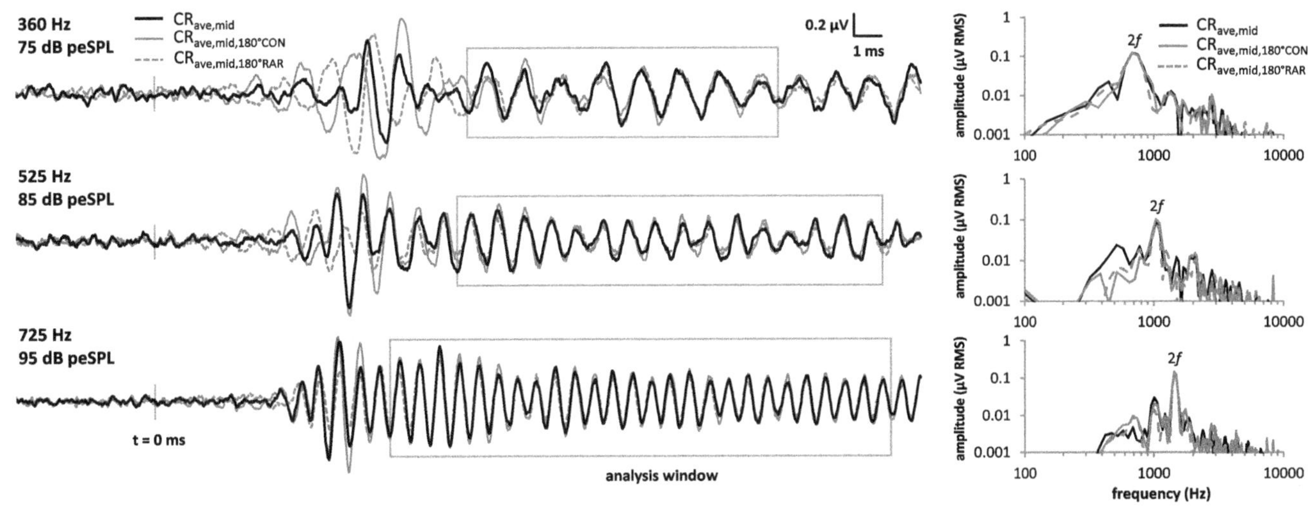

FIGURE 3 | Comparison of the $CR_{ave,mid}$ processing strategies at the 3 frequencies tested. Responses were obtained by averaging CON and RAR alternating stimuli as in standard ECochG ("$CR_{ave,mid}$", black solid traces), and also by presenting only CON tonebursts, and using a 180° group-delayed version of CON response to replace the RAR responses during the processing ("$CR_{ave,mid,180°CON}$", gray solid traces). Similarly, the "$CR_{ave,mid,180°RAR}$" responses (gray dotted traces) were obtained by presenting only RAR tonebursts and using a 180° group-delayed version of the RAR response to replace the CON response during the processing. Although, the onset CAPs differ in latency for these three methods, these fall outside our $CR_{ave,mid}$ analysis window. Within the analysis window (gray boxes), the $CR_{ave,mid}$, $CR_{ave,mid,180°CON}$ and $CR_{ave,mid,180°RAR}$ waveforms mostly overlie. Similarly, the spectra of the three waveforms (right) within these analysis windows also overlie.

The three waveforms do not overlie at the beginning of the tone burst, because the transient onset components differ in latency between condensation and rarefaction responses (Peake and Kiang, 1962). However, the onset-CAP falls outside the analysis window used in our and previous studies. Within the analysis window the three waveforms mostly overlie, as do their amplitude spectra calculated over this same window.

DISCUSSION

The results of the present study have been obtained using variations on the methods and post-processing strategies described by Henry (1995, 1997), Adrian (1930), and Lichtenhan et al. (2013, 2014). The novel averaging strategy presented here halved the averaging time without substantially changing the response for this participant (**Figure 3**), and within-tone-burst averaging improved the signal-to-noise ratio by a factor proportional to the number of analyzed cycles. Ideally, the length of these tone bursts could be greatly increased, thereby lengthening the usable analysis window and further improving the signal-to-noise ratio. This measure would further reduce the averaging time if using a fixed SNR criterion for response detection. It would also improve the frequency specificity of the stimulus by reducing spectral splatter often present in short-duration tone-bursts. These advantages may outweigh the reduction in response amplitude that may result from excluding the pre-plateau components from the analysis window.

We and others are interested in the neurophonic waveform as an objective indicator of low-frequency cochlear sensitivity that can be added to existing ECochG protocols. The waveform may be of particular use for i) objective measurement of low-frequency thresholds/cochlear function in the clinic, and ii) intraoperative monitoring during ear surgery for patients with serviceable low-frequency hearing (e.g., CI recipients). CM recordings during implantation may prove a useful indicator of generalized damage to the organ of Corti (Campbell et al., 2016), and may also provide information regarding OHC operating point shifts caused by cochlear pressure and fluid balance changes (Patuzzi and Moleirinho, 1998). However, the CM is an assay of local OHC function only; a reliable frequency-specific assay of cochlear nerve sensitivity would be useful.

Unfortunately, we cannot conclude that the $CR_{ave,mid}$ waveforms presented here were purely neural, nor that they originated solely from the cochlear apex. This is because (a) no post-processing strategy can distinguish between cochlear microphonic and neurophonic, because the two responses will have varying degrees of both symmetric and asymmetric distortion, depending on sound level and pathology; (b) no additional procedure to assess the neural component (e.g., forward masking) was performed; and (c) our participant did not have normal hearing. The last point means we cannot rely on evidence from previous studies illustrating the reliability of the $CR_{ave,mid}$ as a measure of neural function for stimuli presented below certain sound levels.

The issue of the separation of CM and neurophonic is not new (see, for example, Marsh et al., 1970; Snyder and Schreiner, 1984; Chimento and Schreiner, 1990; Forgues et al., 2014), and must be considered in any future studies of neurophonic waveforms, because the neurophonic and the CM occur concomitantly in cochlear recordings to varying degrees depending on recording location, electrode montage and pathology. Even for differential recordings along the cochlear nerve at the internal auditory meatus (e.g., Snyder and Schreiner, 1984), the CM may be present to a degree because of the proximity of the electrode locations to the cochlear fluids (see Stegeman et al., 1997, Pastras, under review).

Ideally then, to improve the reliability of the $CR_{ave,mid}$ as an estimate of low-frequency sensitivity of the cochlear nerve, recordings should be performed with an electrode placement or montage that limits the contribution of cochlear hair cell potentials and maximizes the contribution of the cochlear nerve electrical activity. For example, we would expect that placing the non-inverting electrode on the promontory rather than the RW would reduce the amplitude of the CM, with little attenuation of the neurophonic. This assumes that the neurophonic, like the CAP, is a field-potential whose dipole is localized to the internal auditory meatus (Brown and Patuzzi, 2010; Rattay and Danner, 2014), whereas the CM is a field potential whose dipole spans the basilar membrane, and which electrically partially cancels at locations such as the bony regions of the middle ear. That is, by utilizing differences in the electrotonic spread of the VIIIth nerve field potential and cochlear hair cell field potential, it should be possible to choose a recording location that has an optimal nerve:hair cell contribution, in regards to their electrical activity. We have not compared recording locations in this study, and we do not suggest that the promontory is by any means the optimal recording location for neurophonic potentials, but the promontory should have a better neural:CM ratio than the RW. This issue should be considered in future measurements, because any reduction in the hair cell component of the response would reduce averaging time and increase certainty about the neural threshold, both of which are crucial considerations for real-time intraoperative monitoring of peripheral sensitivity. It is important to note that optimal electrode recording location will reduce but not eliminate possible "contamination" of neural responses by CM.

Methods for Separating Hair Cell and Neural Contributions

Averaging of responses to alternating polarity stimuli is routinely used in ECochG and provides "good enough" cancelation of CM for detection of onset-CAP. However, it will not cancel the CM unless the CM waveform is symmetric. It has been proposed that CM and neural components could be separated using spectral analysis of the $CR_{ave,mid}$ waveform, assuming asymmetric distortion of CM and half-wave rectification of neural responses (Choudhury et al., 2012; Forgues et al., 2014). This method is unreliable, however, because the CM can distort symmetrically *or* asymmetrically, depending on the operating point of the non-linear transfer curve relating the opening probability of the mechanoelectrical transduction channels and the flow of current into the OHCs (Patuzzi and Moleirinho, 1998). Furthermore, OHC operating point is labile, particularly as a result of exposure to (intense) low-frequency tones (O'Beirne, 2005) or as a result of cochlear pathology such as Menière's syndrome or endolymphatic hydrops (Sirjani et al., 2004; Brown et al., 2013). Similarly, neural response phase varies with sound level (e.g., "peak-splitting"; Kiang, 1990) and following acoustic trauma (Patuzzi and Sellick, 1983). Thus, it is not possible to isolate the underlying cause of changes in the magnitude or phase of spectral components in any given participant, without application of additional measurement techniques, or *a priori* knowledge of the underlying physiology. In animal experiments, Henry (1995, 1997) and Lichtenhan et al. (2014) used tetrodotoxin to block neural responses and reported that, at least in their experiments, a significant proportion of the response measured at the RW was neural in origin. Nevertheless, the question remains whether the source of a response obtained with a human participant in a clinical setting is predominantly neural or OHC, particularly because any given participant will have their own individual pattern of OHC and/or neural hearing loss.

Forward masking presents one potentially useful clinical method of separating CM and neurophonic. Henry (1995, 1997) has demonstrated the use of forward masking of neural responses in RW measurements to obtain "pure" CM waveforms that could be subtracted from the raw waveform to produce a "pure" ANN. This process is analogous to the masking protocol presented by Chimento and Schreiner (1990) for removing CM from scalp-recorded FFR, and has the advantage that the resultant waveform retains the large amplitude response at the stimulus frequency (Chimento and Schreiner, 1990), unlike the summing of responses to alternating polarity stimuli.

$CR_{ave,mid}$ and Audiometric Thresholds

We were not able to compare audiometric thresholds to $CR_{ave,mid}$ threshold here, because (i) the $CR_{ave,mid}$ was obtained at non-standard frequencies (for which audiometric thresholds were not measured) in order to avoid harmonics of 50 Hz mains interference, and (ii) because of the limited amount of data obtained (3 frequencies only). Approximate audiometric thresholds at 360, 525, and 725 Hz (obtained by interpolating from the audiogram data—see Section Methods) did not show a clear relationship to $CR_{ave,mid}$ thresholds, nor did onset-CAP thresholds obtained from the SUM waveforms in **Figure 2**. Audiometric thresholds, together with onset-CAP and $CR_{ave,mid}$ input-output functions should be obtained in a large number of both normal and hearing-impaired participants to determine the relationship between $CR_{ave,mid}$ and audiometric threshold.

Neurophonic Frequency Specificity

Another issue that must be considered in interpreting $CR_{ave,mid}$ amplitudes is the basal-ward recruitment of neural firing at high sound levels (Snyder and Schreiner, 1985). $CR_{ave,mid}$ measurements in (normal hearing) guinea pigs show a significant neural component originating in the cochlear apex only for sound levels of 70 dB SPL or less (Lichtenhan et al., 2014). This issue is further complicated for individuals with hearing loss: the low-frequency tuning curve tails of high characteristic frequency neurons can become hypersensitive with particular patterns of neural/inner hair cell and OHC damage (Liberman and Dodds, 1984; also reviewed in Patuzzi and Robertson, 1988). That tail hypersensitivity also occurs with temporary threshold shift after acoustic trauma (Patuzzi and Sellick,

1983) is a salient point if measuring neurophonic responses intraoperatively before and after temporal bone drilling. High characteristic frequency neuron tail responses could be reduced by masking.

CONCLUSIONS

Incorporating neurophonic measurement into standard ECochG protocols may offer an attractive method for objectively estimating the sensitivity of the apical portions of the cochlea. However, the fact that the CM *and* neurophonic can have varying degrees of both symmetric and asymmetric distortion in any given participant means that no post-processing algorithm can reliably separate these two components (either in the time- or frequency-domains). Before the relationship between the neurophonic and audiometric threshold can be established in normal hearing and pathological ears, future research in humans must determine optimal electrode montages that reduce CM contamination of neurophonic responses at the "front-end", and most importantly, pursue masking techniques that ensure reliable separation of neural and hair cell responses, and which increase the frequency selectivity of the measured neurophonic waveform. These issues must be addressed in a timely manner given the growing interest in the use of the neurophonic as an objective measure of low-frequency cochlear function.

AUTHOR CONTRIBUTIONS

This study was designed by GO. Measurements were made by GO and AA with assistance from Jeremy Hornibrook and Gurjoat Vraich. GO, AA, and AC conducted data analysis. AC and GO wrote the manuscript.

FUNDING

This study was funded by the Oticon Foundation in New Zealand.

ACKNOWLEDGMENTS

The authors would like to thank Dr. Robert Patuzzi, Dr. Daniel Brown, Dr. Hedwig Gockel, and Prof Brian Moore, for their helpful comments and feedback on the manuscript, and Mr. Jeremy Hornibrook, Mr. Phil Bird, and Mr. Gurjoat Vraich, for their assistance with patient recruitment and data acquisition.

REFERENCES

Adrian, E. (1930). The microphonic action of the cochlea: an interpretation of Wever and Bray's experiments. *J. Physiol.* 71, 28–29.

Adrian, E. D., Bronk, D. W., and Phillips, G. (1931). The nervous origin of the Wever and Bray effect. *J. Physiol.* 73, 2P-3.

Adunka, O. F., Dillon, M. T., Adunka, M. C., King, E. R., Pillsbury, H. C., and Buchman, C. A. (2013). Hearing preservation and speech perception outcomes with electric-acoustic stimulation after 12 months of listening experience. *Laryngoscope* 123, 2509–2515. doi: 10.1002/lary.23741

Allsop, A. J. (2016). *Electrophysiological Monitoring of Low Frequency Auditory Thresholds in Humans using the Auditory Nerve Overlapped Waveform.* MAud thesis, University of Canterbury, Christchurch. Available online at: http://hdl.handle.net/10092/12249

ANSI (2004). S3. 6-2004, *Specification for Audiometers.* New York, NY: American National Standards Institute.

Boudreau, J. C., and Tsuchitani, C. (1964). Frequency-following in the superior-olivary complex of the cat. *J. Acoust. Soc. Am.* 36, 1017–1017. doi: 10.1121/1.2143202

Brown, D. J., Chihara, Y., Curthoys, I. S., Wang, Y., and Bos, M. (2013). Changes in cochlear function during acute endolymphatic hydrops development in guinea pigs. *Hear. Res.* 296, 96–106. doi: 10.1016/j.heares.2012.12.004

Brown, D. J., and Patuzzi, R. B. (2010). Evidence that the compound action potential (CAP) from the auditory nerve is a stationary potential generated across dura mater. *Hear. Res.* 267, 12–26. doi: 10.1016/j.heares.2010.03.091

Campbell, L., Kaicer, A., Sly, D., Iseli, C., Wei, B., Briggs, R., et al. (2016). Intraoperative real-time cochlear response telemetry predicts hearing preservation in cochlear implantation. *Otol. Neurotol.* 37, 332–338. doi: 10.1097/MAO.0000000000000972

Chimento, T. C., and Schreiner, C. E. (1990). Selectively eliminating cochlear microphonic contamination from the frequency-following response. *Electroencephalogr. Clin. Neurophysiol.* 75, 88–96. doi: 10.1016/0013-4694(90)90156-E

Choudhury, B., Fitzpatrick, D. C., Buchman, C. A., Wei, B. P., Dillon, M. T., He, S., et al. (2012). Intraoperative round window recordings to acoustic stimuli from cochlear implant patients. *Otol. Neurotol.* 33, 1507. doi: 10.1097/MAO.0b013e31826dbc80

Derbyshire, A. J., and Davis, H. (1935). The action potentials of the auditory nerve. *Am. J. Physiol.* 113, 476–504.

Dorman, M. F., and Gifford, R. H. (2010). Combining acoustic and electric stimulation in the service of speech recognition. *Int. J. Audiol.* 49, 912–919. doi: 10.3109/14992027.2010.509113

Forgues, M., Koehn, H. A., Dunnon, A. K., Pulver, S. H., Buchman, C. A., Adunka, O. F., et al. (2014). Distinguishing hair cell from neural potentials recorded at the round window. *J. Neurophysiol.* 111, 580–593. doi: 10.1152/jn.00446.2013

Gantz, B. J., Turner, C., Gfeller, K. E., and Lowder, M. W. (2005). Preservation of hearing in cochlear implant surgery: advantages of combined electrical and acoustical speech processing. *Laryngoscope* 115, 796–802. doi: 10.1097/01.MLG.0000157695.07536.D2

Henry, K. R. (1995). Auditory nerve neurophonic recorded from the round window of the Mongolian gerbil. *Hear. Res.* 90, 176–184. doi: 10.1016/0378-5955(95)00162-6

Henry, K. R. (1997). Auditory nerve neurophonic tuning curves produced by masking of round window responses. *Hear. Res.* 104, 167–176. doi: 10.1016/S0378-5955(96)00195-5

Hornibrook, J., Kalin, C., Lin, E., O'Beirne, G. A., and Gourley, J. (2012). Transtympanic electrocochleography for the diagnosis of Ménière's disease. *Int. J. Otolaryngol.* 2012:852714. doi: 10.1155/2012/852714

Kiang, N. Y. S. (1990). Curious oddments of auditory-nerve studies. *Hear. Res.* 49, 1–16. doi: 10.1016/0378-5955(90)90091-3

Liberman, M. C., and Dodds, L. W. (1984). Single-neuron labeling and chronic cochlear pathology. III. Stereocilia damage and alterations of threshold tuning curves. *Hear. Res.* 16, 55–74. doi: 10.1016/0378-5955(84)90025-X

Lichtenhan, J. T., Hartsock, J. J., Gill, R. M., Guinan, J. Jr., and Salt, A. N. (2014). The auditory nerve overlapped waveform (ANOW) originates in the cochlear apex. *J. Assoc. Res. Otolaryngol.* 15, 395–411. doi: 10.1007/s10162-014-0447-y

Lichtenhan, J. T., Cooper, N. P., and Guinan, J. J. (2013). A new auditory threshold estimation technique for low frequencies: proof of concept. *Ear Hear.* 34, 42–51. doi: 10.1097/AUD.0b013e31825f9bd3

Mandalà, M., Colletti, L., Tonoli, G., and Colletti, V. (2012). Electrocochleography during cochlear implantation for hearing preservation. *Otolaryngol. Head Neck Surg.* 146, 774–781. doi: 10.1177/0194599811435895

Marsh, J. T., Worden, F. G., and Smith, J. C. (1970). Auditory frequency-following response: Neural or artifact? *Science* 169, 1222–1223. doi: 10.1126/science.169.3951.1222

O'Beirne, G. A. (2005). *Mathematical Modelling and Electrophysiological Monitoring of the Regulation of Cochlear Amplification.* Ph. D. thesis, University of Western Australia, Crawley. Available online at: http://hdl.handle.net/10092/7365

Patuzzi, R. B., Yates, G. K., and Johnstone, B. M. (1989). The origin of the low-frequency microphonic in the first cochlear turn of guinea-pig. *Hear. Res.* 39, 177–188. doi: 10.1016/0378-5955(89)90089-0

Patuzzi, R., and Moleirinho, A. (1998). Automatic monitoring of mechano-electrical transduction in the guinea pig cochlea. *Hear. Res.* 125, 1–16. doi: 10.1016/S0378-5955(98)00125-7

Patuzzi, R., and Robertson, D. (1988). Tuning in the mammalian cochlea. *Physiol. Rev.* 68, 1009–1082.

Patuzzi, R., and Sellick, P. M. (1983). The alteration of the low frequency response of primary auditory afferents by cochlear trauma. *Hear. Res.* 11, 125–132. doi: 10.1016/0378-5955(83)90075-8

Peake, W. T., and Kiang, N. Y.-S. (1962). Cochlear responses to condensation and rarefaction clicks. *Biophys. J.* 2, 23–34. doi: 10.1016/S0006-3495(62)86838-6

Poulsen, T., and Legarth, S. V. (2008). Reference hearing threshold levels for short duration signals. *Int. J. Audiol.* 47, 665–674. doi: 10.1080/14992020802203330

Radeloff, A., Shehata-Dieler, W., Scherzed, A., Rak, K., Harnisch, W., Hagen, R., et al. (2012). Intraoperative monitoring using cochlear microphonics in cochlear implant patients with residual hearing. *Otol. Neurotol.* 33, 348–354. doi: 10.1097/MAO.0b013e318248ea86

Rattay, F., and Danner, S. M. (2014). Peak I of the human auditory brainstem response results from the somatic regions of type I spiral ganglion cells: evidence from computer modeling. *Hear. Res.* 315, 67–79. doi: 10.1016/j.heares.2014.07.001

Sellick, P., Patuzzi, R., and Robertson, D. (2003). Primary afferent and cochlear nucleus contributions to extracellular potentials during tone-bursts. *Hear. Res.* 176, 42–58. doi: 10.1016/S0378-5955(02)00716-5

Sirjani, D. B., Salt, A. N., Gill, R. M., and Hale, S. A. (2004). The influence of transducer operating point on distortion generation in the cochlea. *J. Acoust. Soc. Am.* 115, 1219–1229. doi: 10.1121/1.1647479

Snyder, R. L., and Schreiner, C. E. (1984). The auditory neurophonic: basic properties. *Hear. Res.* 15, 261–280. doi: 10.1016/0378-5955(84)90033-9

Snyder, R. L., and Schreiner, C. E. (1985). Forward masking of the auditory nerve neurophonic (ANN) and the frequency following response (FFR). *Hear. Res.* 20, 45–62. doi: 10.1016/0378-5955(85)90058-9

Stegeman, D. F., Dumitru, D., King, J. C., and Roeleveld, K. (1997). Near-and far-fields: source characteristics and the conducting medium in neurophysiology. *J. Clin. Neurophysiol.* 14, 429–442. doi: 10.1097/00004691-199709000-00009

Weinberger, N., Kitzes, L., and Goodman, D. (1970). Some characteristics of the 'auditory neurophonic'. *Cell. Mol. Life Sci.* 26, 46–48. doi: 10.1007/BF01900383

Wever, E. G., and Bray, C. W. (1930). Action currents in the auditory nerve in response to acoustical stimulation. *Proc. Natl. Acad. Sci. U.S.A.* 16, 344–350. doi: 10.1073/pnas.16.5.344

Worden, F. G., and Marsh, J. T. (1968). Frequency-following (microphonic-like) neural responses evoked by sound. *Electroencephalogr. Clin. Neurophysiol.* 25, 42–52. doi: 10.1016/0013-4694(68)90085-0

13

The Auditory Nerve Overlapped Waveform (ANOW) Detects Small Endolymphatic Manipulations that May Go Undetected by Conventional Measurements

Jeffery T. Lichtenhan[1], Choongheon Lee[1], Farah Dubaybo[1], Kaitlyn A. Wenrich[1] and Uzma S. Wilson[2]*

[1] Department of Otolaryngology Washington University School of Medicine, Saint Louis, MO, United States, [2] Department of Communication Sciences and Disorders, Northwestern University, Evanston, IL, United States

***Correspondence:**
Jeffery T. Lichtenhan
jlichtenhan@wustl.edu

Electrocochleography (ECochG) has been used to assess Ménière's disease, a pathology associated with endolymphatic hydrops and low-frequency sensorineural hearing loss. However, the current ECochG techniques are limited for use at high-frequencies only ($\geq$1 kHz) and cannot be used to assess and understand the low-frequency sensorineural hearing loss in ears with Ménière's disease. In the current study, we use a relatively new ECochG technique to make measurements that originate from afferent auditory nerve fibers in the apical half of the cochlear spiral to assess effects of endolymphatic hydrops in guinea pig ears. These measurements are made from the Auditory Nerve Overlapped Waveform (ANOW). Hydrops was induced with artificial endolymph injections, iontophoretically applied Ca^{2+} to endolymph, and exposure to 200 Hz tones. The manipulations used in this study were far smaller than those used in previous investigations on hydrops. In response to all hydropic manipulations, ANOW amplitude to moderate level stimuli was markedly reduced but conventional ECochG measurements of compound action potential thresholds were unaffected (i.e., a less than 2 dB threshold shift). Given the origin of the ANOW, changes in ANOW amplitude likely reflect acute volume disturbances accumulate in the distensible cochlear apex. These results suggest that the ANOW could be used to advance our ability to identify initial stages of dysfunction in ears with Ménière's disease before the pathology progresses to an extent that can be detected with conventional measures.

Keywords: electrocochleography, cochlear response, auditory nerve neurophonic, endolymphatic space, scala media, endolymphatic hydrops, Ménière's disease, cochlea

INTRODUCTION

The Auditory Nerve Overlapped Waveform (ANOW) originates in the apical half of the cochlear spiral from afferent neural fibers tuned to low-frequencies (Lichtenhan et al., 2013, 2014, 2016). Conventional electrocochleography (ECochG) measurements such as the compound action potential (CAP) do not work adequately at low frequencies (Spoor and Eggermont, 1976; Picton, 2007; Sininger, 2007). The ANOW is derived from the cochlear response recorded from the auditory periphery. The cochlear response is an electrical measurement originating from the cochlear microphonic of inner and outer hair cells, changes to the lateral wall potential from slow or sustained current through hair cells, summating potential, excitatory postsynaptic potentials, CAPs from onset or phase locked neural excitation, and spontaneous excitation of single-auditory-nerve-fibers (Lichtenhan, 2012; Chertoff et al., 2015). When cochlear responses to alternating low frequency tones are averaged, the fundamental component and odd harmonics are canceled and the even harmonics are preserved. At low and moderate stimulus levels, the even harmonics originate from phase locked neural excitation. The result is a waveform with oscillation at twice the probe frequency. The ANOW technique advanced the work done with the auditory nerve neurophonic, which is simply a cochlear response evoked from low-frequency tones (Henry, 1995; Choudhury et al., 2012; Verschooten et al., 2012; Forgues et al., 2014; Verschooten and Joris, 2014; Koka et al., 2017). In particular, Lichtenhan et al. (2014) identified when the origin of the cochlear responses to low-frequency tones is, and is not, neural excitation from the apical cochlear half when stimulus level and recording location are varied.

The approaches used for the experiments reported here were three scala media manipulations that have been classically used to create, and study, endolymphatic hydrops. We found that the ANOW is considerably more sensitive to all of these manipulations than traditional objective measures of CAP thresholds and the endocochlear potential (EP): the amplitude of the ANOW was altered by each manipulation, while there were minimal changes to CAP thresholds or the EP. Hydrops induced by the small manipulations would not be accurately detectable by imaging techniques (Klis et al., 1990; Salt and DeMott, 1994a; Salt et al., 1995)-a consequence of fixative causing Reissner's membrane shrinkage and the transient nature of acute cochlear manipulations. These results suggest that measurements of ANOW amplitude have advantages over classically used measurements that are commonly used in the clinic and laboratory to identify and study endolymphatic hydrops.

MATERIALS AND METHODS

Surgical Access of the Endolymphatic Space

To access the guinea pig endolymphatic space, the bony wall overlying the dark pigmentation of the stria vascularis was thinned with a flap knife and then an approximately 30 μm fenestra was made with a 1/3 mm House oval window pick (N1705 80, Bausch and Lomb Storz). Endocochlear potential (EP) measurements were used to verify the placement of the injection pipette into the endolymphatic space of the second cochlear turn. EP measurements used for experimental purposes were recorded from an additional fenestra in the third cochlear turn that accommodated an EP electrode. When a pipette was inserted into endolymph, there was no fluid leakage at the insertion site, suggesting that the site was effectively sealed. Experimental protocols for this study were approved by the Animal Studies Committee of Washington University School of Medicine in St. Louis (protocol numbers 20120113 and 20130069).

Volume Injection of Artificial Endolymph

Ears with chronic endolymphatic hydrops have an enlargement of the scala media cross sectional area. Injection of artificial endolymph can be used to model acute endolymphatic hydrops. Injections were made using double-barreled glass pipettes with tips beveled to an approximate 15–20 μm diameter. The injection barrel was filled with artificial endolymph (140-mM KCl and 25-mM KHCO3) while the second barrel was filled with 500 mM KCl and used to confirm placement in the endolymph with EP measurements. The pipette was mounted on a micro-syringe pump injector controlled with a micro-syringe pump controller (UMP3 and Micro4, respectively, World Precision Instruments). During the injections of artificial endolymph volumes into the second cochlear turn, EP measurements were made in the third cochlear turn. Injections of artificial endolymph were performed at rates of 5–10 nL/min for 15 min. The characteristic frequencies of our access sites to the second and third cochlear turns were estimated to be 2.5 kHz for second cochlear turn and 650 Hz for the third cochlear turn, based on the frequency-place map derived from guinea pig single auditory nerve fibers (Tsuji and Liberman, 1997) adjusted to the 20.8 mm length of the endolymphatic space.

Iontophoretic Ca^{2+} Delivery

Ears with chronic endolymphatic hydrops have been shown to have elevated endolymphatic Ca^{2+} (Ninoyu and Meyer zum Gottesberge, 1986; Meyer zum Gottesberge and Ninoyu, 1987; Salt and DeMott, 1994b, 1997; Fettiplace and Ricci, 2006). Administration of Ca^{2+} into the endolymphatic space can thus model some aspects of chronic endolymphatic hydrops. Ca^{2+} was iontophoresed into the endolymphatic space of the second cochlear turn using positive current. Pipettes for iontophoresis applications were made from single barreled glass with internal fiber. The pipette tip was beveled to a 2–3 μm diameter and filled with 160 mM $CaCl_2$. The electrode tips were then filled with 0.5% agarose gel to prevent volume passive displacement of the electrolyte during the experiment (i.e., leakage of the electrolyte into the cochlea). The electrodes were stored with the tips in $CaCl_2$ solution, allowing the electrolyte to equilibrate with the gel. Ca^{2+} was iontophoresed into endolymph for 15 min with 100 nA of current using a microiontophoresis current programmer (Model 260, World Precision Instruments).

Tonal Exposures

Brief exposures to low frequency tones at high, but non-damaging levels, (e.g., 95–115 dB SPL) have been shown to induce transient endolymphatic hydrops, the origin of the so-called "2-min bounce phenomenon" (Flock and Flock, 2000; Salt, 2004). We presented a 65 dB SPL 200 Hz tone at for 3 min in a closed acoustic assembly with a Sennheiser HD 265. During exposure to the tone, no sound-evoked potentials or acoustic emissions were collected.

Statistics

Statistical analyses were completed in Statistical Analysis System 9.0 (SAS Institute, Cary, NC). A mixed model analysis with autoregressive covariance structure and cases as random factors was used to compare the change between the mean, pre-injection baseline measure (obtained between −10 and −1 min re. injection start) and the post-baseline measure (obtained between 0 and 30 min re. injection start) between the different tone burst frequencies and levels. Estimated marginal means and corresponding 95% confidence intervals were used to report the results of the interaction effect as well as the main effects in the mixed model. All statistical tests were two sided and evaluated at the alpha level of 0.01.

Electrophysiological Measurements

Tucker-Davis System 3 hardware controlled by custom-written software (Visual Basic, Microsoft) on a personal computer was used to make electrophysiologic measurements. A TD-RP2 was used to generate stimuli that were passed through TD-PA5 attenuators, and TD-HB7 headphone amplifiers. Cochlear responses were evoked from 50 tone bursts of alternating polarities. The duration of the tone bursts was 30 ms, and the duration of the linear two-cycle rise and fall times varied with stimulus frequency. Cochlear response measurements were made from 50 averages. An Etymotic ER-10C coupled to the hollow ear bar—a closed sound system—was used to deliver acoustic sound stimuli to the right ear of all guinea pigs. Calibrations were completed in individual ear canals by tracking 70 dB SPL tones from 0.125 to 26 kHz in ¼ octave steps.

Cochlear response measurements were made differentially between an Ag/AgCl ball-tipped electrode near the round window niche and a platinum-needle electrode near the vertex. An Ag/AgCl pellet electrode coupled to exposed soft tissue of the neck with a fluid bridge was used for grounding. ECochG measurements were made with a TD DB4 optically-coupled amplifier (1000x gain, 0.005–15 kHz bandpass filter) routed to an TD-RP2 module for digitization (48.8 kHz) and averaging. No artifact reject was applied.

Measurement names derive from terminology established in Lichtenhan et al. (2014). This terminology was based on stimulus conditions, not assumed cellular origins. The CAP is the commonly used waveform acquired from averaging responses to high-frequency tone bursts of alternating polarity, the $CR_{AVE,ONSET,H}$. CAP thresholds were quantified with an automated procedure that identified the lowest stimulus level yielding a 10 μV N1 to P1 amplitude. The ANOW-AP is the $CR_{AVE,ONSET,L}$, or the amplitude measurement of the two-cycle smoothed waveform (**Figure 1C**) from averaging cochlear responses to alternating polarity low-frequency tones (**Figure 1B**). The ANOW is the amplitude measured in the middle of the waveform resulting from averaging cochlear response to 500 Hz tone bursts of alternating polarity ($CR_{AVE,MID}$, **Figure 1D**). The difference in cochlear responses to low frequency stimuli (CR_{DIF}, **Figure 1A**) were not used in this study. Our previous work demonstrated that this waveform, which is commonly referred to as the "cochlear microphonic," has cellular origins that vary with level and recording location (Lichtenhan et al., 2014), thus limiting the usefulness based on unsatisfactory interpretability.

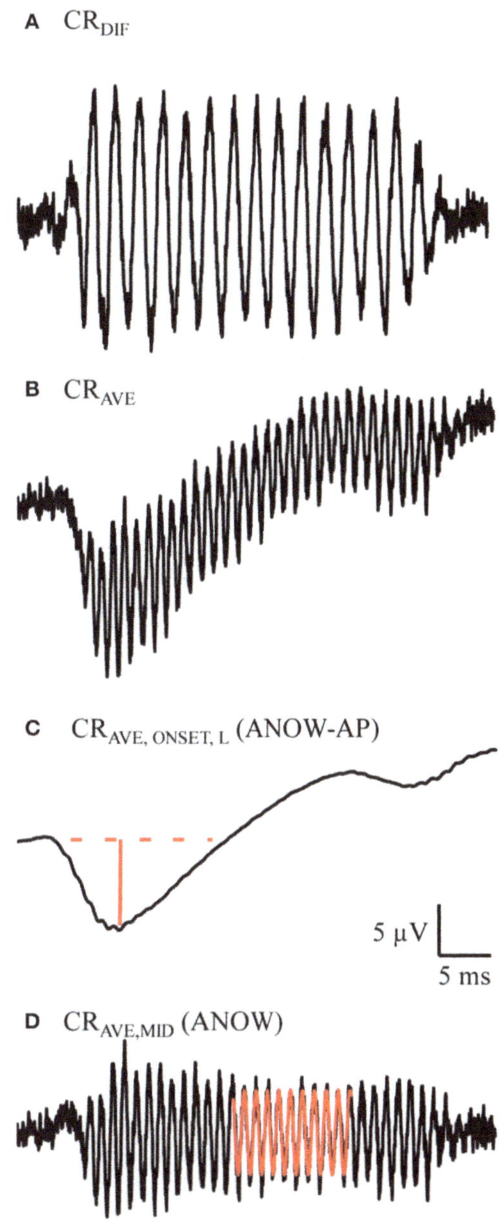

FIGURE 1 | Example measurements used to measure the ANOW-AP and ANOW. These waveforms were evoked from 50 dB SPL 500 Hz tone bursts. Previous work demonstrated that the difference in cochlear responses to alternating tone bursts (CR_{DIF}, **A**) is a blend of both hair cell and neural responses, but has been commonly referred to in the literature as the "cochlear microphonic" (Lichtenhan et al., 2014). Averaging cochlear responses to alternating tone bursts (CR_{AVE}, **B**) and two-cycle smoothing ($CR_{AVE,ONSET,L}$, **C**) yields the onset response to low-frequency stimuli. The amplitude of the ANOW-AP is the solid red line. Subtracting $CR_{AVE,ONSET,L}$ from CR_{AVE} yields the $CR_{AVE,MID}$ **(D)**, the waveform used to quantify the ANOW amplitude (red sinusoid).

RESULTS

Volume Injection of Artificial Endolymph

Volumes of artificial endolymph were injected into the second cochlear turn endolymphatic space at 5 (five ears), 10 (five ears), or 15 (three ears) nL/min for 15 min (75–225 nL total injection). Measurements made during each of these small, though different, injection rates are expressed together in these panels because each rate is very small, and produced similar effects, compared to classical use of artificial endolymph as a model of endolymphatic hydrops. In particular, the volume of artificial endolymph injected in our experiments were up to 16 times smaller than those used in previous contemporary experiments to create endolymphatic hydrops that was detectable by conventional CAP threshold measures (e.g., Sirjani et al., 2004). Laboratory norms for 500 Hz ANOW threshold is 45 dB SPL. Thus, ANOW to 50 dB SPL was 5 dB re. threshold. Volume injections caused significant reductions to the amplitude of the ANOW response to 50 and 65 dB SPL 500 Hz tone bursts between 0 and 30 min after the start of treatment (**Figure 2A**, degrees of freedom (df)(47), $p < 0.01$). Neural onset responses to both ANOW stimuli of either level (ANOW-AP, **Figure 2B**), the traditional CAP to threshold stimuli (**Figure 2C**), and EP measurements (**Figure 2D**) changed significantly (respectively, df(44), $p < 0.01$ df(47), $p < 0.01$, and df(10), $p < 0.01$). While statistically significant, we error on the side of caution and note that the changes to mean ANOW-AP were less than a mere 10%, CAP thresholds were less than 2 dB and EP changed less than 0.5 mV. Moreover, the reduction in ANOW amplitude were consistent and less variable than changes to other measurements. These results show that the amplitude of ANOW response can identify changes that may go undetected by conventional measurements.

Iontophoretic Ca^{2+} delivery

Ca^{2+} was iontophoretically applied into endolymph with 100 nA current. Ca^{2+} was applied nine times to seven ears. That is to say, in two ears Ca^{2+} was applied twice: a second application was made after recovery from the first application. This treatment significantly affected the amplitude of the ANOW response to 50 dB SPL tone bursts of all selected frequencies [**Figure 3A**, $df_{(15)}$, $p < 0.01$], as well as those to 65 dB SPL [**Figure 3C**, $df_{(33)}$, $p < 0.01$]. ANOW onset responses (ANOW-AP) to 50 dB SPL stimuli were significantly affected [**Figure 3B**, $df_{(16)}$, $p < 0.01$], as were ANOW-AP to 65 dB SPL [**Figure 3D**, $df_{(35)}$, $p < 0.01$]. While the effect on ANOW-AP was significant, we note that the magnitude of the effect was to a lesser degree than the effect on ANOW (cf. **Figures 3A,C**). There were significant effects of time, frequency, and an interaction effect on CAP threshold [$df_{(36)}$, $p < 0.01$; $df_{(48)}$, $p < 0.01$; and $df_{(48)}$, $p < 0.01$ respectively]. Pairwise comparison *post hoc* tests found that CAP thresholds to tone burst frequencies associated with cochlear frequency places nearest the administration site (i.e., 2 and 4 kHz) had a significant 10–20 dB threshold shift [**Figure 3E**; $df_{(64)}$, $p < 0.01$ and $df_{(64)}$,

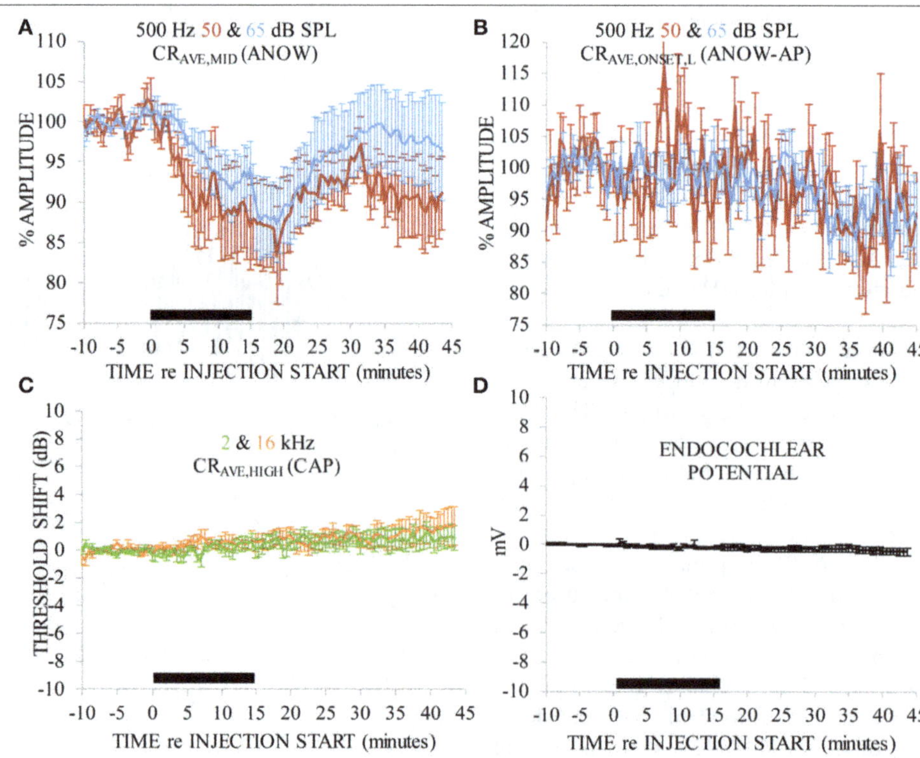

FIGURE 2 | ANOW measurements were markedly affected by 75–225 nL of artificial endolymph injected into the second cochlear turn, but other measurements were not. Data in each panel were normalized to the average of 10 min of pre-injection measurements. Artificial endolymph was injected for 15 min, indicated by the thick black horizontal bar near the x-axis in each panel **(A–D)**. Error bars are standard errors of the mean calculated with measurements across all animals.

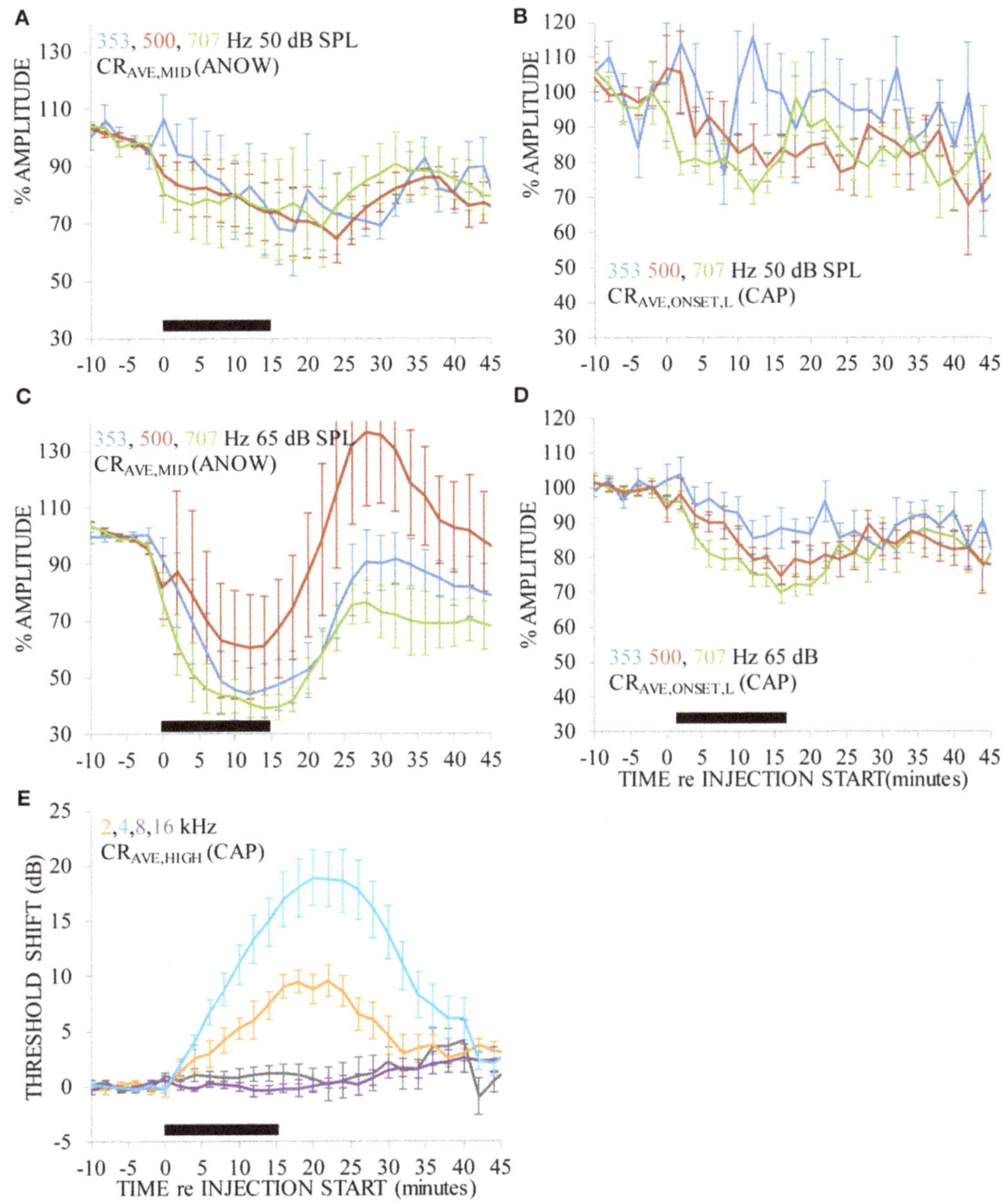

FIGURE 3 | Ca^{2+} applied with 100 nA iontophoresis altered measurements that originate near the second cochlear turn administration site (i.e., CAPs to 2 and 4 kHz, **E**), as would be expected. But, ANOW-based measurements that originate in the apical cochlear half also changed significantly **(A–D)**, and CAP from cochlear regions distant to the administration site (i.e., 8 and 16 kHz) were not affected. Ca^{2+} was applied for 15 min, indicated by the thick black horizontal bar near the x-axis in each panel. Error bars indicate standard errors of the mean calculated with measurements across all guinea pigs.

$p < 0.01$ respectively]. In contrast, CAPs to higher frequency stimuli associated with cochlear frequency places farther away from the administration site were not affected (i.e., 8 and 16 kHz). The close proximity of the second turn endolymphatic iontophoretic site to the spatial origin of 2 and 4 kHz CAPs, and the lack of CAP threshold change to 8 kHz, are consistent with a local and transient disturbance caused by the Ca^{2+} elevation.

It is remarkable that the amplitude of ANOW-based measurements was affected by the Ca^{2+} concentration that declines rapidly with distance from the iontophoretic site. The strong effect of Ca^{2+} on the amplitude of ANOW-based responses suggests it is either very sensitive to small Ca^{2+} disturbances or is sensitive to some other aspect of the Ca^{2+} manipulation, possibly including induced endolymph volume changes. Changes to the amplitude of ANOW-based measurements, but not to CAP thresholds measured away from the administration site, is consistent with volume disturbances in the apical half of the cochlea. Moreover, the amplitude of ANOW-based measurements to the higher 65 dB SPL stimuli detected the change more rapidly than traditional CAP threshold measurements at the same level, suggesting that higher stimulus levels were more sensitive to the induced physiological changes.

200 Hz Exposures

Ears exposed to a 65 dB SPL 200 Hz tone caused the amplitude of the ANOW to "bounce" (i.e., rapidly decrease and then increase) and then slowly recover to pre-exposure measures (**Figure 4A**). These measurements were made from nine exposures to two ears. This effect happed over the first few minutes after the exposure stopped. Changes caused by 200 Hz exposure at this low level went undetected by traditional CAP threshold measurements that originate in the stiffer basal cochlear half to the extent that CAP thresholds did not bounce but the variability of these measurements increased (**Figure 4B**). The 65 dB SPL 200 Hz exposure used here is far less intense than the 115–120 dB SPL exposure that was required in previous experiments for the investigation of the "2-min bounce phenomena." These measurements were made from nine exposures to two ears. Please note that we normalized the x-axis of **Figure 4** differently than **Figures 2**, **3** so that the data could be more easily compared to previous reports on the 2-min bounce phenomena. The time course of the bounce in the amplitude of the ANOW to supra-threshold sounds is similar to that found in measurements originating in the less distensible cochlear base following a 115 dB SPL 200 Hz exposure that has been shown to cause endolymphatic hydrops in guinea pig ears (Salt, 2004). It is therefore possible that changes to ANOW could be caused by fluid volume disturbances in the distensible apical half of the cochlea.

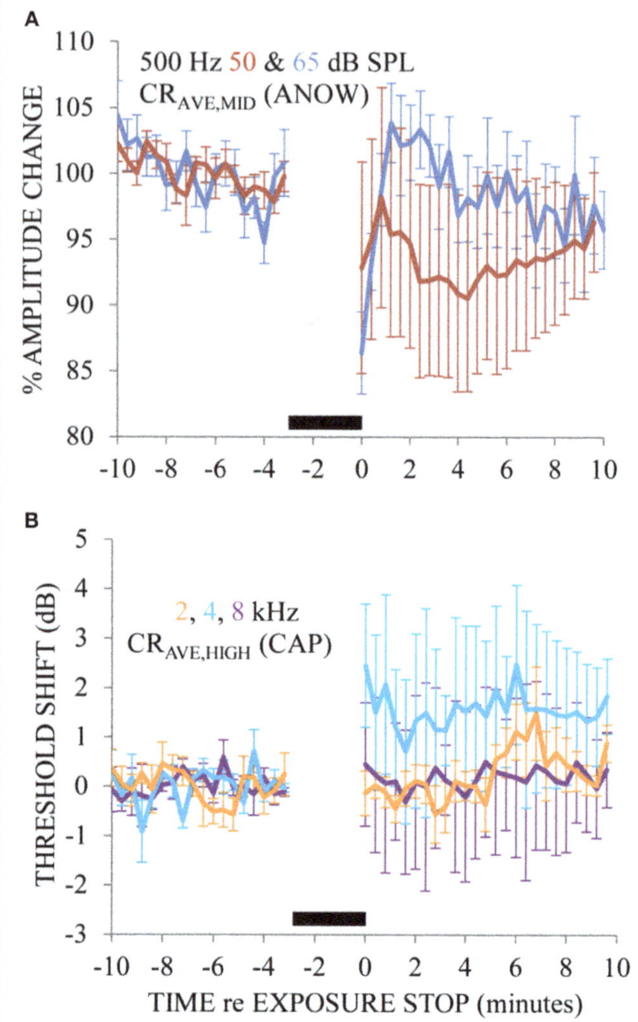

FIGURE 4 | The ANOW amplitude to the 65 dB SPL stimulus level was affected most by 3 min of exposure to 65 dB SPL 200 Hz, and those to 50 dB SPL affected less so **(A)**. CAP thresholds to 2, 4, and 8 kHz were essentially unaffected by the endolymphatic hydrops induced by 200 Hz exposure **(B)**. No physiologic measurements were made during the 3 min of 200 Hz tone exposure, indicated by the thick black horizontal bar near the x-axis in each panel. Error bars are standard error of the mean estimates calculated with measurements across all animals.

DISCUSSION

General

Traditional ECochG techniques do not effectively monitor diseased states in the low-frequency regions of the cochlear spiral. Indeed, it has been suggested that the lack of ECochG-based measures for low-frequency cochlear regions in normal and diseased ears is a likely origin of variable and discrepant findings throughout the literature (Palmer and Shackleton, 2009; Temchin and Ruggero, 2010). In the current study, we used the ANOW to study cochlear manipulations that have been previously used to simulate endolymphatic hydrops. We found that the ANOW could detect subtle dysfunction of the endolymphatic space that was missed by conventional CAP threshold measurements. The transient effects from our acute manipulations would not be detectable with time-intensive, traditional histological approaches used to measure the scala media cross sectional area.

Previous studies have concluded that the low-frequency hearing loss in ears with endolymphatic hydrops did not directly originate from the endolymphatic hydrops (e.g., Klis and Smoorenburg, 1988; Salt, 2004; Chihara et al., 2013), a possible consequence of fixatives causing Reissner's membrane shrinkage such that endolymphatic hydrops is underestimated and lacks correlation with physiologic measurements. But, these previous studies were limited to conventional physiologic measurements that work adequately for the basal cochlear half that is sensitive to high-frequencies. Our results are consistent with the hypothesis that low-frequency disturbances from endolymphatic hydrops would be greater for the more distensible cochlear apex that would partially close mechanoelectric transducer channels. The cochlear apex is one of the most distensible regions of the inner ear (Kimura and Schuknecht, 1965), a likely result of the gradation of basilar membrane width and stiffness. This gradation makes the apical cochlear half more prone to endolymph accumulation than other places along the cochlear length. Previously it was found that slow mechanical biasing of the cochlear partition with low-frequency tones had an effect that was inversely proportional with probe frequency (Lichtenhan, 2012). A related finding was that this "low-frequency biasing" was a sensitive indicator of sustained displacements of the organ of

Corti, such as in ears with endolymphatic hydrops (Salt et al., 2009). Thus, it may be that low-frequency biasing the ANOW could be an even more powerful detector of hydrops than ANOW amplitude alone.

Chronic Endolymphatic Hydrops and Ecochg Assessment

Two features of human Ménière's disease are endolymphatic hydrops and low-frequency sensorineural hearing loss. Endolymphatic hydrops is an enlargement of scala media due to accumulation of endolymph.

The relationship between measures of low-frequency hearing loss and endolymphatic hydrops is of interest because the origin(s) of low-frequency hearing loss in ears with Ménière's disease are still not known. The relationship between the severity of endolymphatic hydrops and low-frequency hearing loss is also not known. Various controversies and theories are fundamental to this interest. For example, (i) endolymphatic hydrops is not always associated with hearing loss in humans nor abnormal physiologic measurements in animals, yet human Ménière's diseased temporal bones with substantial hearing loss always have endolymphatic hydrops (e.g., Klis and Smoorenburg, 1988; Salt, 2004; Merchant et al., 2005; Nadol, 2010; Tagaya et al., 2011; Chihara et al., 2013; Yoshida et al., 2013). In other words, all Ménière's diseased ears have endolymphatic hydrops, but ears with endolymphatic hydrops do not always have symptoms of Meniere's disease. Presumably, there is a lag between the origins of endolymphatic hydrops and the low-frequency sensorineural hearing loss that is associated with Ménière's disease. (ii) A mere 10% of temporal bones from humans with hearing loss from Ménière's disease have sensory cell loss in the cochlear apex so the origin of the low-frequency loss is a mystery (Nadol, 2010). (iii) Acute endolymphatic hydrops increases the endocochlear potential, while chronic hydrops decreases the endocochlear potential (Meyer zum Gottesberge and Ninoyu, 1987; Salt, 2004). (iv) Since acute endolymphatic hydrops decreases the sensitivity of the operating point of the *in vivo* mechanics associated with the transfer of sound into excitement of neuronal membranes, but sustained cochlear partition displacements increase the sensitivity, it may be that mild endolymph accumulation during the early stage of Ménière's disease creates a feedback scenario which causes the diseased state to worsen (cf. Sirjani et al., 2004; Salt et al., 2009). (v) People with Ménière's disease often have word recognition scores that are worse than expected when considering their behavioral audiometric thresholds (Morrison, 1999). An ECochG-based approach to assessing low-frequency physiology in chronically diseased ears may therefore be helpful to address these controversies. ECochG can be minimally invasive and does not always require opening the cranium or cochlea, which could alter endolymphatic hydrops. *The results from our experiments reported here demonstrate that the conventional ECochG CAP thresholds were not as sensitive as ANOW amplitudes from supra-threshold stimuli to acute manipulations to the endolymphatic space. These findings suggest that ANOW may be useful for identifying initial stages of endolymphatic hydrops during the transition from early to late-stage chronic conditions when conventional measures of hearing would be unaffected.*

ANOW Assessment of Acute Models of Endolymphatic Hydrops

ANOW-based measurements, but not conventional CAP thresholds, changed in response to an acute induction of endolymphatic hydrops by injection of small volumes (5–15 nL/min for 15 min) of artificial endolymph to increase the volume of the endolymphatic space (**Figure 2**). The rates of volume injections used here were indeed small, as previous investigations induced endolymphatic hydrops with injection rates of 40–400 nL/min (Sirjani et al., 2004; Brown et al., 2013). The mechanism of endolymphatic hydrops from acute injections of artificial endolymph likely involves the reduction of mechanoelectric transducer current resulting from temporary volume and pressure increases that displace the organ of Corti toward scala tympani (Kakigi and Takeda, 1998; Wit et al., 2000), which is consistent with the recovery of ANOW measurements in **Figure 2A**. Chronic hydrops has traditionally been defined with visual detection of Reissner's membrane distension. But, reticular lamina distension toward the basilar membrane is a likely consequence of endolymphatic hydrops that would not be visible with traditional histological approaches. Changes to the organ of Corti height may occur, but could be misleading with histological measurements with fixatives that can cause hair cell contractions. In any event, a likely origin of the changes to ANOW response amplitudes changes we found could be slight, transient reticular lamina distention toward the basilar membrane, thereby changing hair cell function. A striking finding is that CAP thresholds to 2 kHz did not change while the ANOW measurements did indeed change (**Figure 2**). An injection of artificial endolymph into the second cochlear turn apically displaces the pre-existing volume at the injection site which flows through the 2 kHz region on the path to disrupting the cochlear apex (Salt and DeMott, 1997). This suggests the presence of demarcation region between 2 and 0.5 kHz that separates the stiffer basilar membrane in the basal half of the cochlea from the more distensible sensory structures in the apical half of the cochlea. This may be similar, or even related to, the region of basal-to-apical transition that identifies where cochlear mechanics are drastically different (e.g., Shera and Guinan, 2003; Abdala and Dhar, 2010, 2012; Shera et al., 2010; Temchin and Ruggero, 2010; Dhar et al., 2011; Moleti et al., 2017).

Chronic endolymphatic hydrops is associated with elevated endolymph Ca^{2+} levels, which most likely promotes closure of mechanoelectric transducer channels and contributes to endolymph accumulation (Ninoyu and Meyer zum Gottesberge, 1986; Meyer zum Gottesberge and Ninoyu, 1987; Salt and DeMott, 1994b, 1997; Fettiplace and Ricci, 2006). ANOW measurements changed dramatically in response to acute increases of endolymphatic Ca^{2+} levels, but conventional CAP measurements did not change (**Figures 3B,D**). The endocochlear potential rapidly drives Ca^{2+} out of scala media through non-selective cation channels that are located largely in hair cell stereocilia, as demonstrated by higher endolymphatic Ca^{2+} concentrations in the cochlear apex that has a 20 mV smaller endocochlear potential than in the base (Salt et al., 1989). Iontophoretic application of solutions to manipulate mechanoelectric transduction is a common procedure (e.g., Manley et al., 2004; Manley and Kirk, 2005; Sellick et al., 2006, 2007; Sellick, 2007). But, our approach and results are novel because the ANOW detected changes in response to small manipulations of the endolymphatic space.

The time course of ANOW changes from iontophoretically applied Ca^{2+} (**Figure 3A**) was faster than changes caused by volume injections of artificial endolymph (**Figure 3C**) presumably because Ca^{2+} instantaneously closes mechanoelectric transducer channels, rapidly affecting endolymph homeostasis. In contrast, slow injections of artificial endolymph in volume took longer to initiate flow from the injection site toward the cochlear apex. Maximal changes to 2 and 4 kHz CAP thresholds to iontophoretically applied Ca^{2+} were delayed compared to ANOW measurements to 65 dB SPL. Similarly, additional time was needed for iontophoretically applied Ca^{2+} to affect ANOW measurements to 65 dB SPL than to 50 dB SPL. These delays presumably originate from endolymph accumulation in the distensible apex that gradually affect the stiffer basal half of the cochlear spiral. Another issue regarding the time course of functional changes is that we suspect there are limitations to using volume injections and Ca^{2+} applications to model endolymphatic hydrops. We note that the function of some ears was likely deteriorating after 30 min of volume injection, likely contributing to a secondary decline in measurements in that time frame (cf. **Figure 2**).

Exposure to an intense, low-frequency tone for 3 min can initially cause a hearing threshold shift that is followed by a rapid recovery and finally a maximal shift that gradually recovers (Hirsh and Ward, 1952). The maximal shift occurs around 2 min after the tonal exposure stops, hence the name the "2-min bounce phenomena." Salt (2004) demonstrated that endolymphatic hydrops was the origin of the bounce phenomena. Other findings related to this phenomenon are that the amplitude of reflection-source and distortion-product otoacoustic emissions can bounce (Kemp, 1986; Kirk and Patuzzi, 1997; Drexl et al., 2014, 2016), and that new spontaneous otoacoustic emissions can temporarily emerge from the noise floor (Kugler et al., 2014) but can be reduced in occurrence when the medial olivocochlear efferent system is activated (Kugler et al., 2015; Jeanson et al., 2016). A unique attribute of our findings is that the ANOW amplitude bounced to a low-frequency exposure tone having a sound pressure level as low as 65 dB SPL (**Figure 4A**), which was far less than the traditional exposures that were upwards of 115–120 dB SPL. The time course of the ANOW bounce was similar to bounces reported in other studies, suggesting the origin of the ANOW bounce was the same as that reported previously: endolymphatic hydrops. Bounces after exposure to a moderate-level, low-frequency tonal exposure supports our interpretation that the distensible cochlear apex where the ANOW originates is an ideal region for initial, or acute, hydrops.

CONCLUSIONS

Until now, it has not been known which, if any, of the animal models of endolymphatic hydrops have disturbances in processing low-frequency sounds that would be consistent with the characteristic low-frequency dysfunction found in Ménière's disease. In the current study, we have found that the ANOW measurements from guinea pig, which originate from the auditory nerve fibers of the apical half of the cochlear spiral, are sensitive to manipulations of the endolymphatic space that are known to cause endolymphatic hydrops. ANOW changes were more sensitive than traditional CAP thresholds to the manipulations, suggesting that ANOW may be a useful technique to detect chronic endolymphatic hydrops in its initial stages.

AUTHOR CONTRIBUTIONS

JL performed the experiments. JL, CL, KW, FD, and UW analyzed the data. JL wrote the manuscript.

ACKNOWLEDGMENTS

We thank Spencer B. Smith, Professor Alec N. Salt, and the reviewers for productively criticizing this manuscript. This work was supported by R01 DC014997 (JL) from the National Institutes of Health, National Institute on Deafness and Other Communication Disorders.

REFERENCES

Abdala, C., and Dhar, S. (2010). Distortion product otoacoustic emission phase and component analysis in human newborns. *J. Acoust. Soc. Am.* 127, 316–325. doi: 10.1121/1.3268611

Abdala, C., and Dhar, S. (2012). Maturation and aging of the human cochlea: a view through the DPOAE looking glass. *J. Assoc. Res. Otolaryngol.* 13, 403–421. doi: 10.1007/s10162-012-0319-2

Brown, D. J., Chihara, Y., Curthoys, I. S., Wang, Y., and Bos, M. (2013). Changes in cochlear function during acute endolymphatic hydrops development in guinea pigs. *Hear. Res.* 296, 96–106. doi: 10.1016/j.heares.2012.12.004

Chertoff, M. E., Kamerer, A. M., Peppi, M., and Lichtenhan, J. T. (2015). An analysis of cochlear response harmonics: contribution of neural excitation. *J. Acoust. Soc. Am.* 138, 2957–2963. doi: 10.1121/1.4934556

Chihara, Y., Wong, C., Curthoys, I. S., and Brown, D. J. (2013). The effect of systemic administration of desmopressin on cochlear function in guinea pigs. *Acta Otolaryngol.* 133, 676–684. doi: 10.3109/00016489.2013.771282

Choudhury, B., Fitzpatrick, D. C., Buchman, C. A., Wei, B. P., Dillon, M. T., He, S., et al. (2012). Intraoperative round window recordings to acoustic stimuli from cochlear implant patients. *Otol. Neurotol.* 33, 1507–1515. doi: 10.1097/mao.0b013e31826dbc80

Dhar, S., Rogers, A., and Abdala, C. (2011). Breaking away: violation of distortion emission phase-frequency invariance at low frequencies. *J. Acoust. Soc. Am.* 129, 3115–3122. doi: 10.1121/1.3569732

Drexl, M., Otto, L., Wiegrebe, L., Marquardt, T., Gürkov, R., and Krause, E. (2016). Low-frequency sound exposure causes reversible long-term changes of cochlear transfer characteristics. *Hear. Res.* 332, 87–94. doi: 10.1016/j.heares.2015.12.010

Drexl, M., Uberfuhr, M., Weddell, T. D., Lukashkin, A. N., Wiegrebe, L., et al. (2014). Multiple indices of the 'bounce' phenomenon obtained from the same human ears. *J. Assoc. Res. Otolaryngol.* 15, 57–72. doi: 10.1007/s10162-013-0424-x

Fettiplace, R., and Ricci, A. J. (2006). "Mechanoelectrical transduction in auditory hair cells," in *Vertebrate hair cells. Springer Handbook of Auditory Research*, eds R. A. Eatock, R. R. Fay, and A. N. Popper (New York, NY: Springer), 154–203.

Flock, A., and Flock, B. (2000). Hydrops in the cochlea can be induced by sound as well as by static pressure. *Hear. Res.* 150, 175–188. doi: 10.1016/S0378-5955(00)00198-2

Forgues, M., Koehn, H. A., Dunnon, A. K., Pulver, S. H., Buchman, C. A., Adunka, O. F., et al. (2014). Distinguishing hair cell from neural potentials recorded at the round window. *J. Neurophysiol.* 111, 580–593. doi: 10.1152/jn.00446.2013

Henry, K. R. (1995). Auditory nerve neurophonic recorded from the round window of the *Mongolian gerbil*. *Hear. Res.* 90, 176–184. doi: 10.1016/0378-5955(95)00162-6

Hirsh, I. J., and Ward, W. D. (1952). Recovery of the auditory threshold after strong acoustic stimulation. *J. Acoust. Soc. Am.* 24, 131–141. doi: 10.1121/1.1906867

Jeanson, L., Wiegrebe, L., Gürkov, R., Krause, E., and Drexl, M. (2016). Aftereffects of intense low-frequency sound on spontaneous otoacoustic emissions: effect of frequency and level. *J. Assoc. Res. Otolaryngol.* 18, 111–119. doi: 10.1007/s10162-016-0590-8

Kakigi, A., and Takeda, T. (1998). Effect of artificial endolymph injection into the cochlear duct on the endocochlear potential. *Hear. Res.* 116, 113–118. doi: 10.1016/S0378-5955(97)00209-8

Kemp, D. T. (1986). Otoacoustic emissions, travelling waves and cochlear mechanisms. *Hear. Res.* 22, 95–104. doi: 10.1016/0378-5955(86)90087-0

Kimura, R., and Schuknecht, H. (1965). Membranous hydrops in the inner ear of the guinea pig after obliteration of the endolymphatic sac. *Pract. Otolaryngol.* 27, 343–354. doi: 10.1159/000274693

Kirk, D. L., and Patuzzi, R. B. (1997). Transient changes in cochlear potentials and DPOAEs after low-frequency tones: the 'two-minute bounce' revisited. *Hear. Res.* 112, 49–68. doi: 10.1016/S0378-5955(97)00105-6

Klis, J. F., and Smoorenburg, G. F. (1988). Cochlear potentials and their modulation by low frequency sound in early endolymphatic hydrops. *Hear. Res.* 32, 175–184. doi: 10.1016/0378-5955(88)90089-5

Klis, S. F., Buijs, J., and Smoorenburg, G. F. (1990). Quantification of the relation between electrophysiologic and morphologic changes in experimental endolymphatic hydrops. *Ann. Otol. Rhinol. Laryngol.* 99, 566–570. doi: 10.1177/000348949009900714

Koka, K., Saoji, A. A., and Litvak, L. M. (2017). Electrocochleography in cochlear implant recipients with residual hearing: comparison with audiometric thresholds. *Ear Hear.* 38, e161–e167. doi: 10.1097/AUD.0000000000000385

Kugler, K., Wiegrebe, L., Grothe, B., Kössl, M., Gürkov, R., Krause, E., et al. (2014). Low-frequency sound affects active micromechanics in the human inner ear. *R. Soc. Open Sci.* 1:140166. doi: 10.1098/rsos.140166

Kugler, K., Wiegrebe, L., Gürkov, R., Krause, E., and Drexl, M. (2015). Concurrent acoustic activation of the medial olivocochlear system modifies the after-effects of intense low-frequency sound on the human inner ear. *J. Assoc. Res. Otolaryngol.* 16, 713–725. doi: 10.1007/s10162-015-0538-4

Lichtenhan, J. T. (2012). Effects of low-frequency biasing on otoacoustic and neural measures suggest that stimulus-frequency otoacoustic emissions originate near the peak region of the traveling wave. *J. Assoc. Res. Otolaryngol.* 13, 17–28. doi: 10.1007/s10162-011-0296-x

Lichtenhan, J. T., Cooper, N. P. and Guinan, J. J., Jr. (2013). A new auditory threshold estimation technique for low frequencies: proof of concept. *Ear Hear.* 34, 42–51. doi: 10.1097/AUD.0b013e31825f9bd3

Lichtenhan, J. T., Hartsock, J., Dornhoffer, J. R., Donovan, K. M., and Salt, A. N. (2016). Drug delivery into the cochlear apex: improved control to sequentially affect finely spaced regions along the entire length of the cochlear spiral. *J. Neurosci. Methods* 273, 201–209. doi: 10.1016/j.jneumeth.2016.08.005

Lichtenhan, J. T., Hartsock, J. J., Gill, R. M., Guinan, J. J. Jr, and Salt, A. N. (2014). The auditory nerve overlapped waveform (ANOW) originates in the cochlear apex. *J. Assoc. Res. Otolaryngol.* 15, 395–411. doi: 10.1007/s10162-014-0447-y

Manley, G. A., and Kirk, D. L. (2005). BAPTA induces frequency shifts *in vivo* of spontaneous otoacoustic emissions of the bobtail lizard. *Audiol. Neurootol.* 10, 248–257. doi: 10.1159/000085999

Manley, G. A., Sienknecht, U., and Köppl, C. (2004). Calcium modulates the frequency and amplitude of spontaneous otoacoustic emissions in the bobtail skink. *J. Neurophysiol.* 92, 2685–2693. doi: 10.1152/jn.00267.2004

Merchant, S. N., Adams, J. C., and Nadol, J. B., Jr. (2005). Pathophysiology of Meniere's syndrome: are symptoms caused by endolymphatic hydrops? *Otol. Neurotol.* 26, 74–81. doi: 10.1097/00129492-200501000-00013

Meyer zum Gottesberge, A. M., and Ninoyu, O. (1987). A new aspect in pathogenesis of experimental hydrops: role of calcium. *Aviat. Space Environ. Med.* 58, A240–A246.

Moleti, A. D., Pistilli, D., and Sisto, R. (2017). Evidence for apical-basal transition in the delay of the reflection components of optoacoustic emissions. *J. Acoust. Soc. Am.* 141, 116–126. doi: 10.1121/1.4973866

Morrison, A. W. (1999). "Diagnostic and laboratory evaluation of Ménière's disease," in ed J. P Harris (The Hague: Ménière's disease Kugler Publications), 291–304.

Nadol, J. B. Jr. (2010). "Disorders of unknown or multiple causes," in *Schuknecht's Pathology of the Ear, 3rd Edn.*, eds S. N. Merchant, J. B. Nadol Jr (Shelton, CT: People's Medical Publishing House), 572–630.

Ninoyu, O., and Meyer zum Gottesberge, A. M. (1986). Changes in Ca^{++} activity and DC potential in experimentally induced endolymphatic hydrops. *Arch. Otorhinolaryngol.* 243, 106–107. doi: 10.1007/BF00453759

Palmer, A. R., and Shackleton, T. M. (2009). Variation in the phase of response to low-frequency pure tones in the guinea pig auditory nerve as functions of stimulus level and frequency. *J. Assoc. Res. Otolaryngol.* 10, 233–250. doi: 10.1007/s10162-008-0151-x

Picton, T. W. (2007). "Audiometry using auditory steady-state responses," in *Auditory Evoked Potentials: Basic Principles and Clinical Application,* eds R. F. Burkard, J. J. Eggermont, and M. Don (Baltimore, MD: Lippincott Williams & Wilkins), 441–462.

Salt, A. N. (2004). Acute endolymphatic hydrops generated by exposure of the ear to nontraumatic low-frequency tones. *J. Assoc. Res. Otolaryngol.* 5, 203–214. doi: 10.1007/s10162-003-4032-z

Salt, A. N., Brown, D. J., Hartsock, J. J., and Plontke, S. K. (2009). Displacement of the organ of Corti by gel injections into the cochlear apex. *Hear. Res.* 250, 63–75. doi: 10.1016/j.heares.2009.02.001

Salt, A. N., and DeMott, J. (1994a). Time course of endolymph volume increase in experimental hydrops measured *in vivo* with an ionic volume marker. *Hear. Res.* 74, 165–172. doi: 10.1016/0378-5955(94)90184-8

Salt, A. N., and DeMott, J. (1994b). Endolymph calcium increases with time after surgical induction of hydrops in guinea-pigs. *Hear. Res.* 74, 115–121. doi: 10.1016/0378-5955(94)90180-5

Salt, A. N., and DeMott, J. (1997). Longitudinal endolymph flow associated with acute volume increase in the guinea pig cochlea. *Hear. Res.* 107, 29–40. doi: 10.1016/S0378-5955(97)00018-X

Salt, A. N., DeMott, J. E., and Kimura, R. S. (1995). Comparison of endolymph cross-sectional area measured histologically with that measured *in vivo* with an ionic volume marker. *Ann. Otol. Rhinol. Laryngol.* 104, 886–894. doi: 10.1177/000348949510401111

Salt, A. N., Inamura, N., Thalmann, R., and Vora, A. (1989). Calcium gradients in inner ear endolymph. *Am. J. Otolaryngol.* 10, 371–375. doi: 10.1016/0196-0709(89)90030-6

Sellick, P. M. (2007). Long term effects of BAPTA in scala media on cochlear function. *Hear. Res.* 231, 13–22. doi: 10.1016/j.heares.2007.04.001

Sellick, P. M., Kirk, D. L., Patuzzi, R., and Robertson, D. (2007). Does BAPTA leave outer hair cell transduction channels closed? *Hear. Res.* 224, 84–92. doi: 10.1016/j.heares.2006.11.011

Sellick, P. M., Robertson, D., and Patuzzi, R. (2006). The effect of BAPTA and 4AP in scala media on transduction and cochlear gain. *Hear. Res.* 211, 7–15. doi: 10.1016/j.heares.2005.05.016

Shera, C. A., and Guinan, J. J., (2003). Stimulus-frequency-emission group delay: a test of coherent reflection filtering and a window on cochlear tuning. *J. Acoust. Soc. Am.* 113, 2762–2772. doi: 10.1121/1.1557211

Shera, C. A., Guinan, J. J., and Oxenham, A. J. (2010). Otoacoustic estimation of cochlear tuning: validation in the chinchilla. *J. Assoc. Res. Otolaryngol.* 11, 343–365. doi: 10.1007/s10162-010-0217-4

Sininger, Y. S. (2007). "The use of auditory brainstem response in screening for hearing loss and audiometric threshold prediction," in *Auditory Evoked Potentials: Basic Principles and Clinical Application*, eds R. F. Burkard, J. J.

Eggermont, and M. Don (Baltimore, MD: Lippincott Williams & Wilkins), 254–274.

Sirjani, D. B., Salt, A. N., Gill, R. M., and Hale, S. A. (2004). The influence of transducer operating point on distortion generation in the cochlea. *J. Acoust. Soc. Am.* 115, 1219–1229. doi: 10.1121/1.1647479

Spoor, A., and Eggermont, J. J. (1976). "Electrocochleography as a method for objective audiogram determination," in *Hearing and Davis: Essays Honoring Halowell Davis*, eds S. K. Hirsch, D. H. Eldredge, I. J. Hirsch, and S. R. Silverman (Saint Louis, MI: Washington University Press), 411–418.

Tagaya, M., Yamazaki, M., Teranishi, M., Naganawa, S., Yoshida, T., et al. (2011). Endolymphatic hydrops and blood-labyrinth barrier in Ménière's disease. *Acta Otolaryngol.* 131, 474–479. doi: 10.3109/00016489.2010.534114

Temchin, A. N., and Ruggero, M. A. (2010). Phase-locked responses to tones of chinchilla auditory nerve fibers: implications for apical cochlear mechanics. *J. Assoc. Res. Otolaryngol.* 11, 297–318. doi: 10.1007/s10162-009-0197-4

Tsuji, J., and Liberman, M. C. (1997). Intracellular labeling of auditory nerve fibers in guinea pig: central and peripheral projections. *J. Comp. Neurol.* 5, 188–202. doi: 10.1002/(SICI)1096-9861(19970505)381:2<188::AID-CNE6>3.0.CO;2-#

Verschooten, E., and Joris, P. X. (2014). Estimation of neural phase locking from stimulus-evoked potentials. *J. Assoc. Res. Otolaryngol.* 15, 767–787. doi: 10.1007/s10162-014-0465-9

Verschooten, E., Robles, L., Kovačić, D., and Joris, P. X. (2012). Auditory nerve frequency tuning measured with forward-masked compound action potentials. *J. Assoc. Res. Otolaryngol.* 13, 799–817. doi: 10.1007/s10162-012-0346-z

Wit, H. P., Warmerdam, T. J., and Albers, F. W. (2000). Measurement of the mechanical compliance of the endolymphatic compartments in the guinea pig. *Hear. Res.* 145, 82–90. doi: 10.1016/S0378-5955(00)00078-2

Yoshida, T., Teranishi, M., Kato, M., Otake, H., Kato, K., et al. (2013). Endolymphatic hydrops in patients with tinnitus as the major symptom. *Eur. Arch. Otorhinolaryngol.* 270, 3043–3048. doi: 10.1007/s00405-013-2380-9

14

An Objective Estimation of Air-Bone-Gap in Cochlear Implant Recipients with Residual Hearing Using Electrocochleography

Kanthaiah Koka[1], Aniket A. Saoji[1], Joseph Attias[1,2] and Leonid M. Litvak[1]*

[1] Research and Technology, Advanced Bionics, Valencia, CA, USA, [2] Schneider Children's Medical Center of Israel and Rabin Medical Center, Petach Tikva, Israel

Correspondence:
Kanthaiah Koka
kanthaiah.koka@advancedbionics.com

Although, cochlear implants (CI) traditionally have been used to treat individuals with bilateral profound sensorineural hearing loss, a recent trend is to implant individuals with residual low-frequency hearing. Notably, many of these individuals demonstrate an air-bone gap (ABG) in low-frequency, pure-tone thresholds following implantation. An ABG is the difference between audiometric thresholds measured using air conduction (AC) and bone conduction (BC) stimulation. Although, behavioral AC thresholds are straightforward to assess, BC thresholds can be difficult to measure in individuals with severe-to-profound hearing loss because of vibrotactile responses to high-level, low-frequency stimulation and the potential contribution of hearing in the contralateral ear. Because of these technical barriers to measuring behavioral BC thresholds in implanted patients with residual hearing, it would be helpful to have an objective method for determining ABG. This study evaluated an innovative technique for measuring electrocochleographic (ECochG) responses using the cochlear microphonic (CM) response to assess AC and BC thresholds in implanted patients with residual hearing. Results showed high correlations between CM thresholds and behavioral audiograms for AC and BC conditions, thereby demonstrating the feasibility of using ECochG as an objective tool for quantifying ABG in CI recipients.

Keywords: cochlear implant, electrocochleography, cochlear microphonic, air conduction, bone conduction, air-bone gap

INTRODUCTION

Cochlear implants traditionally have been used to treat individuals with bilateral profound sensorineural hearing loss. However, given the evolution of electrode and signal-processing technology and improved surgical techniques, individuals with low-frequency residual hearing also are able to experience benefit from a cochlear implant (Balkany et al., 2006; Fraysse et al., 2006). Moreover, by combining electrical and acoustic stimulation (EAS), benefit exceeds that of using a hearing aid or a cochlear implant alone (Von Ilberg et al., 1999; Turner et al., 2008).

In order to benefit optimally from EAS technologies, residual hearing in these subjects must be preserved. However, at least 50% of subjects lose their residual hearing after surgery (James et al., 2005; Balkany et al., 2006; Brown et al., 2010; Lenarz et al., 2013; Roland et al., 2016). The loss of residual hearing is attributed mainly to, direct trauma to the basilar membrane (Roland and Wright, 2006; Li et al., 2007) and not due to any potential interference produced by the presence of the electrode in the cochlea(Donnelly et al., 2009; Huber et al., 2010; Greene et al., 2015; Banakis et al., 2016). But several researchers have reported increased air-bone gaps (ABG) post-operatively in a subset of subjects after cochlear implantation despite using surgical techniques to reduce trauma (Attias et al., 2012; Chole et al., 2014; Raveh et al., 2014; Mattingly et al., 2016), thus suggesting that conductive components may be involved that can be attributed to the changes in middle ear mechanics and/or the presence of electrode in the cochlea.

Figure 1 shows an example audiogram from a CI recipient with residual hearing showing large ABGs. These ABGs are difficult to quantify because post-operative hearing sensitivity is exclusively measured with air-conduction (AC) thresholds because bone-conduction (BC) thresholds are technically difficult to assess in individuals with severe-to-profound hearing loss. Specifically, high levels of bone oscillator stimulation in the low frequencies can result in vibrotactile sensations mistakenly reported as audible, thereby contributing to a false increase in ABG. Also, due to smaller transcranial attenuation unmasked BC thresholds may be measured due to the stimulation of the cochlea in the non-test ear. Typically, the contralateral ear is masked with a band of noise to facilitate measurement of BC thresholds in the test ear. However, limited hearing in the contralateral ear may limit the ability to measure masked BC thresholds and lead to inaccurate ABG measurement. Also, it is not possible to accurately measure BC thresholds in patients and children who cannot provide accurate responses to BC stimulation.

Because of these technical barriers to evaluating behavioral BC thresholds, it would be helpful to have an objective method to measure AC and BC thresholds for estimating ABG in implant patients with residual hearing. Koka et al. (2016) and Abbas et al. (2017) used the intra-cochlear electrodes from the implant array to measure electrocochleography (ECochG) in patients with residual hearing. Different electrical potentials such as cochlear microphonics (CM), compound action potential (CAP), summating potential (SP), and auditory nerve neurophonics (ANN) together constitute ECochG responses. The CM represents the combination of transducer currents primarily through the outer hair cell stereocilia (Dallos, 1973) and is known to follow the fine structure of the stimulus waveform. The ANN is assumed to reflect the phase locking activity of the auditory nerve fibers (Snyder and Schreiner, 1984; Lichtenhan et al., 2013; Fitzpatrick et al., 2014; Forgues et al., 2014). The CAP is generated by the auditory nerve in response to the onset and offset of the acoustic stimulus, and the SP is the direct current part of the response with multiple generators. The present study focuses on the alternating current components of the ongoing, or steady state, response to tones. The difference response, which is the difference between alternating polarities, emphasizes responses at odd harmonics of the tone frequency, which are those components of the response that change with stimulus phase. Thus, the difference response is dominated by the CM, but also includes the largest part of the ANN that is periodic with the signal. Current study focused mainly on CM responses. The summation response, which is the summation of alternating polarities, emphasizes responses at even harmonics of the tone frequency, and include the components of the response that do not change with stimulus phase. Thus, the summation response includes the asymmetric distortions present in the CM and ANN. Because these distortions are greater in the ANN than the CM, the ongoing component of the summation response can be dominated by the ANN, when it is present. However, this part of the ANN is only the distortions, and so is smaller than the part that appears in the difference response. That there is some ANN present in the difference response was shown by Forgues et al. (2014), who demonstrated a decrease in difference response by introducing a neurotoxin used to suppress auditory nerve response.

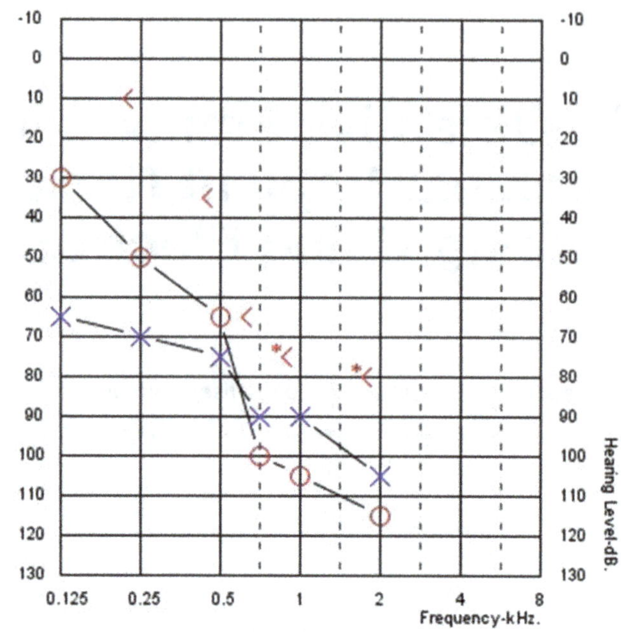

FIGURE 1 | Typical audiogram for a cochlear implant recipient with residual hearing and an air-bone gap (Subject CI04).

This study extends the (Koka et al., 2016) study to evaluate whether CM (which is the difference response) can be used to estimate BC thresholds in implanted patients with residual hearing. Because CM necessarily rules out any vibrotactile responses and contributions from the contralateral ear, it may be applicable for estimating BC thresholds at low frequencies. Thus, this study assessed CM responses for AC and BC stimuli in cochlear implant recipients with residual hearing.

METHODS

Subjects

Four implant recipients with HiRes 90 K® cochlear implants (Advanced Bionics LLC, Valencia, CA) and HiFocus MidScala® electrode arrays with residual hearing participated in this study. **Table 1** shows their ages and duration of implant use. The subjects were recruited based on observation of ABG with CIs. The pre-op ABGs were not available to the authors as part of

TABLE 1 | Subject demographics.

Subject id	Implant type	Electrode type	Implant usage (years))	Age (years)
CI04R	HiRes90K Advantage	MidScala	2	59
CI13	HiRes90K Advantage	MidScala	0.5	61
CI25	HiRes90K Advantage	MidScala	0.25	54
CI20	HiRes90K Advantage	MidScala	0.16	66

this study. The etiology of the hearing loss is unknown for this group. All subjects provided written informed consent prior to participation. The study protocol (#20121035) was approved by the Western Institutional Review Board (WIRB).

Equipment

The AC and BC stimulus delivery and measurement system for assessing behavioral thresholds and ECochG responses was the same as that described in Koka et al. (2016). The Bionic Ear Data Collection System (BEDCS) research software of Advanced Bionics was used to control stimulus delivery and ECochG measurement. The acoustic stimuli were generated by an NI DAQ system (NI DAQ 6216, National Instruments Corporation,, Austin, TX) along with an audio amplifier (Sony PHA-2, Sony Corporation, New York, NY, USA) and presented through a ER-3A insert earphone (Etymotic Research, Inc., Elk Grove Village, IL USA) for AC and through a B-71 bone vibrator for BC. The AC and BC levels were calibrated according to ANSI S3.6 Specifications for Audiometers using clinical audiometric calibration services provided by Audiometrics (Arcadia, CA, USA). ECochG was measured using an Advanced Bionics Clinical Programming Interface (CPI-II), Platinum Series Sound Processor (PSP), and Universal Headpiece (HP). The CPI-II delivered an external trigger to synchronize acoustic/bone vibration stimulus generation and ECochG measurement through the implant.

Pure Tone Audiometry and Tympanometry Procedures

Behavioral AC and BC pure-tone thresholds were measured at 125, 250, 500, 750, 1,000, 1,500, and 2,000 Hz using a stimulus duration of 200 ms and a step size of 2 dB using equipment described above. For each test frequency, thresholds were assessed using an ascending and descending track. The initial stimulus level for the ascending track was below the subject's audible threshold, whereas the initial stimulus level for the descending track was above the subject's behavioral threshold. The final threshold was defined as the average of the ascending and descending values. Masking was used for estimating bone conduction thresholds. Any response reported as vibrotactile or questionably vibrotactile was considered as no response.

Tympanometry was used to understand the condition of middle ear and to rule out conductive hearing loss (GSI Tympstar, Grason-Stadler Inc, Eden Prairie, MN 55344).

Ecochg Recording Procedure

ECochG stimuli consisted of 50-ms tone bursts with ramp duration of 5 ms (Hanning window) presented at each subject's most comfortable level (MCL). For each frequency (125, 250, 500, 750, 1,000, 1,500, and 2,000 Hz), ECochG responses were recorded using 240 presentations with alternating polarity (120 rarefaction and 120 condensation). From the responses to alternating polarities, the difference response (CM) was extracted.

The most apical electrode contact (electrode 1) was used as the active electrode and the ring electrode, located on the electrode lead outside of the cochlea, served as the return electrode. The amplifier on the HiRes90 k implant was configured to have a gain of 1,000 and its output was digitized (9-bits) at 9,280 samples/s. The low-pass filter cutoff was set to 5,000 Hz. With these settings, the Advanced Bionics implant offers a relatively long recording window of 54.4 ms, enabling ECochG recording for low-frequency stimuli down to 125 Hz.

Control Experiments

ECochG recordings can be affected by the stimulus artifact. The bone vibrator contains a relatively strong electromagnet. It is possible that the energy generated by the electromagnet may be coupled to the implant electronics. Two control experiments were conducted to identify and quantify any artifacts that may have occurred.

First, BC ECochG waveforms were compared between stimuli delivered when the ear canal was occluded (foam plug insertion) and unoccluded. The assumption here was that due to occlusion effect, the ECochG will be increased when ear canal was occluded. The absence of stimulus artifacts was confirmed when larger ECochG responses were observed for the occluded condition compared to the unoccluded condition. These control measurements were made for all subjects.

Second, ECochG recordings were made with the bone vibrator placed close, but not touching the mastoid, to determine if any direct electromagnetic coupling occurred. A custom-built holder was used to hold the bone vibrator close to the mastoid consistently across subjects. A template subtraction technique was used to remove electromagnetic coupling artifacts from the ECochG responses if they were detected when the bone vibrator was not touching the mastoid.

Data Analysis

CM response waveforms elicited separately by AC and BC stimulation were obtained from the rarefaction and condensation waveforms by subtracting alternating polarities and computing the average. Fast Fourier Transform (FFT) analysis estimated amplitudes for each stimulus level. CM thresholds were estimated by comparing the amplitude at each stimulus level with a constant noise floor, which was constant across all subjects. Finally, CM thresholds were compared with behavioral AC and BC acoustic thresholds to determine if a correlation existed.

RESULTS

Behavioral Air-Bone Gaps (ABG)

All the subjects in the study demonstrated behaviorally-based ABGs despite tympanometry indicating normal middle ear function. The ABGs varied between 14 to 59 dB with a mean of 36 dB.

Ecochg Responses for BC

Figure 2 shows typical ECochG waveforms in response to BC stimulation of 750 Hz at 50 dB HL (subject CI25). The upper plots show the raw waveforms for rarefaction and condensation stimulation in the time domain (**Figure 2A**) and frequency domain (**Figure 2C**). The lower plots show in the time (**Figure 2B**) and frequency domains (**Figure 2D**) the difference waveforms computed from the responses to the alternating polarity stimuli. These responses were recorded with an occluded ear for which the subject reported an increase in loudness. **Figure 3** shows CM responses from the same subject for an occluded and unoccluded ear in the time domain (**Figure 3A**) and frequency domain (**Figure 3B**). The occluded ear responses clearly show a 6 dB, doubling of amplitude compared to the unoccluded ear.

Control Experiments

No electromagnetic artifacts were observed for these subjects when stimulus levels did not elicit a vibrotactile response. Nonetheless, direct coupling electromagnetic artifacts were observed when stimulus levels were above vibrotactile thresholds, thereby indicating that artifacts exist at high levels. The template subtraction technique removed the stimulus artifact contamination at high levels.

Ecochg vs. Behavioral Thresholds (AC and BC)

Figure 4 shows behavioral and CM thresholds for all frequencies for which hearing was measureable. For all four subjects, the CM threshold profiles followed the behavioral audiometric threshold profiles. The mean and standard deviation of the difference between audiometric and CM thresholds for AC across all frequencies was −9 (±5) dB. The difference between audiometric and CM thresholds for BC across all frequencies was 6 (±6) dB.

Figure 5 plots CM thresholds as a function of audiometric thresholds for both AC and BC. The correlation between CM and audiometric thresholds is highly significant across all frequencies for both AC and BC ($r^2 = 0.84$, $n = 21$, $p < 0.001$ for AC; $r^2 = 0.68$, $n = 15$, $p < 0.001$ for BC). The ABG for behavioral responses was 36 (±12) dB and for CM thresholds was 43 (±12) dB. There was no significant difference between ABG measured using audiometry or ECochG ($p = 0.115$, $n = 15$).

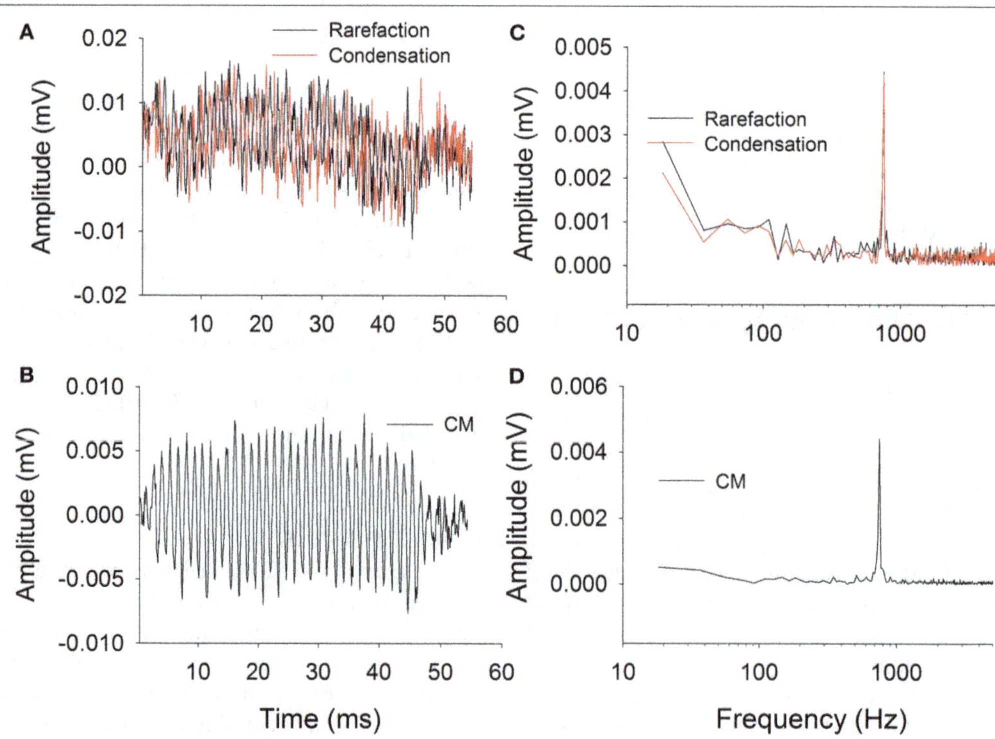

FIGURE 2 | Electrocochleography waveforms recorded with bone vibrator stimulation. (A): Raw waveforms recorded for alternating polarity stimulation. **(B)**: Difference CM response obtained by subtracting responses between alternating polarities. **(C)**: Frequency spectra of the responses to alternating polarities. **(D)**: Frequency spectrum of the difference CM response.

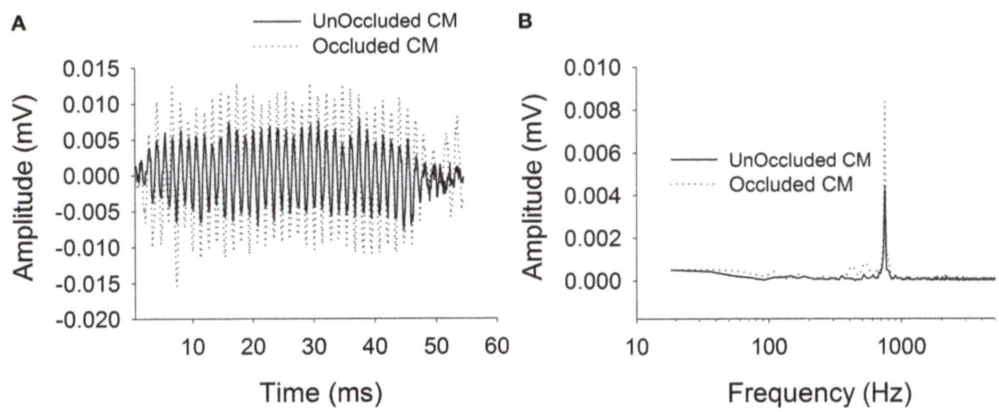

FIGURE 3 | CM responses for bone vibrator stimulation with and without occluded ear canal. (A): Time domain waveforms. **(B)**: Frequency spectra.

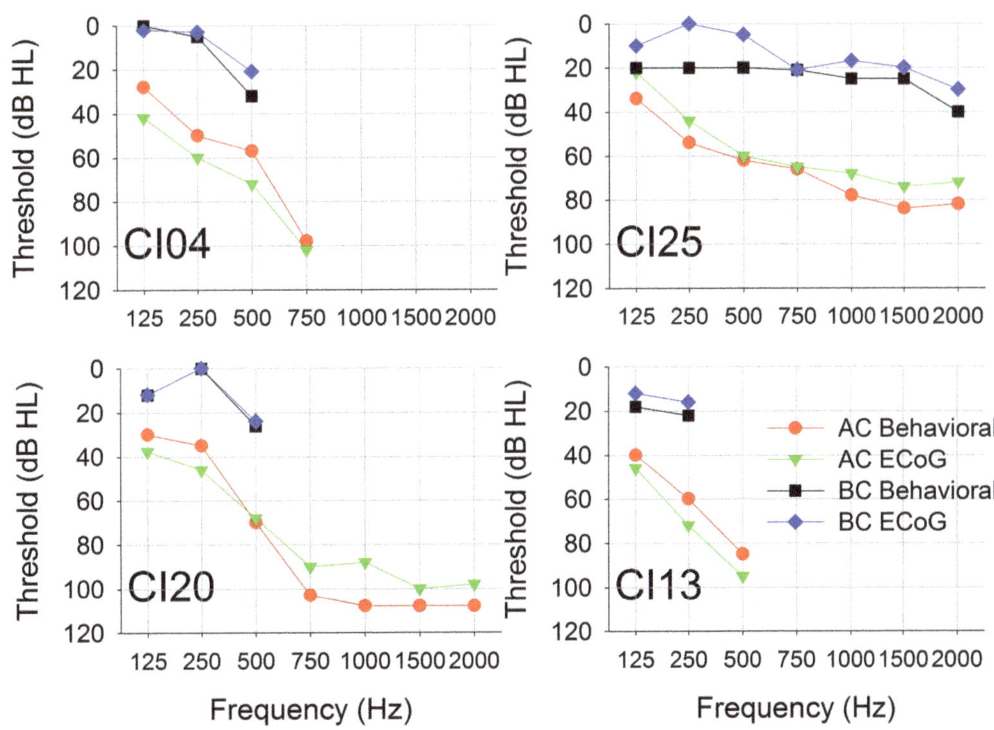

FIGURE 4 | Pure-tone AC and BC thresholds measured using conventional behavioral audiometry and ECochG. Each panel represents data from a single subject.

DISCUSSION

This study measured pure-tone audiometric thresholds and CM thresholds for AC and BC stimulation in four implanted individuals with residual hearing. Across the range of test frequencies, behavioral sensitivity and CM thresholds were highly correlated for both AC and BC stimulation. Moreover, the ABG estimated by the ECochG responses provided a reliable surrogate for behavioral ABG in these subjects.

These results are similar to Koka et al. (2016) for AC thresholds and to Abbas et al. (2017) who showed that CM thresholds approximated behavioral AC thresholds better than auditory nerve neurophonics or compound action potential thresholds. Unique to this study is the demonstration that ECochG responses to BC stimulation can provide an objective indicator of BC thresholds that are not corrupted by vibrotactile responses and does not require contralateral masking. One caveat is that care should be taken to limit BC vibrator output so as not to create electromagnetic artifacts at high stimulus levels. These

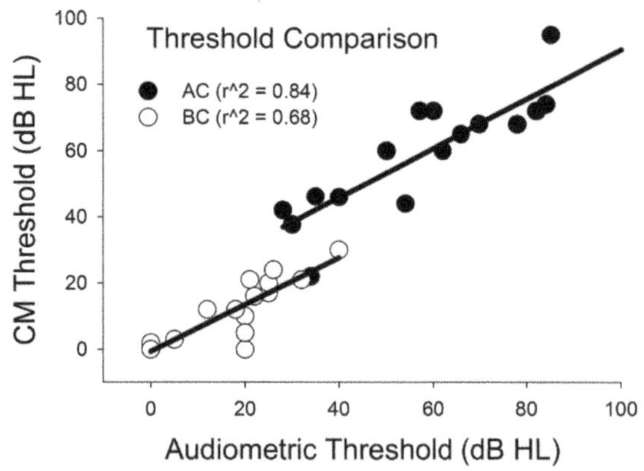

FIGURE 5 | Comparison of CM vs. audiometric thresholds across all subjects and across all frequencies for AC and BC stimulation.

results suggest that ECochG can be used as an objective tool to verify behavioral BC thresholds in CI patients with residual hearing and ABG. In implant patients, intra-cochlear electrode is used to measure ECochG which simplifies the measurement of evoked potentials especially in pediatric patients.

With the observation that ABG may exist after implantation of patients with residual hearing (Chole et al., 2014; Raveh et al., 2014; Mattingly et al., 2016) and in normal-hearing animals after implantation (Hod et al., 2016), this ECochG method can provide an objective tool to estimate reliable ABG without technical issues of measuring behavioral BC thresholds in CI subjects. The fact that this group of subjects had ABG in the presence of normal tympanometry suggests that the ABG originated in the inner ear rather than the middle ear. On the other hand acute studies looking at effect of electrode in the cochlea did show only less than 5 dB differences between air and bone conduction in temporal bones (Donnelly et al., 2009; Huber et al., 2010; Greene et al., 2015; Banakis et al., 2016). Quesnel et al. (2016) suggested that the changes in residual hearing after initial preservation may be due to intracochlear fibrosis and new bone formation changing the compliance of round window and not due to degeneration of hair cells. The current EcochG measurement may acts a tool to monitor ABG chronically and understand whether the increased ABG is due to chronic changes in the cochlea.

CONCLUSION

ECochG responses can provide an objective method for estimating ABG in cochlear implant recipients with residual hearing in the implanted ear.

AUTHOR CONTRIBUTIONS

Authors equally contributed to conception and design, drafting the article; and final approval of the version to be published and KK and AS contributed for acquisition of data, analysis and interpretation of data.

ACKNOWLEDGMENTS

The authors thank the subjects who participated in the study, and Lupe Navarro and Maria Holloway for organizing their visits. This study was funded by Advanced Bionics LLC.

REFERENCES

Abbas, P. J., Tejani, V. D., Scheperle, R. A., and Brown, C. J. (2017). Using neural response telemetry to monitor physiological responses to acoustic stimulation in hybrid cochlear implant users. *Ear Hear.* doi: 10.1097/AUD.0000000000000400. [Epub ahead of print].

Attias, J., Ulanovski, D., Shemesh, R., Kornreich, L., Nageris, B., Preis, M., et al. (2012). Air-Bone gap component of inner-ear origin in audiograms of cochlear implant candidates. *Otol. Neurotol.* 33, 512–517. doi: 10.1097/MAO.0b013e3182544cba

Balkany, T. J., Connell, S. S., Hodges, A. V., Payne, S. L., Telischi, F. F., Eshraghi, A. A., et al. (2006). Conservation of residual acoustic hearing after cochlear implantation. *Otol. Neurotol.* 27, 1083–1088. doi: 10.1097/01.mao.0000244355.34577.85

Banakis, Ã. R. M., Mattingly, Ã. J. K., Greene, Ã. N. T., Jenkins, Ã. H. A., Cass, Ã. S. P., and Tollin, Ã. D. J. (2016). A preliminary investigation of the air-bone gap changes in intracochlear sound pressure with air- and bone-conducted stimuli after cochlear implantation. *Otol. Neurotol.* 37, 1291–1299. doi: 10.1097/MAO.0000000000001184

Brown, R. F., Hullar, T. E., Cadieux, J. H., and Chole, R. A. (2010). Residual hearing preservation after pediatric cochlear implantation. *Otol. Neurotol.* 31, 1221–1226. doi: 10.1097/MAO.0b013e3181f0c649

Chole, R., Hullar, T., and Potts, L. (2014). Conductive component after cochlear implantation in patients with residual hearing conservation. *Am. J. Audiol.* 23, 359–3564. doi: 10.1097/MAO.0b013e3181f0c649

Dallos, P. (1973). *The Auditory Periphery: Biophysics and Physiology.* New York, NY: Academic Press,

Donnelly, N., Bibas, A., Jiang, D., Bamiou, D. E., Santulli, C., Jeronimidis, G., et al. (2009). Effect of cochlear implant electrode insertion on middle-ear function as measured by intra- operative laser Doppler vibrometry. *J. Laryngol. Otol.* 123, 723–729. doi: 10.1017/S0022215109004290

Fitzpatrick, D. C., Campbell, A. T., Choudhury, B., Dillon, M. T., Forgues, M., Buchman, C. A., et al. (2014). Round window electrocochleography just before cochlear implantation: relationship to word recognition outcomes in adults. *Otol. Neurotol.* 35, 64–71. doi: 10.1097/MAO.0000000000000219

Forgues, M., Koehn, H. A., Dunnon, A. K., Pulver, S. H., Buchman, C. A., Adunka, O. F., et al. (2014). Distinguishing hair cell from neural potentials recorded at the round window. *J. Neurophysiol.* 111, 580–593. doi: 10.1152/jn.00446.2013

Fraysse, B., Macías, A. R., Sterkers, O., Burdo, S., Ramsden, R., Deguine, O., et al. (2006). Residual hearing conservation and electroacoustic stimulation with the nucleus 24 contour advance cochlear implant. *Otol. Neurotol.* 27, 624–633. doi: 10.1097/01.mao.0000226289.04048.0f

Greene, N. T., Mattingly, J. K., Jenkins, H. A., Tollin, D. J., Easter, J. R., and Cass, S. P. (2015). Cochlear implant electrode effect on sound energy transfer within the cochlea during acoustic stimulation. *Otol. Neurotol.* 36, 1554–1561. doi: 10.1097/MAO.0000000000000838

Hod, R., Attias, J., Raveh, E., and Nageris, B. I. (2016). Cochlear implantation via round window or cochleostomy: effect on hearing in an animal model. *Laryngoscope* 126, E375–E378. doi: 10.1002/lary.26033

Huber, A. M., Hoon, S. J., Sharouz, B., Daniel, B., and Albrecht, E. (2010). The influence of a cochlear implant electrode on the mechanical func- tion of the inner ear. *Otol. Neurotol.* 31, 512–518. doi: 10.1097/MAO.0b013e3181ca372b

James, C., Albegger, K., Battmer, R., Burdo, S., Deggouj, N., Deguine, O., et al. (2005). Preservation of residual hearing with cochlear implantation: how and why. *Acta Otolaryngol.* 125, 481–491.

Koka, K., Saoji, A. A., and Litvak, L. M. (2016). Electrocochleography in cochlear implant recipients with residual hearing: comparison with audiometric thresholds. *Ear Hear.* doi: 10.1097/AUD.0000000000000385. [Epub ahead of print].

Lenarz, T., James, C., Cuda, D., Fitzgerald O'Connor, A., Frachet, B., Frijns, J. H., et al. (2013). European multi-centre study of the Nucleus Hybrid L24 cochlear implant. *Int. J. Audiol.* 52, 838–848. doi: 10.3109/14992027.2013.802032

Li, P. M., Somdas, M. A., Eddington, D. K., and Nadol, J. B. Jr. (2007). Analysis of intracochlear new bone and fibrous tissue formation in human subjects with cochlear implants. *Ann. Otol. Rhinol. Laryngol.* 116, 731–738. doi: 10.1177/000348940711601004

Lichtenhan, J. T., Cooper, N. P., and Guinan, J. J. Jr. (2013). A new auditory threshold estimation technique for low frequencies: proof of concept. *Ear Hear.* 34, 42–51. doi: 10.1097/AUD.0b013e31825f9bd3

Mattingly, J. K., Uhler, K. M., and Cass, S. P. (2016). Air-bone gaps contribute to functional hearing preservation in cochlear implantation. *Otol. Neurotol.* 37, 1255–1262. doi: 10.1097/MAO.0000000000001171

Quesnel, A. M., Nakajima, H. H., Rosowski, J. J., Hansen, M. R., Gantz, B. J., and Nadol, J. B. (2016). Delayed loss of hearing after hearing preservation cochlear implantation: human temporal bone pathology and implications for etiology. *Hear. Res.* 333, 225–234. doi: 10.1016/j.heares.2015.08.018

Raveh, E., Attias, J., Nageris, B., Kornreich, L., and Ulanovski, D. (2014). Pattern of hearing loss following cochlear implantation. *Eur. Arch Otorhinolaryngol.* 272, 2261–2266. doi: 10.1097/MAO.0b013e3181f0c649

Roland, J. T. Jr., Gantz, B. J., Waltzman, S. B., and Parkinson, A. J. (2016). The Multi- center Clinical Trial Group. United States multicenter clinical trial of the Cochlear Nucleus Hybrid implant system. *Laryngoscope* 126, 175–181. doi: 10.1002/lary.25451

Roland, P. S., and Wright, C. G. (2006). Surgical aspects of cochlear implantation: mechanism of insertional trauma. *Adv. Otorhinolaryngol.* 64, 11–30. doi: 10.1159/000094642

Snyder, R. L., and Schreiner, C. E. (1984). The auditory neurophonic: basic properties. *Hear. Res.* 15, 261–280.

Turner, C. W., Reiss, L. A. J., and Gantz, B. J. (2008). Combined acoustic and electric hearing: preserving residual acoustic hearing. *Hear. Res.* 242, 164–171. doi: 10.1016/j.heares.2007.11.008

Von Ilberg, C., Keifer, J., Tillein, J., Pfenningdorff, T., Hartmann, R., Sturzebecher, E., et al. (1999). Electro-acoustic stimulation of the auditory system, *ORL J. Otorhinolaryngol. Relat. Spec.* 61, 334–340. doi: 10.1159/0000 27695

15

Outer Hair Cell and Auditory Nerve Function in Speech Recognition in Quiet and in Background Noise

*Richard Hoben[1], Gifty Easow[1], Sofia Pevzner[1] and Mark A. Parker[1,2]**

[1] Department of Otolaryngology, Steward St. Elizabeth's Medical Center, Boston, MA, USA, [2] Department of Otolaryngology, Head and Neck Surgery, Tufts University School of Medicine, Boston, MA, USA

Correspondence:
Mark A. Parker
mark_allen.parker@tufts.edu

The goal of this study was to describe the contribution of outer hair cells (OHCs) and the auditory nerve (AN) to speech understanding in quiet and in the presence of background noise. Fifty-three human subjects with hearing ranging from normal to moderate sensorineural hearing loss were assayed for both speech in quiet (Word Recognition) and speech in noise (QuickSIN test) performance. Their scores were correlated with OHC function as assessed via distortion product otoacoustic emissions, and AN function as measured by amplitude, latency, and threshold of the VIIIth cranial nerve Compound Action Potential (CAP) recorded during electrocochleography (ECochG). Speech and ECochG stimuli were presented at equivalent sensation levels in order to control for the degree of hearing sensitivity across patients. The results indicated that (1) OHC dysfunction was evident in the lower range of normal audiometric thresholds, which demonstrates that OHC damage can produce "Hidden Hearing Loss," (2) AN dysfunction was evident beginning at mild levels of hearing loss, (3) when controlled for normal OHC function, persons exhibiting either high or low ECochG amplitudes exhibited no statistically significant differences in neither speech in quiet nor speech in noise performance, (4) speech in noise performance was correlated with OHC function, (5) hearing impaired subjects with OHC dysfunction exhibited better speech in quiet performance at or near threshold when stimuli were presented at equivalent sensation levels. These results show that OHC dysfunction contributes to hidden hearing loss, OHC function is required for optimum speech in noise performance, and those persons with sensorineural hearing loss exhibit better word discrimination in quiet at or near their audiometric thresholds than normal listeners.

Keywords: hidden hearing loss, QuickSIN, outer hair cell, auditory nerve, electrocochleography (ECochG), compound action potential (CAP), wave I auditory brainstem response (ABR), distortion product otoacoustic emission

INTRODUCTION

It is clear that the audiogram, which is the standard metric of audition in humans, is inadequate in identifying otopathologies that contribute to hearing impairment (Moore, 2002; Makary et al., 2011; Liberman et al., 2016). In part, this is because of an incomplete understanding of the cellular basis of decoding complex stimuli, such as speech comprehension in the presence of background noise, and defining the functional roles of cochlear cell types involved in audition may lead to better clinical assessment. Speech recognition in the presence of background noise is a primary complaint of the hearing impaired, and auditory neuroscience seems to have come full circle regarding the understanding of the cellular basis of this function in the cochlea. As early as the 1950s, the auditory nerve (AN) was proposed to play the primary role in the ability to understand speech (Schuknecht and Woellner, 1953). This led to the development of the cochlear implant (House, 1974). However, the discovery of otoacoustic emissions in the 1970s (Kemp, 1978), and later discovery of the motile abilities of outer hair cells (OHCs) in the 1980s (Brownell et al., 1985), led to a paradigm shift in focus that OHCs play a primary role amplifying the speech signal for the fine tuning that is essential for understanding spoken language. OHC function has been described as both a cochlear amplifier (Davis, 1983), where OHCs amplify the passive motion of the basilar membrane (BM), and as a bank of frequency-specific filters that fine tune the acoustic signal (Goldstein et al., 1971; Ruggero, 1994). While these models are correct from a theoretical perspective, translating these functions to a clinical perspective is essential in our understanding of how OHC function contributes to audition. For example, whether OHCs function as cochlear amplifiers that amplify signals at threshold and/or a series of band-width filters to aid speech recognition in the presence of background noise is unknown.

More recently, evidence in animal models have re-examined the functional roles of the AN in quiet and in the presence of background noise (Kujawa and Liberman, 2006, 2009; Furman et al., 2013). Much of this work is based on the observation in animals that the AN is comprised of distinct populations of AN fibers based on their spontaneous firing rate (Liberman, 1978). AN fibers with low spontaneous rates function in increasing background noise, and AN fibers with high spontaneous rates function in quiet backgrounds at or near thresholds (Furman et al., 2013). Low-level noise exposure studies where normal OHC function has been preserved (Kujawa and Liberman, 2009; Lin et al., 2011) suggest that low spontaneous rate AN fibers are selectively damaged leaving high spontaneous rate fibers intact (Furman et al., 2013). The hypothesis derived from these studies is that if humans exhibit similar damage of the low spontaneous rate fibers, the ability to hear in complex listening situations such as speech in the presence of background noise would be diminished. Unfortunately, speech discrimination is very difficult to measure in laboratory animals, so confirmation of this hypothesis in humans has been a recent focus of investigation (Bramhall et al., 2015, 2017; Liberman et al., 2016; Prendergast et al., 2017).

Using loss of function data collected from normal and hearing impaired humans, the aim of this study was to describe the individual and combined contributions of OHCs and the AN in speech discrimination. OHC function was measured using distortion product otoacoustic emissions (DPOAEs), and AN function was measured using the amplitude, latency, and threshold of the VIIIth cranial nerve Compound Action Potential (CAP) measured during ECochG. These responses were correlated to human subject variables that included age, degree of sensorineural hearing loss (SNHL), as well as speech discrimination performances in quiet (SIQ) or in the presence of competing background noise (SIN). Previous research has demonstrated that SNHL has a strong correlation with both SIN performance and CAP amplitude (Bramhall et al., 2015). In order to control for the degree of SNHL, the stimuli for speech testing and AN analyses were presented in the sensation level (SL) scale, which incorporates an individual's threshold as the reference for the intensity scale of the stimuli.

The results demonstrate that OHC dysfunction is detected in the normal diagnostic range of a standard audiogram, optimum SIN performance is correlated with OHC function, and those persons with SNHL exhibit better word discrimination in quiet at or near their audiometric thresholds than normal listeners. The results are best described using linear systems theory where OHCs function as a bank of frequency and intensity filters. These results not only help define to cellular basis of audition, but will also focus the direction of future hearing loss therapies.

MATERIALS AND METHODS

Subjects

Fifty-three English speaking adults (14 males and 39 females) age range 22–71 (mean of 46.0 years old) were recruited from our clinic at St. Elizabeth's Medical Center in Boston, MA to participate in this study. All study procedures were performed and approved by the St. Elizabeth's Institutional Review Board and all participants in the study provided informed consent. An audiological evaluation including tympanometry, air and bone conduction thresholds, speech reception threshold (SRT), and Word Recognition in Quiet using NU-6 word lists was completed for each subject. The inclusion criteria consisted of a high-frequency pure tone average (hfPTA = mean of thresholds at 1, 2, and 4 kHz) of 50 dB HL or less, normal (Type A) tympanometry using a 226 Hz probe tone (Jerger et al., 1972), no conductive pathology, no pure tone asymmetry >10 dB HL between ears, and no documented otological disease. All of the following measurements were recorded from the best ear based on their hfPTA. The entire procedure took ~2 h and most subjects broke these into two 1 h sessions.

Audiometry

A Madsen Astera audiometer was used to generate the pure tone and speech stimuli and the responses were recorded on GN Otometrics Otosuite V 4.70.00 software. Behavioral threshold was obtained at 0.025, 0.05, 1, 2, 3, 4, 6, and 8 kHz using a modified Hughson-Westlake procedure (Carhart and Jerger, 1959) in 5 dB HL steps under a calibrated insert earphone in a audiometric sound booth. SRT using recorded materials was obtained this same procedure using spondee words rather than pure tone stimuli.

Word Recognition Score (WRS) in Quiet

Subjects were presented with a unique and randomized NU-6 wordlist (25 words) using recorded materials presented at 0, 10, 20, and 40 dB Sensation Level (SL; above SRT) under headphones in quiet in an audiometric sound booth and the percent of correct responses were recorded for each presentation level.

Quick Speech-In-Noise (QSIN)

Quick Speech-In-Noise (QSIN) test (Killion et al., 2004) was used to asses speech recognition in the presence of background noise. Sentences were presented at 0, 10, 20, and 40 dB SL (relative to SRT) in the presence of multi-talker babble varying in signal-to-noise (SNR) ratio from 0 to 25 dB. HL Subjects were familiarized with the task using one practice list and then presented with 2 scored lists for each ear. Scores were averaged and reported as mean SNR loss, with larger positive numbers indicating poorer performance.

Distortion Product Otoacoustic Emission (DPOAE)

Distortion Product Otoacoustic Emission (DPOAE) amplitudes and thresholds were evoked using a Madsen Capella II Otoacoustic system and recorded using Otosuite software (version 4.70.00). DPOAE SNRs were measured using an 8 to 1 kHz F2 frequency sweep where L1 was set to 65 dB SPL and L2 was set to 55 dB SPL (F2/F1 ratio = 1.22; Kujawa and Liberman, 2009). The acceptance criterion was set to minimum DPOAE level of −5 dB SPL and SNR of 6 dB SPL or more. These recordings were repeated three times, and DPOAE SNRs were averaged to obtain mean SNR amplitude per F2. DPOAE thresholds were obtained using a 75 dB SPL to 25 dB SPL (L1 = L2) intensity sweep in 5 dB SPL steps at audiometric frequencies using the same acceptance criteria. Threshold was defined as the lowest intensity that elicited a DPOAE above the noise floor. Threshold was set at 20 dB SPL in cases where the DPOAE was present at the lowest presentation level (25 dB SPL), and was set to 80 dB SPL in cases where there was no repeatable DP present at the highest presentation level (75 dB SPL).

Electrocochleagraphy (ECochG)

Electrocochleagraphy (ECochG) waveforms were obtained using the Bio-logic Navigator Pro auditory evoked potentials system and incorporating Lilly wick tympanic membrane electrodes (Intelligent Hearing Systems) coupled with Bio-logic insert earphones. Electrodes were soaked in sterile normal saline solution at room temperature for 20 min, and then inserted into the external auditory meatus by an experienced audiologist so that the electrode rested on the tympanic membrane. An insert earphone was then placed in the same ear canal to deliver the acoustic stimuli and help stabilize the electrode. The reference electrode was place on the contralateral mastoid and the ground electrode was place on the high forehead (horizontal montage). An alternating polarity 4,000 Hz toneburst stimulus (Blackman ramp with a four cycle rise and fall) was presented at a repetition rate of 13.3/s with a 10–1,500 Hz filter and an amplifier gain of 50,000 and digitized in a 10.66 ms time window. The average waveform was generated from 1,000 sweeps. Acoustic stimuli were presented at 0, 30, 40, 50, 60, and 70 dB SL (in dB nHL relative to the hfPTA). Since behavioral detection thresholds are 25 dB lower than ABR thresholds (Ngan and May, 2001; Henry et al., 2011), the choice was made to base the SL scale on audiometric thresholds rather than ABR thresholds. Average ECochG waveforms were analyzed by an experienced audiologist with a clinical Certification in Neurophysiological Interoperate Monitoring (CNIM). The CAP was identified as the largest peak occurring at ~2.0–3.5 ms after stimulus onset and the amplitude was measured with the Bio-logic Auditory Evoked Potential software (version 6.2.0) as the difference in voltage between the peak of the CAP and the following trough (Lasky, 1984; Bramhall et al., 2015). At least three waveforms were generated for each ear and the average amplitudes, latencies, and thresholds for each presentation level were obtained and used for further analysis (**Figure 1**). The lowest presentation level to elicit a repeatable CAP was defined as threshold.

Linear Mixed Effects Modeling

The collected data was modeled as described in detail by Bramhall et al. (2015), with the exception that this current paper used SPSS (IBM SPSS Statistics version 23, release 23.0.0.0) rather than R to generate the models. Deidentified subject number was used as the random effects variable; covariates included subject age, DPOAE amplitudes and thresholds at all F2 frequencies, CAP amplitudes and latencies at all presentation levels, and CAP thresholds; the

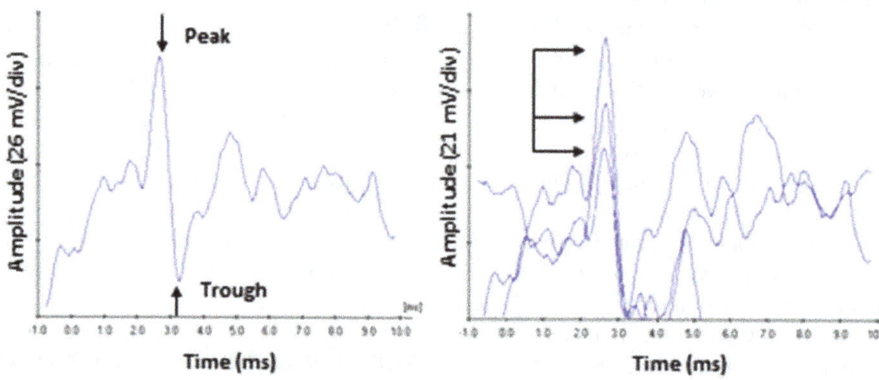

FIGURE 1 | ECochG recording of the compound action potential. (Left) Representative tracing of a 60 dB SL presentation to a subject in the Normal Hearing group. Amplitude was measured from the peak of CAP to the following trough. **(Right)** Responses were recorded three times, and the average peak amplitudes and latencies were calculated. Arrows highlight the variability on amplitude characteristic of this recording in unanaesthetized human subjects. By comparison, CAP peak latency values (read off the abscissa) exhibited less variability.

subjects hfPTA was used as the residual weighted variable; and the subjects QSIN scores were used as the dependent variable.

Analysis

After data collection, patient responses were rank ordered and divided into groups as described in the text. Power analyses using an alpha of 0.05 determined the power to be >0.8 for analyses between the groups described in the text. A test of normalcy indicated that these results were not normally distributed so non-parametric statistical analyses were utilized. Correlations between group variables were conducted using Kendall's tau-b (τ_b) correlation coefficient, which is a non-parametric measure of the strength and direction of an association between variables ranked in either ordinal or continuous scales using SPSS. The τ_b correlation coefficient was calculated for each condition (i.e., presentation level, frequency) as described, however only the strongest correlations were described in the text for clarity. SPSS also calculates the p-value of the τ_b correlation coefficient, which are plotted in appropriate figures. With the exception of the word recognition in quiet analyses, statistically significant trends between groups were measured by the non-parametric Jonckheere–Terpstra (J–T) test (Bewick et al., 2004). For clinically significant differences of word recognition in quiet, statistically significant differences in performance were based on previously published binomial modeling of word recognition scores (Thornton and Raffin, 1978). Three graphical methods are used to visualize the data in the main text. Data are plotted either as scatter plots of individual data points for correlational analysis; box and whisker plots using upper and lower quartiles (upper and lower ends of the box), median (line within the box), range of scores (error bars), and suspected outliers (either less than the lower quartile or higher than the upper quartile by 1.5 times the inter quartile range, open circles accompanied by subject identification number) in order to better visualize the variance within each group; or mean values with error bars representing the standard error of the mean to visuals the statistically significant differences between groups. For all figures, asterisks represent a $p < 0.05$.

RESULTS

SNHL Is Correlated with SIN

The results show statistically significant correlations between SNHL (measured by hfPTA) and subject age, SIN performance (measured by QSIN SNR Loss), and OHC function (measured by DPAOE amplitude and threshold; **Figure 2**). In order to visualize these correlations, subjects were ranked by hfPTA and divided into one of four groups based on their degree of high frequency SNHL (Normal Hearing < 15 dB HL, $n = 7$ males and 22 females; Minimal SNHL = 15–24 dB HL, $n = 1$ male and 3 females; Mild SNHL = 25–39 dB HL, $n = 6$ males and 4 females; Moderate SNHL = 40–50 dB HL, $n = 6$ males and 4 females; **Figure 3**). In clinical audiometry, the Minimal SNHL group represents the lower end of the Normal range and is most often used in pediatric rather than adult audiometry. There was a statistically significant positive correlation between SNHL (hfPTA) and age ($\tau b = 0.636$, $p = 0.000$; **Figure 2A**). The non-parametric J–T test for ordered alternatives showed that there was a statistically significant trend of increased age with increasing hearing loss (**Figure 3B**). Specifically, there was a statistically significant increase in age between the Normal hearing (33.7 ± 1.97 years) and Mild (59.6 ± 2.79 years) and Moderate SNHL groups ($p = 0.00$).

SIQ testing between 10 and 40 dB SL showed no clinically significant differences between any of these groups (**Figure 4**). Interestingly, persons with normal hfPTAs exhibited a decrease on WRS (11.0 ± 2.57% correct) compared to subjects with moderate SNHL (19.6 ± 2.57% correct) when the word lists were presented at or near threshold (0 dB SL). While this difference was not significant on a clinical level, this trend will be explored in detail below.

There were no statistically significant differences in SIN testing between any groups analyzed in this study for 0, 10, and 20 dB SL presentation levels, so only 40 dB SL presentation levels are shown in the following figures. Similar to SIQ, SIN testing at 40 dB SL also showed a statistically significant direct correlation between hfPTA and QSIN score ($\tau_b = 0.518$, $p = 0.000$; **Figure 2B**). J–T testing showed subjects in the Mild (2.4 ± 0.79 SNR loss, $p = 0.002$) and Moderate (and 4.8 ± 0.49 SNR loss, $p = 0.000$) SNHL groups exhibited statistically significant higher QSIN scores than persons in the Normal hfPTA group (−0.2 ± 1.08 SNR loss; **Figure 3C**). There was also a statistically significant increase in QSIN scores between the Minimal (1.0 ± 0.82 SNR loss) and Moderate SNHL groups ($p = 0.007$). Since higher QSIN scores represent poorer SIN performance (Killion et al., 2004), these results suggest that SIN performance worsens as hfPTA increases.

Characteristics of OHC Dysfunction in SNHL

OHC function was also correlated with the degree of SNHL. High frequency PTA was negatively (inversely) correlated with DPOAE amplitude (measured as DPAOE SNR) with a maximum correlation value at 4 kHz ($\tau_b = -0.601$, $p = 0.000$; **Figure 2C**). J–T testing showed that even subjects in the Minimal SNHL group exhibited statistically significant decreases in DPOAE SNR at 3–6 kHz compared to subjects in the Normal hfPTA group (**Figure 5A**). Furthermore, there was a statistically significant decrease in DPOAE SNR as the degree of SNHL progressed from the Normal group at 1–6 kHz. The largest decrease in amplitude between consecutive groups occurred between the Normal hfPTA and Minimal SNHL groups (−11.49 dB SNR at 4 kHz). Similarly, subjects in the Moderate SNHL group exhibited statistically significantly diminished DPOAE SNRs compared to subjects in the Minimal group at 1–2 and 4 kHz, and to the Mild SNHL group at 1.5–2 kHz (p-values are listed in **Figure 5A**).

High Frequency PTA was directly correlated with DPOAE threshold with the strongest correlation coefficient at 3 kHz ($\tau_b = 0.564$, $p = 0.000$; **Figure 2D**), and J–T testing showed an elevation on DPOAE threshold as hfPTA increased (**Figure 5B**). The Minimal SNHL group exhibited a statistically significant DPOAE threshold shift at 2–4 kHz compared to the Normal hfPTA group. Although the DPOAE threshold elevation progressed

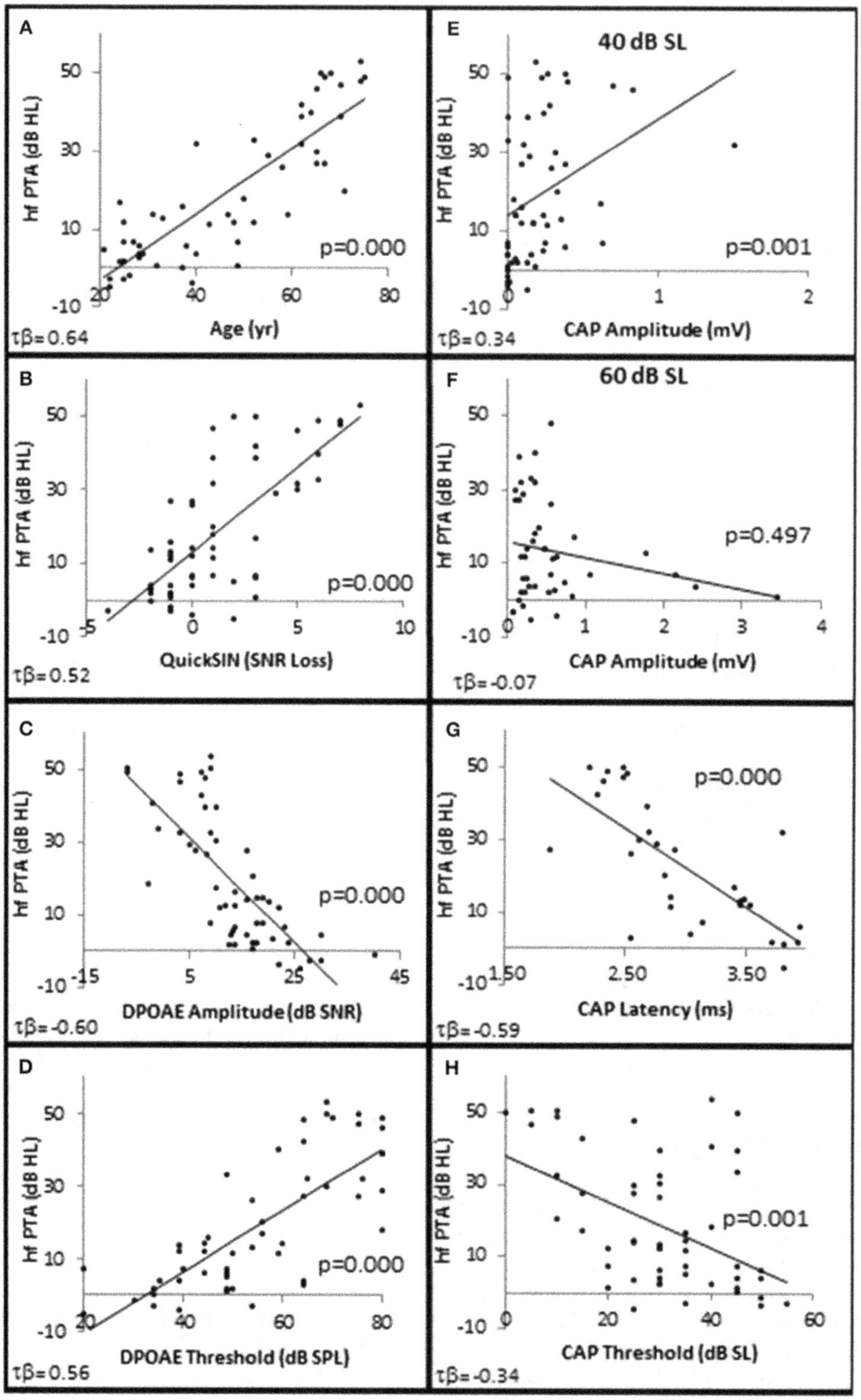

FIGURE 2 | SNHL is Correlated with age, speech in noise performance, and OHC function. Distribution of SNHL (hfPTA) as a function of age **(A)**, SIN performance (Quick SIN) with better performance in noise corresponding to lower values of SNR loss **(B)**, OHC function measured by DPAOE amplitude **(C)**, and DPAOE threshold **(D)** at 4 kHz, AN function measured by CAP amplitude in response to 4 kHz tone pips presented at 40 dB SL **(E)** and 60 dB SL **(F)**, CAP latency in response to 4 kHz tone pips presented at 30 dB SL **(G)** and CAP thresholds **(H)**. Lines represent best fit (linear).

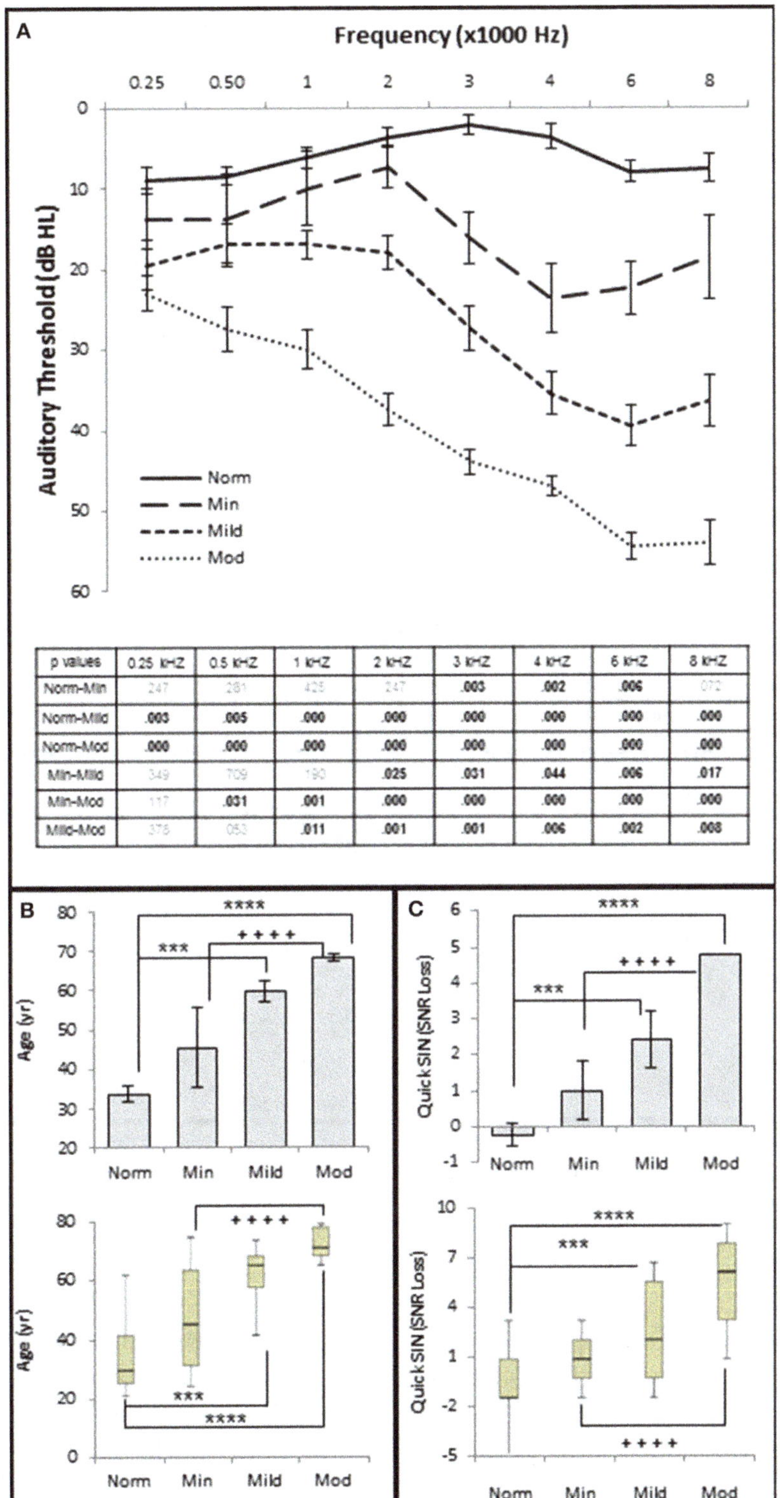

p values	0.25 kHZ	0.5 kHZ	1 kHZ	2 kHZ	3 kHZ	4 kHZ	6 kHZ	8 kHZ
Norm-Min	247	281	425	247	**.003**	**.002**	**.006**	072
Norm-Mild	**.003**	**.005**	**.000**	**.000**	**.000**	**.000**	**.000**	**.000**
Norm-Mod	**.000**	**.000**	**.000**	**.000**	**.000**	**.000**	**.000**	**.000**
Min-Mild	349	709	190	**.025**	**.031**	**.044**	**.006**	**.017**
Min-Mod	117	**.031**	**.001**	**.000**	**.000**	**.000**	**.000**	**.000**
Mild-Mod	376	053	**.011**	**.001**	**.001**	**.006**	**.002**	**.008**

FIGURE 3 | Increasing SNHL is correlated with decreased speech in noise performance. (A) Mean pure tone audiograms from each group. The table lists the *p*-values between each group by stimulus frequency. Bold text indicates a $p < 0.05$. **(B)** Distribution of the subject age (years) in each group. Top graph plots mean values +/1 s.e.m. Bottom graph plots this same data using upper and lower quartiles (box), median values (line within box), maximum and minimum scores (error bars). **(C)** Speech in noise performance from each group where lower SNR Loss corresponds to better performance in the presence of background noise. Top graph plots mean values ± 1 s.e.m. Bottom graph plots this same data using box and whisker plots. Norm, Normal Hearing Group; Min, Minimal SNHL; Mild, Mild SNHL; Mod, Moderate SNHL; *** statistically significant difference between Normal and Mild SNHL groups; ****statistically significant difference between Normal and Moderate SNHL groups; ++++statistically significant difference between Minimal SNHL and Moderate SNHL groups.

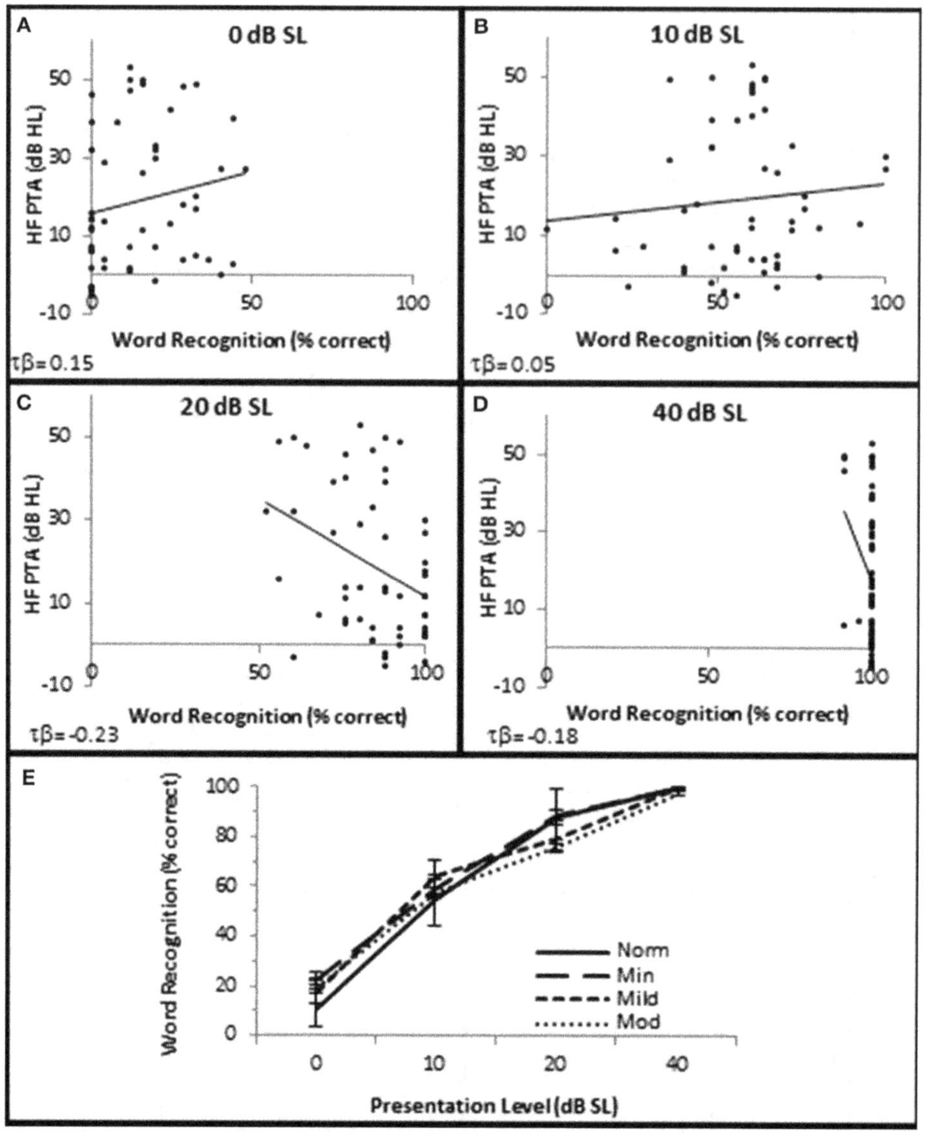

FIGURE 4 | SNHL is not clinically correlated with speech in quiet performance. Distribution of individual WRS scores plotted as a function of SNHL (hfPTA) for 0 **(A)**, 10 **(B)**, 20 **(C)**, and 40 dB **(D)** sensation levels (dB above SRT). **(E)** Performance-intensity functions plotting the mean data from each SNHL group. Error bars = s.e.m. Norm, Normal Hearing Group; Min, Minimal SNHL; Mild, Mild SNHL; Mod, Moderate SNHL. Lines represent best fit (linear). Clinically statistically significant differences were based on Thornton and Raffin (1978).

through the Mild and Moderate groups, the largest statistically significant threshold shift between consecutive groups occurred between the Normal and Minimal groups (17.38 dB SPL at 4 kHz).

Taken together, these results suggest that OHC function is correlated with pure tone audiometry, and that even subjects with minimal high frequency SNHL may exhibit statistically significant OHC damage. Since a PTA between 15 and 25 dB HL is often considered within the normal range in adult humans, this finding illustrates an example of an otopathology undetected in a standard audiogram commonly known as "Hidden Hearing Loss."

Characteristics of AN Dysfunction in SNHL

Next, CAP amplitude, latency, and thresholds were analyzed to study AN function within these groups. There was a direct correlation between hfPTA and CAP amplitude when 4 kHz tone pips were presented at 30 dB SL (τ_b = 0.209, p = 0.038; data not shown) and 40 dB SL (τ_b = 0.336, p = 0.001; **Figure 2E**) presentation levels. However, there was a difference in amplitude-intensity function between these groups (**Figure 6A**). The Normal hfPTA group exhibited small CAP amplitudes at low stimulus presentation levels (30–40 dB SL; R^2 = 0.82, y = 0.0708x, intercept = 0.00) and a steep growth function in amplitude at 50–70 dB SL (R^2 = 0.87, y = 0.3307x, intercept

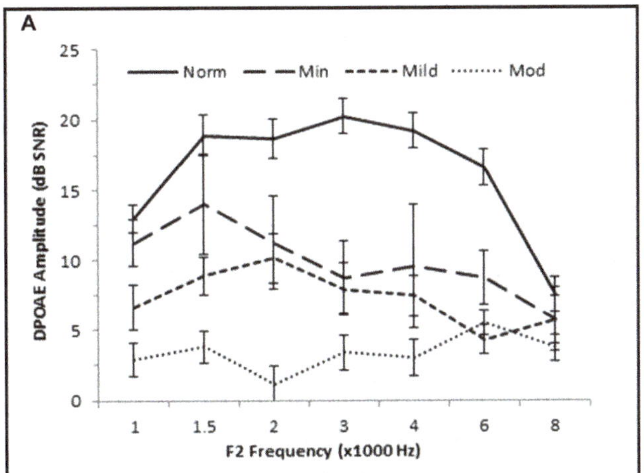

P values	1 kHZ	1.5 kHZ	2 kHZ	3 kHZ	4 kHZ	6 kHZ	8 kHZ
Norm-Min	.542	.224	.060	**.005**	**.038**	**.001**	.782
Norm-Mild	**.005**	**.001**	**.001**	**.000**	**.000**	**.000**	.332
Norm-Mod	**.000**	**.000**	**.000**	**.000**	**.000**	**.000**	.105
Min-Mild	.156	.172	.668	.944	.320	.100	.477
Min-Mod	**.009**	**.002**	**.004**	.109	**.028**	.346	.370
Mild-Mod	.111	**.024**	**.007**	.140	.103	.509	.494

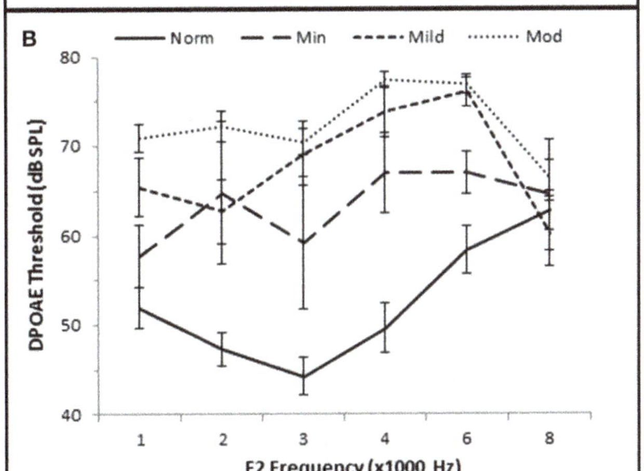

P values	1 kHZ	2 kHZ	3 kHZ	4 kHZ	6 kHZ	8 kHZ
Norm-Min	.291	**.033**	**.046**	**.025**	.293	.978
Norm-Mild	**.005**	**.001**	**.000**	**.000**	**.000**	.643
Norm-Mod	**.000**	**.000**	**.000**	**.000**	**.000**	.653
Min-Mild	.282	.670	.283	.154	**.016**	.857
Min-Mod	**.022**	.125	.333	.959	**.035**	.342
Mild-Mod	.157	**.047**	.939	.331	.709	.196

FIGURE 5 | OHC dysfunction occurs in minimal to moderate SNHL. (A) DPOAE SNR (amplitude) and threshold **(B)** from each group. The tables list the *p*-values between each group by stimulus frequency. Bold text indicates a $p < 0.05$. Norm, Normal Hearing Group; Min, Minimal SNHL; Mild, Mild SNHL; Mod, Moderate SNHL.

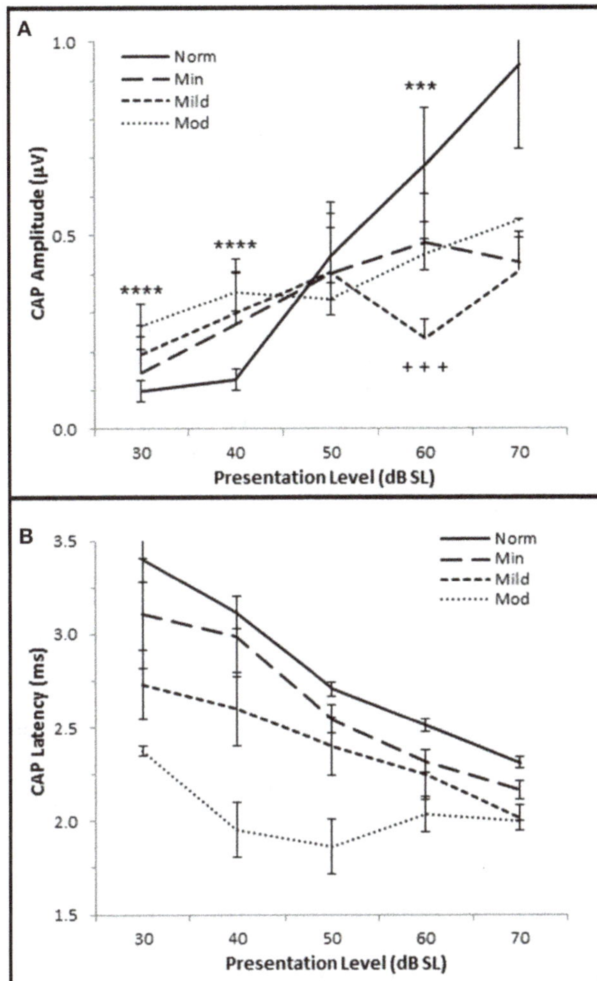

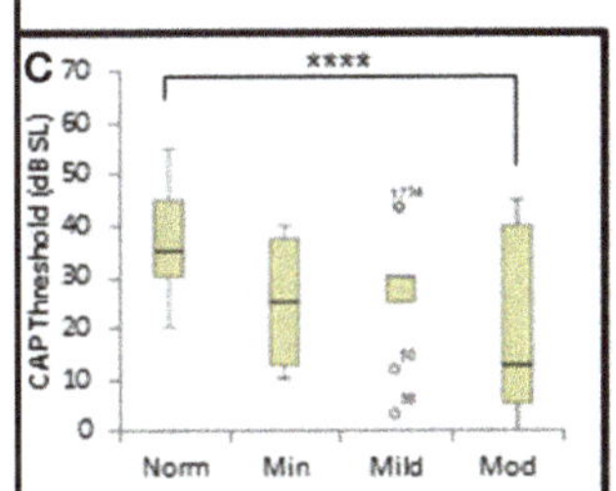

P values	30 dBSL	40 dBSL	50 dBSL	60 dBSL	70 dBSL
Norm-Min	.203	.670	.162	**.041**	.092
Norm-Mild	**.004**	**.014**	**.003**	**.001**	**.000**
Norm-Mod	**.000**	**.000**	**.000**	**.000**	**.000**
Min-Mild	.192	.174	.108	.395	.065
Min-Mod	**.003**	**.001**	**.005**	.277	.052
Mild-Mod	**.015**	**.011**	.068	.537	.617

FIGURE 6 | AN dysfunction occurs in mild to moderate SNHL. (A) Mean CAP amplitude from each group based on presentation level (dB SL). **(B)** CAP latency-intensity functions from each group. The table lists the *p*-values of CAP latency between each group by stimulus frequency. Bold text indicates a $p < 0.05$. **(C)** Box and whisker plots illustrating the median and range values of CAP thresholds for each group. Open circles represent suspected outliers, and numbers indicate the subject identification of the suspected outlier. Norm, Normal Hearing Group; Min, Minimal SNHL; Mild, Mild SNHL; Mod, Moderate SNHL; ***statistically significant difference between Normal and Mild SNHL groups; ****statistically significant difference between Normal and Moderate SNHL groups; +++statistically significant difference between Minimal SNHL and Mild SNHL groups.

= 0.00) at higher presentation levels. In contrast, subjects in the Minimum, Mild, and Moderate SNHL groups exhibited a steeper growth function at low intensity levels, and flatter growth function at 50 dB SL and above. J-T testing between groups showed that presentation levels below 50 dB SL elicited progressive increases in CAP amplitude between Normal hfPTA and Moderate SNHL groups. Specifically, the Moderate SNHL group exhibited a statistically significant ($p = 0.033$) 0.17 µV increase over the Normal hfPTA group at 30 dB SL, and a statistically significant ($p = 0.003$) 0.23 µV increase over the Normal hfPTA group at 40 dB SL. Interestingly, tone pip presentation levels >50 dB SL resulted in a statistically non-significant ($\tau\beta = -0.072$, $p = 0.497$; **Figure 2F**) trend in the opposite direction whereby the hearing impaired groups exhibited diminished CAP amplitudes compared to those in the Normal hfPTA group (**Figure 6A**). As can be seen by the error bars in **Figure 6A**, the group with better hearing exhibited increased amplitude variability at louder presentation levels. The only statistically significant difference between groups at louder presentation levels occurred at 60 dB SL between the Normal hfPTA and Mild SNHL groups (−0.45 μV difference, $p = 0.003$) and between Minimum and Mild SNHL groups (−0.23 μV difference, $p = 0.045$). Also unlike lower presentation levels, there was not a graded decrease in amplitude as a function of hfPTA at presentation levels above 50 dB SL. This may be due to the fact that many persons in the Moderate SNHL group had hfPTAs so great that the stimuli could either not be generated at such a high level (i.e., 105 dB SPL), or that these presentation levels were intolerably loud for the subjects.

In contrast to the variability observed in CAP amplitude, CAP latency-intensity functions exhibited a more consistent trend across groups. High frequency SNHL correlated with a statistically significant decrease in CAP latency at all presentation levels, with a maximum correlation coefficient at 30 dB SL (τ_b = 0–0.592, $p = 0.000$; **Figure 2G**). The J–T test (**Figure 6B**) showed that CAP latency-intensity functions exhibited a progressive and statistically significant decrease between Normal hfPTA groups and Mild SNHL (maximum latency shift at 30 dB SL of 0.67 ms, $p = 0.004$), and between Normal hfPTA and Moderate SNHL groups (maximum latency shift at 40 dB SL of 1.17 ms $p = 0.000$) at all intensity levels. Similarly, there was a statistically significant decrease in latency-intensity functions at lower levels of intensity between the Minimal and Moderate SNHL groups (−0.74 ms at 30 dB SL, $p = 0.003$; −1.04 ms at 40 dB SL, $p = 0.001$; −0.69 ms at 50 dB SL, $p = 0.001$), and the Mild and Moderate SNHL groups (−0.36 ms at 30 dB SL, $p = 0.015$; −0.65 ms at 40 dB SL, $p =$ 0.011).

In addition to CAP amplitude and latency, there was a statistically significant inverse correlation between hfPTA and CAP threshold ($\tau_b = -0.343$, $p = 0.001$; **Figure 2H**). J–T testing showed a statistically significant decrease in CAP threshold between the Normal hfPTA and Moderate SNHL groups (−15.7 dB SL difference, $p = 0.011$; **Figure 6C**). Although there was a significant correlation of decreased CAP threshold with high frequency SNHL, no other groups exhibited statistically significant differences between them.

Contrary to stimuli played at the same overall level dB SPL, stimuli played at equivalent SPL respective to pure tone average show that increased hearing loss leads to a general trend of lower CAP thresholds, shorter CAP latencies, and smaller CAP amplitudes at low presentation levels. At higher presentation levels, there was a general trend that hearing loss resulted in the expected results of decreases CAP amplitudes, however the trend that SNHL correlated with shorter CAP latencies was still evident. It should be noted that unlike the DPOAE results, there were no significant differences between the Normal hfPTA and Minimal SNHL groups in terms of CAP amplitude or threshold. In terms of CAP latency, the only statistically significant difference between these two groups was a −0.19 μV ($p = 0.041$) decrease that occurred at 60 dB SL presentation levels. Given these results, it is difficult to say there is a statistically significant difference between Normal hfPTA and Minimal SNHL in terms of AN activity. However, there is a statistically significant graded decrease in latency as SNHL increases from Mild to Moderate severity.

SIN Is Positively Correlated with OHC Function

Next, the data was analyzed to determine whether AN density, measured by CAP amplitude (Kujawa and Liberman, 2009), contributed to SIN performance. Since diminished DPOAE SNRs and increased DPOAE thresholds existed in the Minimal-Moderate SNHL groups (**Figure 5B**) only the Normal group (n = 29) was used in this analysis in order to control for OHC loss. The Normal group was ranked by CAP amplitudes at the 40 dB SL presentation level, and divided into high and low CAP amplitude groups based on whether their CAP amplitudes were either 1 s.e.m higher or 1 s.e.m lower than the Normal SNHL group mean of 156 μV (Low CAP < 156 μV < High CAP; **Figure 7A**). J–T testing indicated that persons with normal hfPTAs and normal OHC function who also exhibited higher CAP amplitudes exhibited statistically significantly shorter CAP latencies at higher presentation levels (maximum difference of −0.206 ms, $p = 0.002$; **Figure 7B**). This data suggest a general trend of an inverse relationship between CAP amplitude and latency at both low and high presentation levels when OHC function is normal. The data further showed there was no statistically significant differences in DPOAE SNRs between these two groups at most frequencies, however there was a statistically insignificant difference in DPOAE SNR at 4 k Hz (−5.1 dB SPL difference at 40 dB SL, $p = 0.048$; **Figure 7C**), while there were no statistically significant differences in DPOAE threshold between these groups (**Figure 7D**). Next, SIN and SIQ scores between these groups were analyzed to determine whether AN function played a solitary role in speech recognition. There were no significant differences in either SIQ (**Figure 7E**) or SIN (**Figure 7F**) performance in persons with diminished CAP amplitudes and normal OHC function. This data suggests that AN function by itself does not play a significant role in speech recognition in quiet or in the presence of background noise.

In order to determine which cell types play a role in speech discrimination in the presence of background noise, all of the subjects from each group were used to correlate SIN performance with OHC and AN function (**Figure 8**). The results indicated that SIN performance was correlated with DPOAE function, where lower QSIN scores (better performance in noise) inversely correlated with DPOAE SNR (maximum $\tau_b = -0.522$, $p = 0.000$ at 4 kHz; **Figure 8A**) and a directly correlated with DPOAE thresholds (maximum $\tau_b = 0.378$, $p = 0.000$ at 3 kHz; **Figure 8B**). To further investigate these correlations, subjects were ranked by QuickSIN scores, and were divided into either Normal SIN (QSIN < 1 dB SNR loss) or Poorer SIN (QSIN > 0 dB SNR loss) groups. It should be noted that the manufactures' QSIN

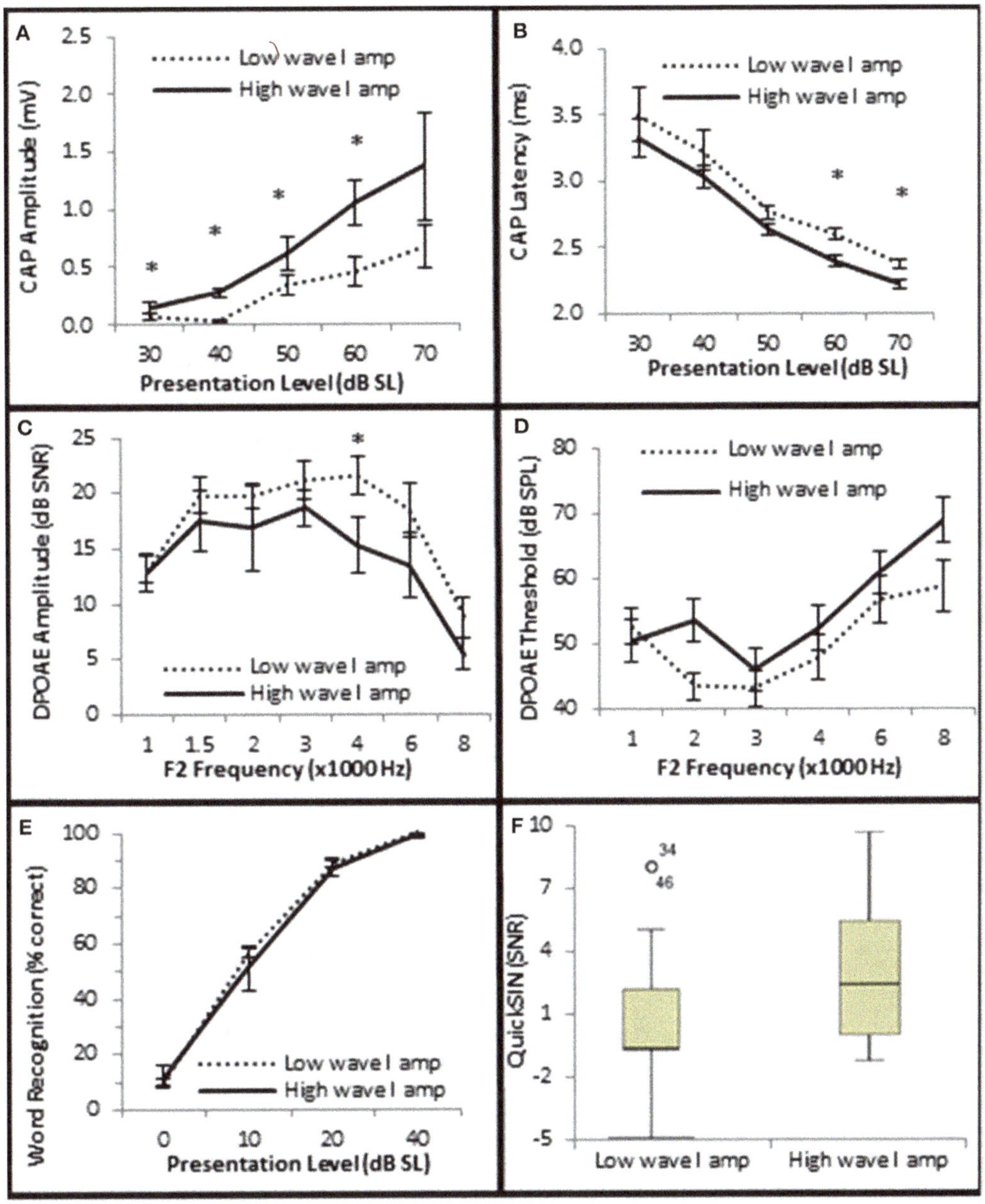

FIGURE 7 | Subjects with larger CAP amplitudes exhibited no significant improvement in SIQ or SIN when OHC function is normal. (A) Persons exhibiting normal OHC function (Normal Group) were subdivided into two groups (Low and High) based on whether their CAP amplitudes were either higher or lower than the group mean ± 1 s.e.m. Persons exhibiting normal OHC function and high CAP amplitudes exhibited statistically significant shorter CAP latencies at high presentation levels **(B)**, but failed to exhibit statistically significant differences in DPOAE SNRs **(C)** or DPOAE thresholds **(D)** at most frequencies. Speech testing showed no clinically significant differences in word recognition in quiet **(E)** or speech recognition ion the presence of background noise **(F)** between these groups. Panels **(A–E)** represent mean data +/1 1 s.e.m. Panel **(F)** is a box and whisker plot showing the median data (line within the box). Open circle represents suspected outliers, and numbers indicate the subject identification of the suspected outlier. *Statistically significant difference between groups.

cutoff score between normal and mild SIN impairment is 2 dB SNR loss, with 3 dB SNR loss representing "near normal." However, the new data presented in **Figure 5** demonstrates that OHC damage can occur in a person with a hfPTA as low as 15 dB HL, and **Figure 3C** shows that the QSIN cutoff for normal OHC function is -0.2 ± 0.3 dB SNR loss. Therefore, in order control for hidden hearing loss that was not accounted for by the manufactures of the QSIN, this paper will use a QSIN score of <1 dB SNR loss to differentiate between SIN performance in a non-pathological ear and a QSIN score >0 dB SNR loss to correspond to an SIN performance in a pathological ear.

The distribution of QSIN scores were roughly divided in half at 0 SNR Loss (**Figure 9A**), where 25 subjects performed better

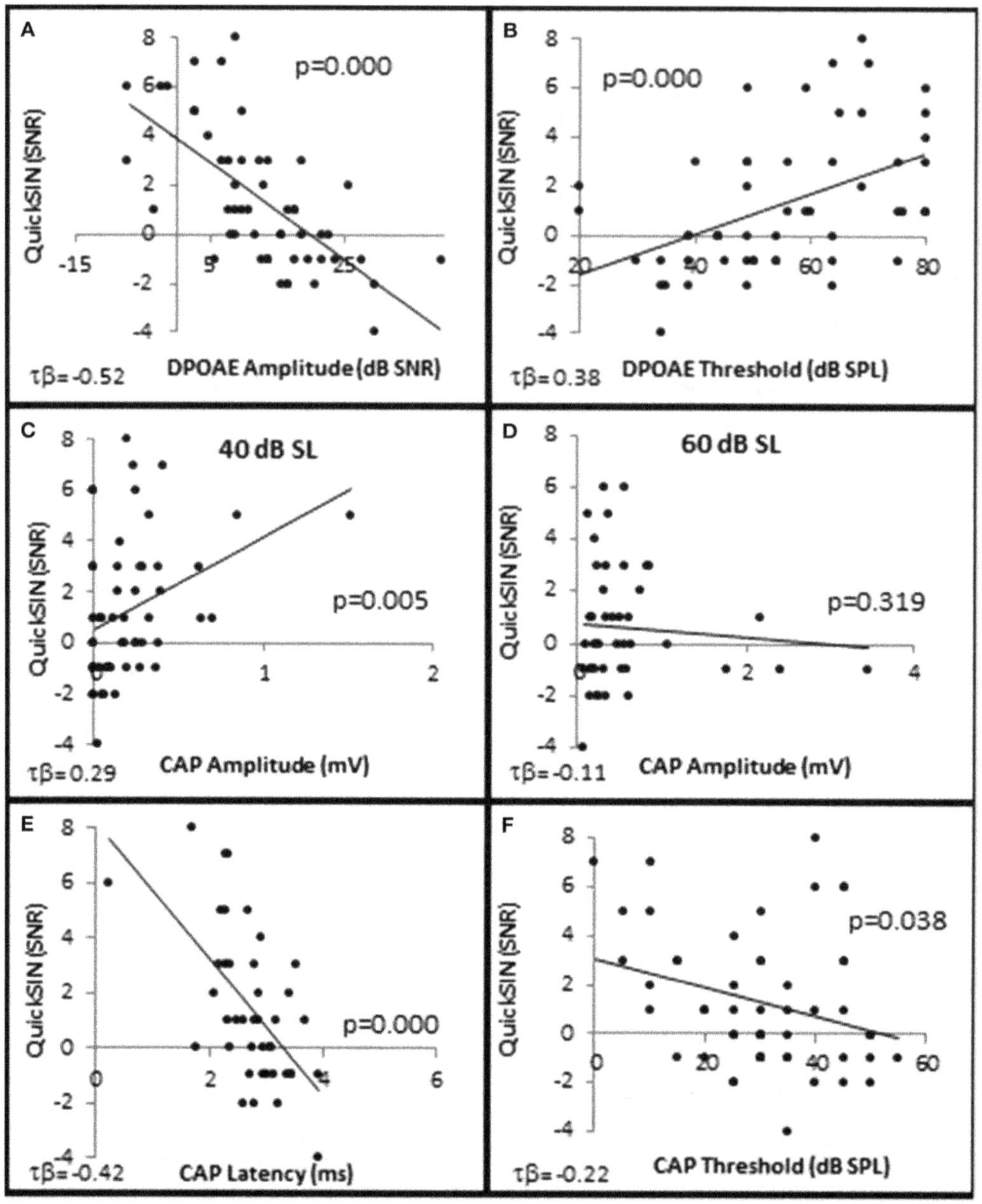

FIGURE 8 | Speech in noise performance is correlated with OHC function. Distribution of individual QuickSIN scores plotted as a function DPAOE amplitude **(A)**, DPAOE threshold **(B)**, CAP amplitude when the 4 kHz tone pip is presented at 40 dB SL **(C)**, and 60 dB SL **(D)**, CAP latency at 40 dB SL **(E)**, and CAP threshold **(F)**. As noted in the text, all correlations were statistically significant with the exception of **(D)**. Lines represent best fit (linear).

in background noise (Normal SIN) and 28 subjects performed worse in background noise (Poorer SIN). J-T testing showed that the group performing better in background noise had statistically significantly lower QuickSIN scores (QSIN $= -1.0 \pm 0.19$ SNR loss vs. 3.4 ± 0.43 SNR loss), which provides confidence that there is a statistically significant difference ($p = 0.000$) in performance in background noise between these groups (**Figure 9B**). Subjects performing better in background noise were statistically significantly younger (mean $= 39.7 \pm 2.71$ years vs. 52.6 ± 3.71 years, $p = 0.022$; **Figure 9C**) and had statistically significantly lower audiometric thresholds (hfPTA $= 10.0 \pm 2.29$ dB HL) compared to subjects with poorer performance in background noise (mean $= 33.6 \pm 2.71$ dB HL PTA, $p = 0.00$), with the latter group exhibiting a mild sloping SNHL above 1 kHz (**Figure 9D**). There were no clinically significant differences in word recognition in quiet between these two groups when NU-6 word lists were presented at any sensation levels (**Figure 9E**).

J-T testing showed that subjects exhibiting better speech discrimination in the presence of background noise also exhibited statistically significantly greater DPOAE SNRs from 1 to 6 kHz (maximum difference of 10.77 dB SNR at 4 kHz, $p = 0.00$; **Figure 9F**) and lower DPOAE thresholds from 1

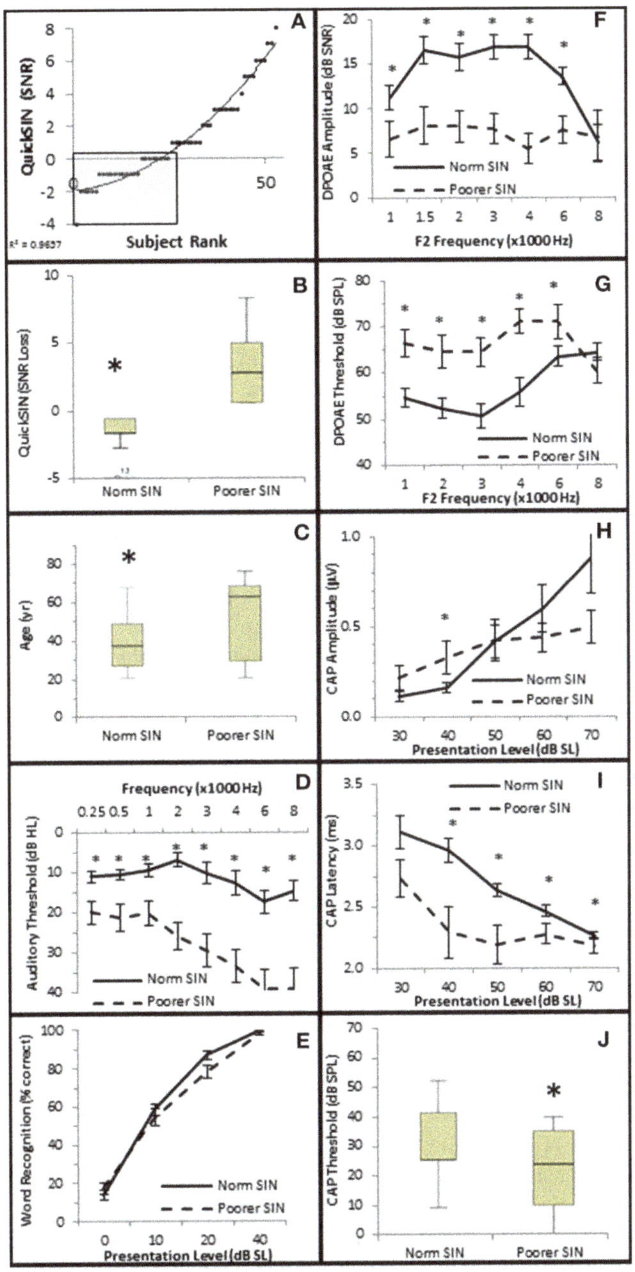

FIGURE 9 | Subjects performing better in noise were younger with better audiometric thresholds and better OHC functions. (A) Subjects were ranked by QuickSIN scores, and divided into either Normal SIN (QSIN < 1 dB SNR loss, shaded box) or Poorer SIN (QSIN > 0 dB SNR loss) groups as described in the text. Line represents best fit. **(B)** Box and whisker plots show statistically significant differences between these groups. Open circle represents suspected outliers, and numbers indicate the subject identification of the suspected outlier. Further comparison between these groups showed that those performing better in nose were younger **(C)** and exhibited better (lower) pure tone thresholds **(D)**. There were no clinically significant differences word recognition in quiet between these groups **(E)**. Persons performing better in the presence of background noise also exhibited more robust DPOAE SNRs **(F)** and lower DPOAE thresholds **(G)**. This group also exhibited lower CAP amplitude at 40 dB SL (**H**; compare with the normal line in **Figure 6A**), longer CAP latencies **(I)**, and lower CAP thresholds **(J)**. *Statistically significant difference between groups.

to 4 kHz (maximum difference of 15.11 dB SPL at 3 kHz, $p = 0.00$; **Figure 9G**) compared to subjects performing poorer in background noise. This data indicates that persons who performed better in background noise exhibited more robust DPOAE responses and suggests that loss of OHC function may diminish speech recognition in the presence of background noise.

Interestingly, the results suggest that the AN may also play a role in speech discrimination in the presence of background noise when OHC function is also abnormal. Similar to the Normal group in **Figure 6**, the Normal SIN group exhibited a statistically significant direct correlation between QSIN scores and CAP amplitude at presentation levels below 50 dB SL ($\tau_b = 0.285$, $p = 0.005$ at 40 dB SL; **Figure 8C**), and a non-significant inverse correlation at higher presentation levels (maximum $\tau_b = -0.111$, $p = 0.319$ at 60 dB SL; **Figure 8D**). J-T testing showed that while on average, those individuals performing better in background noise (i.e., lower QSIN scores) exhibited higher CAP amplitudes at louder presentation levels (above 50 dB SL), the variability in CAP amplitude also increased at higher presentation levels, particularly in the Normal group, so that no statistically significant differences in CAP amplitude existed between these groups (**Figure 9H**). In contrast, those individuals who performed better in background noise exhibited smaller CAP amplitudes when the tone pips were presented at lower presentation levels (below 50 dB SL), although this difference was only significant at 40 dB SL presentation levels (-0.178 µV difference, $p = 0.01$).

SIN performance exhibited a statistically significant inverse correlation with CAP latency (maximum $\tau_b = -0.423$, $p = 0.000$ at 40 dB SL; **Figure 8E**) and CAP threshold (maximum $\tau_\beta = -0.215$, $p = 0.038$ at 40 dB SL; **Figure 8D**). J-T testing demonstrated that those persons performing better in background noise exhibited statistically significantly longer CAP absolute latencies at presentation levels ranging from 40 to 70 dB SL (maximum difference of 0.553 ms at 40 dB SL, $p = 0.07$; **Figure 9I**) and statistically significantly higher CAP thresholds (mean = 34.8 dB SL) compared to those performing poorer in background noise (25.9 dB SL, $p = 0.03$; **Figure 9J**).

Therefore, the general pattern of AN function for persons with poor SIN performance (higher CAP amplitude at low presentation levels, shorter latencies, lower threshold) more closely resembled the AN dysfunction observed in the Minimal-Moderate hfPTA groups in **Figure 6** where the OHCs were damaged rather than the AN response measured from cochleas with normal OHC function (higher CAP amplitudes, longer CAP latencies) shown in **Figures 7A,B**. Taken together, this data suggests that the those subjects with poor SIN performance may exhibit AN dysfunction as well as OHC dysfunction.

To test this theory, a linear mixed effects model (Bramhall et al., 2015) was generated to predict the relative contributions of OHC and AN activity on SIN performance. This model predicted that the main effects of DPOAE amplitude and DPOAE threshold had significant effects on QSIN scores ($p = 0.01$ and $p = 0.04$, respectively; **Table 1**), but the main effects of CAP amplitude did not ($p = 0.25$). Furthermore, this model also predicted that the interaction between DPOAE and CAP amplitudes did not have a significant effect on QSIN scores ($p = 0.37$), nor did the

TABLE 1 | Linear mixed effects model of speech perception in noise.

Dependent variable	Predictor (Fixed effects)	Coefficient	Standard error	*p*-values
QuickSIN (SNR loss)	Intercept	2.661 (dB SNR Loss)	1.081103	**0.03**
	DOPAE amplitude (4 kHz)	−0.222 (dB SNR Loss/dB SNR)	0.073916	**0.01**
	DOPAE threshold (3 kHz)	0.071 (dB SNR Loss/dB SPL)	0.032974	**0.04**
	CAP amplitude (40 dB SL)	1.846 (dB SNR Loss/μV)	1.533834	0.25
	DPOAE * CAP amplitudes	0.159 (dB SNR Loss/dB SNR * μV)	0.168321	0.37
	DPOAE threshold * CAP amplitude	−0.589 (dB SNR Loss/dB SPL * μV)	0.083386	0.49

Bold text indicates a statistically significant p-value ≤ 0.05.

interaction between DPAOE thresholds and CAP amplitudes ($p = 0.49$). Furthermore, there were no statistically significant main effects or interaction effects on QSIN scores when factoring in CAP amplitudes at higher presentation levels (i.e., 60 dB SL), CAP latencies at any presentation level, or CAP thresholds into this model (data not shown). These results suggest that OHC function, rather than AN function, is a statistically significant predictor of SIN.

SIQ at or Near Threshold Is Correlated with OHC Function

In order to examine whether OHC and or AN function played a role in speech recognition in quiet, subjects were presented NU-6 word lists at equivalent SLs and the subjects' WRSs were correlated with OHC and AN function. The results showed that presentation Levels between 10 and 40 dB SL failed to yield clinically significant differences in any metric (data not shown). However, WRS presented at or near threshold was correlated with OHC function (**Figure 10**).

To further investigate this, subjects were divided into one of two groups depending upon their performance on the NU-6 word list presented at or near their individual thresholds (0 dB SL). Based on the 95% critical difference limits of the measured results listed in Thornton and Raffin (1978) (see in Table 5 of this reference), subjects were divided into either a poorer performing group who either scored 0% or 4% (one word) correct (Poorer WRS group, $n = 21$), or a better performing group who scored between 8 and 48% correct (Better WRS group, $n = 32$; **Figure 11A**). The 95% critical difference limits of Thornton and Raffin (1978) revealed a statistically significant performance gap between the Poorer WRS and Better WRS groups at presentation levels of 0 dB SL (0.8 ± 0.35% correct vs. 24.0 ± 1.2% correct). J–T testing of this same data similarly revealed a statistically significant difference between these groups ($p = 0.000$; **Figure 11B**). J–T testing between these groups at 10 dB SL also showed a difference between the Poorer WRS and Better WRS groups (43.8 ± 4.3 vs. 62.8 ± 2.9% correct), however, these results were not clinically significant when using the binomial modeling of speech discrimination typically used in the clinic (Thornton and Raffin, 1978).

Those subjects performing poorer in quiet near threshold were statistically significantly younger subjects (40.3 ± 3.38 years vs. 49.8 ± 3.27 years, $p = 0.047$; **Figure 11C**), with better high frequency hearing thresholds (maximum difference at 6 kHz of 14.5 dB HL, $p = 0.027$; **Figure 11D**). These two groups also exhibited statistically significant differences in hearing in the presence of background noise. Those subjects exhibiting poorer WRS at or near threshold performed better on the QSIN (0.2 ± 0.45 SNR loss) than those exhibiting better WRS in quiet at or near threshold (2.0 ± 0.53 SNR loss, $p = 0.045$; **Figure 11E**), suggesting that different mechanisms may be involved in speech perception in quiet at or near threshold and in the presence of background noise.

SIQ at or near threshold was inversely correlated with OHC function, where WRS was negatively correlated with DPAOE SNR (maximum $\tau b = -0.237$, $p = 0.019$ at 4 kHz; **Figure 10A**) and positively correlated with DPAOE threshold (maximum $\tau b = 0.216$, $p = 0.035$ at 2 kHz; **Figure 10B**). J–T testing showed statistically significant differences in OHC function between these groups with the Better WRS group exhibiting lower DPOAE amplitudes (maximum difference of −6.38 dB SNR at 4 kHz, $p = 0.005$; **Figure 11F**) and higher DPOAE thresholds (maximum difference of 9.43 dB SNR at 4 kHz, $p = 0.009$; **Figure 11G**) than their poorer performing counterparts.

While Better WRS performing groups on average exhibited larger CAP amplitudes (**Figure 11H**) and lower CAP thresholds (**Figure 11J**), neither of these effects were statistically significant. However, one component of the AN response correlated with word recognition at or near threshold in quiet. There was a statistically significant inverse correlation between WRS and CAP latency (maximum $\tau_b = -0.334$, $p = 0.003$ at 40 dB SL; **Figure 10D**). J–T testing showed that the Better WRS group exhibited shorter wave I absolute latencies (maximum difference of 0.74 ms at 40 dB SL, $p = 0.000$; **Figure 11I**) than the group performing poorer on WRS at or near threshold. This data suggests that persons with diminished OHC activity may perform better in quiet at or near thresholds when stimuli are presented at equivalent SLs.

DISCUSSION

The overall goal of this study was to investigate OHC and AN function in regards to speech discrimination in quiet and in presence of background noise. Animal studies have speculated that the multiple AN fiber innervation of individual IHCs may

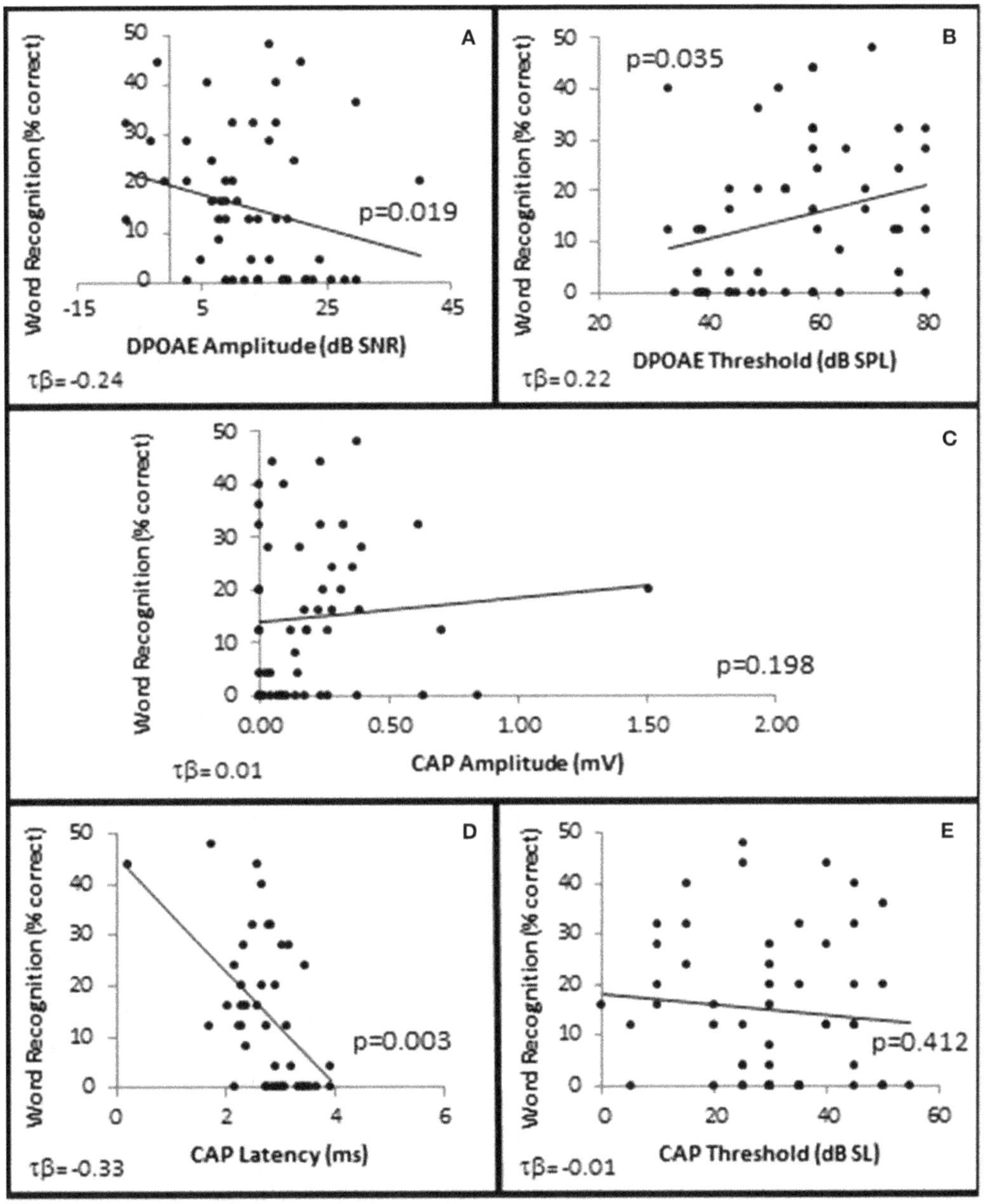

FIGURE 10 | SIQ at or near threshold is correlated with OHC function. Distribution of WRSs in quiet from all subjects presented at 0 dB SL as a function of DPAOE amplitude **(A)** and DPAOE threshold **(B)** at 4 k Hz; as well as AN function measured by CAP amplitude **(C)**, and latency **(D)** in response to 4 kHz tone pips presented at 40 dB SL, and CAP thresholds **(E)**. Lines represent best fit (linear).

function in complex listening situations such as speech detection in the presence of background noise (Schuknecht and Woellner, 1953; Kujawa and Liberman, 2009; Makary et al., 2011; Furman et al., 2013), however this theory is difficult to test using animal models. Furthermore, AN fiber density has been correlated to the wave I amplitude of the auditory brainstem response (ABR) in animal studies where OHC integrity has been preserved (Kujawa and Liberman, 2009; Lin et al., 2011), suggesting that wave I amplitude may be used as a tool to measure AN density. This paper attempted to determine whether ECochG CAP amplitude, which is synonymous with wave I of the ABR, correlated with SIN or SIQ in human subjects, and also to determine whether OHC function measured by DPOAEs contributed to these complex listening tasks.

A previous study using linear mixed effects models in humans similarly found that SIN was correlated to an inverse interaction between ECochG CAP amplitude and SNHL, while ECochG CAP amplitude had no effect on SIQ (Bramhall et al., 2015). This current study supports the later observation (**Figures 10C, 11H**). The aforementioned study used a 4 kHz tone pip presented at 70 dB SPL to evoke the CAP and found that subjects exhibiting both better audiometric thresholds and high ECochG CAP

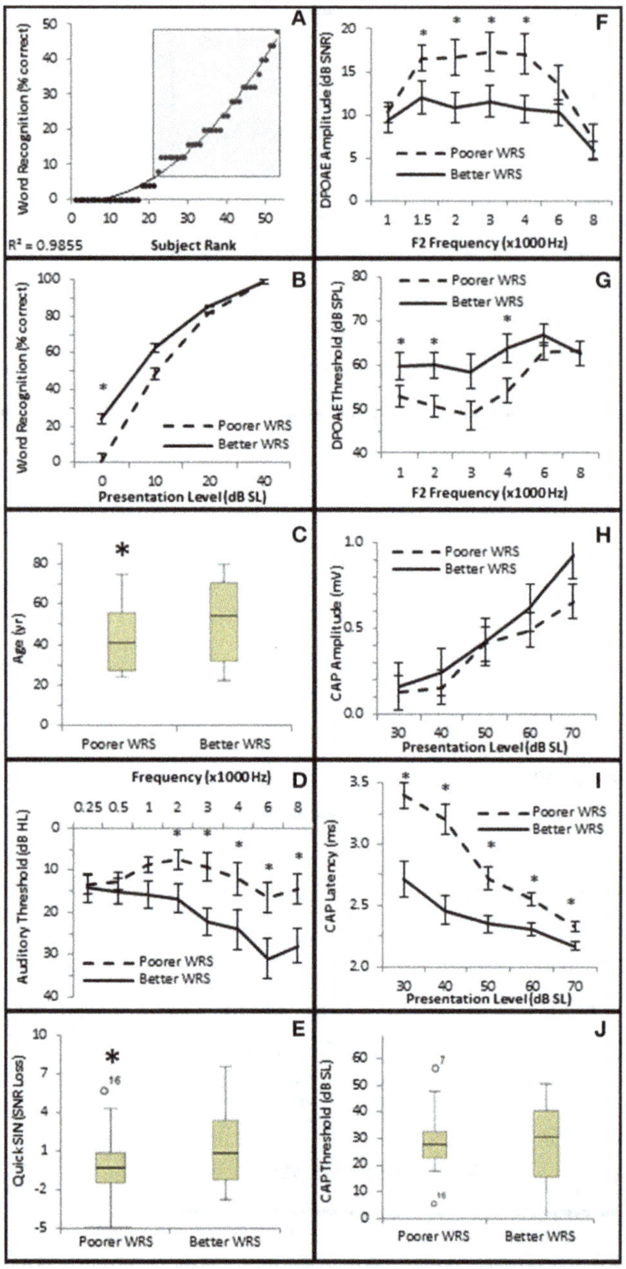

FIGURE 11 | Subjects with better SIQ performance at or near threshold exhibit OHC dysfunction. **(A)** Subjects were ranked by Word Recognition scores presented at 0 dB SL, and were divided into either Poorer (WRS < 8% correct) or Better (WRS > 4% correct, shaded box) groups as described in the text. Diagonal line represents best fit. Comparison between these groups showed that those performing better in quiet at or near threshold exhibited statistically significant improved WRS at low presentation levels **(B)**, were older **(C)**, with poorer (higher) pure tone thresholds **(D)**, and poorer (higher SNR Loss) speech in noise performance **(E)**. Persons performing better in quiet at or near threshold also exhibited diminished DPOAE SNRs **(F)** and higher DPOAE thresholds **(G)**, suggesting the OHC function plays a role in speech in quiet at or near threshold. This group failed to exhibit statistically significant differences in CAP amplitude **(H)** or threshold **(J)**. However, this same group exhibited statistically significantly lower CAP latencies **(J)**. Open circles in **(E,J)** represents suspected outliers, and numbers indicate the subject identification of the suspected outlier. *Statistically significant difference between groups.

amplitudes performed better on the QSIN. That study found inverse correlations between age and CAP amplitude, SNHL and CAP amplitude, SIN performance, and SNHL, however that study found no direct correlation between ECochG CAP amplitude and SIN performance. Rather, SIN performance was dependent on the inverse interaction between SNHL and ECochG CAP amplitude, where persons who exhibited both lower CAP amplitudes and poorer audiometric thresholds were found to have performed poorly in the presence of background noise. One possible reason why Bramhall et al. (2015) failed to find statistically significant differences between ECochG CAP amplitudes and SIN performance was the high variability in CAP amplitude, particularly among persons with PTAs <12.5 dB HL. Another possible factor could have been that both SIN performance and ECochG CAP amplitude were so strongly correlated with SNHL that the degree of hearing loss could mask differences in these variables. A third possibility could be that CAP amplitudes are not correlated with SIN in humans.

This current paper used graded SL presentations in order to correct for the effect of the degree of SNHL on ECochG CAP amplitude. These results suggest that a loss of tuning in pathological ears leads to level dependent changes in ECochG CAP amplitudes, shorter CAP latencies, and lower (better) CAP thresholds when stimuli were presented at equivalent SLs. Furthermore, these results indicate that normal OHC function is required for optimal SIN performance.

Effects of Diminished Cochlear Tuning on ECochG CAP Amplitudes

There were contrasting results related to ECochG CAP amplitude in this study depending on the intensity level of the tone pip used to evoke the CAP and the degree of SNHL exhibited by the subjects. On average, increased SNHL resulted in diminished ECochG CAP amplitudes at higher stimulus levels, however the opposite effect was observed at presentation levels below 50 dB SL (**Figure 6A**). There could be different causes for this observation. Considering first the Normal hfPTA group (solid line in **Figure 6A**), increasing presentation level likely increased the frequency spectrum of the stimuli, which may in turn affect the CAP amplitude (**Figure 12**). At lower presentation levels, the stimuli consisted of tone pips with limited frequency spectrum, but as the presentation intensity increased above 40 dB SL (Normal group) the frequency spectrum of the stimulus and the population of AN fibers activated by that stimulus would be expected to increase to more closely resemble a click (Pfeiffer and Kim, 1975). Therefore, higher presentation levels would recruit more AN fibers and increase the CAP amplitude and variability, which is seen in the normal group in **Figure 6A**. Placing the variability in CAP amplitude aside for the time being, it could be assumed that an increase in AN fiber activation would lead to increased CAP amplitudes at louder presentation levels, which is the general trend in this figure. This may explain the observation in **Figure 9H**, where persons with normal SIN performances who also have normal hfPTAs (**Figure 3C**) and normal OHC function (**Figure 5**) exhibit higher CAP amplitudes at louder presentation levels than persons with SNHL.

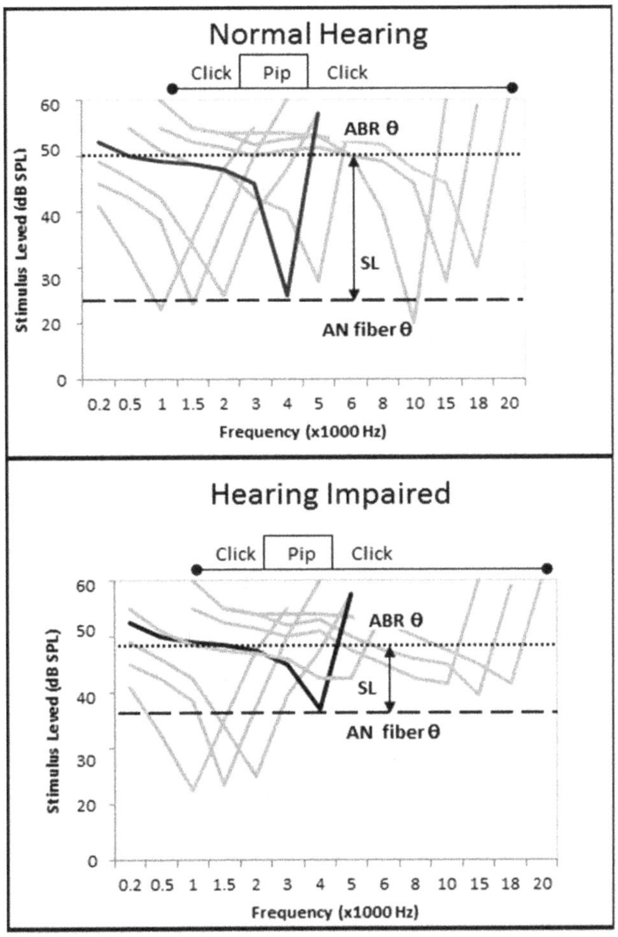

FIGURE 12 | Loss of cochlear tuning results in SL-dependent changes in CAP amplitude, shorter CAP latencies, and lower CAP thresholds. (Top) Hypothetical AN fiber tuning curves in a listener without otopathology illustrating the CF of a fiber tuned to 4 kHz (black) and off-tuned fibers (gray). The difference between the AN fiber threshold and ECochG threshold, which can be imagined as a subject's SL, occurs because the level must be raised by 25 dB SPL to recruit enough off-tuned AN fibers to evoke a CAP. When the tone pip is presented at a low level, relatively few AN fibers are recruited, so CAP amplitude is low. When the tone pip is presented at a higher level, the stimulus acquires the acoustic characteristics of a click and more off-fibers are recruited and CAP amplitude increases (compare with **Figure 6A**). **(Bottom)** OHC damage leads to increased audiometric thresholds, micromechanical distortions to BM vibrations, and changes in AN fiber tuning that include an elevation of AN fiber threshold and a broadening of off-fiber tuning. When a 4 kHz tone pip stimulus is presented at a low SL, the net effect of this otopathology is a hypersensitivity of off-fiber tuning that leads to recruitment of more off-tuned ANF fibers, lower CAP thresholds, shorter CAP latencies, and higher CAP amplitudes. At higher presentation levels where the stimuli acquires characteristics of a click, the otopathology leads to a decrease in the number off-tuned AN fibers that can be recruited so the CAP amplitude does not increase as drastically as seen in the non-pathological ear (**Figure 6A**), and a CAP amplitude decreases in comparison to the non-pathological ear.

On the other hand, lower presentation levels suggest the opposite effect. In these cases, persons in the Normal hfPTA group exhibited lower CAP amplitudes than those with moderate SNHL (**Figure 6A**), and also performed better in noise (**Figure 9H**), the latter of which is expected clinically in a person with normal hearing. This data shows that as hearing impairment increased from minimal to moderate SNHL, the amplitude of CAP increased and the SIN performance decreased in response to lower SL presentations. This increase in CAP amplitude at low SL exhibited by persons with SNHL may be attributed to a combination of two factors. First, a loss of tuning caused by OHC dysfunction would be expected to lead to a broadening of the BM vibration at a given frequency (Liberman and Dodds, 1984). This loss of tuning, or loss of the cochlear amplifier, should result in a change of AN fiber tuning, where the characteristic frequency (CF) of a given AN fiber becomes elevated (threshold elevation) and its tuning curve becomes broader and exhibits a hypersensitivity in adjacent AN fibers with higher CFs (Liberman and Dodds, 1984). Since auditory evoked responses are more sensitive (lower thresholds) in the high frequency regions of the cochlea (Goldstein et al., 1971), this shift in tuning to a higher frequency may recruit more AN fibers to fire for a given stimulus (Pfeiffer and Kim, 1975), and would increase CAP amplitude (**Figure 6A**), decrease CAP latency (**Figure 6B**), and lower CAP threshold (**Figure 6C**). One way to explain this data is with linear systems theory (Goldstein et al., 1971; Liberman and Dodds, 1984; Ruggero, 1994; Henry et al., 2011), where the OHCs function as a bank of frequency filters that fine-tune the response of not only the BM, but the AN fibers as well. This fine-tuning means that fewer AN fibers are recruited in a non-pathological ear for a low SL presentation, and the CAP amplitude is relatively lower, CAP latency is relatively longer, and CAP threshold is relatively higher. Loss of the OHC filter function results in a broadening of the region of AN activation even for low SL presentations that is reflected in the increase in CAP amplitude in those persons with OHC damage (i.e., Minimal to Moderate SNHL groups in **Figure 6A**).

The second process causing the increase in CAP amplitude at low SL exhibited by persons with SNHL may be due to the SPL of the stimuli needed to elicit an AN response. For a normal cochlea, a 4 kHz tone pip presented at 40 dB SL (i.e., 40 dB HL in a normal ear) would elicit activation of a select population of AN fibers whose CFs are close to this place of resonance on the BM. The loss of OHCs would lead to a broadening of BM resonance, a change in AN tuning, and a decrease in PTA. In these patients, a tone pip presented at 40 dB HL may be sub-threshold and not activate enough AN fibers to elicit a CAP, and so the intensity level would have to be raised to reach CAP threshold. In such cases, those persons with a moderate SNHL would need a 40 dB SL stimulus that is presented at a higher SPL (i.e., 70 dB HL) to recruit enough AN fibers to elicit a CAP. This loud presentation level would lead to a broader area of BM resonance and would activate a larger population of AN fibers (Pfeiffer and Kim, 1975) that would result in higher CAP amplitudes. In this case, the fact that they are low presentation levels on the SL scale may obfuscate the fact that a more intense signal is required to elicit a response. This observation is born out in **Figure 6A** where persons exhibiting SNHL have a comparatively more linear growth function than the non-linear function of the Normal hfPTA group.

The CAP amplitude-intensity function, therefore, can be used to estimate two different sites of lesions of the 8th cranial nerve. At lower presentation levels, the 4 kHz tone pip may be measuring specific damage to cells that affect the tuning to this frequency, while at higher presentation levels, this stimulus loses its frequency specificity but measures the activity of a greater population of the AN fibers. Therefore, measuring AN activity using the SL based CAP amplitude-intensity function is a way to measure both site specific and more global AN dysfunction. That being said, measuring CAP amplitude in humans has some inherent complications.

Unlike laboratory animals, ECochG CAP, and ABR amplitudes are notoriously variable in humans (Gorga et al., 1985; Winzenburg et al., 1993; Burkhard et al., 2007; Hall, 2007). Causes of this variability include placement of the recording electrode and physiological noise inherent in these recordings. The typical ECochG recording methods include a trans-tympanically needle electrode placed on the base of the cochleae, a wick electrode placed on or near the tympanic membrane as in this current study, or gold foil wrapped triptodes placed near the opening of the external auditory meatus. Bramhall et al. (2015) used triptodes and also found a large variability in ECochG CAP amplitude, and the decision to move to a wick electrode near the tympanic membrane for this study was an attempt to address this variability. While the magnitude of the amplitudes had increased as the recording was conducted closer to the cochlea in the paper presented here, there were no statistically significant changes in the variability of the amplitude between triptodes and wick electrode methods (data not shown). This observation is born out in the literature as well (Winzenburg et al., 1993). Another source of variability has been attributed to the presence intrasubject noise consisting of both electromyographical and electroencephalographical artifacts (Zvonar et al., 1974), which is diminished in animal studies because animals are normally sedated during ABR testing while humans are typically not sedated. Further studies on sedated humans could be conducted to determine whether sedation leads to a lower variability in CAP amplitude as observed in animal studies. Sex genotype also plays a role in ABR amplitude and latency (Don et al., 1993). However, differences in sex should not affect this analysis because the subjects were divided in groups based on their behavioral or physiological responses irrespective of their sex. Regardless, the intake questionnaire of this study didn't differentiate between gender identity and sex genotype, the latter of which presumably exerts a stronger effect on CAP amplitudes than the former. Therefore, a complete analysis of sex genotype/gender effects on these findings would be warranted in future studies.

Finally, a recent study has proposed using the ratio between the summating potential (SP) and action potential (AP) of ECochG CAP to estimate AN dysfunction in humans (Liberman et al., 2016). Reanalysis of the data presented in this paper utilizing the AP/SP analysis described in Liberman et al. (2016) showed that SP/AP ratio had no significant correlations to either SIN or SIQ described in this paper (data not shown). The difference between this current paper and the aforementioned paper could be due to the different methods of SIN testing. Here, the QSIN, which consisted of target sentences presented in increasing levels of background speech babble, was used because it has face validity for clinical applications. However, Liberman et al. (2016) saw significant differences in SIN performance between musicians and non-musicians when using a more complex SIN protocol consisting of 45% or 65% time compressed NU 6 word lists presented with 0.3 s reverberation and in ipsilateral narrowband noise. This is a more complex task that may be required to detect changes in AN dysfunction and which may or may not have translational correlations related to noise exposure or AN integrity. A comparative analysis between these different SIN assessments is warranted in future experiments.

Effects of Diminished Cochlear Tuning on CAP Latency and Threshold

In contrast to amplitude, absolute or inter-peak latency is a less variable metric and is used clinically for ABR analysis in humans (Hecox and Galambos, 1974). Factors that contribute to ECochG CAP latency include the cochlear transport time (Don et al., 1993), which is influenced by passive properties of the basilar membrane such as the stiffness gradient and mass loading; cochlear filter build-up time, which involves the "cochlear amplifier" processes (Davis, 1983), where OHC depolarization sharpens the tuning of the basilar membrane and shifts the frequency of resonance more apically; the neurotransmission time that involves the summation potential, AN synchrony, and frequency characteristics of the AN fibers; and frequency and intensity characteristics of the acoustic stimuli which would influence all of these processes (reviewed in Don et al., 1998). It has been proposed that OHC dysfunction results in the loss of the cochlear filter build-up time, which would result in the decrease in ABR latency observed in patients with cochlear (sensory), as opposed to retrocochlear, hearing loss (Don et al., 1998; Lichtenhan and Chertoff, 2008; Henry et al., 2011). As mentioned previously, OHC damage is also known to cause hyper-sensitivity in the tail regions of AN fiber tuning curves (Liberman and Dodds, 1984), which is theorized to lead to a shift in AN fiber tuning to higher frequencies that would decrease the latency in hearing impaired individuals (Goldstein et al., 1971; Lichtenhan and Chertoff, 2008; Strelcyk et al., 2009; Henry et al., 2011). As mentioned above, increasing the stimulus intensity may also increase the population of active AN fibers, which would be expected to decrease the latency as well. Therefore, CAP latency may be affected by OHC dysfunction, altered AN tuning, and stimulus variables.

The data presented in **Figure 6B** indicates that ECochG CAP latency decreases with increasing SNHL when the stimulus is presented at equivalent SLs. This data is the opposite of many studies that found either increased age or increased SNHL resulted in an increase in ABR wave latency in response to click evoked stimuli (Attias and Pratt, 1984; Gorga et al., 1985; Gourevitch et al., 2009). However, those studies used broad band stimuli presented at a constant presentation level and did not control for the effect of hearing loss on the stimulus level. In order to correct for an individual's hearing threshold on stimulus intensity, this current study presented stimuli relative to their individual audiometric thresholds, or SL. The results presented in this paper indicate that CAP latency is inversely proportional to an individual's hearing loss when the stimulus is presented at equivalent SLs. This observation is similar to previous studies where sensory hearing loss was correlated with a decrease in absolute CAP (Lichtenhan and Chertoff, 2008) and ABR wave V latency in humans (Don et al., 1998; Strelcyk et al., 2009; Scheidt et al., 2010) and a decrease in absolute wave I amplitudes and latencies in chinchillas (Henry et al., 2011) when narrow band stimuli (derived-band ABR and tone burst, respectively) were presented at equivalent SLs.

Our data indicates a general trend of an inverse relationship between ECochG CAP amplitude and latency at both low and high presentation levels (**Figures 6A,B**) when OHC function is normal. These data also suggests that ECochG CAP latency is a more reliable metric than CAP amplitude to differentiate between normal and abnormal SIN (**Figure 9I**) and SIQ (**Figure 11I**) performance. ECochG CAP amplitude is more variable compared to CAP latency (**Figure 1**), and different presentation levels result in changes in relative amplitude (**Figures 6A**, **9H**, **11H**). In comparison, ECochG CAP latency is a more reliable predictor of SNHL, SIN, and SIQ. However, while wave I amplitude has been correlated to AN density in animal models, the contribution of AN fiber density on wave I latency has not been determined and further animals studies examining this are warranted.

Similar to latency, ABR thresholds, rather than amplitudes, are routinely used clinically in humans but not without criticism (Eggermont, 1982). Here, we demonstrated that ECochG CAP thresholds decreased with increasing hearing loss at equivalent presentation levels (**Figure 6C**). As explained in the preceding discussion, stimulus effects, and decreased tuning would explain the decrease in ECochG CAP thresholds when constant stimulus intensity is used. In non-pathological ears, there is typically a 25 dB SPL difference between AN fiber threshold and CAP threshold (Ngan and May, 2001; Henry et al., 2011). Animal data has shown that hearing impairment causes an upward compression of both AN fiber thresholds (Liberman, 1978) and ABR threshold range (Ngan and May, 2001) that may reduce the difference between AN fiber and CAP thresholds and act to lower ABR thresholds in hearing impaired subjects. Support for this theory is presented in this paper when considering that hearing impaired subjects (older subjects with poorer audiometric thresholds and poorer OHC function) exhibit lower CAP thresholds that their normal hearing counterparts when stimuli are presented on an SL scale (**Figure 9J**).

Anatomical Correlates of SIN and SIQ

The effect of SIN performance on ECochG CAP amplitude was not as initially expected. The initial hypothesis was that CAP amplitude, which correlates with AN fiber density when using click stimuli, would directly correlate with SIN performance. However, when controlled for normal OHC function, those individuals with higher CAP amplitudes (**Figure 7A**) failed to exhibit statistically significant differences in either SIQ (**Figure 7E**) or SIN (**Figure 7F**) performance compared to those exhibiting lower CAP amplitudes. This suggests that SIN performance is not correlated with CAP amplitude, and therefore SIN is not correlated to AN fiber density. Alternatively, it could be that the differences in amplitude between these two groups is too similar and needs to be greater than we defined in this paper to show a statistically significant difference in SIN performance. Further studies in a larger population of persons with normal DPOAEs and diminished CAP amplitudes may be required to definitively determine whether reduced CAP amplitudes correlated with reduced SIN performance. As mentioned previously, it could be that more challenging SIN assessments, such as time compressed speech in reverberation, may find a statistically significant difference between these groups. However, these current results suggest that when controlled for OHC damage, CAP amplitude by itself is not a predictor of either SIN or SIQ performance.

Since ECochG CAP latency includes components of OHC function and neural transmission, comparing CAP latency and DPOAE results may help to determine whether OHCs or the AN contribute to the behavioral response. For instance, the data presented in **Figure 6B** indicates there is not a significant difference in latency between the Normal and Minimal SNHL groups, whereas **Figure 5** indicates that OHC amplitudes and OHC thresholds are diminished in the Minimal SNHL group. This suggests that persons exhibiting minimal SNHL exhibit OHC dysfunction rather than statistically significant AN dysfunction. The data also suggests that speech in noise performance is correlated with both OHC function (**Figures 8A,B**, **9F,G**) and CAP latency (**Figures 8E**, **9I**), with persons performing better in the presence of background noise (lower QSIN score) exhibiting more robust OHC responses (higher DPOAE SNRs and lower DPOAE thresholds), and longer CAP latencies (Normal group) than those performing poorer in background noise. These results suggest that the AN may play a role in SIN, however as mentioned above, several variables contribute to CAP latency and so it cannot be concluded that AN dysfunction contributes to SIN by analyzing CAP latency alone.

These results provide scant evidence that AN integrity is a major variable contributing to SIN performance. The observation that persons performing better in noise also exhibit both lower CAP amplitudes at lower SLs (**Figures 8C**, **9H**) and lower CAP thresholds (**Figures 8F**, **9J**), which are profiles consistent with normal hearing, bolster the hypothesis that the AN also plays a role in SIN, however the CAP amplitude data was only significant at one low presentation level (40 dB SL; **Figure 9H**). Further evidence of both OHC and AN involvement in SIN performance can be seen when analyzing loss of function in SNHL patients. These results suggest that OHC dysfunction may occur in minimal degrees of SNHL (**Figure 5**), while AN dysfunction may not be statistically significant until greater degrees of SNHL (mid SNHL for CAP latency effects, and moderate SNHL for CAP amplitude and threshold effects; **Figure 6**). Furthermore, there are no statistically significant differences in SIN between Normal hfPTA and Minimal SNHL groups (**Figure 3C**), but statistically significant differences in SIN performance first appear in the Mild SNHL group. These results suggest the possibility that AN dysfunction may play a role in decreased SIN performance. However, the linear mixed effects model, which is a statistical approach that incorporated the variances associated with every variable measured in this study into a single statistical model, showed that CAP amplitude failed to have a statistically significant correlation with SIN performance

(**Table 1**). Furthermore, this model showed that both DPOAE amplitude and DPAOE thresholds are correlated with QSIN scores, which suggests that OHC function is a primary variable contributing to SIN performance using the QuickSIN.

Similarly, results from the SIQ study can be used to differentiate between the OHC and AN components in CAP latency measures. As shown in **Figure 10**, persons with better WRS in quiet at or near threshold exhibited poorer OHC function (**Figures 10A,B, 11F,G**) and shorter CAP latencies (**Figures 10D, 11I**), but exhibit equivocal CAP amplitudes (**Figures 10C, 11H**) and thresholds (**Figures 10H, 11J**). Since ECochG CAP latency encompasses both OHC and AN functions, and there are no differences in CAP threshold or amplitude between these groups, one conclusion could be that OHC dysfunction rather than AN (dys)function enhances SIQ performance at or near threshold. This can be explained by the normally sharp tuning of the BM and subsequent sharp tuning of the AN fibers through normal OHC function, which act as a bank of filters with an end result that limits SIQ performance at or near threshold. OHCs may act more like a filter bank at low presentation levels that enhances frequency sensitivity measured by pure tone thresholds (**Figure 11D**) but diminishes speech discrimination performance in quiet at or near threshold (**Figure 11E**). Another explanation for improved SIQ performance may be due to the increased presentation levels to those persons exhibiting SNHL. As can be seen in **Figure 11D**, on average those persons performing better in quiet also exhibit a sloping SNHL. Therefore, it could be that these persons utilize low frequency information for speech recognition in quiet at or near threshold. It is possible that both processes, OHC damaged filter function coupled with the increased stimulus levels, leads to enhanced SIQ performance at or near threshold. Further studies analyzing the correlation between slope and degree of SNHL would be helpful in describing the contributions of OHC dysfunction and signal level in SIQ performance.

There may be a behavioral correlate for this in humans. Some persons with SNHL also exhibit an unusual growth in the perception of loudness, termed loudness recruitment (Dix et al., 1948). The data presented here suggests that loudness recruitment may be acting at the level of the inner ear. Previous studies and have shown that OHC damage causes hypersensitivity in the tail region of the damaged AN fiber tuning curve, which has been interpreted to mean that one role of the OHC is to decrease the sensitivity of AN fibers tuned to adjacent CFs (Liberman and Dodds, 1984). In this sense, individual OHCs may function as a band-pass filter to dampen the stimulation of adjacent AN fibers. Loss of this function would lead to recruitment of adjacent AN fibers, which is consistent with the hypothesis that loudness recruitment is caused by OHC dysfunction (Moore, 2002). Furthermore, it may be that AN dysfunction also plays a role in this phenomenon. Since low spontaneous rate fibers are more susceptible to damage, they may be missing in this population and high spontaneous rate fibers, which function in quite backgrounds, are likely left intact (Furman et al., 2013). Therefore, it could be that the neural pathway in persons with SNHL is optimized for speech understanding in quiet at or near threshold.

Unhidden Hearing Loss: Profile of SNHL

It is well-documented that the standard audiogram in insufficient to adequately describe the underlying otopathology that causes SNHL (Merchant and Nadol, 2010). Proper definition of the functional roles of inner hair cells (IHCs), OHCs, and AN fibers is essential for the understanding of the cellular basis of audition. As important, biotechnologies using drug, cell based, or gene therapies aimed at regenerating hair cells or AN fibers (reviewed in Parker, 2011) will depend upon proper assessment of these cell types in order to identify the underlying otopathologies involved in SNHL. Improvements on hearing aid and cochlear implant technologies can also be made if the functions of the OHCs and AN fibers are known and are incorporated into their signal processing algorithms.

The data presented in **Figure 5A** suggests that OHC function is correlated with pure tone audiometry, and that even subjects with minimal high frequency SNHL may exhibit significant OHC damage. However, since a PTA between 15 and 25 dB HL is often considered within the normal range in adult humans, this finding illustrates an example of an undetected otopathology commonly known as "Hidden Hearing Loss (HHL)," which can be defined as an otopathology that is not recorded by the standard audiogram. Several subtypes of HHL have been described including auditory synaptopathy (Furman et al., 2013), auditory neuropathy (Starr et al., 1996; Makary et al., 2011), and OHC dysfunction (Gorga et al., 1997). This latter study examined DPOAEs in 806 subjects and found that OHC dysfunction was evident with a PTA of 20 dB HL or greater, which is within the 10–25 dB HL range typically used as clinically normal in human hearing. The data presented here argues for a lowering of the normative range cut-off from 20 dB HL (Gorga et al., 1997) to 15 dB HL and suggests that a minimal SNHL is a clinical presentation of an underlying OHC otopathology. As previously mentioned, recent studies have suggested that synaptopathy/auditory neuropathy can also occur in persons with PTAs below 25 dB HL (Liberman et al., 2016; Bramhall et al., 2017), even if the degree of impairment in this group is debatable (Prendergast et al., 2017). Therefore, there is growing evidence that the standard audiogram is a poor representation of the underlying otopathologies that cause SNHL and a holistic assessment may be more appropriate to better target future treatments.

From the data presented in this paper, the profile of SNHL can be defined as follows; a typically older person with a higher hfPTA, poorer OHC function (lower DPOAE SNR, higher DPOAE thresholds), poorer AN function (higher CAP amplitude at low presentation levels, lower CAP amplitude at higher presentation levels, shorter CAP latencies, lower CAP thresholds when controlled for SNHL), poorer SIN performance, and better SIQ performance at or near threshold. All of these characteristics can be easily measured using standard audiometric techniques presented in this paper. The data presented here indicates that those persons exhibiting SNHL perform better in quiet at or near threshold and may shed light on the anatomical correlates associated with increased sensitivity to loud sounds experienced by those afflicted with SNHL.

Rather than use a standard SPL scale, this paper used a SL scale in order to correct for the degree of SNHL. This scale is useful when considering the perception of the individual with hearing loss and may be useful in assessing therapies from the patient's perspective. For instance, while a 40 dB HL stimulus presented to a person with normal hearing is perceived, this same stimulus presented to a person with SNHL may be imperceived because it may be presented at a sub-threshold level. Therefore, the stimulus level must be increased in order for the hearing impaired listener to detect this signal; however, the signal being detected may be distorted, the loss of OHCs would lead to a broader region of the BM being deflected, and a larger population of AN fibers with modified tuning may be recruited to elicit a CAP. This may lead to a different listening experience between those with normal and pathological ears, which can be particularly problematic in terms in terms of amplification provided by hearing aids. The observation that persons with OHC dysfunction may actually perform better in quiet at or near threshold may be exploited in future technologies where speech in noise detection, rather than amplification, would be the targeted therapy.

AUTHOR CONTRIBUTIONS

RH assisted in experimental design and performed Electroacoustic measurements. GE and SP assisted in experimental design, recruited subjects, and collected audiometric and DPAOE data. MP designed all experiments, wrote the IRB application, analyzed the data, and wrote the manuscript.

FUNDING

This work was supported by departmental funds from the Department of Otolaryngology, Head and Neck Surgery at Steward St. Elizabeth's Medical Center in Boston, MA.

ACKNOWLEDGMENTS

The authors would like to thank Stephane Maison for reviewing and editing this manuscript prior to submission.

REFERENCES

Attias, J., and Pratt, H. (1984). Auditory evoked potentials and audiological follow-up of subjects developing noise-induced permanent threshold shift. *Audiology* 23, 498–508. doi: 10.3109/00206098409070089

Bewick, V., Cheek, L., and Ball, J. (2004). Statistics review 10: further nonparametric methods. *Crit. Care* 8, 196–199. doi: 10.1186/cc2857

Bramhall, N. F., Konrad-Martin, D., McMillan, G. P., and Griest, S. E. (2017). Auditory brainstem response altered in humans with noise exposure despite normal outer hair cell function. *Ear Hear.* 38, e1–e12. doi: 10.1097/AUD.0000000000000370

Bramhall, N., Ong, B., Ko, J., and Parker, M. (2015). Speech perception ability in noise is correlated with auditory brainstem response wave I amplitude. *J. Am. Acad. Audiol.* 26, 509–517. doi: 10.3766/jaaa.14100

Brownell, W. E., Bader, C. R., Bertrand, D., and de Ribaupierre, Y. (1985). Evoked mechanical responses of isolated cochlear outer hair cells. *Science* 227, 194–196. doi: 10.1126/science.3966153

Burkhard, R., Don, M., and Eggermont, J. J. (2007). *Auditory Evoked Potentials.* Baltimore, MD: Lippincott Williams & Wilkins.

Carhart, R., and Jerger, J. (1959). Preferred methods for clinical determination of pure-tone thresholds. *J. Speech Hear. Disord.* 24, 330–345. doi: 10.1044/jshd.2404.330

Davis, H. (1983). An active process in cochlear mechanics. *Hear. Res.* 9, 79–90. doi: 10.1016/0378-5955(83)90136-3

Dix, M. R., Hallpike, C. S., and Hood, J. D. (1948). Observations upon the loudness recruitment phenomenon, with especial reference to the differential diagnosis of disorders of the internal ear and 8th nerve. *J. Laryngol. Otol.* 62, 671–686. doi: 10.1017/S0022215100009518

Don, M., Ponton, C. W., Eggermont, J. J., and Kwong, B. (1998). The effects of sensory hearing loss on cochlear filter times estimated from auditory brainstem response latencies. *J. Acoust. Soc. Am.* 104, 2280–2289. doi: 10.1121/1.423741

Don, M., Ponton, C. W., Eggermont, J. J., and Masuda, A. (1993). Gender differences in cochlear response time: an explanation for gender amplitude differences in the unmasked auditory brain-stem response. *J. Acoust. Soc. Am.* 94, 2135–2148. doi: 10.1121/1.407485

Eggermont, J. J. (1982). The inadequacy of click-evoked auditory brainstem responses in audiological applications. *Ann. N.Y. Acad. Sci.* 388, 707–709. doi: 10.1111/j.1749-6632.1982.tb50839.x

Furman, A. C., Kujawa, S. G., and Liberman, M. C. (2013). Noise-induced cochlear neuropathy is selective for fibers with low spontaneous rates. *J. Neurophysiol.* 110, 577–586. doi: 10.1152/jn.00164.2013

Goldstein, J. L., Baer, T., and Kiang, N. Y. S. (1971). "A theoretical treatment of latency, group delay, and tuning characteristics for auditory-nerve responses to clicks and tones," in *Physiology of the Auditory System,* ed M. B. Sachs (Baltimore, MD: National Education Consultants), 133–141.

Gorga, M. P., Neely, S. T., Ohlrich, B., Hoover, B., Redner, J., and Peters, J. (1997). From laboratory to clinic: a large scale study of distortion product otoacoustic emissions in ears with normal hearing and ears with hearing loss. *Ear Hear.* 18, 440–455. doi: 10.1097/00003446-199712000-00003

Gorga, M. P., Worthington, D. W., Reiland, J. K., Beauchaine, K. A., and Goldgar, D. E. (1985). Some comparisons between auditory brain stem response thresholds, latencies, and the pure-tone audiogram. *Ear Hear.* 6, 105–112. doi: 10.1097/00003446-198503000-00008

Gourevitch, B., Doisy, T., Avillac, M., and Edeline, J. M. (2009). Follow-up of latency and threshold shifts of auditory brainstem responses after single and interrupted acoustic trauma in guinea pig. *Brain Res.* 1304, 66–79. doi: 10.1016/j.brainres.2009.09.041

Hall, J. W. (2007). *New Handbook of Auditory Evoked Responses.* Boston, MA: Pearson.

Hecox, K., and Galambos, R. (1974). Brain stem auditory evoked responses in human infants and adults. *Arch. Otolaryngol.* 99, 30–33. doi: 10.1001/archotol.1974.00780030034006

Henry, K. S., Kale, S., Scheidt, R. E., and Heinz, M. G. (2011). Auditory brainstem responses predict auditory nerve fiber thresholds and frequency selectivity in hearing impaired chinchillas. *Hear. Res.* 280, 236–244. doi: 10.1016/j.heares.2011.06.002

House, W. F. (1974). Goals of the cochlear implant. *Laryngoscope* 84, 1883–1887. doi: 10.1002/lary.5540841104

Jerger, J., Jerger, S., and Mauldin, L. (1972). Studies in impedance audiometry. I. Normal and sensorineural ears. *Arch. Otolaryngol.* 96, 513–523. doi: 10.1001/archotol.1972.00770090791004

Kemp, D. T. (1978). Stimulated acoustic emissions from within the human auditory system. *J. Acoust. Soc. Am.* 64, 1386–1391. doi: 10.1121/1.382104

Killion, M. C., Niquette, P. A., Gudmundsen, G. I., Revit, L. J., and Banerjee, S. (2004). Development of a quick speech-in-noise test for measuring signal-to-noise ratio loss in normal-hearing and hearing-impaired listeners. *J. Acoust. Soc. Am.* 116, 2395–2405. doi: 10.1121/1.1784440

Kujawa, S. G., and Liberman, M. C. (2006). Acceleration of age-related hearing loss by early noise exposure: evidence of a misspent youth. *J. Neurosci.* 26, 2115–2123. doi: 10.1523/JNEUROSCI.4985-05.2006

Kujawa, S. G., and Liberman, M. C. (2009). Adding insult to injury: cochlear nerve degeneration after "temporary" noise-induced hearing loss. *J. Neurosci.* 29, 14077–14085. doi: 10.1523/JNEUROSCI.2845-09.2009

Lasky, R. E. (1984). A developmental study on the effect of stimulus rate on the auditory evoked brain-stem response. *Electroencephalogr. Clin. Neurophysiol.* 59, 411–419. doi: 10.1016/0168-5597(84)90042-X

Liberman, M. C. (1978). Auditory-nerve response from cats raised in a low-noise chamber. *J. Acoust. Soc. Am.* 63, 442–455. doi: 10.1121/1.381736

Liberman, M. C., and Dodds, L. W. (1984). Single-neuron labeling and chronic cochlear pathology. III. Stereocilia damage and alterations of threshold tuning curves. *Hear Res* 16, 55–74. doi: 10.1016/0378-5955(84)90025-X

Liberman, M. C., Epstein, M. J., Cleveland, S. S., Wang, H., and Maison, S. F. (2016). Toward a differential diagnosis of hidden hearing loss in humans. *PLoS ONE* 11:e0162726. doi: 10.1371/journal.pone.0162726

Lichtenhan, J. T., and Chertoff, M. E. (2008). Temporary hearing loss influences post-stimulus time histogram and single neuron action potential estimates from human compound action potentials. *J. Acoust. Soc. Am.* 123, 2200–2212. doi: 10.1121/1.2885748

Lin, H. W., Furman, A. C., Kujawa, S. G., and Liberman, M. C. (2011). Primary neural degeneration in the Guinea pig cochlea after reversible noise-induced threshold shift. *J. Assoc. Res. Otolaryngol.* 12, 605–616. doi: 10.1007/s10162-011-0277-0

Makary, C. A., Shin, J., Kujawa, S. G., Liberman, M. C., and Merchant, S. N. (2011). Age-related primary cochlear neuronal degeneration in human temporal bones. *J. Assoc. Res. Otolaryngol.* 12, 711–717. doi: 10.1007/s10162-011-0283-2

Merchant, S. N., and Nadol, J. B. (2010). *Schuknecht's Pathology of the Ear, 3rd Edition*. Shelton, CT: PMPH-USA.

Moore, B. C. (2002). Psychoacoustics of normal and impaired hearing. *Br. Med. Bull.* 63, 121–134. doi: 10.1093/bmb/63.1.121

Ngan, E. M., and May, B. J. (2001). Relationship between the auditory brainstem response and auditory nerve thresholds in cats with hearing loss. *Hear. Res.* 156, 44–52. doi: 10.1016/S0378-5955(01)00264-7

Parker, M. A. (2011). Biotechnology in the treatment of sensorineural hearing loss: foundations and future of hair cell regeneration. *J. Speech Lang. Hear. Res.* 54, 1709–1732. doi: 10.1044/1092-4388(2011/10-0149)

Pfeiffer, R. R., and Kim, D. O. (1975). Cochlear nerve fiber responses: distribution along the cochlear partition. *J. Acoust. Soc. Am.* 58, 867–869. doi: 10.1121/1.380735

Prendergast, G., Guest, H., Munro, K. J., Kluk, K., Leger, A., Hall, D. A., et al. (2017). Effects of noise exposure on young adults with normal audiograms I: electrophysiology. *Hear. Res.* 344, 68–81. doi: 10.1016/j.heares.2016.10.028

Ruggero, M. A. (1994). Cochlear delays and traveling waves: comments on 'Experimental look at cochlear mechanics.' *Audiology* 33, 131–142. doi: 10.3109/00206099409071874

Scheidt, R. E., Kale, S., and Heinz, M. G. (2010). Noise-induced hearing loss alters the temporal dynamics of auditory-nerve responses. *Hear. Res.* 269, 23–33. doi: 10.1016/j.heares.2010.07.009

Schuknecht, H. F., and Woellner, R. C. (1953). Hearing losses following partial section of the cochlear nerve. *Laryngoscope* 63, 441–465. doi: 10.1288/00005537-195306000-00001

Starr, A., Picton, T. W., Sininger, Y., Hood, L. J., and Berlin, C. I. (1996). Auditory neuropathy. *Brain* 119(Pt 3), 741–753. doi: 10.1093/brain/119.3.741

Strelcyk, O., Christoforidis, D., and Dau, T. (2009). Relation between derived-band auditory brainstem response latencies and behavioral frequency selectivity. *J. Acoust. Soc. Am.* 126, 1878–1888. doi: 10.1121/1.3203310

Thornton, A. R., and Raffin, M. J. (1978). Speech-discrimination scores modeled as a binomial variable. *J. Speech Hear. Res.* 21, 507–518. doi: 10.1044/jshr.2103.507

Winzenburg, S. M., Margolis, R. H., Levine, S. C., Haines, S. J., and Fournier, E. M. (1993). Tympanic and transtympanic electrocochleography in acoustic neuroma and vestibular nerve section surgery. *Am. J. Otol.* 14, 63–69.

Zvonar, M., Zvonar-Kuhndl, B., and Odenthal, D. W. (1974). Anaesthesia and Sedation For Electrocochleography. *Acta. Otolaryngol.* 77(Suppl. 316), 37–38. doi: 10.1080/16512251.1974.11675745

16

Intraoperative Electrocochleographic Characteristics of Auditory Neuropathy Spectrum Disorder in Cochlear Implant Subjects

*William J. Riggs[1], Joseph P. Roche[2], Christopher K. Giardina[3], Michael S. Harris[1], Zachary J. Bastian[3], Tatyana E. Fontenot[3], Craig A. Buchman[4], Kevin D. Brown[3], Oliver F. Adunka[1] and Douglas C. Fitzpatrick[3]**

[1] Department of Otolaryngology/Head and Neck Surgery, Ohio State University College of Medicine, Columbus, OH, United States, [2] Lab Department of Otolaryngology/Head and Neck Surgery, University of Wisconsin School of Medicine, Madison, WI, United States, [3] Department of Otolaryngology/Head and Neck Surgery, The University of North Carolina at Chapel Hill School of Medicine, Chapel Hill, NC, United States, [4] Department of Otolaryngology/Head and Neck Surgery, Washington University School of Medicine in St. Louis, St. Louis, MO, United States

***Correspondence:**
Douglas C. Fitzpatrick
douglas_fitzpatrick@med.unc.edu

Auditory neuropathy spectrum disorder (ANSD) is characterized by an apparent discrepancy between measures of cochlear and neural function based on auditory brainstem response (ABR) testing. Clinical indicators of ANSD are a present cochlear microphonic (CM) with small or absent wave V. Many identified ANSD patients have speech impairment severe enough that cochlear implantation (CI) is indicated. To better understand the cochleae identified with ANSD that lead to a CI, we performed intraoperative round window electrocochleography (ECochG) to tone bursts in children (n = 167) and adults (n = 163). Magnitudes of the responses to tones of different frequencies were summed to measure the "total response" (ECochG-TR), a metric often dominated by hair cell activity, and auditory nerve activity was estimated visually from the compound action potential (CAP) and auditory nerve neurophonic (ANN) as a ranked "Nerve Score". Subjects identified as ANSD (45 ears in children, 3 in adults) had higher values of ECochG-TR than adult and pediatric subjects also receiving CIs not identified as ANSD. However, nerve scores of the ANSD group were similar to the other cohorts, although dominated by the ANN to low frequencies more than in the non-ANSD groups. To high frequencies, the common morphology of ANSD cases was a large CM and summating potential, and small or absent CAP. Common morphologies in other groups were either only a CM, or a combination of CM and CAP. These results indicate that responses to high frequencies, derived primarily from hair cells, are the main source of the CM used to evaluate ANSD in the clinical setting. However, the clinical tests do not capture the wide range of neural activity seen to low frequency sounds.

Keywords: cochlear implants, electrocochleography, auditory neuropathy spectrum disorder, intraoperative, pediatrics, cochlear microphonic

INTRODUCTION

Auditory neuropathy spectrum disorder (ANSD) is a hearing dysfunction characterized by an apparent discrepancy between the measures of cochlear and neural function when viewed by surface electrode auditory brainstem response (ABR) testing. Relatively healthy hair cells are identified by the presence of otoacoustic emissions (OAEs) and/or cochlear microphonic (CM) in ABR testing, coupled with small or absent wave V (Kaga et al., 1996; Starr et al., 1996; Berlin et al., 1998; Rance et al., 1999; Teagle et al., 2010). A wide range of etiologies and associations for ANSD has been identified, including perinatal hyperbilirubinemia, mechanical ventilation, infection (measles, mumps), mutations in the otoferlin gene and cochlear nerve deficiency (Starr et al., 2001; Varga et al., 2003; Buchman et al., 2006; Bielecki et al., 2012). Proposed sites of lesion include the inner hair cells (IHCs), the synapse between the IHCs and the type I afferents of the auditory nerve, the auditory nerve itself, and the synapse between the auditory nerve fibers and their targets in the cochlear nucleus (Starr et al., 1996; Doyle et al., 1998; Zeng et al., 1999; Berlin et al., 2003; Fuchs et al., 2003; Rapin and Gravel, 2003). Many subjects with ANSD have hearing loss and/or speech perception deficits severe enough that treatment with a cochlear implant (CI) is indicated. A number of studies of the electrocochleography (ECochG) of ANSD subjects receiving CIs have been done, however these studies used acoustic stimuli specialized for this group such as high frequency 8 kHz tone pips or clicks (McMahon et al., 2008; Santarelli et al., 2008; Santarelli, 2010; Stuermer et al., 2015). While high frequencies may be useful in diagnosis, most of the ECochG responses in CI subjects, in both children and adults, are in fact to low frequencies (Fitzpatrick et al., 2014; McClellan et al., 2014; Formeister et al., 2015). Thus, to compare ANSD with non-ANSD subjects, responses to both high and low frequencies must be obtained. For this study, we recorded responses to tones across the frequency range in CI subjects, both children and adults, with and without ANSD.

Speech perception outcomes with cochlear implantation, including those with ANSD, demonstrate wide variations from patient to patient (Cohen et al., 1991; Gantz et al., 1993; Firszt et al., 2004; Holden et al., 2013). Most studies have failed to demonstrate specific factors or combinations of factors that account for more than about 25% of the variance in outcomes (Shea et al., 1990; Fayad et al., 1991, 2006; Gantz et al., 1993; Shipp and Nedzelski, 1995; Blamey, 1997; Nadol, 1997; Shipp et al., 1997; Rubinstein et al., 1999; Friedland et al., 2003; Lazard et al., 2012; Blamey et al., 2013). A recent measure used in both adults and children is the "total response" seen in the ECochG responses (ECochG-TR), which is the sum of the spectral peaks in response to tones of different frequencies. In adults, the ECochG-TR has been shown to account for about 40–50% of the variance in speech perception outcomes (Fitzpatrick et al., 2014; McClellan et al., 2014). In a specific group of children old enough for word test scores to be administered, the ECochG-TR accounted for 32% of the variance (Formeister et al., 2015). Thus, ECochG-TR provides a description of residual cochlear physiology that could prove useful in providing counseling and rehabilitation on the basis of patient-specific factors.

When using low frequency tones, the "on-going response" (continuous steady state response to tones) of the ECochG signal, which is used to calculate the ECochG-TR, is typically composed of the cochlear microphonic (CM) and the auditory nerve neurophonic (ANN). The CM is derived from currents through mechano-sensitive transduction channels in the stereocilia of hair cells (Dallos, 1973), and the ANN is the evoked potential correlate of phase-locking in auditory nerve fibers (Snyder and Schreiner, 1984; Henry, 1995). It is similar to the frequency-following response recorded from the scalp, except that the phase-locking represented is dominated by the auditory nerve rather that brainstem sources. Potentials more commonly seen to high frequencies include the compound action potential (CAP) and summating potential (SP). The CAP represents synchronous firing of auditory nerve fibers to the onsets of sounds, and the SP is derived from complex mixture of sources that roughly follows the envelope, which to tones is a sustained baseline offset. In short, the CM is a hair cell potential, the ANN and CAP are neural potentials, and the SP is affected by hair cell and neural sources capable of envelope-following. Unfortunately, methods to quantify the contributions of the different sources to each potential are lacking, particularly in CI subjects. The major contributor to the TR is the CM, but to low frequencies in many cases the ANN is also present. Although, the presence of the ANN affects the patterns of distortions and spectral components in the recording, a quantitative separation is not currently available. In addition, the morphology of the CAP in CI subjects is highly variable (Scott et al., 2016), and to low frequencies it is mixed with the CM while to high frequencies it can be mixed with the SP, so quantification is difficult. Thus, there is at present no method for determining the proportion of the ECochG that can be considered neural. However, the presence and to an approximation the strength of the ANN and CAP are visually apparent in the recordings, so the approach used here was to score these components individually and add the results to produce a "nerve score" in each case. The CM and SP to high frequencies were also measured as clues to the relative contributions of hair cells to the ECochG.

METHODS

Data in this study include 296 ears from 267 subjects (29 were second sides). Of these, 285 ears were studied under the approval of the Institutional Review Board (IRB) at the University of North Carolina at Chapel Hill (#05-2616) and 11 ears from the Ohio State University (OSU) and Nationwide Children's Hospital (Ohio State University IRB approval #2015H0045). Adults and pediatric (<18 years of age) CI recipients who were English speaking or whose parents were English speaking, and whose ear for implantation was not atretic, were offered enrollment in the study. Written informed consent was obtained from all adults, and parental/guardian consent was obtained for all pediatric subjects. Children who had attained 7 years of age were also asked to assent to participate in the study. In the situation where both ears were implanted and recorded, each ear was considered separately.

ANSD Subjects

A total of 48 ears (39 subjects) were in the ANSD group, 45 ears from children and 3 from adults. The evaluation and management paradigm for children with ANSD is the same between participating study institutions, which for UNC has been published previously (Buchman et al., 2006; Roche et al., 2010; Teagle et al., 2010; Hang et al., 2012). The diagnosis of ANSD was established by the finding of absent or disordered auditory neural activity in the setting of preserved cochlear function, typically established with ABR and OAE testing. Preserved cochlear function was determined when OAEs were present or the early part of the ABR waveforms demonstrated reversal of polarity with alternation of the stimulus polarity in either click or pure tone testing- representing a present CM. Most children were diagnosed with ANSD in our tertiary institutions though some were referred for treatment after a diagnosis was established. All available diagnostic tests were reviewed to confirm the electrophysiological phenotype and diagnosis. The adults all underwent routine CI evaluation, and were tested with a "click" ABR to confirm CM presence. Other groups used for comparison included children (119 ears, 101 subjects) and adults (163 ears, 158 subjects) undergoing cochlear implantation who were not classified as having ANSD.

Surgical and Recording Setup

All ECochG recordings were made to acoustic stimulation from the round window (RW) intraoperatively during CI surgery. For the purposes of this study, a foam insert earphone was placed and secured in a manner to prevent occlusion of the sound tubing. The inverting and common electrodes were placed behind the contralateral mastoid and on the glabella, respectively. A standard transmastoid facial recess approach was employed. The anterosuperior portion of the RW overhang was drilled to provide better access to the RW niche. A monopolar electrode (Neurosign, Magstim Co., Wales, UK or Neuro-Kartush raspatory probe instrument, Integra, Plainsboro, NJ, U.S.A.) was then placed with the tip situated immediately within the RW niche. Impedance of the RW and surface electrodes were measured and recordings were terminated if any had impedances of greater than 16 kilo-ohms (kΩ) that could not be reduced below this point. Saline was introduced into the RW niche if the monopolar electrode impedance was high; this was typically enough to bring the impedance measurement to an acceptable level. The Bio-logic Navigator Pro (Natus Medical Inc., San Carlos, CA) system was used to generate acoustic stimuli and record responses. Acoustic stimuli were delivered from Etymotic speaker (ER-3b) through sound tubing and insert earphones. Responses to a frequency series were performed in all subjects, and in most subjects a level series was then performed at the frequency which elicited the strongest response during the prior sweep (typically 500 Hz). The frequency series consisted of 250, 500, 750, 1,000, 2,000, and 4,000 Hz tone bursts presented in alternating phase at 90 dB nHL (101–112 dB SPL). A Blackman window was used to shape the tone bursts which had 1–4 ms rise and fall times with plateaus ranging from 5 to 20 ms (lower frequencies 250–750 Hz had shorter rise and fall times with longer plateaus compared to higher frequencies). Next the level series began at 90 dB nHL and was typically performed in 10 dB decrements until no response was seen during the recordings. Condensation, rarefaction, as well as the difference and sums of pairs of these were stored as averages in separate buffers. A final trial was included where the sound tubing was occluded with a surgical clamp to ensure the recorded responses were not speaker artifact.

Physiologic Analysis

The ECochG results were processed and analyzed using custom software routines written in MATLAB. The condensation and rarefaction traces were extracted and used to calculate the sum and difference waveforms. To evaluate the overall residual response magnitude from each cochlea we measured the "total response," or ECochG-TR, from the ongoing, steady-state part of the response to the tones (Fitzpatrick et al., 2014). To estimate the proportion of the neural as opposed to hair cell activity we developed a "nerve score" based on visual analysis of the CAP and ANN.

ECochG-TR

For each frequency a window (4–12 cycles per window dependent on frequency with bin widths ranging from 62 Hz at 250–331 Hz at 4,000 Hz) that isolated the ongoing portion, which occurs after the CAP and prior to the end of the stimulus, was selected for a fast Fourier transform (FFT) to analyze the spectral characteristics of the response. A significant response at a given stimulus frequency or harmonic was present if it exceeded the noise level by three standard deviations. The noise and its variance were determined from up to 6 bins, 3 on each side of the peak that were outside the ranges of response to the stimulus frequency. Responses that were not significant were given a value of 0.02 μV, which is the limit of our detection threshold, when included in summary data. The ECochG-TR was calculated as the sum of the magnitudes of the significant responses at the first, second and third harmonics across all 6 stimulus frequencies, all presented at 90 dB nHL. The first and third harmonics were measured from the difference of the two phases, and the second harmonic from the sum.

Nerve Score

In the Introduction, we described some of the issues related to measuring and separating the different potentials in the ECochG. Here, we will describe the presumed sources for each potential and describe in more detail the issues with more quantitative measurements that lead to the development of the nerve score. In **Figures 1A–C** we show schematics of the sources of the CM, ANN and CAP, respectively. The CM is derived from the opening and closing of transduction channels in the stereocilia of hair cells that follows the sinusoidal motion of the basilar membrane. However, the input/output function of each hair cell has limits based on saturation of channel openings or closings, so the CM is only nearly sinusoidal to low intensities (**Figure 1A**; see Russell, 2008 for a review). In addition, the saturation in

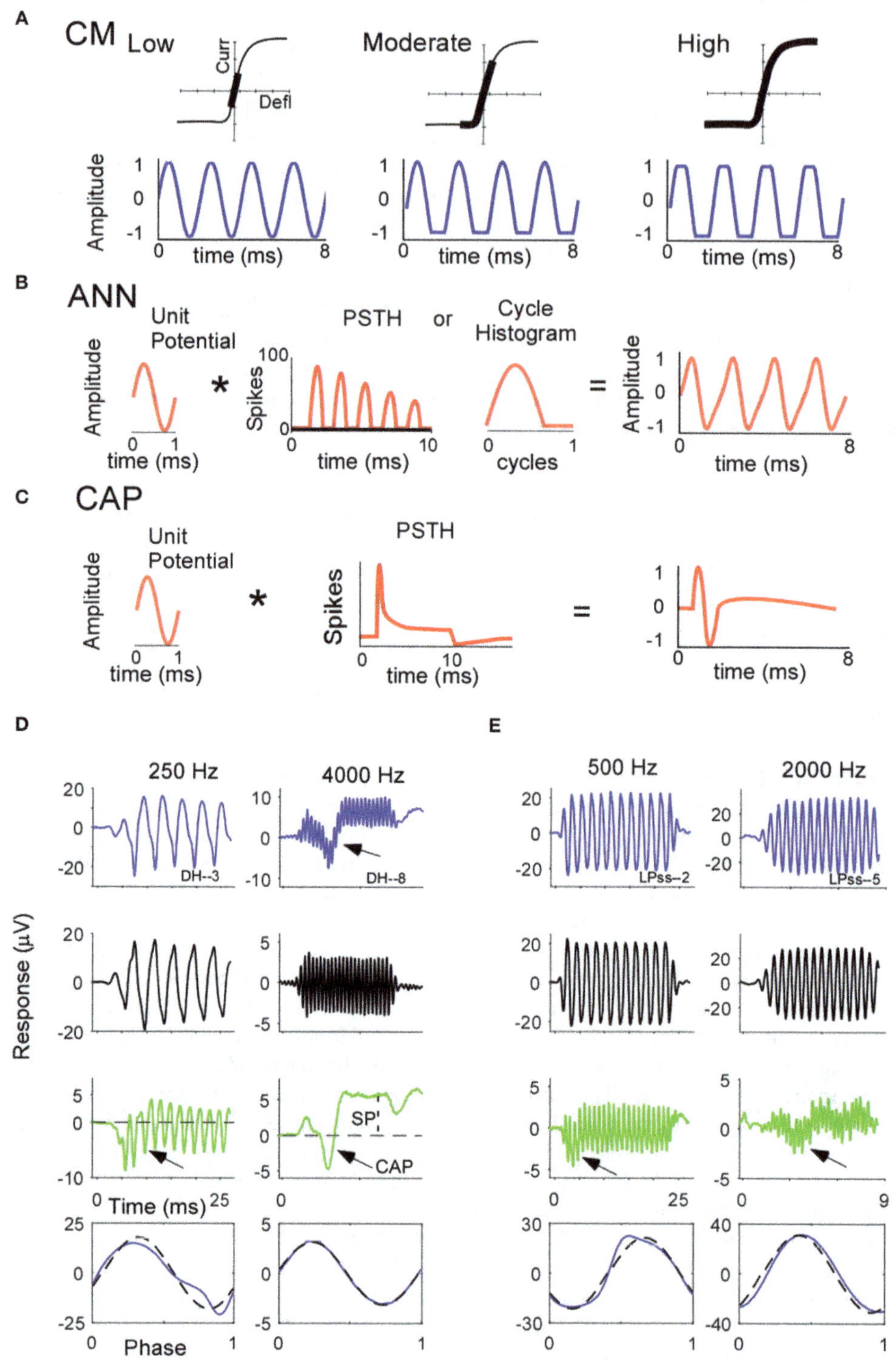

FIGURE 1 | Schematics of the sources of the CM, ANN, and CAP **(A–C)** and examples of ECochG responses obtained from two CI subjects **(D,E)**. **(A)** Typical input-output function of hair cell transduction (top row) producing asymmetries in saturation points as a function of intensity (bottom row). **(B)** The ANN is produced by the convolution (*) of a unit potential, or shape of an action potential as it appears at the round window, and the cyclic response to a low frequency in the population of unit responses, which is equivalent to the cycle histogram. The waveform expected is shown to the right. **(C)** The CAP is produced by the convolution (*) of the unit potential and well-timed onset responses in the population. **(D,E)** Responses from two subjects to a low and a high frequency tones. For each subject and frequency, the first three rows are, respectively, the responses to condensation phase of stimulation, the difference between the responses to condensation and rarefaction phases (not shown), and the sum of the responses to the two phases. The fourth row depicts an "average cycle" which is the average of all cycles from condensation phase stimuli in a window after the CAP, and from rarefaction stimuli after flipping and shifting the response in time to match that of the condensation phase. See text for further explanation of features identified in these examples.

the two directions of motion can be asymmetric, with the operating point, or proportion of channels open at rest, typically <50%. Thus, to moderate intensities there will be asymmetric saturation, and then to high intensities there will be a symmetric component as saturation occurs to both directions of motion. The distortions produced by these limits, in the absence of higher order features such as adaptation, would be expected to produce a flattening of the peaks in the ECochG from the CM. Spectrally, the asymmetric component of the saturation produces even harmonics of the fundamental, including zero or DC, while the symmetric component produces odd harmonics (Teich et al., 1989). For moderate and high intensities the population recording will be from regions with various degrees of saturation as the excitation spreads basally. The function shown is generic to illustrate these basic points; *in vivo* IHCs are thought to have more asymmetric input/output functions than OHCs, and basal IHCs are more asymmetric than apical. In recordings from the round window in a noise-damaged cochlea the degree of hair cell asymmetry contributing to the population response is difficult to predict.

The ANN is the evoked potential correlate of neural phase-locking to low frequency stimuli, which is the firing of action potentials over restricted portions of a stimulus cycle. Like the CAP (Goldstein and Kiang, 1958; Wang, 1979; Chertoff, 2004), the ANN can be considered to be the result of a convolution of a unit potential with the post-stimulus time histogram (PSTH) from the population of neural responses (**Figure 1B**). The unit potential is the representation of a single action potential observed at the round window, which has been described using spike-triggered averaging (Kiang et al., 1976; Prijs, 1986; Versnel et al., 1992). To low frequencies, the PSTH of single neurons contains peaks separated by the stimulus period, which can be folded into the cycle histogram (Rose et al., 1967; Johnson, 1980; Palmer and Russell, 1986). The cycle histogram shows rectification since the firing rate cannot go below zero. The population cycle histogram is less well-understood, but would presumably include some smearing in time and phase when averaged across multiple fibers. The smearing must be relatively small, because the ANN is a prominent feature of the responses to low frequency sounds (Snyder and Schreiner, 1984; Henry, 1995; Forgues et al., 2014; Lichtenhan et al., 2014; Verschooten et al., 2015).

As mentioned, the CAP is produced by the convolution of the unit potential and the population PSTH of auditory nerve fibers (**Figure 1C**). The CAP is a prominent feature because of the synchronous firing of action potentials that occur to the onset of sounds. These onset responses are timed most precisely to broad band stimuli produced by fast rise times. Thus, the CAP is stronger to high than to low frequency sounds, where the rise time is limited by the stimulus period.

The SP (not shown) is produced by multiple sources capable of producing a DC response to tones. These include the asymmetry in hair cell transduction, which is likely to different between inner and outer hair cells, which also differ in their membrane properties (Kros, 2007). The auditory nerve has also been shown to contribute to the SP in several studies (van Emst et al., 1995; Sellick et al., 2003; Forgues et al., 2014). For the auditory nerve, the DC is unlikely to be due to timing in PST, which, unlike the CAP and ANN is asynchronous to high frequencies and intensities. However, an asymmetry in the unit potential, even if small, could produce a DC given the large number of action potentials produced in response to even moderate levels of sound. Such asymmetry in the unit potential has not yet been shown.

With these features of the ECochG signal in mind, the goal of this study is to subjectively characterize the presence of neural compared to hair cells components in the responses to tones of children with and without ANSD who are receiving CIs. The neural components are the ANN and the CAP, with some neural contribution to the SP a possibility as well. The descriptions of the sources of these potential provided above helps to explain why the ANN and CAP are difficult to quantify, such that only a qualitative method was used. That is, the ANN is always mixed with the CM in the ongoing part of the response to the low frequency tone. However, the ANN is generally the more distorted signal, because the shape of the unit potential is unrelated to the stimulus, and the cycle histogram is roughly half-wave rectified. So the presence of strong harmonics, both even and odd, is evidence of the presence of the ANN. However, due to its periodicity the ANN's magnitude cannot be known because some or most will be in the first harmonic, where the largest part of the CM also resides. Furthermore, some of the CM can be in the higher harmonics due to the asymmetric and symmetric distortions described in **Figure 1A**, so the simple presence of higher harmonics of either even or odd order is not proof that the ANN is present. Thus, there is no simple method to objectively identify or quantify the CM and ANN contributions to the ongoing response.

In many CI subjects the CAP is obvious and can be measured using accepted methods. However, in a recent study (Scott et al., 2016) only 50% of CI subjects showed a CAP, and the difficulties in measurements were described, including (1) most CI subjects have responses only to low frequencies where the CAP is small compared to high frequencies; (2) the frequency content of the CAP, centered near 1,000 Hz, overlaps that of the stimulus frequencies that produce the largest responses in CI subjects, preventing the use of filtering to separating the CAP and CM, and (3) some CI subjects have an SP that is strong and rising (or falling) relative to the CAP, so that determining the strength of the CAP is problematic even when one is visually apparent.

The SP is relatively easily quantified as a sustained shift in the baseline. Here the problem is one of interpretation, since the sources of the SP are less than fully clear. However, we will present data from ANSD subjects that suggests there is a neural contribution to the SP.

For these reasons we have not yet found an acceptable objective means of identifying neural activity in each case. That is, although many features, such as large CAP or large harmonic distortions clearly correlate with neural activity, each metric has issues with false positive or negatives. In most cases, the reasons for the results can be observed in the responses themselves when further examined. In **Figures 1D,E**, we present examples of the data subsequently used to determine the "nerve score," based on the presence and approximate strength of the ANN and CAP. For each case the responses to a low and to a high frequency are presented, with low defined as in the range of strong phase-locking and high as above that range as defined in animal studies (Weiss and Rose, 1988). The first three rows in the figures are, respectively, the responses to condensation phase of stimulation (top), the difference between the responses to condensation and rarefaction phases (second row), and the sum of the responses to the two phases (third row). The responses to the condensation phase stimulus are the "raw" data, while the difference curves represent the part of the responses that changes with the change of polarity of the stimulus, and the summed curves represents the parts of the responses that don't change with the stimulus phase. These features make the difference curve contain predominantly odd-order harmonics, dominated by the first harmonic at the stimulus frequency, while the summed curve contains predominantly the even-order harmonics, particularly the second which is at twice the stimulus frequency. The CAP (arrows) is usually most visible in the summed curve when present, as is the SP. The bottom row shows the "average cycle" obtained from the cycles of response after the CAP and prior to the stimulus offset. This average cycle is where the distinct types of distortions characteristic of the CM and ANN can best be seen.

The example in D is a case with both a strong ANN and a strong CAP. A strong ANN is suggested by the prominent response at twice the stimulus frequency seen in the summed curve to the 250 Hz stimulus, and is clearly seen in the "average cycle" (lower left, solid curve). This curve is the average of all cycles from condensation phase stimuli in a window after the CAP, and from rarefaction stimuli after shifting the response in time to match that of the condensation phase. The average curve in this case is highly distorted compared to a sinusoid representing the stimulus (dashed line) that has been shifted in phase to have the best fit to the response. The lack of an ANN to the high frequency stimulus is shown by the lack of an AC component in the summed curve, and to a purely sinusoidal average cycle. The CAP (arrows) is most clearly seen to the high frequency stimulus in the summed curve, but is also readily visible in the response to condensation phase stimuli. However, it is embedded in an SP that is rising during the same time period, making its measurement problematic.

The example in E is a case where the ANN and CAP were small relative to the CM. To the low frequency stimulus there was still an AC component in the summed curve, but inspection of the average cycle showed a peak-flattened shape that is consistent with rectification of the CM as much as the presence of an ANN. There is also some AC response to twice the stimulus frequency in the summed curve to the high frequency stimulus, representing asymmetry in the CM rather than the ANN. To both frequencies a CAP is present but small CAP (arrows).

Because of these difficulties in measurement of the ANN and CAP we devised a subjective scale termed the "nerve score." To classify the presence and strength of the ANN we examine the average cycle of the ongoing response to low frequency tones (1,000 Hz and less). An ANN was considered present when the response appeared as a distorted version of a sinusoid, and the distortion was not compatible with a simple rectification or saturation of the CM. Our previous animal experiments where the neural responses were removed with kainic acid (Forgues et al., 2014) demonstrated that removing the neural activity removes these complex distortions, but leaves the peak-flattening type typical of the CM. The CAP was identified primarily in the summed curves, but in some responses to low frequencies the CAP shifts when the phase is changed by a time interval similar to the stimulus period, such that it shows up either exclusively or partially in the difference curve. The strength of *each neural potential* was defined on a scale of 0–2, where a score of 0 indicated there was no identifiable neural contribution across any frequency, 1 indicated small but clear evidence for the component and 2 indicated a large CAP or ANN to one or more frequencies. Once the CAP and ANN were individually scored, *their scores were then added* to produce a nerve score, with a range of 0 (no CAP or ANN) to 4 (CAP and ANN both strong). The case in D was given a nerve score of 4 because both the ANN and CAP were 2's, while the case in E had a nerve score of 1 because of the small but CAP but no definitive evidence of an ANN. Additional examples of data leading to particular nerve scores are provided in the results.

The SP

To tones, the SP is a baseline shift that persists for the duration of the tone (**Figure 1D**). Using the summed curve, this shift was measured by averaging points in the 2 ms prior to stimulus onset (i.e., the baseline) and offset (i.e., during the response), and computing the difference.

RESULTS

ECochG-TR

The ECochG-TR magnitudes as a function of age for the entire cohort are depicted in **Figure 2A**. The cases with ANSD (**Figure 2A**, triangles) were found at the upper end of the magnitude distribution. The overall distributions of ECochG-TR for the ANSD subjects, non-ANSD children, and non-ASND adults are shown in **Figure 2B**. The ANSD cohort had the highest median ECochG-TR, followed by the adults and the non-ANSD children. The differences were significant both as a main effect of group (Kruskal–Wallis, df $= 2$, chi-sq $= 61.1$, $p < 0.0001$), and for each comparison ($p < 0.01$).

The proportion of significant responses obtained at each frequency was also different among the groups (**Figure 2C**). For frequencies of 1,000 Hz and lower, the proportions of ears with significant responses were nearly universal for ANSD cases, and were ~80% of ears in the other groups. Above 1,000 Hz, the proportion of ears with responses declined in all groups, but ANSD subjects had a smaller decline. When present, the magnitudes of the responses (**Figure 2D**) were higher to all frequencies in the ANSD ears compared to the others.

Pediatric Cohort

Most of the ANSD cases were children, who have a distinct mix of hearing loss etiologies that leads to CI use. As expected from the results in **Figure 2**, when evaluating the distribution of ECochG-TR across etiologies for the pediatric ears, the ANSD group demonstrated larger overall magnitudes compared to all other etiologies (**Figure 3**) The ANSD children almost universally had

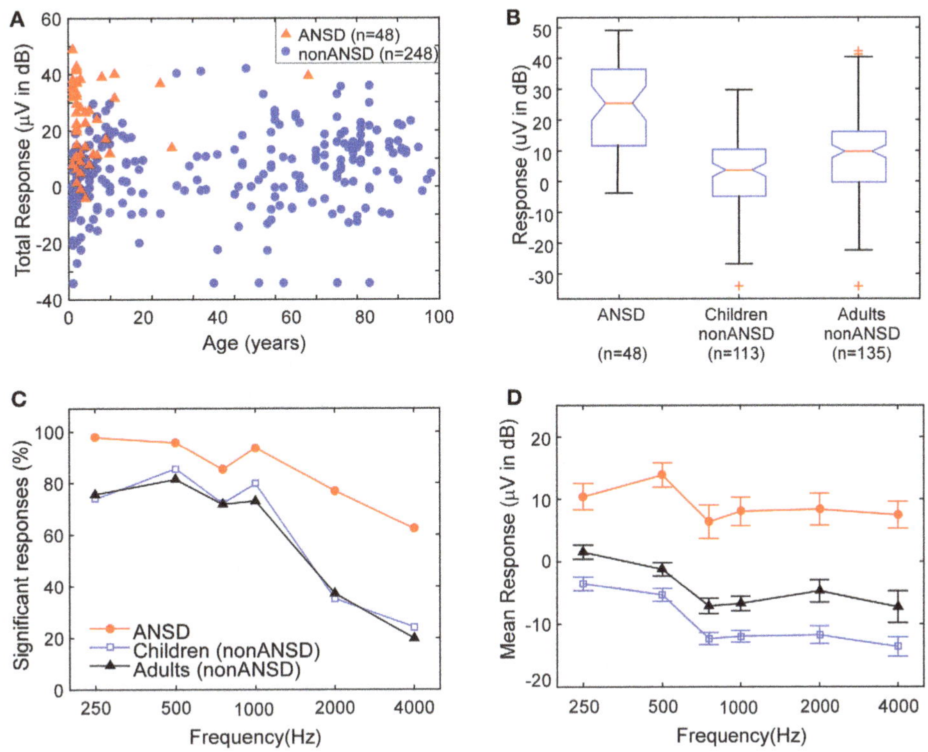

FIGURE 2 | RW ECochG-TR for all CI ears. **(A)** Scatter plot of ECochG-TR vs. Age. **(B)** Distributions of ECochG-TR for three groups. **(C)** Percent of cases with significant responses across frequency for the three groups. **(D)** Magnitude of significant responses across frequency for the three groups.

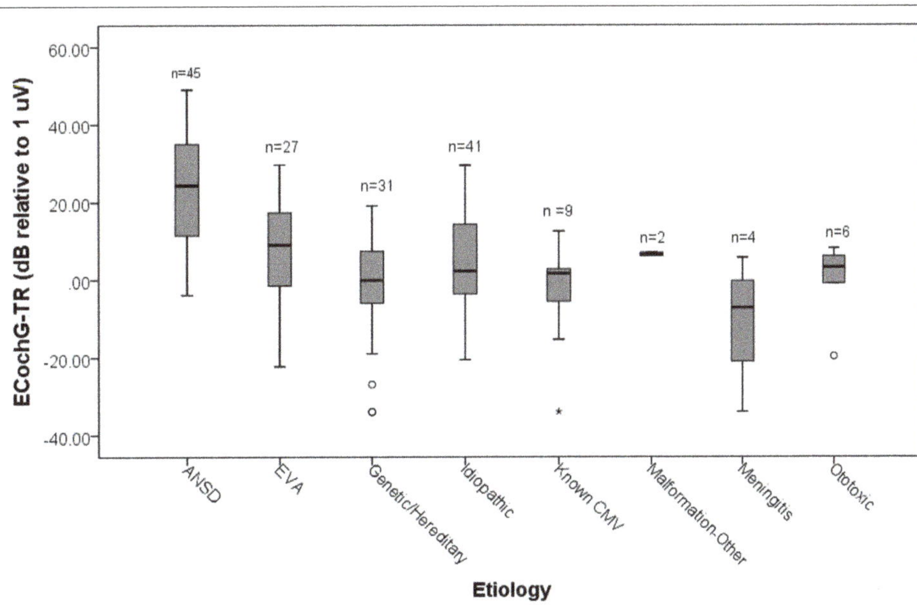

FIGURE 3 | Distributions of ECochG-TR by etiology in children. ANSD subjects had the highest ECochG-TR magnitudes. Outliers: o, Close extreme; *, Far extreme.

an ECochG-TR >1 µV (0 dB in the graph) with a mean magnitude of 23.6 ± 13.6 dB (standard deviation). A large fraction of the ANSD subjects had responses greater than 10 µV (20 dB on the graph). In contrast, for the non-ANSD etiologies a significant fraction had an ECochG-TR of <1 µV and few had values larger than 10 µV. Etiologies associated with widespread cochlear inflammation and fibrosis (meningitis and CMV) had among the lowest ECochG-TRs.

Degrees of Neural Activity in ANSD Subjects

It might be expected that the large responses seen in the ANSD cohort would be associated with relatively low nerve activity. However, we found a wide spectrum of neural responses, which spanned the full range of "nerve scores." Examples of ANSD cases with nerve scores demonstrating a high degree of neural activity, in the form of a CAP and/or ANN, are shown in **Figure 4**. The left panels show the summed responses to a low frequency stimulus, and the middle panels show each cycle plotted individually (dotted lines) to produce an "average cycle"(thick line). The black line in the middle panels represents the best fit sinusoid to each case, which was used for the visual analysis of the ANN (see Section Methods). The right panels of **Figure 4** show the summed responses to the alternated stimulus phases. These curves emphasize the CAP which is used in the nerve score, and also help visualize the SP, which has a strong hair cell component, and will be described further in later sections.

The case in **Figure 4A** showed strong distortions in the ANN as well as a prominent CAP, so the ANN and CAP were both individually scored a 2 for a total nerve score of 4. The other cases (**Figures 4B–E**) had nerve scores of 2 or 3, derived through different combinations of the ANN and CAP, as indicated.

Examples of cases with nerve scores demonstrating a low degree of neural activity (nerve score $\leq$1) are shown in **Figure 5**. The case in **Figure 5A** showed a small ANN (middle panel with arrow), and no CAP (right panel), so the nerve score was 1. The case in **Figure 5B** showed no ANN but a small CAP, so the nerve

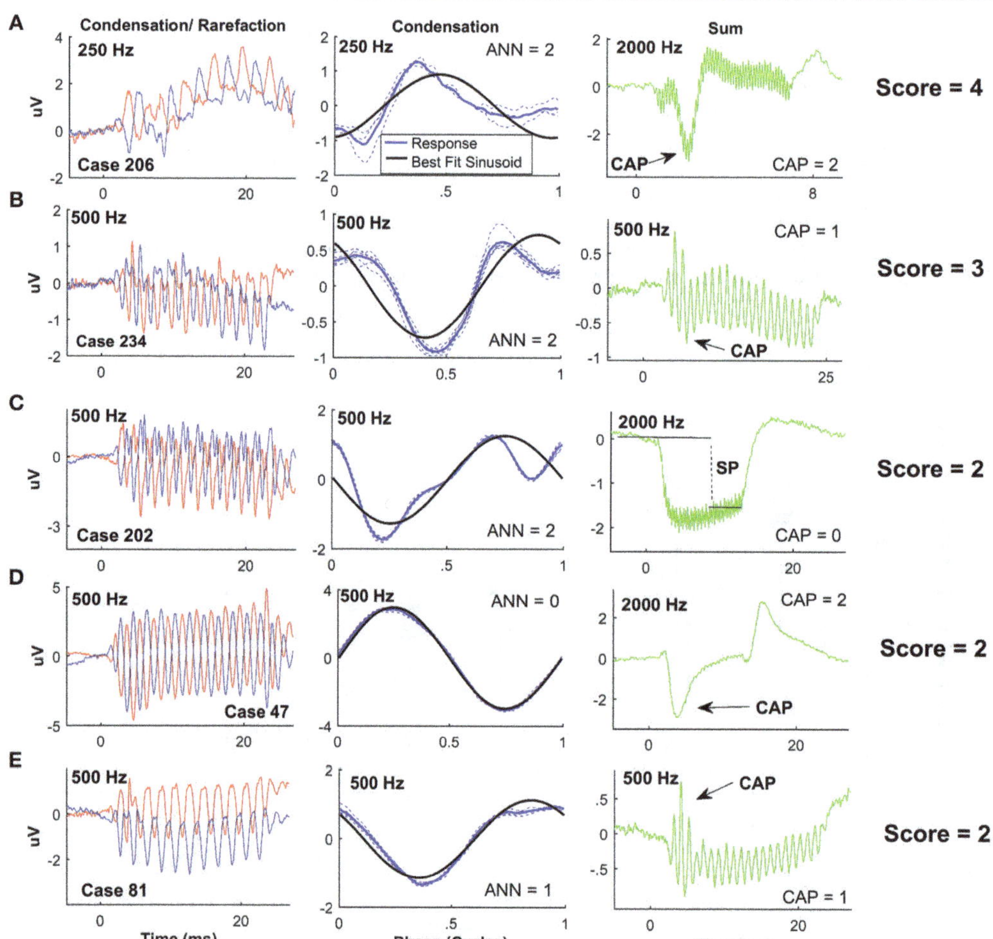

FIGURE 4 | ECochG examples of ANSD subjects with considerable evidence of neural activity. For each case the response to condensation and rarefaction phase of a low frequency stimulus is shown on the left. The middle panels show the individual (dotted lines) and average cycles (thick line) to condensation phase stimuli taken from a window (8–20 ms) intended to isolate the ongoing, or steady state portion of the response. The solid black line is the best fit sinusoid. The right panels show the sum of responses to the two phases, for the frequencies as shown, which isolates the CAP and SP. **(A)** Phenotype demonstrating a score of 4, with a strong ANN shown by the distortions on the average cycles, and a strong CAP to 2,000 Hz. **(B)** This case had a nerve score of 3 with a strong ANN and small but clear CAP. **(C)** A case with a nerve score of 2, and a phenotype demonstrating a strong, ANN but no CAP, and a large negative SP. **(D)** Another case with a nerve score of two with no apparent ANN but a strong CAP. Here the SP was small. **(E)** Another nerve score of two with a phenotype showing a small CAP and ANN.

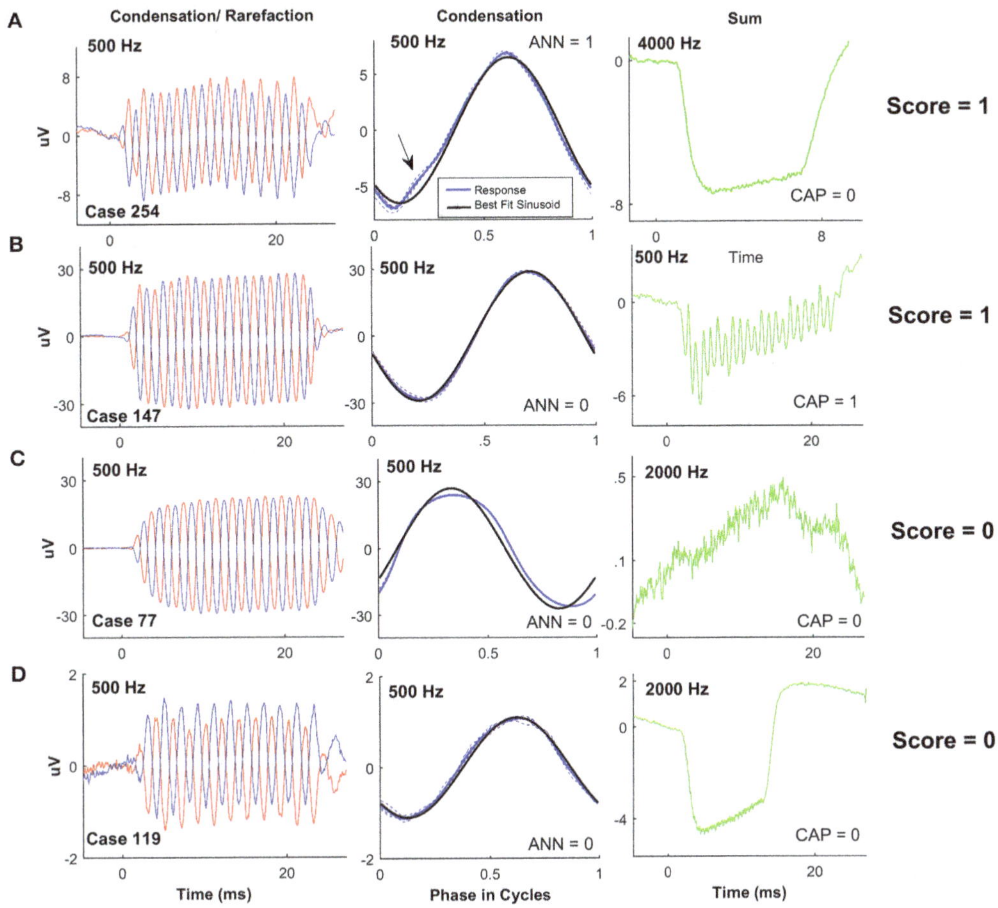

FIGURE 5 | ECochG examples with minimal neural activity. **(A)** A case with a nerve score of 1, showing a small ANN (arrow) and no CAP, and a large negative SP. **(B)** Another case with a nerve score of 1, that had a phenotype with no ANN and a small CAP. **(C)** A case with no ANN or CAP, and no SP either. **(D)** Another case with no ANN or CAP, but a large negative SP.

score was also 1. In **Figures 5C,D** there was no CAP or ANN, so the nerve scores were both zero. However, the SPs were markedly different in these cases.

Two additional cases in ANSD subjects help to show the sensitivity of the method to identify neural activity even in cases where it is expected to be small. One of the cases was a 1 year old with a mutation in the gene for otoferlin, a protein required for docking of vesicles containing neurotransmitter. This was the only one of our sample with this etiology. This presynaptic site of lesion should block the ANN but not affect transduction, so the phenotype expected is a large CM with no ANN. The case did show a very large CM to all frequencies as expected. However, there was also evidence for neural activity in the average cycle to a 250 Hz tone (**Figure 6A**). The deviation from the sinusoid (arrows) is small, but in a signal this large all of the individual cycles lie on top of each other and each shows this same feature, so it is not attributable to noise. This type of distortion also has no clear correlate in the CM (see **Figure 1A**, and so instead is most likely to be due to neural activity). The second case was of cochlear nerve deficiency, and was the only one of these cases ($n = 4$) where the ANN was apparent in the average cycle to 250

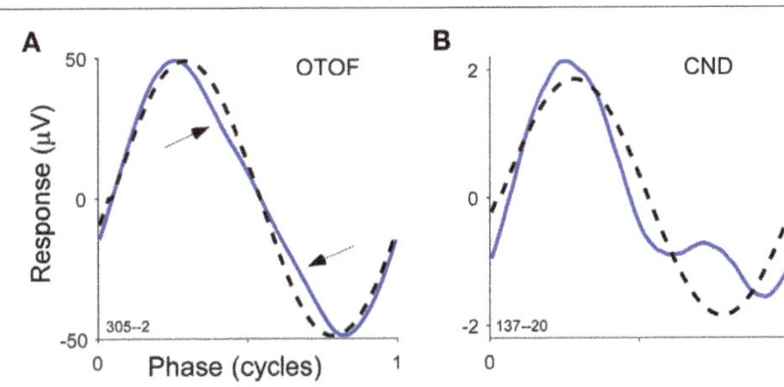

FIGURE 6 | Average 500 Hz cycle for two different known etiologies of the ANSD group. **(A)** Subject had confirmed otoferlin gene mutation. To 500 Hz distortions (arrows) due to the ANN can be identified. **(B)** Subject had cochlear nerve deficiency as identified by neuroimaging but has strong ANN distortions in the 500 Hz average cycle. These examples illustrate the sensitivity of ECochG for detecting neural activity when little is expected to be present.

(**Figure 6B**). These examples help to illustrate that the responses of tones to low frequencies can provide a highly sensitive means of assessing neural activity.

Distributions of Nerve Scores

The distributions of the different patterns of ANN and CAP are shown in **Table 1**. There was a wide spectrum of nerve scores, with scores of 2 or higher seen in 29 ears while 19 had nerve scores ≤1. An ANN score of 2 was seen in 20 ears compared to only 8 for the CAP, and the ANN scores were higher than the CAP for 23 cases compared to only 9 where the CAP had the higher score.

To compare the nerve scores among the different groups, only those where the ECochG-TR was >0.5 μV were used for the non-ANSD groups. The nerve score for responses smaller than this were always 0 because components other than the CM could not be visually distinguished. All of the ANSD subjects had and ECochG-TR >0.5 μV. Nerve scores were not significantly different among subjects with different etiologies of hearing loss (**Figure 7**) including ANSD (Kruskal–Wallis, df = 2, chi-sq = 5.88, p = 0.053). The near-significant p-value is due to the relatively high nerve scores among subjects with idiopathic hearing loss compared to subjects with known non-ANSD etiologies. The median nerve scores among subjects with ANSD were in-between the two non-ANSD groups.

A Negative SP and a Phenomenon of "Offset Overshoot" May Be Related to a Lack of Neural Activity

To frequencies of 1,000 Hz or greater the SP could be prominent, but to lower frequencies it was typically small. In response to the higher frequencies, three morphologies of the SP were observed, as illustrated in **Figures 4**, **5**. One morphology was a large, negative SP (right panels in **Figures 4C**, **5A,D**). This morphology was associated with either no CAP or only a small CAP. In cases with a large CAP (**Figures 4A,D**), the SP was small, and could be negative or positive. Finally, some cases had a large CM but no SP (**Figure 5C**). These latter two cases (**Figures 5C,D**) are interesting because they are both cases of cochlear nerve deficiency, and the difference in SP magnitude may be indicative of different sites of lesion (see Section Discussion).

The distributions of SP polarity and magnitude differed among ANSD and non-ANSD groups. The frequency where these differences were most clearly seen was 2,000 Hz as in **Figures 4**, **5**. As shown in **Table 2**, most of the ANSD cases (17/27) had a negative SP and no CAP to 2,000 Hz. Only 3 cases had a CAP to 2,000 Hz, so in the calculation of the nerve score, most of the CAPs were seen to frequencies of 1,000 Hz and below. In contrast, cases with the features of no CAP and a negative SP were uncommon in the two non-ANSD groups (6/32 combined). The number of cases included in the two-non ANSD are relatively reduced compared to the ANSD group, because of the few cases with good responses to this high frequency (**Figure 2**).

Illustration of the differences in the values of SP for ANSD and non-ANSD subjects is shown in **Figure 8**. In **Figure 8**, the magnitude and polarity of the SP to 2,000 Hz at 90 dB nHL are plotted against the magnitude of the ongoing response. The dotted lines are shown at ±2 μV, to highlight that most of the cases with negative SPs were ANSD subjects, while most non-ANSD cases had SPs near zero. One ANSD and one adult non-ANSD case had positive SPs >2 μV. The ANSD case had no CAP

TABLE 1 | Distribution of nerve scores in ANSD subjects.

CAP	+	ANN	=	Nerve score	No. of cases
2		2		4	6
1		2		3	12
2		1		3	0
0		2		2	2
2		0		2	2
1		1		2	7
1		0		1	7
0		1		1	9
0		0		0	3
			Total		48

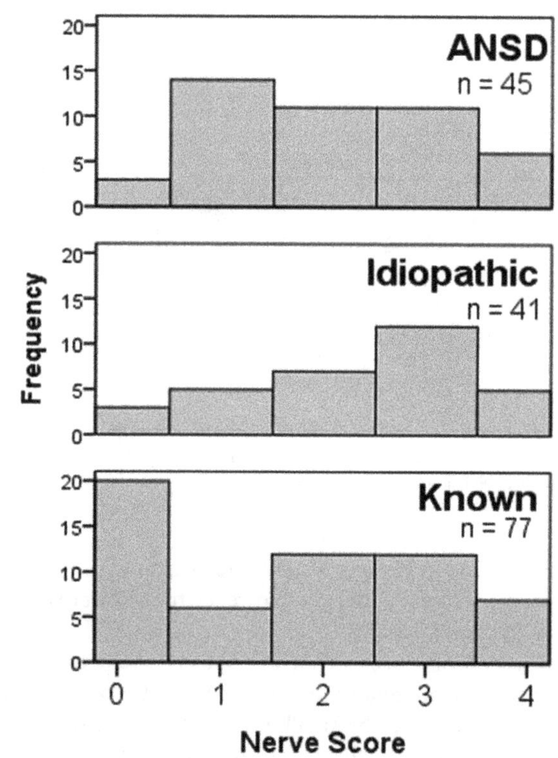

FIGURE 7 | Nerve score distributions for children with different etiologies of hearing loss. All groups showed the full range of nerve scores, and the distribution in the ANSD group was not significantly different from the others.

TABLE 2 | SP morphologies to 2,000 Hz at 90 dB nHL in ANSD and non-ANSD subjects.

SP morphologies	ANSD	Children non-ANSD	Adults non-ANSD	Total
No SP	7	5	8	20
CAP, small SP	3	3	10	16
Negative SP, no CAP	17	1	5	23
Total	27	9	23	59

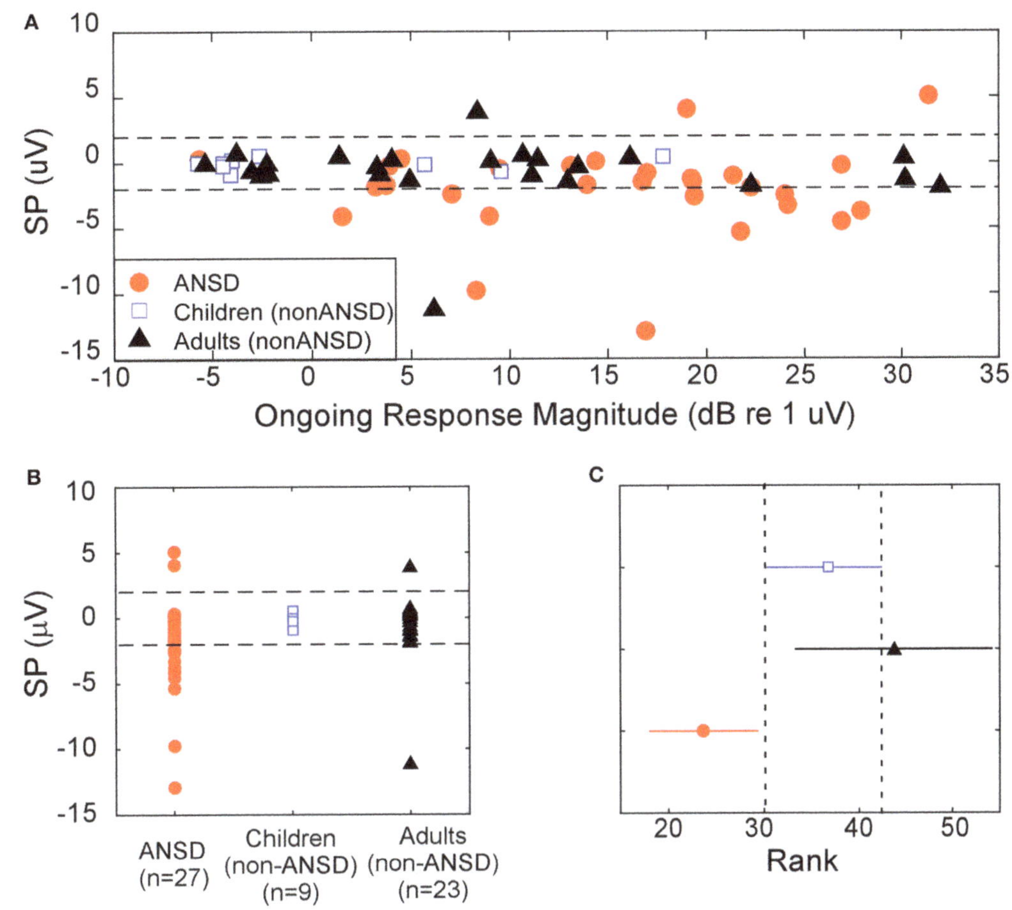

FIGURE 8 | Distributions of the SP to 2,000 Hz at 90 dB nHL among the three groups. **(A)** SP distribution among the groups as a function of the ongoing response. **(B)** Distributions of the SP by group. **(C)** Mean SP rank by group. Dotted lines are the 95% confidence interval around the non-ANSD children.

and the morphology of the SP was similar to those with negative SPs, but reversed. The non-ANSD case with a large, positive SP had a large CAP. The distributions of the SP values are shown in **Figure 7B**. There was a main effect of group (Kruskal–Wallis test, dfs = 2, chi-sq = 11.4, $p = 0.003$) and multiple comparisons of the mean ranks showed the ANSD group to have a significantly more negative SP overall compared to the other groups, which did not differ between themselves (**Figure 8C**).

In addition to the SP, a number of ANSD cases ($n = 5$) were seen which demonstrated an offset overshoot to 2,000 Hz (**Figures 9A–C**, right panel). No identifiable onset CAP was discernable in any of the ears where this overshoot was observed. In addition, a similar overshoot is often seen in gerbil responses after a neurotoxin has been applied (personal observations). Tentatively therefore, we consider this overshoot to be related to the SP. The SP is a complex mixture of sources with different polarities and time courses, so complex phenomena can be expected under different hearing conditions.

Adult Cohort

Three adults with ANSD were identified by the presence of CM on ABR, after audiological testing had suggested ANSD. As with the children, the ECochG-TRs in adults were large (**Figure 2**) and the degree of neural activity varied considerably even in this small group, with nerve scores of 1–3, demonstrating a mix of ANN and CAP involvement.

DISCUSSION

Our expectation was that ANSD subjects would have a large cochlear response and relatively little neural activity compared to other CI subjects. The results were that ANSD cases had on average a larger ECochG-TR; the responses extended more often to high frequencies; and responses to each frequency were on average larger in ANSD compared to non-ANSD cases. However, in the ANSD cases there was a full range of "nerve scores," derived from CAPs and the ANN, with the scores dominated by the presence of the ANN. Thus, to low frequencies there was little difference in neural activity in ANSD compared to non-ANSD cases. In contrast, to high frequencies the majority of ANSD cases showed no CAP and a strongly negative SP, while this pattern was rare in the non-ANSD groups. Thus, the hallmark of ECochG in subjects with a clinical report of ANSD is of large responses

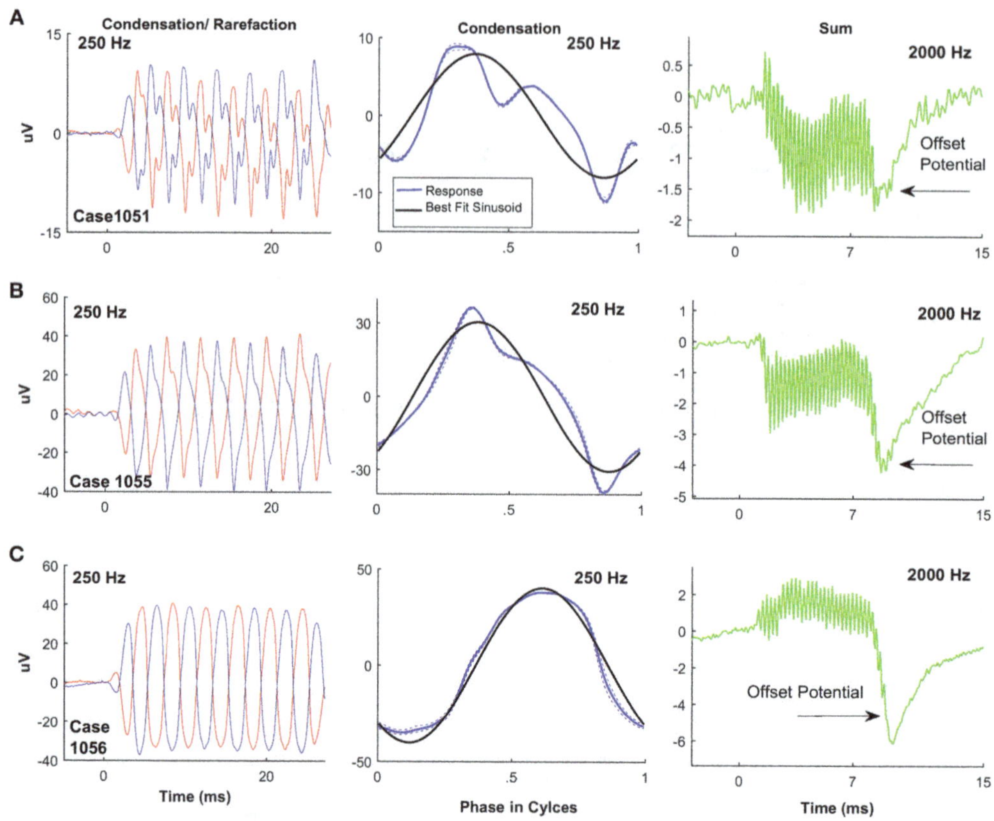

FIGURE 9 | Overshoot potential in some ANSD children reflected in the "sum" tracing. **(A–C)** Three different cases showing the offset overshoot. Note that there is no onset CAP, so this overshoot is unlikely to be related to a CAP to the offset.

with a lack of neural activity to high frequencies, combined with responses to low frequencies that have the same distribution of neural activity as found in non-ANSD cases. In the following, we will describe how these attributes are fully compatible with the main clinical findings of a CM with small or absent wave V in ABR results.

The Cochlear Microphonic in ANSD Subjects

To high frequency stimuli the cyclic response to tones consists purely of the CM, since it is above the range of phase-locking in the auditory nerve. The main distinction of ANSD compared to other CI subjects is the large CM to high frequencies, which accounts for the appearance of the CM in ABR recordings from these subjects. We did not fully explore the upper end of the frequency range, since in most subjects the highest frequency used was 4 kHz, where most ANSD subjects still had robust responses, in contrast to the non-ANSD groups, where responses to 2 and 4 kHz were relatively rare.

To low frequencies the responses in ECochG are still primarily the CM, even though they can be mixed with the ANN, when present. Thus, the larger overall responses to low frequencies in ANSD compared to non-ANSD subjects could indicate greater CM from the apex than in the non-ANSD groups. However, a more likely cause is the additional CM from higher CF regions of the cochlea that respond to low frequency stimuli as well.

The presence of the CM indicates the integrity of hair cells, but it cannot be specifically localized to outer hair cells, as is generally understood to be the case in studies of normal hearing animals (Dallos, 1973). This determination is difficult because both inner and outer hair cells produce a CM, and the pattern of hair cell loss in an individual subject is unknown. The presence of OAEs would be a more direct measure of functional outer hair cells, but a CM could be derived from the low CF cochlear regions where OAEs are not tested, and/or damaged hair cells that generate a CM but do not produce a functioning cochlear amplifier. Other responses features, in particular the SP, might be able to contribute to the determination of OHC vs. IHC activity.

Neural Activity in ECochG: The Compound Action Potential and ANN in ANSD Subjects

The CAP is a highly variable feature in CI subjects (Scott et al., 2016), including those with ANSD, as documented here. When present, it is a clear indication of neural activity. However, its absence does not fully assess neural activity, since the ANN was more prevalent than the CAP. We tried numerous methods to quantify the ANN prior to adopting the subjective method ultimately used. The ANN contributes to a 2nd harmonic in the response (Henry, 1995; Lichtenhan et al., 2013; Forgues et al., 2014), but the amount of the 2nd harmonic is not directly related to the size of the ANN because (1) most of its energy is at the first harmonic, where it is mixed with energy from the CM, (2) phase relationships between the ANN and CM can cause the net magnitudes in each harmonic to vary independent of their strength, and (3) the CM can produce harmonics of both even and odd order as well, so the simple presence of distortions in the spectrum is not a reliable indication of the ANN. Instead, the shape of the distortions in the average cycle must be examined to determine if the harmonics could plausibly be attributed to hair cells. In addition to harmonic analysis we have tried a number of different measurements to quantify the strength of the neural activity in our responses, such as correlation with a sine wave or power-line analysis such as form factor and crest factor. Unfortunately, none has proven adequate to capture the variety of responses seen. Our qualitative approach was therefore to note the presence of the ANN in the shape of the cyclic waveform, and to estimate its strength over a narrow range. We are currently investigating modeling methods to quantify the relative contribution of the CM and ANN.

The finding of a large degree of neural activity to low frequencies seems at odds with the clinical understanding of ANSD as representing an underlying etiology that affects the chain from IHCs to the CNS differently than in non-ANSD cases. However, the main difference between the clinical definitions of ANSD used here is the presence of a CM; both groups are receiving a CI and thus have a small or absent wave V. So, as previously discussed, the presence of a CM is well accounted for by the ECochG results showing greater hair cell activity to high frequencies, and the small but measurable neural activity primarily to low frequencies across all groups accounts for the reduced magnitudes of later waves in the ABR.

The SP in ANSD Subjects

Despite its first description in the 1950s (Davis et al., 1950, 1958), the origin of the SP is still a matter of considerable debate in terms of contributions from inner and outer hair cells and neural sources. Early work suggested outer hair cell sources predominate (Dallos and Cheatham, 1976) but later studies that removed inner hair cells in chinchillas showed a large effect on the CM (Zheng et al., 1997; Durrant et al., 1998). Furthermore, animal work in gerbils using the neurotoxin kainic acid recently showed a neural contribution to the SP (Forgues et al., 2014), which had also been reported previously using other species and compounds for blocking neural activity (van Emst et al., 1995; Sellick et al., 2003). In addition to the complexity of sources, the geometry between sources and recording sites will affect the polarity of the SP, contributing to complex changes across frequency and intensity as sites of generation within the cochlea shift. With these caveats, the phenotype of a large, negative SP (positive in one case) was correlated with the absence of a CAP, and therefore presumably of sustained neural activity as well. In ANSD subjects this phenotype predominated, while it was uncommon in the other groups. Furthermore, in both ANSD and non-ANSD groups, when a large CAP did exist the morphology of the SP was distinctly different, being close to zero in most cases with no preference for polarity. These findings of a relatively reduced CAP and enhanced SP closely parallel those reported previously for ANSD subjects using high frequency stimuli such as clicks and 8 kHz tone bursts (McMahon et al., 2008; Santarelli et al., 2008; Stuermer et al., 2015).

Two cases with cochlear nerve deficiency, an extreme example of ANSD (**Figures 5C,D**), had distinctly different SPs, that may, or may not, be related to different sites of lesion. Both cases had large CMs and no evident neural activity, but one case had no SP, while the other had a large negative SP. The presence of the large, negative SP typical of this and other ANSD cases may be due to the presence of IHCs, which are thought to have much more asymmetrical operating point, or proportion of open channels at rest, than OHCs (Russell, 2008). Thus, the presence of the negative SP could indicate the presences of functioning IHCs, and the lack of the negative SP, combined with no neural activity, could indicate the lack of IHCs. Alternatively, however, the operating point in the IHCs and OHCs in given case may be less asymmetric than in other cases, or the "effective intensity" of the stimulus in the face of hearing loss may produce basilar membrane movement too small for any asymmetry to be evident in the ECochG. Finally, the SP in one case and not the other could be due to presence of currents related to the dendritic potential, or the sum of excitatory post synaptic currents from the terminals of auditory nerve dendrites. These possibilities show that the SP could reveal considerable insights regarding sources of residual physiology in individual cases, as its sources become better understood.

In some cases, a large transient potential was observed to the stimulus offset to high frequencies. There was no CAP at stimulus onset in these cases, so the offset potential is unlikely to be a CAP to the offset. These responses were scored as "no SP" but a small or absent SP can also indicate a balance of contributions from outer hair cells, inner hair cells, and the auditory nerve. That is, different sources of sustained potentials can sum to be near zero at the steady state, while different time courses for each source allow them to be revealed when the stimulus changes.

Current Study in Relation to Previous Studies of ECochG in ANSD Children

Most previous studies of ECochG in ANSD children undergoing cochlear implantation used 8 kHz tone pips or clicks as stimuli (Gibson and Sanli, 2007; McMahon et al., 2008; Santarelli et al., 2008; Stuermer et al., 2015). These are primarily high frequency stimuli, which is an appropriate choice for many ANSD subjects who typically have good responses to high frequencies. However, to characterize ANSD subjects in the context of the general pediatric population, tone bursts that can transmit concentrated energy to low frequencies are needed because many CI subjects have no residual responses to high frequencies. Nearly all subjects, adult and pediatric, show responses to low frequency tone bursts with high signal to noise ratio when recorded at the RW (**Figure 2** and Choudhury et al., 2012; Fitzpatrick et al., 2014; McClellan et al., 2014; Dalbert et al., 2015).

The focus of much of the previous work with ECochG in ANSD subjects has been to identify phenotypes showing different sites of lesion that may result in different speech perception outcomes (Gibson and Sanli, 2007; McMahon et al., 2008). Sites can be identified as pre-synaptic by the absence of dendritic or spiking nerve activity and post-synaptic if either of these exist (McMahon et al., 2008). The idea is that if the lesion is presynaptic there is insufficient neurotransmitter release and thus a lack of neural spiking, but if there is spiking the lesion must be post-synaptic, e.g., demyelination causing asynchrony, central deficits, or loss of a fraction of synaptic connections due to excitotoxicity at the nerve terminal. Results in the current study showed that only a small number of ANSD cases did not demonstrate any evidence of a CAP or ANN, and hence had no evidence of neural spiking activity. However, rather than interpreting all of the cases with spiking activity as "post-synaptic" we think it is likely that in many instances there are still some residual neural connections primarily in low frequency regions of the cochlea, even in cases that should be considered a pre-synaptic etiology, such as otoferlin (see **Figure 6**). In general, therefore, the presence of neural activity in the ECochG does not necessarily indicate a post-synaptic site of lesion.

Non-ANSD and Unknown Etiologies

In both adult and pediatric non-ANSD cases the ECochG-TR was on average lower than in ANSD cases. In children, those with inflammatory reactions including CMV or meningitis had the lowest ECochG-TR. For those with the smallest responses there were no detectable CAPs, ANNs or SPs that could be distinguished from a sinusoidal CM. However, to the majority of cases where these additional potentials could be detected, the neural involvement covered the full spectrum of nerve scores, similar to the ANSD group. Previously, it was noted that adults and children had similar ranges of ECochG-TR, and a similar distribution of frequencies that contributed to the responses, as also reported here in **Figure 2** (Fitzpatrick et al., 2014). However, here we report that in children the upper end of the ECochG-TR distribution is mostly filled by ANSD cases, which represents a large difference from adults, in whom ANSD is uncommon.

CONCLUSIONS

The difference between ANSD and non-ANSD subjects lies primarily in the high frequency regions of the cochlea. These regions produce a larger CM and SP, and are less likely to produce a CAP, compared to non-ANSD subjects. These features are consistent with a large hair cell response combined with a limited neural response expected for ANSD. In contrast, for responses to low frequencies the neural components, primarily in the form of the ANN, are similar between ANSD and non-ANSD subjects, and vary from no evidence of neural contributions to clear evidence of CAP and/or ANN. Therefore, responses from low frequency parts of the cochlea produce a similarly wide distribution of evidence for neural activity between ANSD and non-ANSD subjects. It remains to be determined if the levels of neural activity seen using acoustic stimuli by ECochG are important in speech perception outcomes with the CIs.

AUTHOR CONTRIBUTIONS

WR, JR, CG, MH, ZB, TF, CB, KB, DF, OA contributed to data collection and manuscript preparation. WR, JR, DF, and OA contributed to analysis of data.

FUNDING

This project was funded by NIH through NIDCD (5T32DC005360-12 and 1-F30-DC-015168-01A1) and by a research contract with MED-EL Corporation.

REFERENCES

Berlin, C. I., Bordelon, J., St John, P., Wilensky, D., Hurley, A., Kluka, E., et al. (1998). Reversing click polarity may uncover auditory neuropathy in infants. *Ear Hear.* 19, 37–47. doi: 10.1097/00003446-199802000-00002

Berlin, C. I., Morlet, T., and Hood, L. J. (2003). Auditory neuropathy/dyssynchrony: its diagnosis and management. *Pediatr. Clin. North Am.* 50, 331–340. doi: 10.1016/S0031-3955(03)00031-2

Bielecki, I., Horbulewicz, A., and Wolan, T. (2012). Prevalence and risk factors for auditory neuropathy spectrum disorder in a screened newborn population at risk for hearing loss. *Int. J. Pediatr. Otorhinolaryngol.* 76, 1668–1670. doi: 10.1016/j.ijporl.2012.08.001

Blamey, P. (1997). Are spiral ganglion cell numbers important for speech perception with a cochlear implant? *Am. J. Otol.* 18, S11–S12.

Blamey, P., Artieres, F., Baskent, D., Bergeron, F., Beynon, A., Burke, E. et al. (2013). Factors affecting auditory performance of postlinguistically deaf adults using cochlear implants: an update with 2251 patients. *Audiol. Neurootol.* 18, 36–47. doi: 10.1159/000343189

Buchman, C. A., Roush, P. A., Teagle, H. F., Brown, C. J., Zdanski, C. J., and Grose, J. H. (2006). Auditory neuropathy characteristics in children with cochlear nerve deficiency. *Ear Hear.* 27, 399–408. doi: 10.1097/01.aud.0000224100.30525.ab

Chertoff, M. E. (2004). Analytic treatment of the compound action potential: estimating the summed post-stimulus time histogram and unit response. *J. Acoust. Soc. Am.* 116, 3022–3030. doi: 10.1121/1.1791911

Choudhury, B., Fitzpatrick, D. C., Buchman, C. A., Wei, B. P., Dillon, M. T., He, S., et al. (2012). Intraoperative round window recordings to acoustic stimuli from cochlear implant patients. *Otol. Neurotol.* 33, 1507–1515. doi: 10.1097/MAO.0b013e31826dbc80

Cohen, N. L., Waltzman, S. B., and Fisher, S. G. (1991). Prospective randomized clinical trial of advanced cochlear implants: preliminary results of a department of veterans affairs cooperative study. *Ann. Otol. Rhinol. Laryngol.* 100, 823–829. doi: 10.1177/000348949110001007

Dalbert, A., Pfiffner, F., Roosli, C., Thoele, K., Sim, J. H., Gerig, R., et al. (2015). Extra- and intracochlear electrocochleography in cochlear implant recipients. *Audiol. Neurootol.* 20, 339–348. doi: 10.1159/000438742

Dallos, P. (1973). *The Auditory Periphery Biophysics and Physiology.* New York, NY: Academic Press, Inc.

Dallos, P., and Cheatham, M. A. (1976). Production of cochlear potentials by inner and outer hair cells. *J. Acoust. Soc. Am.* 60, 510–512. doi: 10.1121/1.381086

Davis, H., Deatherage, B. H., Eldredge, D. H., and Smith, C. A. (1958). Summating potentials of the cochlea. *Am. J. Physiol.* 195, 251–261.

Davis, H., Fernandez, C., and McAuliffe, D. R. (1950). The excitatory process in the cochlea. *Proc. Natl. Acad. Sci. U.S.A.* 36, 580–587. doi: 10.1073/pnas.36.10.580

Doyle, K. J., Sininger, Y., and Starr, A. (1998). Auditory neuropathy in childhood. *Laryngoscope* 108, 1374–1377. doi: 10.1097/00005537-199809000-00022

Durrant, J. D., Wang, J., Ding, D. L., and Salvi, R. J. (1998). Are inner or outer hair cells the source of summating potentials recorded from the round window? *J. Acoust. Soc. Am.* 104, 370–377. doi: 10.1121/1.423293

Fayad, J., Linthicum, F. H. Jr., Otto, S. R., Galey, F. R., and House, W. F. (1991). Cochlear implants: histopathologic findings related to performance in 16 human temporal bones. *Ann. Otol. Rhinol. Laryngol.* 100, 807–811. doi: 10.1177/000348949110001004

Fayad, J. N., Don, M., and Linthicum, F. H. Jr. (2006). Distribution of low-frequency nerve fibers in the auditory nerve: temporal bone findings and clinical implications. *Otol. Neurotol.* 27, 1074–1077. doi: 10.1097/01.mao.0000235964.00109.00

Firszt, J. B., Holden, L. K., Skinner, M. W., Tobey, E. A., Peterson, A., Gaggl, W., et al. (2004). Recognition of speech presented at soft to loud levels by adult cochlear implant recipients of three cochlear implant systems. *Ear Hear.* 25, 375–387. doi: 10.1097/01.AUD.0000134552.22205.EE

Fitzpatrick, D. C., Campbell, A. T., Choudhury, B., Dillon, M. P., Forgues, M., Buchman, C. A., et al. (2014). Round window electrocochleography just before cochlear implantation: relationship to word recognition outcomes in adults. *Otol. Neurotol.* 35, 64–71. doi: 10.1097/MAO.0000000000000219

Forgues, M., Koehn, H. A., Dunnon, A. K., Pulver, S. H., Buchman, C. A., Adunka, O. F., et al. (2014). Distinguishing hair cell from neural potentials recorded at the round window. *J. Neurophysiol.* 111, 580–593. doi: 10.1152/jn.00446.2013

Formeister, E. J., McClellan, J. H., Merwin, W. H. III, Iseli, C. E., Calloway, N. H., Teagle, H. F., et al. (2015). Intraoperative round window electrocochleography and speech perception outcomes in pediatric cochlear implant recipients. *Ear Hear.* 36, 249–260. doi: 10.1097/AUD.0000000000000106

Friedland, D. R., Venick, H. S., and Niparko, J. K. (2003). Choice of ear for cochlear implantation: the effect of history and residual hearing on predicted postoperative performance. *Otol. Neurotol.* 24, 582–589. doi: 10.1097/00129492-200307000-00009

Fuchs, P. A., Glowatzki, E., and Moser, T. (2003). The afferent synapse of cochlear hair cells. *Curr. Opin. Neurobiol.* 13, 452–458. doi: 10.1016/S0959-4388(03)00098-9

Gantz, B. J., Woodworth, G. G., Knutson, J. F., Abbas, P. J., and Tyler, R. S. (1993). Multivariate predictors of audiological success with multichannel cochlear implants. *Ann. Otol. Rhinol. Laryngol.* 102, 909–916. doi: 10.1177/000348949310201201

Gibson, W. P., and Sanli, H. (2007). Auditory neuropathy: an update. *Ear Hear.* 28, 102S–106S. doi: 10.1097/AUD.0b013e3180315392

Goldstein, M. H., and Kiang, N. Y. S. (1958). Synchrony of neural activity in electric responses evoked by transient acoustic stimuli. *J. Acoust. Soc. Am.*30, 107–114. doi: 10.1121/1.1909497

Hang, A. X., Kim, G. G., and Zdanski, C. J. (2012). Cochlear implantation in unique pediatric populations. *Curr. Opin. Otolaryngol. Head Neck Surg.* 20, 507–517. doi: 10.1097/MOO.0b013e328359eea4

Henry, K. R. (1995). Auditory nerve neurophonic recorded from the round window of the Mongolian gerbil. *Hear. Res.* 90, 176–184. doi: 10.1016/0378-5955(95)00162-6

Holden, L. K., Finley, C. C., Firszt, J. B., Holden, T. A., Brenner, C., Potts, L. G., et al. (2013). Factors affecting open-set word recognition in adults with cochlear implants. *Ear Hear.* 34, 342–360. doi: 10.1097/AUD.0b013e3182741aa7

Johnson, D. H. (1980). The relationship between spike rate and synchrony in responses of auditory-nerve fibers to single tones. *J. Acoust. Soc. Am.* 68, 1115–1122. doi: 10.1121/1.384982

Kaga, K., Nakamura, M., Shinogami, M., Tsuzuku, T., Yamada, K., and Shindo, M. (1996). Auditory nerve disease of both ears revealed by auditory brainstem responses, electrocochleography and otoacoustic emissions. *Scand. Audiol.* 25, 233–238. doi: 10.3109/01050399609074960

Kiang, N. Y. S., Moxon, E. C., and Kakn, A. R. (1976). "The relations of gross potentials recorded from the cochlea to single unit activity in the auditory nerve," in *Electrocochleography*, eds R. J. Ruben, C. Elberling, and G. Salomon (Baltimore, MD: University Park Press), 95–115.

Kros, C. J. (2007). How to build an inner hair cell: challenges for regeneration. *Hear. Res.* 227, 3–10. doi: 10.1016/j.heares.2006.12.005

Lazard, D. S., Vincent, C., Venail, F., Van de Heyning, P., Truy, E., Sterkers, O., et al. (2012). Pre-, per- and postoperative factors affecting performance of postlinguistically deaf adults using cochlear implants: a new conceptual model over time. *PLoS ONE* 7:e48739. doi: 10.1371/journal.pone.0048739

Lichtenhan, J. T., Cooper, N. P., and Guinan, J. J. Jr. (2013). A new auditory threshold estimation technique for low frequencies: proof of concept. *Ear Hear.* 34, 42–51. doi: 10.1097/AUD.0b013e31825f9bd3

Lichtenhan, J. T., Hartsock, J. J., Gill, R. M., Guinan, J. J. Jr., and Salt, A. N. (2014). The Auditory nerve overlapped waveform (ANOW) originates in the Cochlear apex. *J. Assoc. Res. Otolaryngol.* 15, 395–411. doi: 10.1007/s10162-014-0447-y

McClellan, J. H., Formeister, E. J., Merwin, W. H. III, Dillon, M. T., Calloway, N., Iseli, C., et al. (2014). Round window electrocochleography and speech perception outcomes in adult cochlear implant subjects: comparison with audiometric and biographical information. *Otol. Neurotol.* 35, e245–e252. doi: 10.1097/MAO.0000000000000557

McMahon, C. M., Patuzzi, R. B., Gibson, W. P., and Sanli, H. (2008). Frequency-specific electrocochleography indicates that presynaptic and postsynaptic mechanisms of auditory neuropathy exist. *Ear Hear.* 29, 314–325. doi: 10.1097/AUD.0b013e3181662c2a

Nadol, J. B. Jr. (1997). Patterns of neural degeneration in the human cochlea and auditory nerve: implications for cochlear implantation. *Otolaryngol. Head Neck Surg.* 117, 220–228. doi: 10.1016/S0194-5998(97)70178-5

Palmer, A. R., and Russell, I. J. (1986). Phase-locking in the cochlear nerve of the guinea-pig and its relation to the receptor potential of inner hair-cells. *Hear. Res.*24, 1–15. doi: 10.1016/0378-5955(86)90002-x

Prijs, V. F. (1986). Single-unit response at the round window of the guinea pig. *Hear. Res.* 21, 127–133. doi: 10.1016/0378-5955(86)90034-1

Rance, G., Beer, D. E., Cone-Wesson, B., Shepherd, R. K., Dowell, R. C., King, A. M., et al. (1999). Clinical findings for a group of infants and young children with auditory neuropathy. *Ear Hear.* 20, 238–252. doi: 10.1097/00003446-199906000-00006

Rapin, I., and Gravel, J. (2003). "Auditory neuropathy": physiologic and pathologic evidence calls for more diagnostic specificity. *Int. J. Pediatr. Otorhinolaryngol.* 67, 707–728. doi: 10.1016/S0165-5876(03)00103-4

Roche, J. P., Huang, B. Y., Castillo, M., Bassim, M. K., Adunka, O. F., and Buchman, C. A. (2010). Imaging characteristics of children with auditory neuropathy spectrum disorder. *Otol. Neurotol.* 31, 780–788. doi: 10.1097/MAO.0b013e3181d8d528

Rose, J. E., Brugge, J. F., Anderson, D. J., and Hind, J. E. (1967). Phase-locked response to low-frequency tones in single auditory nerve fibers of the squirrel monkey. *J. Neurophysiol.* 30, 769–793.

Rubinstein, J. T., Parkinson, W. S., Tyler, R. S., and Gantz, B. J. (1999). Residual speech recognition and cochlear implant performance: effects of implantation criteria. *Am. J. Otolaryngol.* 20, 445–452.

Russell, I. J. (2008). "Cochlear receptor potentials," in *The Senses, A Comprehensive Reference*, eds A. I. Basbaum, A. Kaneko, G. M. Shepherd, G. Westheimer, T. D. Albright, R. H. Masland, P. Dallos, D. Oertel, S. Firestein, G. K. Beauchamp, M. C. Bushnell, J. H. Kaas, and E. Gardner (San Diego, CA: Elsevier), 319–358.

Santarelli, R. (2010). Information from cochlear potentials and genetic mutations helps localize the lesion site in auditory neuropathy. *Genome Med.* 2:91. doi: 10.1186/gm212

Santarelli, R., Starr, A., Michalewski, H. J., and Arslan, E. (2008). Neural and receptor cochlear potentials obtained by transtympanic electrocochleography in auditory neuropathy. *Clin. Neurophysiol.* 119, 1028–1041. doi: 10.1016/j.clinph.2008.01.018

Scott, W. C., Giardina, C. K., Pappa, A. K., Fontenot, T. E., Anderson, M. L., Dillon, M. T., et al. (2016). The compound action potential in subjects receiving a cochlear implant. *Otol. Neurotol.* 37, 1654–1661. doi: 10.1097/MAO.0000000000001224

Sellick, P., Patuzzi, R., and Robertson, D. (2003). Primary afferent and cochlear nucleus contributions to extracellular potentials during tone-bursts. *Hear. Res.* 176, 42–58. doi: 10.1016/S0378-5955(02)00716-5

Shea, J. J. III, Domico, E. H., and Orchik, D. J. (1990). Speech recognition ability as a function of duration of deafness in multichannel cochlear implant patients. *Laryngoscope* 100, 223–226. doi: 10.1288/00005537-199003000-00002

Shipp, D. B., and Nedzelski, J. M. (1995). Prognostic indicators of speech recognition performance in adult cochlear implant users: a prospective analysis. *Ann. Otol. Rhinol. Laryngol. Suppl.* 166, 194–196.

Shipp, D., Nedzelski, J., Chen, J., and Hanusaik, L. (1997). Prognostic indicators of speech recognition performance in postlinguistically deafened adult cochlear implant users. *Adv. Otorhinolaryngol.* 52, 74–77. doi: 10.1159/000059010

Snyder, R. L., and Schreiner, C. E. (1984). The auditory neurophonic: basic properties. *Hear. Res.* 15, 261–280. doi: 10.1016/0378-5955(84)90033-9

Starr, A., Picton, T. W., Sininger, Y., Hood, L. J., and Berlin, C. I. (1996). Auditory neuropathy. *Brain* 119(Pt 3), 741–753. doi: 10.1093/brain/119.3.741

Starr, A., Sininger, Y., Nguyen, T., Michalewski, H. J., Oba, S., and Abdala, C. (2001). Cochlear receptor (microphonic and summating potentials, otoacoustic emissions) and auditory pathway (auditory brain stem potentials) activity in auditory neuropathy. *Ear Hear.* 22, 91–99. doi: 10.1097/00003446-200104000-00002

Stuermer, K. J., Beutner, D., Foerst, A., Hahn, M., Lang-Roth, R., and Walger, M. (2015). Electrocochleography in children with auditory synaptopathy/neuropathy: diagnostic findings and characteristic parameters. *Int. J. Pediatr. Otorhinolaryngol.* 79, 139–145. doi: 10.1016/j.ijporl.2014.11.025

Teagle, H. F. B., Roush, P. A., Woodard, J. S., Hatch, D. R., Zdanski, C. J., Buss, E., et al. (2010). Cochlear implantation in children with auditory neuropathy spectrum disorder. *Ear Hear.* 31, 325–335. doi: 10.1097/AUD.0b013e3181ce693b

Teich, M. C., Keilson, S. E., and Khanna, S. M. (1989). Rectification models in cochlear transduction. *Acta Oto-Laryngol.* 467, 235–240. doi: 10.3109/00016488909138343

van Emst, M. G., Klis, S. F., and Smoorenburg, G. F. (1995). Tetraethylammonium effects on cochlear potentials in the guinea pig. *Hear. Res.* 88, 27–35. doi: 10.1016/0378-5955(95)00095-L

Varga, R., Kelley, P. M., Keats, B. J., Starr, A., Leal, S. M., Cohn, E., et al. (2003). Non-syndromic recessive auditory neuropathy is the result of mutations in the otoferlin (OTOF) gene. *J. Med. Genet.* 40, 45–50. doi: 10.1136/jmg.40.1.45

Verschooten, E., Robles, L., and Joris, P. X. (2015). Assessment of the limits of neural phase-locking using mass potentials. *J. Neurosci.* 35, 2255–2268. doi: 10.1523/JNEUROSCI.2979-14.2015

Versnel, H., Prijs, V. F., and Schoonhoven, R. (1992). Round-window recorded potential of single-fibre discharge (unit response) in normal and noise-damaged cochleas. *Hear. Res.* 59, 157–170. doi: 10.1016/0378-5955(92)90112-Z

Wang, B. (1979). *The Relation between the Compound Action Potential and Unit Discharges of the Auditory Nerve.* Boston, MA: Massachusetts Institute of Technology.

Weiss, T. F., and Rose, C. (1988). A comparison of synchronization filters in different auditory receptor organs. *Hear. Res.* 33, 175–179. doi: 10.1016/0378-5955(88)90030-5

Zeng, F. G., Oba, S., Garde, S., Sininger, Y., and Starr, A. (1999). Temporal and speech processing deficits in auditory neuropathy. *Neuroreport* 10, 3429–3435. doi: 10.1097/00001756-199911080-00031

Zheng, X. Y., Ding, D. L., McFadden, S. L., and Henderson, D. (1997). Evidence that inner hair cells are the major source of cochlear summating potentials. *Hear. Res.* 113, 76–88. doi: 10.1016/S0378-5955(97)00127-5

17

Human Summating Potential Using Continuous Loop Averaging Deconvolution: Response Amplitudes Vary with Tone Burst Repetition Rate and Duration

Alana E. Kennedy[1], Wafaa A. Kaf[1], John A. Ferraro[2], Rafael E. Delgado[3] and Jeffery T. Lichtenhan[4]*

[1] Department of Communication Sciences and Disorders, Missouri State University, Springfield, MO, United States,
[2] Department of Hearing and Speech, University of Kansas Medical Center, Kansas City, KS, United States, [3] Department of Biomedical Engineering, University of Miami, Coral Gables, FL, United States, [4] Department of Otolaryngology, Washington University School of Medicine, St. Louis, MO, United States

***Correspondence:**
Wafaa A. Kaf
wafaakaf@missouristate.edu

Electrocochleography (ECochG) to high repetition rate tone bursts may have advantages over ECochG to clicks with standard slow rates. Tone burst stimuli presented at a high repetition rate may enhance summating potential (SP) measurements by reducing neural contributions resulting from neural adaptation to high stimulus repetition rates. To allow for the analysis of the complex ECochG responses to high rates, we deconvolved responses using the Continuous Loop Averaging Deconvolution (CLAD) technique. We examined the effect of high stimulus repetition rate and stimulus duration on SP amplitude measurements made with extratympanic ECochG to tone bursts in 20 adult females with normal hearing. We used 500 and 2,000 Hz tone bursts of various stimulus durations (12, 6, 3 ms) and repetition rates (five rates ranging from 7.1 to 234.38/s). A within-subject repeated measures (rate x duration) analysis of variance was conducted. We found that, for both 500 and 2,000 Hz stimuli, the mean deconvolved SP amplitudes were larger at faster repetition rates (58.59 and 97.66/s) compared to slower repetition rates (7.1 and 19.53/s), and larger at shorter stimulus duration compared longer stimulus duration. Our concluding hypothesis is that large SP amplitude to short duration stimuli may originate primarily from neural excitation, and large SP amplitudes to long duration, fast repetition rate stimuli may originate from hair cell responses. While the hair cell or neural origins of the SP to various stimulus parameters remains to be validated, our results nevertheless provide normative data as a step toward applying the CLAD technique to understanding diseased ears.

Keywords: cochlea, auditory nerve, phase locking, tone burst, high stimulus rate, continuous loop averaging deconvolution

INTRODUCTION

Electrocochleography (ECochG) is a technique that can be used to objectively assess physiologic properties of the auditory periphery. The application of ECochG to both clinical and research purposes is extensive and its use as a diagnostic tool for Ménière's disease has long been considered. While specific criteria have been examined, such as the use of the summating potential (SP)/compound action potential (AP) amplitude ratio, the relatively low sensitivity of this measure alone has limited its diagnostic value for Ménière's disease (Ferraro and Tibbils, 1999; Ferraro and Durrant, 2006; Al-momani et al., 2009). The lack of sensitivity of the SP/AP ratio measure obtained from click stimuli, and the unknown origins of the disease, has led to the continued refinement of ECochG uses to advance the differential diagnosis of Ménière's disease.

One such method has been the use of tone burst stimuli to assess the SP across frequencies. As Ménière's disease typically presents with fluctuating hearing loss, initially affecting the low frequencies, physiologic measurements from throughout the length of the cochlear spiral may help provide new insight into the disease. While the origins of various components of the SP and AP components are still being sought after and understood, both have been shown to vary greatly with stimulus parameters. While the SP and AP can interleave in a given measurement, the amplitude of the SP appears to sustain for the duration of the response and makes it an attractive attribute to study.

Gibson (1993) was one of the first to develop criteria for the use of tone burst ECochG measurements to assess of Ménière's disease with the SP amplitude. Gibson (1993) determined that the most effective frequencies when evaluating the disorder were 500 and 1,000 Hz, while 4,000 Hz was the least effective. Gibson (2009) repeated the study with matched hearing loss controls (ears without Ménière's disease, but with sensorineural hearing loss) and found that 500, 1,000, and 2,000 Hz were most sensitive, while significant overlap in responses between groups occurred at 4,000 and 8,000 Hz. (Gibson, 1993, 2009) also compared the results to click stimuli SP/AP amplitude ratio measurements, and determined the use of tone burst SP amplitude was a sensitive measure to Ménière's disease. Others have found increased sensitivity with SP amplitudes obtained from 1,000 Hz tone burst stimuli when compared to click evoked SP/AP amplitude ratios (Conlon and Gibson, 2000; Iseli and Gibson, 2010). These findings support the use of frequency specific stimuli in ECochG measures when examining the effects of Ménière's disease.

At present time, the majority of tone burst ECochG studies designed to examine the SP have used relatively long stimulus durations (≥12 ms). While this approach allows for clearer observation of the SP after the AP amplitude has adapted, it limits the stimulus repetition rate at which tone burst stimuli can be presented without overlaying of the signal. Wuyts et al. (2001) examined the effect of 1,000 Hz repetition rate on the SP amplitude in subjects with and without Ménière's disease. Stimulus repetition rate was varied between 8.4 and 37.4 tone bursts/second and the investigators found that that SP amplitude increased with increased rate, regardless of the presence or absence of the disease, with larger SP amplitude found in those with the disease. While Wuyts et al. (2001) studied the effect varying stimulus repetition rate using transtympanic ECochG, there is limited research focused on the use of extratympanic ECochG measurements to tone burst with various repetition rates, particularly above 37 tone bursts/second.

The use of high stimulus repetition rates face limitations as rate increases to the point where the responses overlay, obscuring one another. As measurements to high rates are significantly degraded and difficult to interpret using the standard measure analysis technique, ECochG to very high repetition rates requires a special technique to help analyze the complex, overlain responses (Delgado and Ozdamar, 2004). This complex waveform occurs as the response from one eliciting stimulus has not ended before the presentation of the next. Recently, a new technique, continuous loop averaging deconvolution (CLAD), has been designed to employ algorithmic formulas to deconvolve or "unmix" waveforms collected at very high rates. The application of CLAD to ECochG measurements obtained with high stimulus repetition rates has been utilized successfully. Kaf et al. (2017) quantified normative ECochG and ABR measures to click at rates up to 507 clicks/s using this novel technique. The CLAD technique has also shown promise in the assessment of Ménière's disease through the use of high, 780 clicks/s, repetition rates (Bohorquez et al., 2009).

The present study was designed to investigate the effects of high rate and stimulus duration on SP amplitude of 500 and 2,000 Hz tone burst ECochG in adults with normal hearing. This research is the first step in understanding the physiological effect of high rate on tone burst ECochG in subjects without a history of inner ear pathology, and in establishing normative SP amplitude data upon which further research can build. The goals of this study are to (1) establish normative SP amplitude data for high repetition rate 500 and 2,000 Hz tone bursts, and (2) quantify the effect of stimulus duration on measurements to various stimulus repetition rates.

METHODS

Participants

This study was approved by the Missouri State University Institutional Review Board and written informed consent was obtained from each participant. Twenty-one female adults between the ages of 20–35 years with normal hearing sensitivity were recruited for participation in this study. However, due to poor replicability of tone burst waveforms from one participant, only the data of 20 participants was analyzed in this study. Criteria for participation in the study included: (1) otoscopic evaluation revealing ear canals clear of cerumen and debris, (2) normal hearing sensitivity determined by pure tone air conduction audiometry, with thresholds ≤25 dB HL from 250 to 8,000 Hz (Goodman, 1965); (3) normal middle ear status as confirmed by 226 Hz tympanometry and the presence of normal static compensated admittance, tympanometric pressure, and ear canal volume (American Speech-Language-Hearing Association, 1988); and (4) a recordable SP and AP with standard click ECochG measurements. Female participants were recruited for participation in this study. Although gender differences were not assessed during this study, previous research has not demonstrated significant differences in ECochG responses between male and female subjects (Wilson and Bowker, 2002).

Equipment

All participants were tested in the sound booth at the Missouri State University auditory research laboratory. The Intelligent Hearing Systems SmartAudiometer was used to assess hearing thresholds from 250 to 8,000 Hz using pure tone stimuli presented via ER-3A insert earphones under sound booth conditions. The Intelligent Hearing System Smart–Evoked Potential equipment was used for the extratympanic ECochG recordings; with ER-3A insert earphones used to deliver the stimuli. The equipment was calibrated according to manufacturer specifications, using a precision sound level meter (Quest, Model 155), microphone (Bruel and Kjaer, Model 4144), and a 2-cc (HA-2) coupler (Bruel and Kjaer, Model DB-0138) and followed the IEC standard for peSPL (0 dBnHL = 32 dB peSPL ±3 dB). A homemade tympanic electrode (Ferraro and Durrant, 2006) was used as the inverting electrode placed on the tympanic membrane. The materials used to construct the electrodes included bare silver wire (0.008 inch diameter), silicon tubing (0.0077 inch outer diameter; 0.058 inch inner diameter), cotton balls, electrode conducting gel, and a needle syringe. A microalligator clip was used to connect the wire end of the tympanic membrane electrode to the pre-amplifier.

Stimulus and Recording Parameters

A one channel montage was used for ECochG recording from the test (right) ear of each participant. The inverting tympanic membrane electrode was placed on the tympanic membrane of the right ear, the non-inverting electrode was placed on the ipsilateral (right) mastoid, and the ground electrode was placed on the contralateral (left) mastoid. Ferraro et al. (1994a) suggest the use of an ipsilateral montage in order to reduce the contribution of later waves associated with ABR in the response. Electrode impedance was kept ≤7 Ω at each electrode site.

Prior to the collection of tone burst ECochG at high rate, standard, slow rate click ECochG was performed for the right ear. This step allowed for a clear observation of the SP and AP components in the waveform to ensure these potentials were present under standard ECochG parameters prior to the implementation of the experimental test protocol. Hundred microsecond broad-band click stimuli were presented at 75 dB nHL, with alternating polarity at a rate of 7.1/s. The recording epoch was set for 5 ms. A band-pass filter setting of 10–3,000 Hz and a gain setting of 100,000 were utilized. Two traces were collected, each recorded for 1,000 sweeps.

For the present study, the rate values examined included 7.1, 19.53, 58.59, 97.66, and 234.38/s. All rates, with the exception of 7.1/s, are CLAD rate sequences that were developed and evaluated by the Intelligent Hearing Systems for their ability to deconvolve the recorded response using the CLAD algorithm. These four CLAD stimulus rates were chosen based on the stimulus durations of the tone burst stimuli in order to ensure no overlap occurred in the eliciting signal. As stimulus rate is limited by the stimulus duration, higher rates could not be used without the potential of overlap in the stimulus signal which would be detrimental to the recordings. Loopback recordings of the 500 and 2,000 Hz stimuli were performed at each rate to ensure no overlap occurred within the stimulus.

Each trace was repeated to ensure replicability, with the 2,000 sweeps per trace. The recording epoch was set at 12 ms. As with standard ECochG, recordings were made using an alternating polarity signal a gain of 100,000, and were presented at an intensity level of 75 dB nHL (107 dB SPL). The band-pass filter was set to 3–3,000 Hz; a high pass filter of 3 Hz was used because the SP, as a direct current potential, is particularly sensitive to high pass filter settings. The use of a high pass filter of 3 Hz, is thought to minimize the distortion present in the SP signal (Ferraro et al., 1983).

To examine the effect of rate on SP amplitude response as a function of stimulus duration, recordings were conducted with stimulus durations of 12, 6, and 3 ms for each rate in which no overlap would occur. For example, at 19.53/s all durations (12, 6, and 3 ms) were examined as no overlap occurs at this rate. On the other hand, at the highest rate, 234.38/s, only the 3 ms stimulus duration was examined due to the stimulus overlap that would result from testing using the longer duration stimuli. For both the 500 and 2,000 Hz conditions, 2 ms rise and fall times with an 8 ms plateau was used for the 12 ms duration stimuli and 2 ms rise and fall times with a 2 ms plateau was applied for the 6 ms duration stimuli. For the 3 ms duration stimuli, rise and fall times of 1.5 ms were used, with no plateau.

Procedures

Standard click ECochG was performed on the right ear for all participants. Though not formally analyzed, standard ECochG was performed on all participants to ensure reliable and replicable click ECochG could be obtained prior to the collection of tone burst ECochG. **Figure 1** displays standard click ECochG traces for one of the participants (P9). Two traces were recorded, averaged and assessed to ensure the presence of both the SP and AP waveform components before proceeding with the experimental, tone burst ECochG protocol. In a laboratory environment, participants were comfortably seated in a reclining chair. The participant's skin was scrubbed gently with Nu-Prep gel on the electrode site areas, the participant's right (M2) and left (M1) mastoids. Disposable surface electrodes were then placed and attached to these sites. Next, the tympanic membrane electrode was inserted along ear canal and slowly moved toward the tympanic membrane. The patient was informed that they would feel a slight pressure as the electrode came in contact with the tympanic membrane. The patient was instructed to provide verbal feedback regarding their comfort and the pressure sensation accompanying the contact of electrode with their tympanic membrane. The electrode placement was guided by otoscopy, patient report of tympanic membrane contact, and electrode impedance measure of less than 7kΩ. Following placement of the tympanic membrane electrode, an ER-3A insert earphone was placed in the ear canal to hold the electrode in place and deliver the sound stimuli. The portion of the electrode protruding from the ear canal was taped down to the side of the participant's face and attached to a microalligator clip. Participants were reclined, instructed to relax, and encouraged to take a nap during standard click ECochG and experimental tone burst ECochG testing to 500 and 2,000 Hz.

Following recording of standard click ECochG, tone burst ECochG to 500 and 2,000 Hz were recorded. The order of the tone burst stimuli and the repetition rates were randomized a priori to eliminate any order effect. At each repetition rate, the appropriate stimulus durations were adjusted from long to short

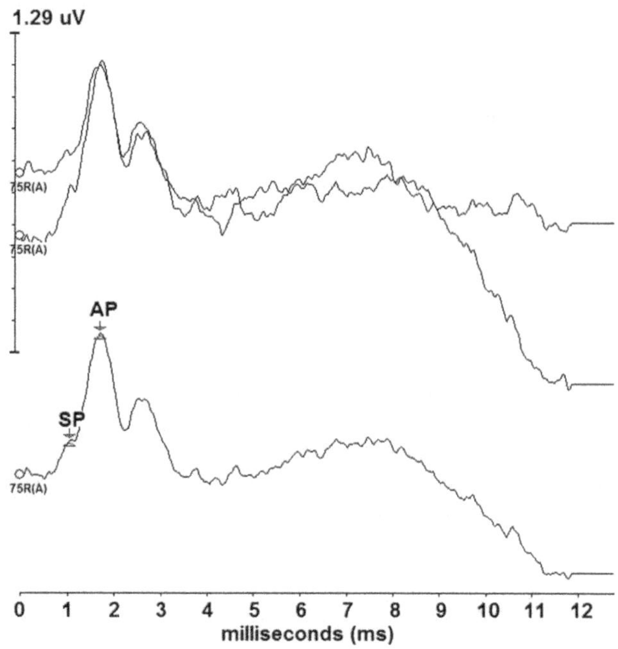

FIGURE 1 | Standard click ECochG responses from one of the participants (P9). Two traces (top) were recorded and averaged (bottom) depicting a typical ECochG response. The SP and AP are labeled on the averaged tracing, though standard ECochG data was not formally assessed during this study.

duration as applicable. With each duration and rate, two traces of 2,000 sweeps each were recorded. Once all recordings from the right ear at both 500 and 2,000 Hz were completed, the tympanic membrane electrode was removed from the participant's ear and otoscopy was performed to rule out any sign of injury to the ear canal and tympanic membrane as a result of tympanic membrane placement and to assess tympanic membrane contact location.

Data Analysis

Recordings were completed on 21 participants; however, only data from 20 participants were included in the analysis. Data from one of the participants was excluded due to poor replicability of the tone burst ECochG waveforms. In addition, data from one participant for the 500 Hz, 234.38/s condition was excluded from the analysis due to an incomplete recording for that rate. All other recordings were included in the data analysis. Analysis of the recorded waveforms occurred offline. The two recorded, non-deconvolved traces from each condition were averaged (see Kaf et al., 2017; **Figure 1** non-deconvovled ECochG to high click rates). Because of the complexity of the non-deconvolved waveforms, the averaged waveforms were then deconvolved using the CLAD algorithm, and the resulting deconvolved traces were labeled to determine the SP amplitude. Uniform labeling was used across all deconvolved waveforms according to the frequency and duration of the recording; rate was not a factor in the labeling of the waveforms. The SP amplitude measurements were made from the midpoint of the stimulus duration, beginning at the onset of the response, to the baseline. SP amplitude measurement from the midpoint of the response is a common practice in the recording of tone burst ECochG and is thought to allow for SP measurement to made without contribution from the AP at the onset of the response and prior to SP decay at the end of the response (Gibson, 1993, 2009; Ferraro et al., 1994a,b; Wuyts et al., 2001). For 12, 6, and 3 ms stimulus durations, the midpoints were 6, 3, and 1.5 ms respectively. Each of these midpoint measures were made from the onset, the beginning of the response, in order to maintain a uniform SP midpoint latency from which the SP amplitude was measured. The onset of the response was chosen as the point at which a positive shift from baseline was noted and was defined as a latency of 1.5 ms for the 2,000 Hz condition, and at a latency of 2.5 ms for the 500 Hz condition across the recordings from all participants. These latency differences between frequencies may be associated with cochlear travel time, which is longer at apical, low frequencies than basal, high frequencies (Ferraro et al., 1994a). All baseline measurements were made at a latency of 1 ms to measure SP amplitude from a point prior to the onset of the response.

Repeated measures analysis of variance was conducted to compare the effect of rate, duration, and the combination of the two on SP amplitude for both the 500 and 2,000 Hz conditions. A 3 (rate—7.1, 19.53, 58.59/s) × 3 (duration—12, 6, 3 ms) within-subject design was utilized in order to assess the interaction across the variables. To evaluate the remaining rates 97.66 and 234.38/s rates, separate one-way analysis of variance for each duration was conducted to compare responses as a function of repetition rate for both frequencies examined. This included comparing three rates (7.1, 19.53, 58.59/s) at 12 ms durations, four rates (7.1, 19.53, 58.59, 97.66/s) at 6 ms durations, and five rates (7.1, 19.53, 58.59, 97.66, 234.38/s) for the evaluation of 3 ms durations.

RESULTS

Figure 2 depicts the deconvolved tone burst ECochG responses from one of the participants (P9) for the 500 Hz condition for the 12, 6, and 3 ms durations. The SP onset to 500 Hz began at a ~2.5 ms, the location of a positive shift in amplitude from the baseline, and was defined as the starting latency from which the SP midpoint was measured. SP amplitudes were compared across stimulus duration and rate. As the SP is dependent on stimulus duration, the latency of the SP response varied with duration: SP latencies were progressively shorter with decreasing stimulus durations. The SP with the longest latency was to 12 ms stimulus duration, while the shortest was to 3 ms.

SPs differed with stimulus repetition rate duration, particularly to the slowest and highest rates. Most notably, oscillations in the waveform can be observed across the slower rates. This pattern was most evident to slower stimulus repetition rates, 7.1 and 19.53/s, but was less evident to increasing rates and not apparent to the fastest rates. This result is consistent with SP oscillations originating from phase-locked neural excitation that adapts to increasing stimulus rate. Oscillations in the SP

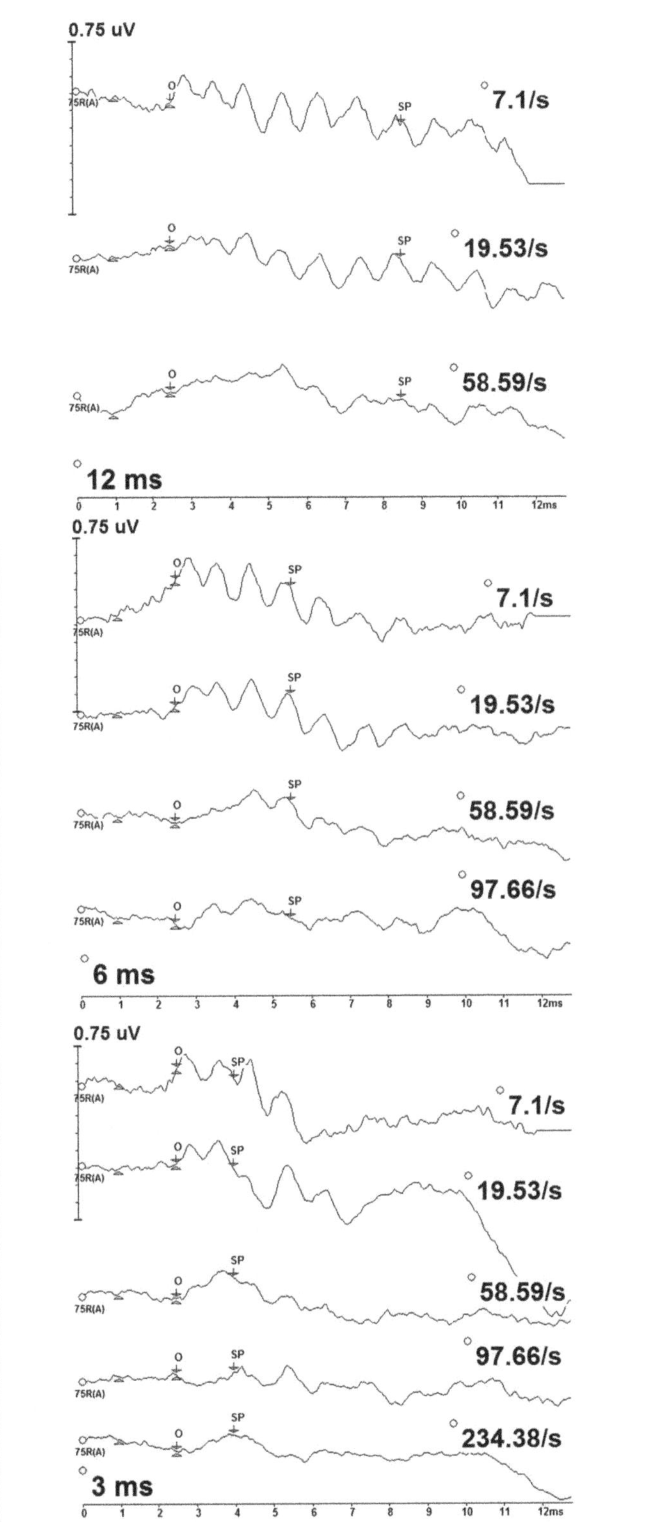

FIGURE 2 | CLAD deconvolved, 500 Hz tone burst ECochG measurements from one participant (P9) across stimulus duration (12 ms—top; 6 ms—middle; 3 ms—bottom). Responses to increasing repetition rate are displayed from top to bottom in each panel. SP amplitude was measured as the baseline at 1 ms to the SP waveform midpoint (SP). The SP waveform midpoint (SP) was measured from onset (O).

waveforms did not cause us to deviate from our methods of quantifying SP amplitudes from various stimulus repetition rates and durations.

Figure 3 shows deconvolved measurements from one participant (P9) to the 12, 6, and 3 ms 2,000 Hz stimulus durations. We identified the SP onset (O) as the point where a positive shift from baseline was observed. SP onset was defined as a 1.5 ms latency to 2,000 Hz, an absolute latency kept constant each stimulus repetition rate and duration for all participants. The length of the SP varied with stimulus duration, with the longest SP response associated with the 12 ms stimulus duration and the shortest with the 3 ms duration.

In contrast to the measurements to 500 Hz stimulus, no oscillating patterns were seen in measurements to 2,000 Hz. Rather, the SP to 2,000 Hz was a notable positive amplitude shift from baseline. The SP latency at peak amplitude varied with stimulus repetition rate and duration, with earlier peak SP amplitude latencies being earlier for slower stimulus repetition rates compared to higher rates. Following this peak the SP amplitude was a gradual decrease in amplitude and increasing latency as the measurement approached baseline. While general amplitude trends were observed over the entirety of the waveform, only the amplitude at midpoint of the SP response was formally assessed.

Group SP amplitudes to 500 Hz varied with stimulus repetition rate (**Figure 4A**) and duration (**Figure 4B**). ANVOA results quantified statistically significant differences for main effect of rate, $F_{(2, 38)} = 6.216, p < 0.05, \eta^2 = 0.246$, and duration, $F_{(2, 38)} = 16.097, p < 0.001, \eta^2 = 0.459$, and a significant rate and duration interaction, $F_{(4, 76)} = 3.461, p < 0.05, \eta^2 = 0.154$. The mean difference between SP amplitude as a function of rate was due to significantly larger SP amplitudes ($p < 0.05$) to 58.59/s (mean = 0.047 μV) than to 7.1/s (mean = 0.00 μV) and 19.53/s (mean = −0.016 μV). No significant difference was found between mean SP amplitudes for the two slowest stimulus repetition rates (7.1 and 19.53/s). The SP amplitude was significantly different ($p < 0.05$) between all stimulus durations. Mean SP amplitude increased with decreasing stimulus duration, in that the smallest mean SP amplitude was found for 12 ms duration and the largest for the 3 ms duration. The SP amplitude trends observed as a function of duration and rate independently indicate significant differences between the applied stimulus parameters in the collection of the SP response, with high rate and short stimulus duration leading to the largest SP amplitude measurements.

SP amplitudes to 2,000 Hz varied with stimulus repetition rate (**Figure 4A**) and duration (**Figure 4B**). We found statistically significant differences for main rate effect $F_{(2, 38)} = 6.774, p < 0.005, \eta^2 = 0.263$, and duration effect $F_{(2, 38)} = 11.379, p < 0.001, \eta^2 = 0.375$, and an interaction between rate and duration, $F_{(4, 76)} = 6.480, p < 0.001, \eta^2 = 0.254$. The mean difference between SP amplitude as a function of rate is due to significantly larger ($p < 0.05$) SP amplitude at 58.59/s rate (mean = 0.190 μV) than at 7.1/s (mean = 0.075 μV) and 19.53/s (mean = 0.117 μV) rates. No significant difference was found between mean SP amplitudes for 7.1 and 19.53/s. The SP amplitude was significantly larger ($p < 0.05$) to 3 ms stimulus duration

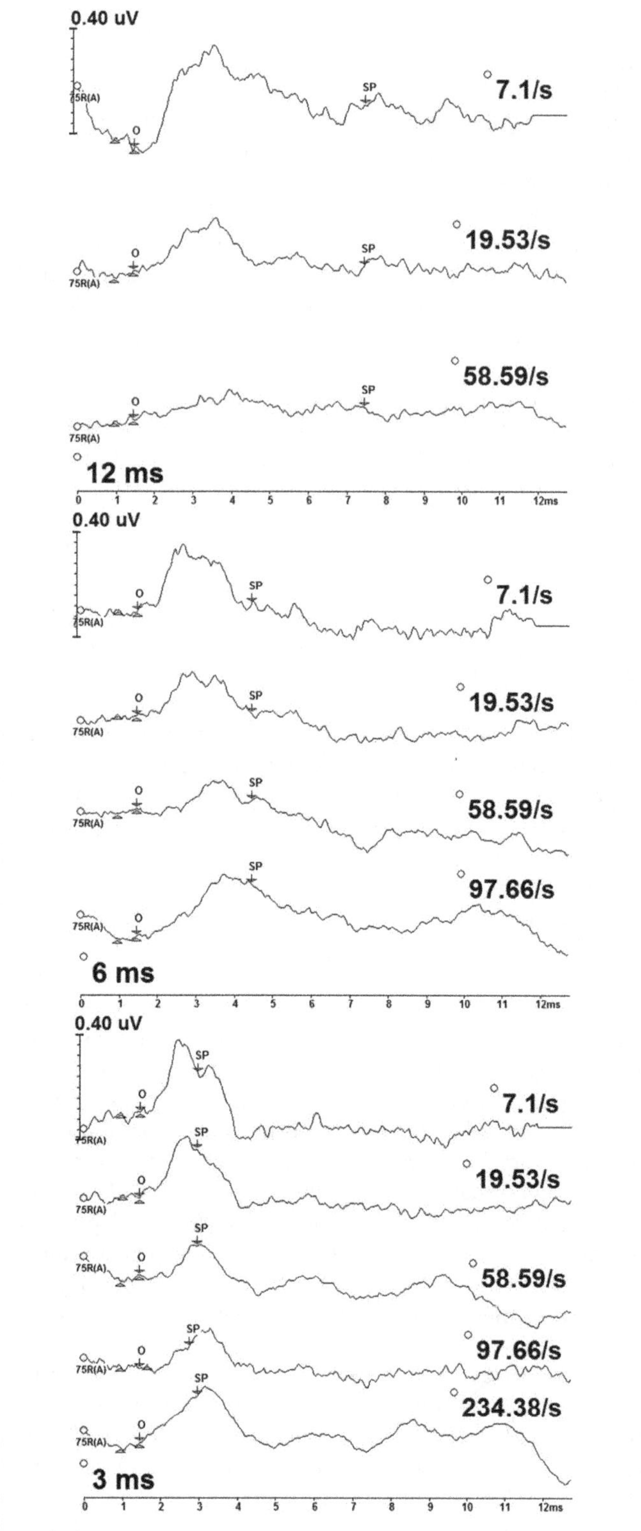

FIGURE 3 | CLAD deconvolved, 2,000 Hz tone burst ECochG measurements from one participant (P9) across stimulus duration (12 ms—top; 6 ms—middle; 3 ms—bottom). Responses to increasing repetition rate are displayed from top to bottom in each panel. SP amplitude was measured as the baseline at 1 ms to the SP waveform midpoint (SP). The SP waveform midpoint (SP) was measured from onset (O).

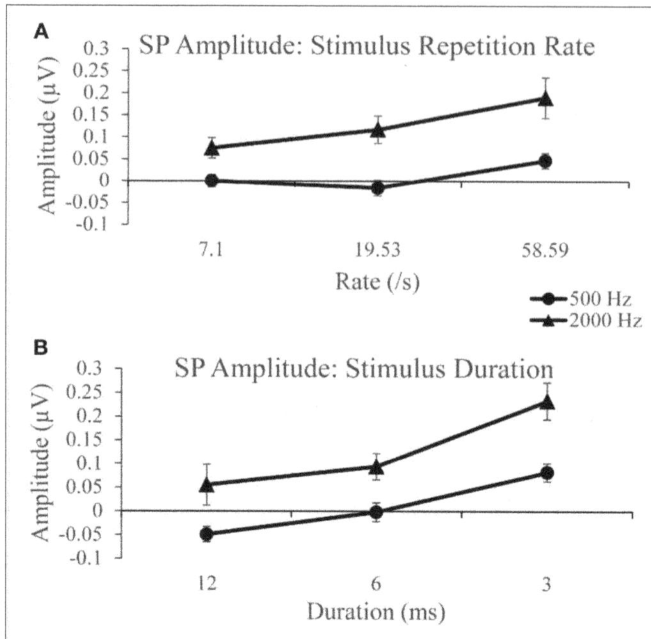

FIGURE 4 | (A) SP amplitudes to 500 and 2,000 Hz varied with stimulus repetition rate (7.1, 19.53, and 58.59/s). SP amplitude to both 500 and 200 Hz were larger for 58.59/s compared to rates 7.1 and 19.53/s. **(B)** SP amplitudes to 500 and 2,000 Hz varied significantly with stimulus duration (12, 6, and 3 ms). SP amplitudes to 500 Hz were significantly larger for 3 ms stimulus duration than for 12 ms durations and 6 ms durations. Likewise, SP amplitudes to 2,000 Hz were significantly larger for the 3 ms stimulus duration than for 12 and 6 ms durations.

compared to the smaller mean amplitudes to 12 and 6 ms. No statistically significant difference was found between the 12 and 6 ms stimulus durations. Again, significant differences across parameters noted, with SP amplitude values significantly larger for short duration and high repetition rates. Further evaluation of SP amplitudes were performed to examine the effect of stimulus repetition rate for each stimulus duration.

Figure 5 shows mean SP amplitude to each duration of 500 Hz. SP amplitude measurements to each stimulus duration was examined independently across each rate. Statistically significant difference, $F_{(2, 38)} = 9.74$, $p < 0.005$, $\eta^2 = 0.339$ was found for the 12 ms duration across rate. *Post-hoc* pairwise comparison revealed significantly larger ($p < 0.05$) SP amplitude to 58.59/s (mean = 0.028 μV) compared to 7.1/s (mean = −0.067 μV) and 19.53/s (mean = −0.107 μV). No significant difference in SP amplitude was found between rates 7.1 and 19.53/s ($p > 0.05$) to 12 ms stimulus duration. The effect of stimulus repetition rate on SP amplitude was also assessed independently for the 6 ms stimulus duration condition, in order to include 97.66/s, and for the 3 ms duration recordings, in order to include 97.66 and 234.38/s. There was no significant effect ($p > 0.05$) across rate for the 6 ms condition. However, a statistically significant difference, $F_{(4, 76)} = 2.499$, $p < 0.05$, $\eta^2 = 0.116$, was found for the SP amplitude across rate for the 3 ms condition. *Post-hoc* pairwise comparison revealed significant differences ($p < 0.05$) between SP amplitude due to significantly larger SP amplitude to 58.59/s (mean = 0.095 μV) and 97.66/s (mean = 0.07 μV), compared

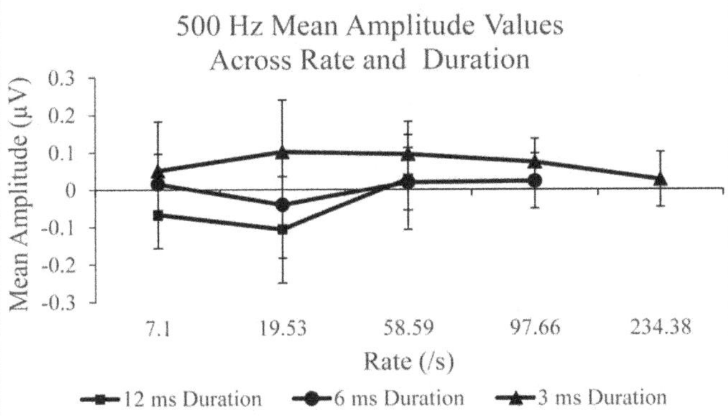

FIGURE 5 | Mean SP amplitude values for the 12 ms duration, 6 ms duration, and 3 ms duration as a function of repetition rate for the 500 Hz condition.

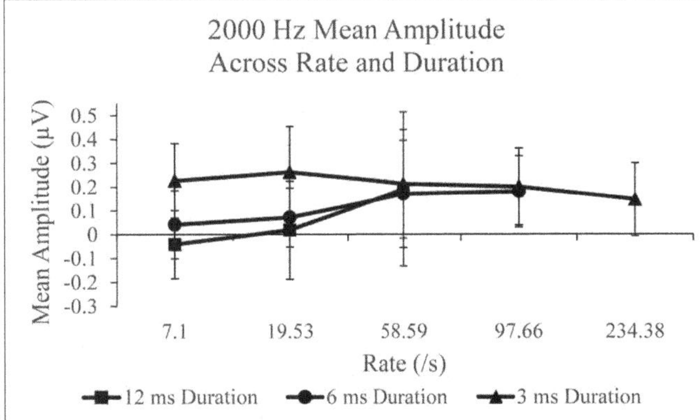

FIGURE 6 | Mean SP amplitude values for the 12 ms duration, 6 ms duration, and 3 ms duration as a function of repetition rate for the 2,000 Hz condition.

to 234.38/s (mean = 0.026 μV). For the long duration stimuli, a significantly larger SP amplitude is collected with higher stimulus rate; however, the opposite trend is observed with the shorter duration stimuli that produces a smaller mean SP amplitude when the fastest rates are used to elicit the response. To evaluate the SP amplitude data of the responses obtained with use of 2,000 Hz eliciting stimuli, identical analysis procedures were applied.

SP amplitudes to 2,000 Hz varied with stimulus rate and duration (**Figure 6**). An independent analysis of the measurements to 12 ms stimulus durations revealed a statistically significant difference across rate $F_{(2, 38)} = 9.936$, $p < 0.005$, $\eta^2 = 0.343$. Significantly larger SP amplitude ($p < 0.05$) was found for 58.59/s (mean = 0.189 μV) compared to 7.1/s (mean = −0.042) and 19.53 (mean = 0.018). No significant difference was found between SP amplitude to 7.1 and 19.53/s ($p > 0.05$) stimulus repetition rates. To examine the remaining rates, 97.66 and 234.38/s, in the analysis, the effect of stimulus rate was assessed independently for the 6 and 3 ms conditions. The 6 ms duration condition revealed a statistically significant difference, $F_{(3, 57)} = 6.009$, $p < 0.005$, $\eta^2 = 0.240$, between SP amplitude across rate. Specifically, a significant difference was found due to larger amplitude at rates 58.56/s (mean = 0.170 μV; $p < 0.05$) and 97.66/s (mean = 0.180 μV; $p < 0.005$), when compared to rate 7.1/s (mean = 0.042 μV). A significantly larger ($p < 0.005$) amplitude was also found for 97.66/s than for 19.53/s (mean = 0.071 μV). No other significant difference ($p > 0.05$) was observed between rates for the 6 ms duration. For the 3 ms condition, a statistically significant difference, $F_{(4, 76)} = 3.384$, $p < 0.05$, $\eta^2 = 0.151$, was noted. Specifically, we found a significantly larger ($p < 0.05$) SP amplitude to 19.53/s (mean = 0.262 μV), than for the two highest rates, 97.66/s (mean = 0.201 μV) and 234.38/s (mean = 0.146 μV). No other significant differences ($p > 0.05$) were found between rates for the 3 ms duration. As was found with the 500 Hz frequency, the application of high rate and long stimulus duration again finds mean SP amplitude that is significantly larger when compared to slow rates, suggesting the use of high rate to elicit a larger SP when long duration stimuli are utilized. Again, the opposite trend was found with the use of short duration stimuli where we observed mean SP amplitude decreasing with increasing rate.

DISCUSSION

The use of ECochG in the assessment of the auditory system has garnered a great deal of evaluation in terms of protocol, parameters, and methodology. While ECochG measurements to tone bursts have been studied for its potential usefulness in objectively assessing Ménière's disease (Gibson, 1993, 2009; Ferraro and Krishnan, 1997; Wuyts et al., 1997; Conlon and Gibson, 2000; Iseli and Gibson, 2010), a condition defined by endolymphatic hydrops (Merchant et al., 2005; Nadol, 2010), fewer studies have examined the usefulness of slow repetition rates (Levine et al., 1992; Ferraro et al., 1994a; Margolis et al., 1995). Ours was a study on a novel assessment of ECochG measurements to tone bursts analyzed with the CLAD technique to quantify SP amplitude at various stimulus repetition rates. Normative data was obtained across frequency, stimulus repetition rate, and stimulus duration to understand the effects of these parameters on the SP.

SP Amplitude

Our study is rooted in the assumption that SP originating from hair cells will sustain throughout the duration of the measurement because hair cells do not habituate, while SP originating from neural excitation will decrease in amplitude because of neural habituation. We found that trends in SP amplitudes to various tone burst repetition rate and durations for both 500 and 2,000 Hz. In particular, SP amplitude was significantly larger for the highest stimulus repetition rate, 58.59/s compared to the slower rates, 7.1 and 19.53/s. Additionally, SP amplitude was significantly larger for the shortest tone burst duration, 3 ms, compared to longer durations, 12 and 6 ms. SP amplitudes were significantly larger for 2,000 Hz than 500 Hz for each stimulus repetition rate and duration.

Overall, the longer duration stimuli evoked larger SP amplitudes with increasing stimulus repetition rate. However, this trend was reversed with the use of short duration stimuli (3 ms), in which mean SP amplitude to 3 ms duration decreased as repetition rate increased. SP amplitudes to 3 ms tone bursts were larger for all repetition rates. While our results are statistically significant, they are not always consistent with that found in previous studies. We flesh out the inconsistencies below in this section.

Slow Repetition Rate

The SP to long duration (12 ms), slow rate (7.1/s) tone bursts had negative amplitude, with −0.067 μV to 500 Hz and −0.042 μV to 2,000 Hz. The direct comparison of the current SP amplitude measures to published research is difficult due to distinct differences in recording and stimulus parameters, as well as differences in methods used to quantify the SP amplitude. Wuyts et al. (1997) performed a meta-analysis of ECochG measurements to click and tone burst stimuli and found that too few reports exist to extract normative SP amplitude data from tone bursts stimuli. Nevertheless, Wuyts et al.'s meta-analysis found a trend that SP from near-baseline levels generally have positive, not negative, amplitudes. Our approach to assigning the non-inverting and inverting electrodes resulted in positive going SP amplitudes, which is consistent with Wuyts et al. (1997) report of negative SP amplitudes. Our findings are consistent with those reported by Ferraro et al. (1994a), though precise stimulus parameter differences exist. Ferraro et al.'s results to 90 dBnHL, 11.3/s, and 2-10-2 duration can be generally compared to our SP amplitudes to slow rate, long duration tone bursts. Ferraro et al. (1994a) found mean SP amplitude values of 0.19 μV to 500 Hz and 0.08 μV to 2,000 Hz, which are comparable to our SP amplitudes when polarity differences from electrode montages are accounted for. While our results are similar to the Ferraro et al. (1994a) study, other reports utilizing long duration tone bursts (15 ms) with slow rate (13/s) obtained larger, positive SP amplitude values in subjects without inner ear disease: Margolis et al. (1995) found respective SP amplitudes of 0.65 and 0.96 μV to 100 and 110 dB SPL 2,000 Hz tone bursts from ears with normal hearing, which are markedly larger than amplitudes found in our study, even when compared to the most positive amplitudes to our 7.1 and 19.53/s stimulus repetition rates.

Our measurements to 500 Hz tone bursts can be informative about the extent to which neural excitation can contribute to recordings made from the auditory periphery. We found oscillations in response waveforms to slower rate, long duration conditions (**Figure 2**), consistent with the contribution of neural excitation that is phase locked to this low frequency stimulus (Lichtenhan et al., 2013, 2014; Chertoff et al., 2015). Oscillations decreased with increasing stimulus repetition rate, further supporting the interpretation of the neural origin of this waveform component, as auditory nerve fibers cannot respond to high-rate stimuli while in their refractory period. As such, it is possible that the oscillations occurring in the slow rate, long duration 500 Hz recordings are contributing to the mean SP amplitude results obtained in the study.

SP amplitude was measured from one pre-defined midpoint along the waveform for all rates and participants and the measurements did not take into account variations associated with the peaks and troughs of the oscillations. As SP amplitudes collected were small, these oscillations may have had a significant impact on the collected amplitude data. For example, the midpoint occurring at a peak of the oscillation for one recording and at a trough for another had the potential to influence the SP amplitude values obtained.

A technique to reduce the contribution of the oscillations within the 500 Hz recordings is to filter the measurements with a low-pass cut-off frequency. Using the Intelligent Hearing Systems software, spectral filtering was applied offline to a single measurement to evaluate this method as a technique to examine the 500 Hz recordings. **Figure 7** displays this technique for a 12 ms, 58.59/s deconvolved trace across four spectral filters: 0–250 Hz, 0–300 Hz, 0–350 Hz, and 0–450 Hz. As more filtering was applied, the smoother the resultant waveform. The labeled SP indicates the pre-defined midpoint for the 12 ms stimulus duration. Filtering the measurements is a possible technique to improve SP detection.

High Repetition Rate

Our negative SP amplitudes to slow repetition rate, 12 ms stimulus duration tone bursts contrast the positive amplitudes we measured to higher rates. SP amplitudes to higher rate (58.59/s), long duration (12 ms) tone bursts were significantly larger than those to slower rates (7.1 and 19.53/s) to both tone burst frequencies. Oscillations in responses to high rate, 500 Hz

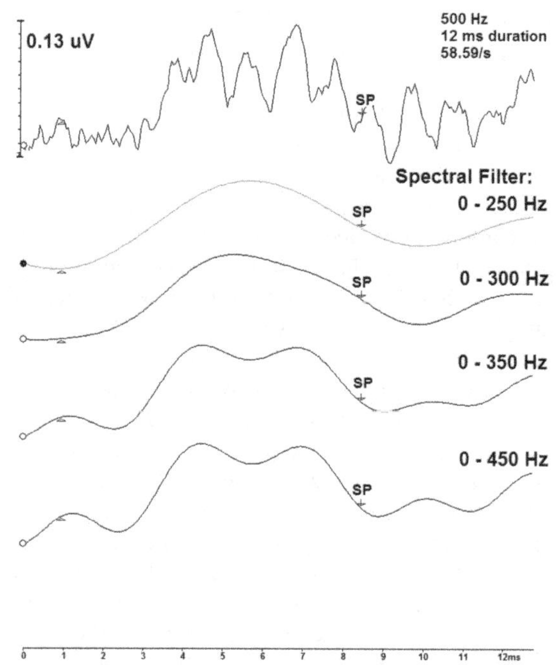

FIGURE 7 | Spectral filtering of a CLAD deconvolved tone burst ECochG waveform (top) for the 500 Hz, 12 ms, 58.59/s condition. Displayed in descending order, four spectral band pass filters were applied: 0–250, 0–300, 0–350, and 0–450 Hz. SP indicates the pre-defined midpoint of the 12 ms duration.

tone bursts were reduced and a positive mean SP amplitude of 0.028 μV was collected for the highest rate. There were no significant differences found among SP amplitudes to 6 ms 500 Hz tone bursts of various repetition rates. These results can inform clinicians and basic investigators on the appropriate parameters needed to assess low-frequency function: use long duration stimuli with a high repetition rate to quantify non-neural SP to 500 Hz.

Also our results showed that SP amplitudes tended to increase with increasing stimulus repetition rate with the use of 2,000 Hz, long duration tone bursts, a common finding in previous studies. Wilson and Bowker (2002), for example, studied ECochG measurements to clicks ranging from 7.1 to 151.1/s, albeit without the CLAD technique. They found that SP amplitudes increased in response to higher stimulus repetition rates. However, their SP amplitudes were overall reduced because of poor frequency specification to their click stimuli and poor morphology and overlying responses that result from not using the CLAD technique. These findings highlight the usefulness of tone burst stimuli and the CLAD technique for measurements to high stimulus rates.

Stimulus Level and Recording Location

We made SP amplitude measurements to higher stimulus repetition rates, shorter stimulus duration, and, perhaps more importantly, to low stimulus intensity. DC responses are generally thought to originate from higher level stimuli that probe the asymmetric regions of the sigmodial, saturating, non-linear function that can describe the transfer of sound from mechanical to electrical mediums in the inner ear. We avoided high-intensity stimuli because of our lengthy test sessions, and presented both the 500 and 2,000 Hz tone bursts at 75 dB nHL (107 dB SPL), a level which may resulted in lower SP amplitudes. It is possible that our lower levels may have evoked a larger SP had we used a transtympanic approach, but a transtympanic approach would increase the measured amplitude of all DC origins, albiet hair cell or neural. Indeed, amplitudes from an extratympanic approach can be ~4–10 times smaller than those from transtympanic approach (Ferraro et al., 1994b; Haapaniemi et al., 2000). Direct microscope visualization for uniform electrode placement on the umbo may provide uniformity in measurements, but straightening the ear canal with the electrode in place can be painful and direct microscopic visualization is challenging because the white cotton tipped electrode soaked in gel reflects a light that obstructs the visualization of electrode placement. The most common way to identify electrode placement is after measurements are done and remaining electrode gel and irritation is visualized with otoscopy. Smith et al. (2016) found that electrode placement mostly affects measurements from low-frequencies when an insert-earphone is used, a possible influence on our measurements to 500 Hz.

High Repetition Rate and Continuous Loop Averaging Deconvolution

Our study demonstrated the use of the CLAD technique applied to ECochG measurements to tone bursts. Several studies have also demonstrated the use of the CLAD technique to ECochG measurements, but those studies focused on the use of click stimuli (Bohorquez et al., 2006, 2009; Bextermueller, 2015; Dixon, 2015; Kaf et al., 2017). Measurements to stimulus repetition rates up to 234.38/s were successfully deconvolved allowing for clear observation of the SP and the AP within the recordings. This novel finding supports the use of CLAD with responses evoked using tone burst stimuli. With close monitoring of the maximum repetition rate in the CLAD sequence, CLAD can be applied to test SP amplitudes at high rates which were previously limited due to the overlain responses.

Limitations and Future Studies

Our results cannot be generalized outside the specific recording analysis techniques. Currently, there is no standardized tone burst parameters for ECochG approaches across research institutions. This is a double edged sword making direct comparison from one study to another quite challenging, but does not restrict investigators' creative use of stimulus parameters to study and understand normal and diseased ears.

We subjectively measured SP amplitudes at mid-point that was relative to a fixed waveform onset to mediate uniform SP amplitude measurement across participants. A limitation of this approach was that SP onset did indeed vary between participants. Our SP amplitude measures may thus have variations that were untethered to a gold standard for the onset of SP measurements. Future research could reassess our data to determine how various definitions of SP onset influences results.

The most pressing research to address in future work on this topic is to use legitimate DC-coupled recordings of SP measurements and validate our interpretations in animal models where the neural origins of SP amplitude measures can be manipulated. Injection of neurotoxic solutions into the cochlear apex is a new approach that can treat the entire length of the cochlear spiral (Lichtenhan et al., 2016). Using the stimulus and analysis approaches of our current study in animals where the apical injection technique can be applied could quantify the extent to which neural excitation contributes to our interpretation of data presented here.

CONCLUSION

We collected normative SP amplitude from females with normal hearing using extratympanic ECochG, tone burst stimuli, and a CLAD analysis technique. SP amplitude measures to 2,000 Hz, long duration stimuli increased with increasing repetition rate, as did SP amplitudes to 500 Hz with the longest stimulus duration (12 ms) and highest stimulus repetition rate (58.59/s). These increased amplitude measures are consistent with SP origins from hair cell responses, not neural excitation, and suggest that high stimulus repetition rate could be used to minimize neural contributions to SP measures. SP amplitude measures to our shortest stimulus duration (3 ms) were consistent with marked contribution of neural excitation, thus identifying a stimulus condition to use when an SP measurement originating from neural responses is desired. Our study also demonstrated the use of the CLAD technique with ECochG measurements to tone bursts presented with high stimulus repetition rates. While the use of tone burst stimuli limited our stimulus repetition rate to 234.38/s, the deconvolved waveforms nevertheless show that the CLAD technique can be used with frequency-specific stimuli. Overall, this research was a step toward understanding how varying stimulus parameters can be used to advance our understanding of the origins of SP amplitude measures, an important step for advancing the use of ECochG in diagnosis of Ménière's disease that mainly affects low frequency hearing early in the disease process.

AUTHOR CONTRIBUTIONS

AK, WK, RD, JL, JF: Meet all criteria for authorship.

FUNDING

This study was supported by the Missouri State University Graduate College Thesis Research Funding. WK received an Emerging Research Grant from the Hearing Health Foundation. JL was supported by R01 DC014997 from the National Institutes of Health, National Institute on Deafness and Other Communication Disorders.

ACKNOWLEDGMENTS

The authors thank Dr. Erdem Yavuz for help during our pilot recording to determine the best stimulus parameters for this research, and the study participants.

REFERENCES

Al-momani, M. O., Ferraro, J. A., Gajewski, B. J., and Ator, G. (2009). Improved sensitivity of electrocochleography in the diagnosis of Ménière's disease. *Int. J. Audiol.* 48, 811–819. doi: 10.3109/14992020903019338

American Speech-Language-Hearing Association (1988). *Tympanometry [Relevant Paper]*. Available online at: www.asha.org/policy.

Bextermueller, K. (2015). *Electrocochleography and Auditory Brainstem Response in Normal Adults and Vestibular Migraine Patients Using Continuous Loop Averaging Deconvolution.* Doctoral thesis, Missouri State University, Springfield.

Bohorquez, J., Morawski, K., Ozdamar, O., and Niemczyk, K. (2006). "High rate transtympanic electrocochleography," in *Meniere's Patients Using Continuous Loop Averaging Deconvolution (CLAD). Poster Presentation.* Available online at: https://umshare.miami.edu/web/wda/engineeringfiles/BME/bohorquez.pdf (Accessed January 30, 2016).

Bohorquez, J., Ozdamar, O., McNeer, R., and Morawski, K. (2009). "Clinical application of evoked potential continuous loop averaging deconvolution (CLAD)," in *25th Southern Biomedical Engineering Conference 2009, IFMBE Proceedings*, eds A. McGoron, C. Li, and W.-C. Lin (Miami, FL), 133–134.

Chertoff, M. E., Kamerer, A. M., Peppi, M., and Lichtenhan, J. T. (2015). An analysis of cochlear response harmonics: contribution of neural excitation. *J. Acoust. Soc. Am.* 138, 2957–2963. doi: 10.1121/1.4934556

Conlon, B. J., and Gibson, W. P. R. (2000). Electrocochleography in the diagnosis of Ménière's disease. *Acta Otolaryngol.* 120, 480–483. doi: 10.1080/000164800750045965

Delgado, R. E., and Ozdamar, O. (2004). Deconvolution of evoked responses obtained at high stimulus rates. *J. Acoust. Soc. Am.* 115, 1242–1251. doi: 10.1121/1.1639327

Dixon, S. (2015). *Fast Stimulus Rate Electrocochleography and Auditory Brainstem Response Using Continuous Loop Averaging Deconvolution in Normal Individuals and Ménière's Patients.* Doctoral thesis, Missouri State University, Springfield.

Ferraro, J. A., Best, L. G., and Arenberg, I. K. (1983). The use of electrocochleography in the diagnosis, assessment, and monitoring of endolymphatic hydrops. *Otolaryngol. Clin. North Am.* 16, 69–82.

Ferraro, J. A., Blackwell, W. L., Mediavilla, S. J., and Thedinger, B. S. (1994a). Normal summating potential to tone bursts recorded from the tympanic membrane in humans. *J. Am. Acad. Audiol.* 5, 17–23.

Ferraro, J. A., and Durrant, J. D. (2006). Electrocochleography in the evaluation of patients with Ménière's disease/endolymphatic hydrops. *J. Am. Acad. Audiol.* 17, 45–68. doi: 10.3766/jaaa.17.1.6

Ferraro, J. A., and Krishnan, G. (1997). Cochlear potentials in clinical audiology. *Audiol. Neurootol.* 2, 241–256. doi: 10.1159/000259251

Ferraro, J. A., Thedinger, B. S., Mediavilla, S. J., and Blackwell, W. L. (1994b). Human summating potential to tone bursts: observation on tympanic membrane versus promontory recordings in the same patients. *J. Am. Acad. Audiol.* 5, 24–29.

Ferraro, J. A., and Tibbils, R. P. (1999). SP/AP area ratio in the diagnosis of Ménière's disease. *Am. J. Audiol.* 8, 1–8. doi: 10.1044/1059-0889(1999/001)

Gibson, W. P. R. (1993). "A comparison of clicks versus tone bursts in the diagnosis of endolymphatic hydrops," in *ECocG, OAE, and Intraoperative Monitoring: Proceedings of the First International Conference, Wurzburg, Germany, September 20-24, 1992,* ed D. Hohmann (Amsterdam: Kugler Publications), 55–59.

Gibson, W. P. R. (2009). A comparison of two methods using transtympanic electrocochleography for the diagnosis of Ménière's disease: click summating potential/action potential ratio measurements and tone burst summating potential measurements. *Acta Otolaryngol.* 129, 38–42. doi: 10.1080/00016480902729843

Goodman, A. (1965). Reference levels for pure-tone audiometer. *ASHA* 7, 262–263.

Haapaniemi, J., Laurikainen, E., Johansson, R., and Karjalainen, S. (2000). Transtympanic versus tympanic membrane electrocochleography in examining cochleovestibular disorders. *Acta Oto-laryngol. Suppl.* 543, 127–129. doi: 10.1080/000164800454189

Iseli, C., and Gibson, W. (2010). A comparison of three methods of using transtympanic electrocochleography for the diagnosis of Ménière's disease: click summating potential measurements, tone burst summating potential measurements, and biasing of the summating potential using a low frequency tone. *Acta Otolaryngol.* 130, 95–101. doi: 10.3109/00016480902858899

Kaf, W. A., Lewis, K. M., Yavuz, E., Dixon, S. M., van Ess, M., Jamos, A. M., et al. (2017). Fast click rate electrocochleography and auditory brainstem response in normal-hearing adults using continuous loop averaging deconvolution. *Ear Hear.* 38, 244–254. doi: 10.1097/AUD.0000000000000381

Levine, S. C., Margolis, R. H., Fournier, E. M., and Winzenburg, S. M. (1992). Tympanic electrocochleography for evaluation of endolymphatic hydrops. *Laryngoscope* 102, 614–622. doi: 10.1288/00005537-199206000-00005

Lichtenhan, J. T., Cooper, N. P., and Guinan, J. J. (2013). A new auditory threshold estimation technique for low frequencies: proof of concept. *Ear Hear.* 34, 42–51. doi: 10.1097/AUD.0b013e31825f9bd3

Lichtenhan, J. T., Hartsock, J. J., Dornhoffer, J., Donovan, K. M., and Salt, A. N. (2016). Drug delivery into the cochlear apex: improved control to sequentially affect finely spaced regions along the entire length of the cochlear spiral. *J. Neurosci. Methods* 1, 201–209. doi: 10.1016/j.jneumeth.2016.08.005

Lichtenhan, J. T., Hartsock, J. J., Gill, R. M., Guinan, J. J., and Salt, A. N. (2014). The Auditory Nerve Overlapped Waveform (ANOW) originates in the cochlear apex. *J. Assoc. Res. Otolaryngol.* 15, 395–411. doi: 10.1007/s10162-014-0447-y

Margolis, R. H., Ricks, D., Fournier, E. M., and Levine, S. E. (1995). Tympanic electrocochleography for diagnosis of Ménière's disease. *Arch. Otolaryngol. Head Neck Surg.* 121, 44–55. doi: 10.1001/archotol.1995.01890010032007

Merchant, S. N., Adams, J. C., and Nadol, J. B. Jr. (2005). Pathophysiology of Meniere's syndrome: are symptoms caused by endolymphatic hydrops? *Otol. Neurotol.* 26, 74–81. doi: 10.1097/00129492-200501000-00013

Nadol, J. B. Jr. (2010). "Disorders of unknown or multiple causes," in *Schuknecht's Pathology of the Ear, 3rd Edn,* eds S. N. Merchant and J. B. Nadol Jr. (Shelton, CT: People's Medical Publishing House), 572–630.

Smith, B. S., Lichtenhan, J. T., and Cone, B. (2016). Behavioral pure tone threshold shifts caused by tympanic membrane electrodes. *Ear Hear.* 37, e273–e275. doi: 10.1097/AUD.0000000000000275

Wilson, W. J., and Bowker, C. A. (2002). The effects of high stimulus rate on the electrocochleogram in normal-hearing subjects. *Int. J. Audiol.* 41, 509–517. doi: 10.3109/14992020209056071

Wuyts, F. L., Van de Heyning, P. H., Van Spaendonck, M. P., and Molenberghs, G. (1997). A review of electrocochleography: instrumentation settings and meta-analysis of criteria for diagnosis of endolymphatic hydrops. *Acta Oto-Laryngol. Suppl.* 526, 14–20. doi: 10.3109/00016489709124014

Wuyts, F. L., Van de Heyning, P. H., Van Spaendonck, M., Van der Stappen, A., D'Haese, P., and Erre, J.-P. (2001). Rate influences on tone burst summating potential amplitude in electrocochleography: clinical and experimental data. *Hear. Res.* 152, 1–9. doi: 10.1016/S0378-5955(00)00207-0

18

Hidden Hearing Loss? No Effect of Common Recreational Noise Exposure on Cochlear Nerve Response Amplitude in Humans

*Sarah K. Grinn[1,2], Kathryn B. Wiseman[1], Jason A. Baker[1] and Colleen G. Le Prell[1]**

[1] School of Behavioral and Brain Sciences, University of Texas at Dallas, Dallas, TX, United States, [2] College of Public Health and Health Professions, University of Florida, Gainesville, FL, United States

***Correspondence:**
Colleen G. Le Prell
colleen.leprell@utdallas.edu

This study tested hypothesized relationships between noise exposure and auditory deficits. Both retrospective assessment of potential associations between noise exposure history and performance on an audiologic test battery and prospective assessment of potential changes in performance after new recreational noise exposure were completed.

Methods: 32 participants (13M, 19F) with normal hearing (25-dB HL or better, 0.25–8 kHz) were asked to participate in 3 pre- and post-exposure sessions including: otoscopy, tympanometry, distortion product otoacoustic emissions (DPOAEs) (f2 frequencies 1–8 kHz), pure-tone audiometry (0.25–8 kHz), Words-in-Noise (WIN) test, and electrocochleography (eCochG) measurements at 70, 80, and 90-dB nHL (click and 2–4 kHz tone-bursts). The first session was used to collect baseline data, the second session was collected the day after a loud recreational event, and the third session was collected 1-week later. Of the 32 participants, 26 completed all 3 sessions.

Results: The retrospective analysis did not reveal statistically significant relationships between noise exposure history and any auditory deficits. The day after new exposure, there was a statistically significant correlation between noise "dose" and WIN performance overall, and within the 4-dB signal-to-babble ratio. In contrast, there were no statistically significant correlations between noise dose and changes in threshold, DPOAE amplitude, or AP amplitude the day after new noise exposure. Additional analyses revealed a statistically significant relationship between TTS and DPOAE amplitude at 6 kHz, with temporarily decreased DPOAE amplitude observed with increasing TTS.

Conclusions: There was no evidence of auditory deficits as a function of previous noise exposure history, and no permanent changes in audiometric, electrophysiologic, or functional measures after new recreational noise exposure. There were very few participants with TTS the day after exposure - a test time selected to be consistent with previous animal studies. The largest observed TTS was approximately 20-dB. The observed pattern of small TTS suggests little risk of synaptopathy from common recreational noise exposure, and that we should not expect to observe changes in evoked potentials for this reason. No such changes were observed in this study. These data do not support suggestions that common, recreational noise exposure is likely to result in "hidden hearing loss".

Keywords: synaptopathy, hidden hearing loss, noise induced hearing loss (NIHL), recreational noise, temporary threshold shift (TTS), speech-in-noise, words in noise (WIN), action potential (AP)

INTRODUCTION

The mammalian auditory system is susceptible to noise exposure injury resulting from damage to cells in the inner ear. Changes in function can be temporary or permanent (for review, see Ryan et al., 2016). The Occupational Safety and Health Administration (OSHA) federal noise regulations define an auditory "standard threshold shift" as a permanent change in hearing threshold, relative to one's baseline audiogram, of an average of 10-dB or more at 2, 3, and 4 kHz in either ear (OSHA, 1983). A temporary threshold shift (TTS), by definition, does not meet this regulatory standard for a workplace-induced noise injury. However, recent findings suggest that large TTS may result in permanent synaptic loss (Kujawa and Liberman, 2009), followed by slow, progressive neural degeneration (Kujawa and Liberman, 2006). Thus, exposures that result in TTS may be more harmful than previously believed (Kujawa and Liberman, 2015).

Noise exposures that result in a relatively robust TTS 24-h after the noise exposure have been accompanied by loss of the synaptic connections between inner hair cells (IHCs) and the afferent neurons in mice (Kujawa and Liberman, 2009; Wang and Ren, 2012; Fernandez et al., 2015) and guinea pigs (Lin et al., 2011; Furman et al., 2013). With this decrease in the neural output of the cochlea, the amplitude of Wave-I of the sound-evoked auditory brainstem response (ABR) is permanently reduced, even though the ABR Wave-I threshold remains unchanged (for reviews, see Kujawa and Liberman, 2015; Liberman and Kujawa, 2017). Because these noise exposures result in damage that cannot be detected by conventional audiometric threshold assessment, this synaptopathic injury has been referred to as "hidden hearing loss", a term originally coined by Schaette and McAlpine (2011). Synaptopathic injury appears to be biased toward low spontaneous firing rate neurons, which have higher response thresholds and are responsible for coding higher intensity (suprathreshold) sounds (Furman et al., 2013). In contrast, synaptic contacts with the high-spontaneous rate neurons, which have lower response thresholds and are responsible for coding lower intensity sounds (i.e., audiometric thresholds), appear to be largely unaffected. This may explain why the threshold audiogram is not sensitive to loss of IHCs (Lobarinas et al., 2013) or afferent synapses (Kujawa and Liberman, 2009).

It has been suggested that noise-induced neuropathic damage may explain the disproportionate difficulties some individuals experience processing speech in noisy environments, despite clinically normal hearing thresholds (Kujawa and Liberman, 2009; Lin et al., 2011; Makary et al., 2011). More recently, there have been several suggestions that recreational noise could induce cochlear synaptopathy manifested as difficulty understanding speech in background noise with deficits "hidden" behind a standard audiogram. Liberman (2015) points to "the loud pop of Fourth of July fireworks or the roar of the crowds at a football game" as not only affecting hair cells, but also damaging the auditory neurons, and suggests that their research finding "raises questions about the risks of routine exposure to loud music at concerts and clubs and via personal listening devices." Jensen et al. (2015) similarly point to the increasing sales of portable listening devices, and suggest that there has been a corresponding "shift of 'at-risk' users from adults to adolescents." Suggestions such as these have led multiple groups to seek evidence that would suggest a potential synaptopathic injury in otherwise normal-hearing young adult cohorts (Stamper and Johnson, 2015a,b; Prendergast et al., 2017; Spankovich et al., 2017; Fulbright et al., in press).

Although Stamper and Johnson (2015a) presented evidence that was interpreted as consistent with a synaptopathic noise injury (reduction in ABR Wave-I amplitude) secondary to recreational noise history in normal-hearing young adults, the investigation did not account for differences in ABR Wave-I amplitude as a function of sex. After controlling for sex, the observed effects were limited to females (Stamper and Johnson, 2015b). More recently, Prendergast et al. (2017), Fulbright et al. (in press), and Spankovich et al. (2017) were unable to provide evidence consistent with noise-induced synaptopathic injury in other young adult populations with varying recreational noise histories. However, failure to detect deficits in ABR Wave-I amplitude in young adults with recreational noise exposure histories is perhaps not that surprising. In animal models, shorter or less intense noise exposures that result in smaller TTS changes do not result in synaptopathic injury, functional deficits, or progressive neuronal loss (Hickox and Liberman, 2014; Fernandez et al., 2015; Jensen et al., 2015; Lobarinas et al., 2017). In studies with rodents, 20–30 dB TTS 24 h post noise generally has not been associated with synaptopathic change, whereas 40–50 dB TTS 24 h post noise clearly has been associated with synaptopathic damage. Thus, typical recreational noise

---

Abbreviations: ABR, Auditory brainstem response; AE, annual exposure; ASSR, Auditory Steady State Response; dB, decibel; dBA, A-weighted decibel; dB HL, decibel hearing level; dB S/B, decibel signal to babble ratio; dB SPL, decibel sound pressure level; DPOAE, distortion product otoacoustic emission; ECochG, Electrocochleography; EHF, extended high frequency; EL, exposure level; Hz, hertz; IHC, inner hair cell; kHz, kilohertz; $L_{Aeq8760}$, A-weighted equivalent sound level 8760 h; NIOSH, National Institute on Occupational Safety and Health; NU-6, Northwestern University Auditory Test Number 6; OHC, outer hair cell; OSHA, Occupational Safety and Health Administration; PTS, permanent threshold shift; SRT, Speech Recognition Threshold; TTS, temporary threshold shift; WRS, Word Recognition Score; WIN, Words-in-Noise.

exposures commonly experienced by young adults likely are not sufficient to result in an acute neural pathology. The lack of deficits observed in studies assessing young adults with a history of recreational noise exposure (Prendergast et al., 2017; Spankovich et al., 2017; Fulbright et al., in press) does not preclude the possibility that damage emerges with louder, longer, or more frequently repeated noise exposures, such as firearm exposure (Bramhall et al., 2017), explosions (Remenschneider et al., 2014), and blast exposure in the course of military service (Helfer et al., 2011; Gallun et al., 2012a,b; Saunders et al., 2015). The data from Bramhall et al. (2017) are compelling in showing reduced ABR Wave-I amplitude in civilians and military personnel with high noise exposure, and the data from Liberman et al. (2016) raise important questions about the potential for hazard for musicians. The issue of unknown damage-risk criteria for synaptopathic injury and hidden hearing loss is a challenge not only for public health hearing loss prevention efforts targeting adolescents, but also for the protection of noise-exposed workers (for discussion, see Dobie and Humes, 2017; Murphy and Le Prell, 2017).

The current investigation is the first to describe prospective monitoring of young adults attending loud recreational venues for potential changes in both auditory evoked potentials and functional performance (tone detection and speech-in-noise testing) as a consequence of acute recreational noise exposure. The unique features of this study were (1) collection of data pre- and post-noise exposure, (2) the use of a sound-pressure-level meter smartphone app to document exposure during loud events attended by participants, and (3) the integration of functional word-in-noise tests with evoked potential measures in assessing effects of recreational noise. These data were collected with the specific goal of generating evidence that will provide insight into the potential hazards of individual recreational events, as a function of the accrued noise dose, so that future investigations can more precisely target at-risk populations. In addition to the use of prospective test design, the current investigation adds data on the relationship between hearing-in-noise and noise exposure history. Distortion product otoacoustic emission (DPOAE) amplitude was assessed in order to differentiate potential damage to the outer hair cell (OHC) and IHC populations.

METHODS

This study was approved by the Institutional Review Board at the University of Texas at Dallas. Signed consent forms were obtained from participants prior to study enrollment. Participants were recruited from the University of Texas at Dallas campus in Richardson, Texas and the Callier Center for Communication Disorders in Dallas, Texas. All study procedures were performed using dedicated clinical research equipment located at the Callier Center for Communication Disorders in Dallas, TX. All study procedures were conducted by students in their third or fourth year of training in the Doctor of Audiology program. Participants were allowed to withdraw at any time; they were compensated for each laboratory visit.

Participants included 32 young adults (13 male, 19 female; mean age 23.5 years, range 21–27 years). Participants were asked to self-identify sex; we are not aware of any participants for whom gender identity was different from biological sex. All participants met the study enrollment criteria, including normal otoscopic examination bilaterally (visualization of the tympanic membranes with no apparent abnormalities), normal tympanometric examination bilaterally (Type A with 226 Hz probe tone), and normal hearing (defined as thresholds of 25 dB HL or better from 0.25 to 8 kHz bilaterally).

Participants were invited to attend three test sessions. In order to avoid enticing participants to attend a loud recreational event, the second session was specified as being either (A) the day after attending a loud recreational event of their choice, or (B) a second baseline session during which the participant would be retested to establish retest reliability in the absence of attending a loud event. The third session was completed 1-week later. Although having plans to attend a loud event was not an enrollment criterion, all participants already had plans to attend common "loud" recreational events at the time of study enrollment (concert, $n = 16$; multi-day music festival, $n = 2$; bar with live music, $n = 3$; bar with digital music, $n = 4$; dance event, $n = 3$; movie, $n = 1$). The participants self-identified events as "loud," and there was no duration requirement; as such, the recreational events varied with respect to type, level, and duration.

Noise levels were estimated using the smartphone app "SPL Graph," installed on each participant's phone prior to event attendance. Data presented by Grinn et al. (2017) showed this app to be accurate within 2-dB of a class 1 sound level meter (SLM) across 25 used (not-new) iPhones (models 5, 5S, 6, 6S, 6S Plus, and 7) for test signals including steady-state broadband noise (90–110 dBA) and five pop songs (85–105 dBA). To assure that individual participants in this study were able to accurately measure sound levels using this app, the app was installed on participant iPhones and accuracy was verified against a class 1 SLM (Brüel and Kjær, type 2250; calibration verified using a Brüel and Kjær Type 4231 calibrator prior to use). At the baseline test session, participants were taught how to use the app and demonstrated the ability to point their phone microphone at a sound source to capture a measurement. Ten instantaneous sound level measurements (dBA) were captured by each participant at various moments throughout their loud event; the average event sound level was estimated using these 10 instantaneous sound level measurements. Event duration was recorded and reported by the participant. Estimated noise dose per individual participant was calculated using 29 CFR 1910.95 Appendix A (OSHA, 1983) based on the measured levels and the reported duration of attendance.

Taken together, the overall design included 3 test sessions completed as follows: (1) baseline test prior to attending a loud event, (2) retest within 24 h after the loud event, (3) retest 1-week after the loud event. Of the 32 participants enrolled in the study, 26 completed all 3 test sessions and their data are included in both the retrospective and prospective analyses. Two additional participants completed the first two test sessions, but not the final 1-week post noise session. Data from these participants was included in the analyses. Three additional participants completed only the baseline test session and their data are included only in the retrospective analysis, as there were no post-noise data to include for these two participants. One additional participant completed the online surveys but did not complete any test sessions; their survey data were excluded as there were no audiologic data for this participant.

Retrospective Noise Survey

Participant demographic information and self-reported retrospective noise exposure history were obtained via online survey using Qualtrics. The online survey was created based on the Noise Exposure Questionnaire (NEQ), which has now been used by a variety of groups to retrospectively assess self-reported exposure to occupational and recreational noise (Megerson, 2010; Stamper and Johnson, 2015a; Spankovich et al., 2017; Fulbright et al., in press). This questionnaire, expanded from a similar survey developed by Neitzel et al. (2004), assesses the self-reported frequency of previous exposures to various noisy activities (e.g., concerts, motorcycles, power tools, firearm use, etc.). From these responses, the total noise exposure within the previous year is calculated (for detailed procedures, see Megerson, 2010; Johnson et al., 2017). In brief, each activity is assigned an Exposure Level (EL) based on measured sound levels in previously reported literature. All hours not "assigned" to a noisy activity are assigned a default value of 60-dBA. For each participant, the total number of annual hours of exposure to each loud activity is divided by the reference duration (the number of hours allowed per year based on typical sound levels). These individual activity-specific doses are then summed to estimate total annual noise dose (Annual Exposure, AE).

From the AE—the total annual accumulated noise dose based on the self-reported activities—the $L_{Aeq8760}$ equivalent noise exposure term is derived. There are 8,760 h in a 1-year period (24 h/day × 365 days/year = 8,760 h); of these, some 2,000 h might be assumed to be spent working at some occupation (8 h/day × 5 days/week × 50 weeks per year = 2,000 h). Thus, the total year over which exposure can accrue is approximately two doublings of the typical occupational window. If using a 3-dB exchange rate and an 85-dB criterion level to set a safe exposure limit (as advocated by NIOSH, 1998), then the allowed exposure over 8,760 h should be approximately 6-dB less than the allowed exposure over the 2,000 work h. Thus, the "safe" exposure over 8,760 h has been derived to be 79 dBA. Therefore, $L_{Aeq8760}$ is calculated using the following equation:

$$L_{Aeq8760} = [10 \times \log(AE/100)] + 79$$

Audiologic Testing

At each test session, the following clinical measures were performed bilaterally:

Otoscopy

Visual examination of the ear canal and tympanic membrane was conducted to assure normal anatomy and no presence of debris. Normal otoscopic outcomes were defined as visualization of the tympanic membrane with no apparent abnormalities.

Tympanometry

Tympanometric measures were used to assess the functional status of the middle ear using a Grason Stadler Instruments TympStar Pro in compliance with *ANSI S3.39* and *IEC 601-1* criteria. Normal middle ear function was defined as Type A 226 Hz tympanograms bilaterally.

Distortion Product Otoacoustic Emissions (DPOAEs)

The 2f1-f2 distortion product was elicited with two simultaneously presented "primary" tones (f1 and f2) at an f2/f1 ratio of 1.2, with f2 frequencies of 1, 2, 3, 4, 6, and 8 kHz (f1: 55-dB SPL; f2: 45-dB SPL). These levels were selected based on previous studies showing temporary noise-induced changes in DPOAE amplitude were greater at these levels than when f1 and f2 were presented at higher levels (65/55) or lower levels (45/35) (Le Prell et al., 2012, 2016). Two runs were performed per ear at each test session to assure repeatability. DPOAE measurements were obtained using the Interacoustics Eclipse DPOAE Module in combination with an ER10C microphone-earphone assembly and a disposable foam ear tip.

Audiometry

Pure-tone air and bone conduction thresholds were obtained at all 3 test sessions (pre-event baseline, the day after the loud event, and 1-week post-noise) using the Modified Hughson-Westlake procedure for frequencies from 0.25 to 8 kHz, with sound levels decreased by 10-dB after each correct detection and increased by 5-dB after each missed stimulus. All audiometric testing was conducted inside a sound-treated booth, using a GSI Audiostar Pro audiometer. ER3-A insert earphones were used for air conduction audiometry and all speech testing. A GSI Audiostar Pro bone oscillator was used for bone conduction audiometry.

Speech Recognition Threshold (SRT)

As part of the standard clinical battery, speech recognition thresholds (SRT) were obtained using a recorded spondee list from the GSI Audiostar Pro audiometer. The spondee words have two syllables which are pronounced with equal emphasis (e.g., "toothbrush"). The SRT is the minimum signal level at which the listener can correctly identify 50% of the speech material presented (Plomp and Mimpen, 1979). Routine clinical tests include SRT primarily for the purpose of validating pure-tone threshold measurements ("cross-check principle"). The relationships between pure-tone average (PTA) threshold at 0.5, 1, and 2 kHz (PTA512) were assessed at baseline as a cross-check (based on the significant correlation described by Dobie and Sakai, 2001); SRT scores were not further analyzed.

Word Recognition Score (WRS)

Word Recognition Score (WRS) testing is supra-threshold testing during which participants attempt to correctly identify monosyllabic words, which are more difficult to identify than the spondee words used in SRT testing. Clinically, WRS is used to evaluate an individual's maximum speech understanding in an ideal listening environment (Dirks et al., 1977; Gelfand, 2001; McArdle and Hnath-Chisolm, 2014). Because understanding sound is more difficult than detecting sound, supra-threshold speech-based tests have been suggested to have the potential to distinguish audibility from intelligibility (Soli, 2008; Brungart et al., 2014). As part of the standard clinical battery used here, WRS was determined based on the number of correctly reported Northwestern University Auditory Test Number 6 (NU-6) words; recorded words were presented in quiet via the GSI Audiostar Pro. The NU-6 word list was presented at 40-dB above the participant's SRT; 25 words were presented to each ear. Although WRS is typically obtained at an intensity level intended to achieve the individual's maximum recognition ability (commonly abbreviated PBmax), this creates a problem with the use of these tests in research studies that include normal hearing participants as there is a ceiling effect in which normal-hearing listeners do uniformly well given the 40 dB SNR (see review by Le Prell and Clavier, 2017). The intensity level for the test is frequently set at a predetermined sensation level relative to the SRT or PTA threshold (Gelfand, 2001), with 40 dB SL being common (Martin et al., 1994). Based on the robust performance across participants and test sessions, there was no effort to systematically analyze the WRS data collected from the participants.

Words-in-Noise (WIN) Test

Speech-in-noise scores were assessed using the Words-in-Noise (WIN) test on the GSI Audiostar Pro following the procedures established by Wilson et al. (2003; for review, see Wilson, 2011). This test uses a subset of the NU-6 words spoken by a female speaker, with words presented in multi-talker babble composed of 6 female voices. The babble is fixed at 80-dB SPL as per Wilson et al. (2003), Wilson (2011). Target word level begins at 104-dB SPL and decreases in 4-dB steps from 104- to 80-dB SPL, providing 5 words at signal-to-babble (S/B) ratios that decrease from 24 (easiest) to 0 (most difficult). The primary performance metric is the 50% correct point, or dB S/B threshold, calculated using the equation dB $S/B = 26 - (0.8 \times N)$, with N defined as the total number of correct words across all conditions (for review, see Wilson, 2011). There are two 35-word lists with established equivalent recognition performance (Wilson and McArdle, 2007; Wilson et al., 2007a). There are 3 different randomization options for each of these lists; the randomization options were varied across the 3 test sessions in order to avoid practice effects. Wilson and McArdle (2007) defined 3.5 dB-S/B as a clinically meaningful difference between scores (corresponding to a difference of approximately 4 words out of the 35 words presented).

Electrophysiology

Two-channel ECochG data were collected using an Interacoustics Eclipse EP25 following the procedures described by Atcherson and Stoody (2012). The most common two-channel setup uses simultaneous ipsilateral and contralateral recording sites, with each ear serving as the inverting input for separate differential amplifiers. However, because the contralateral ear recordings were not analyzed in this study, the data generated via the two-channel setup are essentially equivalent to one-channel data collection; a two-channel setup was used to avoid the introduction of error in switching the electrode montage from right ear recordings to left ear recordings. Waveform repeatability was established during each test session at 70-, 80-, and 90-dB nHL for click, and 2, 3, and 4 kHz tone burst stimuli [Blackman, 5 cycles (termed "sines" within Eclipse stimulus parameters)]. Parameters were configured for alternating polarity, 11.7/s stimulus rate, and 500 sweeps of averaging. Etymotic ER3-26A gold electrodes (tiptrodes) were placed inside the ear canals, and Multipurpose Cloth electrodes (Oaktree Products, Inc.) were positioned in the standard adult diagnostic clinical configuration with non-inverting and ground electrodes stacked with spacing at midline high forehead (Fz). Electrode surface area was prepared with NuPrep and electrodes were prepared with Sanibel Lectron II conductivity gel. Action potential (AP) amplitude and summating potential (SP) amplitude were independently scored for each waveform by two different reviewers, with amplitude automatically calculated by the Interacoustics Eclipse EP25 system after peak marking. Although AP amplitude was easily identified across waveforms with scoring highly consistent across reviewers, SP amplitude was not as readily identified, and scoring was more variable. Variability in SP scoring across reviewers is well documented (see Roland and Roth, 1997). Discrepancies were resolved subsequent to review by a licensed audiologist after limiting the dataset to the 90 dB nHL waveforms, in which SP was clearest. SP was identifiable in all stimulus conditions (click, and 2, 3, and 4 kHz tonebursts) in 44% of left ears and 45% of right ears. The reviewers were masked with respect to $L_{Aeq8760}$ and acute recreational noise dose while analyzing and marking waveforms, but the session at which the waveform was collected (baseline, next day, next week) was not masked.

Statistical Analyses

An initial series of analyses included comparisons of data from the right and left ears. These comparisons typically used two-way ANOVA with ear and frequency as dependent variables, although in the case of the WIN test, the signal to babble ratio (ranging from 0 to 24) was assessed in place of frequency. Statistical tools within SigmaPlot version 13.0 were used. SigmaPlot automatically handles the missing data by using a general linear model approach. This approach constructs hypothesis tests using the marginal sums of squares (also commonly called the Type III or adjusted sums of squares). SigmaPlot tests normality of the data distribution using the Shapiro-Wilk Normality Statistic with a criterion of $p = 0.05$. Equal variance assumptions are also tested using $p = 0.05$. There were cases in which one or both of these criteria were violated during the ANOVA tests. In those cases, one-way ANOVA on ranks was used instead, with analyses completed within frequencies. Because the DPOAE and ABR data were repeated within sessions, the data from the first and second runs were first compared using paired t-tests or Wilcoxon sign tests as appropriate (based on the outcome of the normality tests), and then the average of the two runs was used within the comparisons of the right and left ears. Although there were robust, statistically significant differences across frequencies and across dB S/B conditions, the ears were not systematically different; therefore, the average data values from the right and left ears were used in all subsequent analyses. Use of the average value despite some small right vs. left ear differences was explicitly intended to prevent inappropriate inflation of study power. Genetics, diet, smoking, cardiovascular disease, and most types of recreational noise exposure would be expected to affect both ears relatively equally, and thus the right and left ears are not independent. Although noise exposure might be asymmetric, particularly in the case of firearms, firearm use was rare ($n = 3$ female participants), and there was no evidence of asymmetric function in this small number of participants with a history of firearm use.

The second set of analyses assessed potential differences between males and females; these analyses used the averaged data from the right and left ears. These comparisons typically used two-way ANOVA with sex and frequency as dependent variables, although in the case of the WIN test, the signal to babble ratio (ranging from 0 to 24) was assessed in place of frequency. In those cases in which data were not normally distributed, one-way ANOVA on ranks was used instead, with analyses completed within each frequency. The Shapiro-Wilk test was used to assess normality of the distribution and the Brown-Forsyth Test was used to assess compliance with equal variance requirements. If either test was failed, then non-parametric tests were used. For comparisons of noise exposure, comparisons were via t-test if the normality and variance requirements were met, and were via Mann-Whitney Rank Sum tests if these conditions were not met.

To assess relationships between retrospective noise history ($L_{Aeq8760}$) and auditory function at baseline, a series of correlation analyses were completed. Pearson correlation was used when data were normally distributed, and Spearman correlation was used in those cases where data were not normally distributed, as noted below. The Pearson correlation coefficient (R) is reported for parametric analysis, and the Spearman Rho (ρ) correlation coefficient is reported for non-parametric analysis. Linear regression lines of best fit are shown for data sets that were amenable to parametric analysis, and non-linear regression lines of best fit are shown for data sets that required non-parametric analysis.

Finally, multiple regression was used to assess the potential relationships between previous noise exposure (estimated using $L_{Aeq8760}$) and auditory metrics to determine if functional outcomes could be predicted by noise history and other important variables (e.g., age, sex, and related functional test data). The analysis of the relationship between SP/AP ratio and $L_{Aeq8760}$ was limited to the subset of waveforms in which both SP and AP could be readily identified. Multiple regression was completed within IBM SPSS Statistics version 23.

Statistical significance was defined as $P < 0.05$ for all analyses; when multiple pair-wise comparisons were required, statistical correction for multiple pair-wise comparisons was completed using Bonferroni correction. The Bonferroni correction compensates for the increase in risk of Type I errors associated with multiple pair-wise comparisons by testing each individual pair at a significance level of alpha/mu, where alpha is the desired overall alpha level (here, 0.05) and mu is the number of pair-wise comparisons completed. The Bonferroni correction can be too conservative if there are a large number of comparisons to be made.

RESULTS

Comparisons of Males vs. Females

Previous 12-months Noise Exposure ($L_{Aeq8760}$): No Differences between Males and Females

Across participants, the average $L_{Aeq8760}$ score obtained from the retrospective noise survey was 79.6 (SD = 4.3), with values ranging from 63.9 to 87.1. The mean $L_{Aeq8760}$ score for males was 80.2 (SD = 2.9, range = 74.3–85.0). The mean $L_{Aeq8760}$ score for females was 79.2 (SD = 5.0, range = 63.9–87.1); the female with the $L_{Aeq8760}$ score of 63.9 was an outlier, as all other participants had $L_{Aeq8760}$ scores of 72.4 or greater. Males were compared to females using a Mann-Whitney Rank Sum Test; there was no statistically significant difference with respect to retrospective noise exposure history assessed using $L_{Aeq8760}$.

With the exception of the one female who reported very little noise exposure, the distribution of $L_{Aeq8760}$ scores was highly similar to that reported by others. The range of $L_{Aeq8760}$ noise scores was 64–84 for females and 64–88 for males in Megerson (2010), 67–83 for females and 70–82 for males in Stamper and Johnson (2015a), and 64–84 for females and 68–87 for males in Fulbright et al. (in press). Recent data from Spankovich et al. (2017) are also similar, with a range of scores from 66 to 83 for both male and female participants in this cohort. Taken together, the range of noise exposures experienced by this participant cohort is similar to (generally overlaps with) the range of noise exposures reported for young adult populations recruited on different campuses by different research teams. Although there was no effort to perform a statistical comparison of noise exposures across studies, the similar distributions of the exposure data across studies suggest the current cohort is not systematically different from other samples recruited by others. Individual $L_{Aeq8760}$ scores were used as the basis for all analyses assessing potential effects of noise exposure history on different auditory metrics.

Pure-Tone Threshold Sensitivity: Males Poorer than Females at Baseline

The potential for threshold differences associated with sex was evaluated using two-way ANOVA with sex and frequency as independent variables. Both the normality and equal variance requirements were satisfied. There were statistically significant main effects for sex ($F = 7.292$, $df = 1{,}247$, $P = 0.007$) and frequency ($F = 9.390$, $df = 1{,}7$, $P < 0.001$), with no statistically significant interaction. Male thresholds were approximately 1–3 dB poorer than female thresholds across frequencies (see **Figure 1A**). Although there was adequate power to detect the main effect for sex, none of the Bonferroni-corrected pairwise comparisons were statistically significant when male and female thresholds were compared within frequencies. The overall small but statistically significant main effect for sex observed here replicates small but statistically significant differences in other cohorts in which males have had slightly poorer thresholds than females (Niskar et al., 1998; Serra et al., 2005; Kim et al., 2009; Shah et al., 2009; Shargorodsky et al., 2010; Le Prell et al., 2012, 2016; Spankovich et al., 2014). However, it is possible that the sex differences reported here and by others are an artifact of the

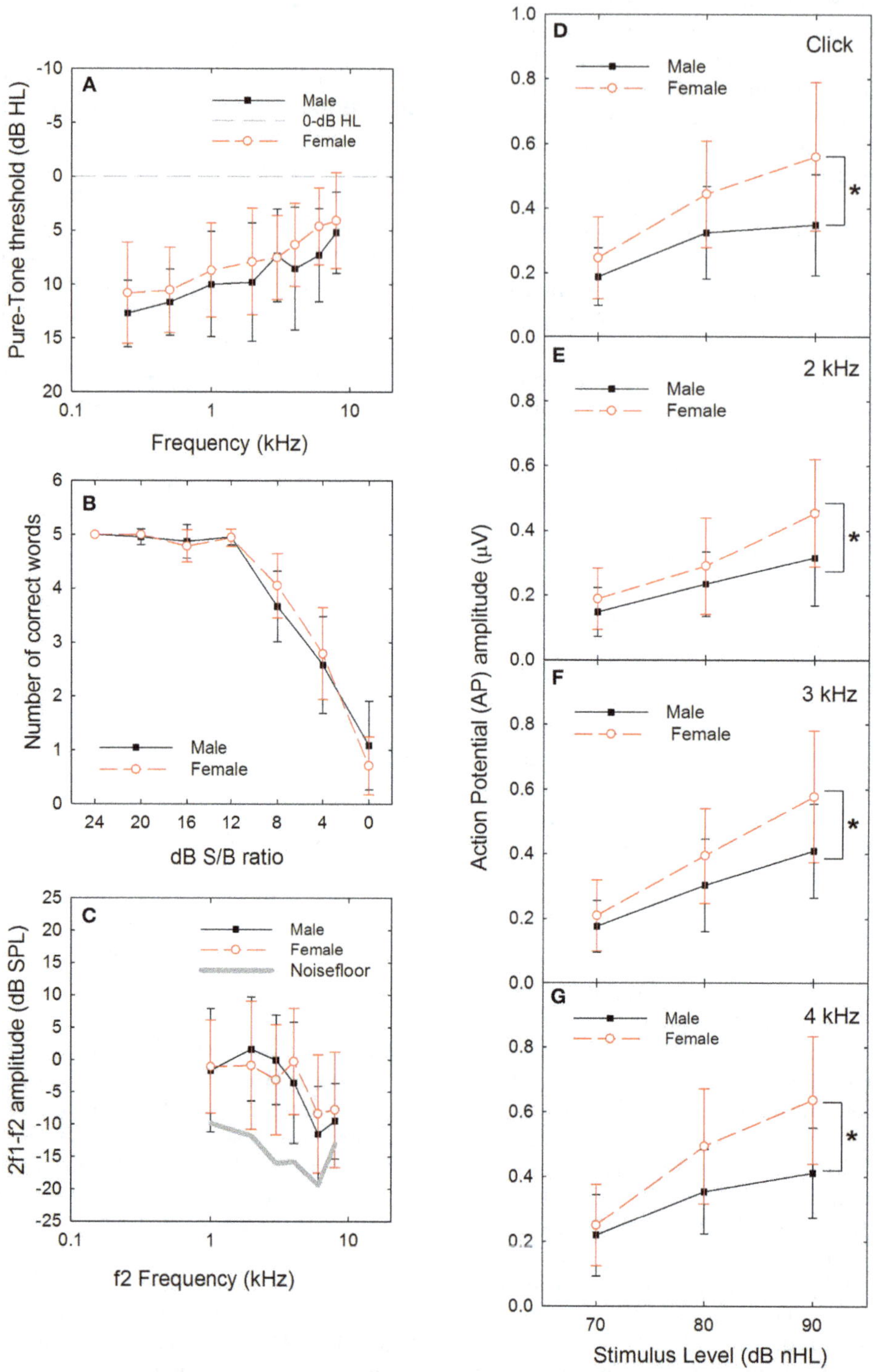

FIGURE 1 | (A) There was a statistically significant difference in threshold at baseline, as a function of sex (male vs. female), with males having slightly poorer thresholds. Dashed line indicates 0-dB HL reference. **(B)** There were no statistically significant differences in performance within any of the signal-to-babble (dB S/B) conditions as a function of sex (male vs. female). **(C)** There was no statistically significant difference in distortion product otoacoustic emission (DPOAE) amplitude as a function of sex (male vs. female). **(D)** There were statistically significant differences in sound-evoked action potential (AP) amplitude as a function of sex (male vs. female), with females having significantly larger amplitudes compared to males with p-values less than 0.01 at 90 dB nHL levels (see asterisks) for clicks (**D**, $P = 0.002$) and tonebursts at 2 kHz (**E**, $P = 0.006$), 3 kHz (**F**, $P = 0.004$), and 4 kHz (**G**, $P < 0.001$). Sex differences at 80 dB nHL were statistically significant with p-values less than 0.05 for click and toneburst stimuli at 3 and 4 kHz, but not 2 kHz (click: $P = 0.021$; 2 kHz: 0.224; 3 kHz: $P = 0.045$; 4 kHz: $P = 0.007$). Data are mean ±1 SD.

study size as other studies have found no statistically significant differences as a function of sex (Henderson et al., 2011; Sekhar et al., 2011).

Words-in-Noise (WIN) Test: No Differences between Males and Females at Baseline

The potential for differences in performance on the WIN test as a function of sex was evaluated using two-way ANOVAs for the total number of words correct and the number of words correct within dB S/B conditions. There was a statistically significant effect of SNR ($F = 299.151$, $df = 6{,}216$, $P < 0.001$), with poorer performance as SNR decreased, but no statistically significant effect of sex ($F = 0.117$, $df = 1{,}6$, $P = 0.733$) was observed, nor were there any statistically significant interactions. Because the normality and equal variance tests were failed, a series of one-way ANOVAs (for data that met normality requirements) and ANOVA on Rank tests (for data that failed to meet normality requirements) were performed to assess potential sex differences within dB S/B conditions. There was no statistically significant effect of sex within 0 dB or 4 dB S/B conditions based on one-way ANOVA, and no statistically significant effect of sex within 8–24 dB S/B conditions based on one-way ANOVA on Rank tests. Participant performance was normally distributed at the most difficult listening conditions, but was skewed toward 100% correct within the easier signal-to-babble conditions (see **Figure 1B**). Similarly, there were no statistically significant sex differences on overall performance measures, including total number of words correct and dB S/B threshold, when one-way ANOVAs were completed (not shown).

Distortion Product Otoacoustic Emission (DPOAE) Amplitude: No Differences between Males and Females at Baseline

After averaging the data across run 1 and run 2, and for the left and right ears, a series of two-way ANOVAs with sex and frequency as independent variables were completed. There was a statistically significant main effect for frequency ($F = 10.571$, $df = 5{,}185$, $P < 0.001$) but not for sex ($F = 0.261$, $df = 5{,}185$, $P = 0.610$; see **Figure 1C**), and there was no statistically significant interaction. In general, Bonferroni-corrected pair-wise comparisons revealed that DPOAE response amplitude was larger at 1, 2, 3, and 4 kHz than at 6 and 8 kHz responses. Both the normality and the equal variance test requirements were met.

Action Potential Amplitude: Statistically Significant Differences between Males and Females at Baseline

Female AP amplitude was consistently larger than male AP amplitude at higher sound levels (see **Figures 1D–G**). To identify the statistical reliability of the differences between males and females, a three-way ANOVA with signal (click, 2, 3, or 4 kHz), level (70, 80, or 90 dB nHL), and sex (male vs. female) was performed. There were statistically significant main effects for signal ($F = 15.480$, $df = 3{,}368$, $p < 0.001$), level ($F = 137.659$, $df = 2{,}368$, $p < 0.001$) and sex ($F = 71.936$, $df = 1{,}368$, $p < 0.001$). In addition, there was a statistically significant interaction between sound level and sex, with males and females being statistically significantly different within the 80 ($t = 4.593$, $p < 0.001$) and 90 ($t = 8.322$, $p < 0.001$) dB nHL levels, but not at the 70 dB nHL level ($t = 1.776$, $p = 0.077$). Because the normality and equal variance tests were failed, a series of one-way ANOVA on ranks were used within signal x level conditions to confirm the statistical significance of the differences as a function of sex. As seen in **Table 1**, there were no statistically significant sex-related differences in ABR amplitude at 70 dB nHL. Statistically significant differences emerged at 80 dB nHL for several stimulus conditions (click: $P = 0.021$, 3 kHz: $P = 0.045$; 4 kHz: $P = 0.007$). Differences between males and females were statistically significant for all stimuli at 90 dB nHL (click: $P = 0.002$, 2 kHz: $P = 0.006$; 3 kHz: $P = 0.004$; 4 kHz: $P < 0.001$). If the statistical criterion is arbitrarily increased from 0.05 to 0.01 given the increased risk of Type I errors within the series of one-way ANOVAs (which are not corrected for pair-wise comparisons), then the statistically significant sex-related differences are generally limited to 90-dB nHL.

Relationships between Previous 12-Months Noise Exposure ($L_{Aeq8760}$) and Function

Multiple linear regression was used to assess whether retrospective noise history (based on the self-reported data used to calculate $L_{Aeq8760}$) reliably predicts functional (audiologic) outcomes at baseline, including threshold, DPOAE amplitude, AP amplitude, SP/AP ratio, and WIN threshold. Each regression model included the specific functional outcome measured at the baseline visit as the dependent variable (DV), with independent variables (IVs) in each model specifically including retrospective self-reported noise history ($L_{Aeq8760}$), age, sex, and related functional tests (i.e., DPOAE amplitude, audiometric threshold) measured at the baseline visit. Ear was not included as a predictor, as the initial analyses did not reveal statistically significant ear-related differences. The results of all models are provided in **Table 2**, with statistically significant models indicated with an asterisk. All statistical analyses were per the following strategy.

First, regression analysis was used to test if retrospective noise history predicted DPOAE amplitude. Each model included DPOAE amplitude (for each frequency 1–8 kHz) as the DV, and noise history ($L_{Aeq8760}$), age, and sex as IVs. Results indicated the models to be non-significant for all frequencies (1–8 kHz), suggesting that none of the variables (noise history, sex, age) reliably predicted DPOAE amplitude. Next, regression was used to determine if retrospective noise history predicted audiometric threshold, using threshold (for each frequency from 1 to 8 kHz) as the DV, and noise history ($L_{Aeq8760}$), age, sex, and DPOAE amplitude, with DPOAE frequency corresponding to the frequency of the threshold as IVs (e.g., 4 kHz threshold DV included when analyzing 4 kHz DPOAE IV). Results showed a statistically significant regression for the 1 kHz DV [$F_{(4,\,21)} = 4.09$, $p = 0.01$ with $R^2 = 0.44$] with DPOAE at 1 kHz as a significant predictor of the DV (see **Table 3**). The model predicting 4 kHz was also significant [$F_{(4,\,21)} = 3.47$, $p = 0.03$ with $R^2 = 0.40$] with DPOAE amplitude at 4 kHz as a significant predictor (see **Table 4**). All other models of

TABLE 1 | ANOVA results for AP amplitude analyses, comparing males versus females.

	70 dB nHL	80 dB nHL	90 dB nHL
Click	$F = 3.541$, $df = 1.30$, $P = 0.07$	$F = 5.977$, $df = 1.30$, $P = 0.021$*	$F = 11.342$, $df = 1.30$, $P = 0.002$*
2 kHz	$F = 2.749$, $df = 1.30$, $P = 0.108$	$H = 1.480$ with 1 degrees of freedom ($P = 0.224$)	$F = 8.699$, $df = 1.30$, $P = 0.006$*
3 kHz	$H = 1.032$ with 1 degrees of freedom. ($P = 0.310$)	$F = 4.382$, $df = 1.29$, $P = 0.045$*	$F = 9.634$, $df = 1.29$, $P = 0.004$*
4 kHz	$F = 0.633$, $df = 1.30$, $P = 0.433$	$F = 8.457$, $df = 1.30$, $P = 0.007$*	$H = 12.167$ with 1 degrees of freedom ($P = <0.001$*)

*The only statistically significant main effect was a main effect of sex, with females having larger AP amplitudes than males at higher presentation levels. Data are one-way ANOVA for those data sets in which normal distribution and equal variance requirements were met and one-way ANOVA on Ranks if parametric test requirements were not met. *$P < 0.05$.*

TABLE 2 | Multiple regression models evaluated are listed below.

Dependent Variable	Independent Variables	*F*	*df*	*P*
DPOAE 1 kHz	Age, Sex, $L_{Aeq8760}$	0.75	3, 22	0.53
DPOAE 2 kHz	Age, Sex, $L_{Aeq8760}$	1.03	3, 22	0.40
DPOAE 3 kHz	Age, Sex, $L_{Aeq8760}$	1.17	3, 22	0.34
DPOAE 4 kHz	Age, Sex, $L_{Aeq8760}$	1.37	3, 22	0.28
DPOAE 6 kHz	Age, Sex, $L_{Aeq8760}$	0.23	3, 22	0.88
DPOAE 8 kHz	Age, Sex, $L_{Aeq8760}$	1.27	3, 22	0.32
1 kHz threshold	Age, Sex, $L_{Aeq8760,}$ DPOAE 1 kHz	4.09	4, 21	0.01*
2 kHz threshold	Age, Sex, $L_{Aeq8760,}$ DPOAE 2 kHz	1.89	4, 21	0.15
3 kHz threshold	Age, Sex, $L_{Aeq8760,}$ DPOAE 3 kHz	1.05	4, 21	0.41
4 kHz threshold	Age, Sex, $L_{Aeq8760,}$ DPOAE 4 kHz	3.47	4, 21	0.03*
6 kHz threshold	Age, Sex, $L_{Aeq8760,}$ DPOAE 6 kHz	1.76	4, 21	0.18
8 kHz threshold	Age, Sex, $L_{Aeq8760,}$ DPOAE 8 kHz	0.58	4, 21	0.68
AP – 2 kHz stimulus	Age, Sex, $L_{Aeq8760,}$ DPOAE 2 kHz, 2 kHz threshold	0.34	5, 20	0.88
AP – 3 kHz stimulus	Age, Sex, $L_{Aeq8760,}$ DPOAE 3 kHz, 3 kHz threshold	0.59	5, 19	0.71
AP – 4 kHz stimulus	Age, Sex, $L_{Aeq8760,}$ DPOAE 4 kHz, 4 kHz threshold	1.55	5, 20	0.22
AP – click stimulus	Age, Sex, $L_{Aeq8760,}$ average DPOAE 2-4 kHz, PTA234	1.44	5, 20	0.25
SP/AP – 2 kHz stimulus	Age, Sex, $L_{Aeq8760,}$ DPOAE 2 kHz, 2 kHz threshold	2.03	5, 8	0.18
SP/AP – 3 kHz stimulus	Age, Sex, $L_{Aeq8760,}$ DPOAE 3 kHz, 3 kHz threshold	0.17	5, 17	0.97
SP/AP – 4 kHz stimulus	Age, Sex, $L_{Aeq8760,}$ DPOAE 4 kHz, 4 kHz threshold	0.42	5, 13	0.83
SP/AP – click stimulus	Age, Sex, $L_{Aeq8760,}$ average DPOAE 2-4 kHz, PTA234	0.87	5, 7	0.55
WIN – 8 dB SNR	Age, Sex, $L_{Aeq8760,}$ DPOAE 4 kHz, PTA1234, AP – click stimulus	0.47	6, 19	0.82
WIN – 4 dB SNR	Age, Sex, $L_{Aeq8760,}$ DPOAE 4 kHz, PTA1234, AP – click stimulus	0.37	6, 19	0.89
WIN – 0 dB SNR	Age, Sex, $L_{Aeq8760,}$ DPOAE 4 kHz, PTA1234, AP – click stimulus	1.89	6, 19	0.14
WIN – Total score	Age, Sex, $L_{Aeq8760,}$ DPOAE 4 kHz, PTA1234, AP – click stimulus	0.95	6, 19	0.48

*There were no statistically significant effects of Sex, Age, or $L_{Aeq8760}$. The models that were statistically significant ($P < 0.05$) are marked with an asterisk and the full results are provided in subsequent tables. *$P < 0.05$.*

audiometric threshold were found to be non-significant for all other frequencies. After correcting for multiple pair-wise comparisons using the Bonferroni procedure, the models in **Tables 3, 4** did not meet the adjusted criteria for statistical significance.

Regression was then utilized to test if noise history predicted AP amplitude. Each model included AP amplitude (for tone burst 2–4 kHz and click at 90 dB nHL input level) as the DV, and noise history ($L_{Aeq89760}$), age, sex, DPOAE amplitude, and audiometric threshold as IVs. DPOAE amplitude and threshold frequency corresponded to frequency of AP input (e.g., 4 kHz AP DV included 4 kHz DPOAE and 4 kHz audiometric threshold IVs). For AP amplitude with click stimulus DV, DPOAE amplitudes and thresholds at 2–4 kHz were averaged and used as IVs, as the click stimulus has a broad frequency spectrum which stimulates the 2–4 kHz region of the cochlea as well as regions tuned to other frequencies (see Hall, 1992). Results indicated that the AP models were non-significant for all stimulus frequencies (see **Figure 2** for correlation and line of best fit data). Additional regression analyses were performed to determine if noise history predicted SP/AP ratio. Each model included SP/AP ratio (for tone burst 2–4 kHz and click at 90 dB nHL input level) as the DV, and the same IVs as the previous analysis of AP. Results indicated that the models were not statistically significant at any stimulus frequencies (see **Table 2**). Because the analysis of the relationship between SP/AP ratio and $L_{Aeq8760}$ was limited to the subset of waveforms in which both SP and AP could be readily identified, the sample size was smaller and power was reduced; as such, the

TABLE 3 | Multiple regression results for 1 kHz audiometric threshold at baseline.

	B	SE	*P*
Constant	–	23.29	0.31
Sex	0.16	2.36	0.56
Age	0.09	0.72	0.74
$L_{Aeq8760}$	0.32	0.21	0.07
DPOAE at 1 kHz	−0.56	0.18	0.004**

*There were no statistically significant effects of Sex, Age, or $L_{Aeq8760}$. The only statistically significant factor associated with 1 kHz audiometric threshold was DPOAE amplitude at 1 kHz. **$P < 0.01$.*

TABLE 4 | Multiple regression results for 4 kHz audiometric threshold at baseline.

	B	SE	*P*
Constant	–	27.17	0.20
Sex	0.07	2.77	0.80
Age	0.33	0.84	0.25
$L_{Aeq87860}$	0.24	0.24	0.18
DPOAE at 4 kHz	−0.49	0.17	0.01*

*There were no statistically significant effects of Sex, Age, or $L_{Aeq8760}$. The only statistically significant factor associated with 4 kHz audiometric threshold was DPOAE amplitude at 4 kHz. *$P < 0.05$.*

lack of statistically significant relationships should be interpreted with caution. In cases in which a potential relationship between SP/AP ratio and function is observed, the interpretation of the SP/AP ratio requires careful consideration of the generators of both the SP and AP (see Discussion).

Finally, regression analysis was used to determine if noise history predicted WIN scores. Each model included WIN score (for each SNR from 0 to 8 dB S/B) as the DV, and noise history ($L_{Aeq8760}$), age, sex, DPOAE amplitude (4 kHz input), audiometric threshold (PTA1234), and AP amplitude (click stimulus) as the IV. PTA1234 was selected based on Wilson et al. (2007b). Results indicated that the models were not statistically significant at any signal to noise ratio (see **Table 2**).

Acute Noise Exposure at Recreational Events

A total of 28 of the original 32 participants attended a recreational event that they deemed "loud," and returned the day after the event for repeat audiometric testing (see **Table 5** for event summary, sound level measurements, and duration of event attendance). Calculated using 29 CFR 1910.95, the average participant noise dose was 168.4 ± 276% (range 3.5–1,230.8%), based on event levels of 93.3 ± 7.8 dBA (range 73.1–104.2 dBA) and durations of 4.2 ± 3.5 h (range 1.5–16.0 h). There were two participants with 16-h attendance at a music festival with sound levels of 103–104 dBA; these two participants (one male, one female) had much higher doses than the other participants (see **Figure 3A**). Excluding these two outliers, the average recreational noise exposure was 92.7 ± 7.7 dBA (range 73.1–104.2 dBA) for 3.3 ± 0.9 h (range 1.5–4.5 h), yielding an event dose of 97.8 ± 92.5% (range 3.5–318.2%). There were 9 participants with doses of less than 50% (4 male, 5 female), 10 participants with doses of 50 to 100% (4 male, 6 female), and 9 participants with doses above 100% (3 male, 6 female). There was no statistically significant difference in OSHA exposure dose for males and females compared via Mann-Whitney Rank Sum Test (Mann-Whiney U statistic = 88.000, $P = 0.814$; Shapiro-Wilk Normality Test failed).

Because NIOSH guidance (NIOSH, 1998) advocates more conservative exposure limits than OSHA regulations require (OSHA, 1983), the noise dose accrued at the event is higher when calculated based on NIOSH recommendations (see **Table 5, Figure 3B**). When noise dose was instead calculated using NIOSH recommendations of an 85-dBA relative exposure limit (REL) and using a 3-dB exchange rate, there were 5 participants with doses of less than 50% (2 male, 3 female), 3 participants with doses of 50 to 100% (1 male, 2 female), and 20 participants with doses above 100% (8 male, 12 female). There was no statistically significant difference in exposure assessed as NIOSH dose for males and females when compared via Mann-Whitney Rank Sum Test (Mann-Whiney U statistic = 88.000, $P = 0.814$; Shapiro-Wilk Normality Test failed).

Dose was converted to time-weighted average (the 8-h equivalent level) as shown in **Figures 3C,D**. OSHA TWA is calculated based on 100% dose being equivalent to 8-h exposure to 90-dBA noise, with a 5-dB exchange rate used for sound levels other than 90-dBA (see dashed line in **Figure 3C**). NIOSH TWA is calculated based on 100% dose being equivalent to 8-h exposure to 85-dBA noise, with a 3-dB exchange rate used for sound levels other than 85-dBA (see dashed line in **Figure 3D**). There was no statistically significant difference in OSHA TWA for males and females when compared via *t*-test ($t = -0.0865$ with 26 degrees of freedom, two-tailed *P*-value = 0.932; both Shapiro-Wilk Normality Test and Brown-Forsythe Equal Variance Test passed). Similarly, there was no statistically significant difference in NIOSH TWA for males and females when compared via *t*-test ($t = -0.0590$ with 26 degrees of freedom, two-tailed *P*-value = 0.953; both Shapiro-Wilk Normality Test and Brown-Forsythe Equal Variance Test passed).

A series of correlation analyses were used to assess potential linear relationships between acute exposure (OSHA TWA) and functional change. OSHA TWA was normally distributed. Pearson correlation was used when all data were normally distributed, and, Spearman correlation was used in those cases where a subset of the data were not normally distributed as noted below.

Acute Noise-Induced Changes in Pure-Tone Threshold Sensitivity

After pre-noise baseline was established (**Figure 1**), most of the participants attended a loud event ($n = 28$). Thresholds were reassessed the day after the event (within 24 h of the event). The timing of the post-noise tests (i.e., the day after the loud event) was explicitly selected to parallel the timing in animal studies (Kujawa and Liberman, 2009; Lin et al., 2011; Wang and Ren, 2012; Hickox and Liberman, 2014; Fernandez et al., 2015; Jensen et al., 2015; Lobarinas et al., 2017). The final test 1-week later was

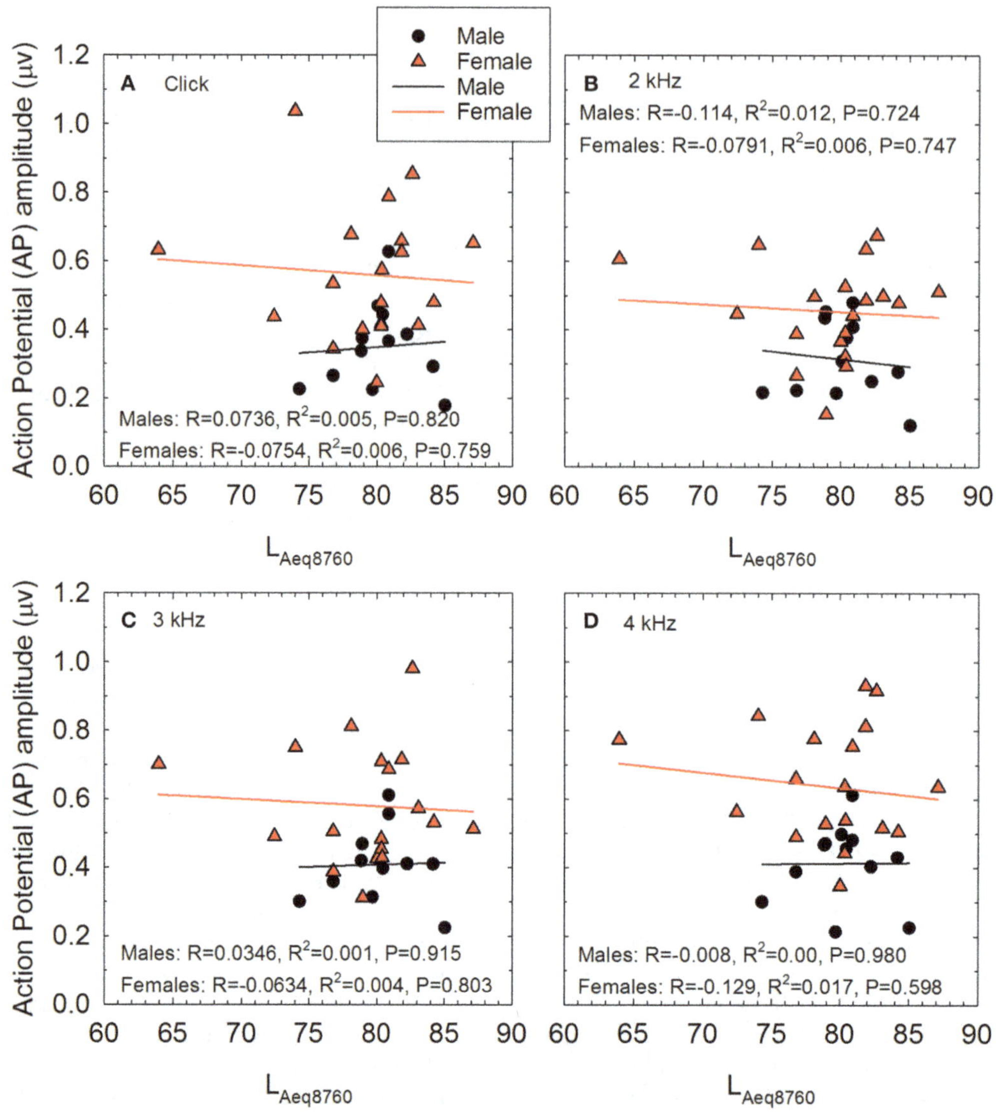

FIGURE 2 | The relationship between self-reported noise exposure (calculated as $L_{Aeq8760}$) and action potential (AP) amplitude is shown for male and female participants for stimuli including **(A)** clicks, **(B)** 2 kHz tone bursts, **(C)** 3 kHz tone bursts, and **(D)** 4 kHz tone bursts. All AP amplitude data were normally distributed. Pearson correlation analysis revealed no statistically significant relationships between self-reported noise history and AP amplitude within males or females. Lines of best fit are shown (Males: black symbols and regression lines; Females: red symbols and regression lines).

used to assess recovery of any changes; 26 of the 28 participants returned for the final test.

TTS (calculated as the difference between the pre-noise threshold and the post-noise threshold) as a function of acute noise exposure is shown in **Figures 4A–F**. There was significant individual variability across participants, and the TTS data were not normally distributed. There was one participant with an average shift of 10 dB and three participants with threshold shifts greater than 10 dB; across these four participants, the frequency at which the shift was observed varied, including 1, 2, 4, and 6 kHz. At the 1-week test session, most participants had thresholds that were within ±5 dB of the original pre-noise baseline, although a small number of data points were more variable and were within ±10 dB relative to baseline (see **Figures 4G–L**). Spearman correlation was used to determine if there were any statistically significant relationships between exposure and threshold shift the day after the recreational activity. None of the correlations were statistically significant (see **Figure 4** for scatterplots and Spearman Rho coefficient of determination).

Acute Noise-Induced Changes in Performance on the Word-in-Noise (WIN) Test

Change in performance on the WIN was calculated as the difference between pre-noise baseline performance (see **Figure 1B**) and post-noise performance. The average change in

TABLE 5 | Acute noise exposure.

Participant ID	Sex	Event	Time (H)	Level	NIOSH Dose (%)	NIOSH TWA	OSHA Dose (%)	OSHA TWA
004	F	Movie	2.25	73.1	1.8	67.5	3.5	65.8
012	M	Bar	3	84.2	31.2	79.9	16.3	76.9
028	M	Bar	3	91.9	185.2	87.7	49.2	84.9
032	M	Bar	2.5	94.9	308.6	89.9	62.5	86.6
008	F	Bar	3	104.2	3157.9	100.0	272.7	97.2
005	F	Bar/live music	3	96	476.2	91.8	85.7	88.9
006	M	Bar/live music	3	96	476.2	91.8	85.7	88.9
019	M	Bar/live music	6	93	476.2	91.8	113.2	90.9
022	F	Concert	3	80	11.8	75.7	9.4	72.9
007	F	Concert	3.5	83.3	29.7	79.7	16.6	77.0
016	M	Concert	3.75	83.6	33.9	80.3	20.4	78.5
014	F	Concert	1.5	89.7	55.6	82.4	18.8	77.9
018	F	Concert	3.75	86.8	71.0	83.5	31.0	81.5
009	M	Concert	3.5	88.2	91.6	84.6	33.0	82.0
003	F	Concert	5	89.4	173.0	87.4	62.5	86.6
020	M	Concert	2.5	93.5	204.9	88.1	54.3	85.6
002	F	Concert	2.5	93.5	223.2	88.5	54.3	85.6
017	M	Concert	3	95.7	441.2	91.4	85.7	88.9
001	F	Concert	4.5	97.5	1022.7	95.1	173.1	94.0
021	M	Concert	4	101.1	2105.3	98.2	235.3	96.2
029	F	Concert	3	102.5	2142.9	98.3	230.8	96.0
026	F	Concert	3	104	3030.3	99.8	272.7	97.2
027	F	Concert	3.5	103.9	3500.0	100.4	318.2	98.3
031	F	Dance event	4.5	91.8	271.1	89.3	73.8	87.8
013	F	Dance event	2.25	95.7	330.9	90.2	64.3	86.8
010	F	Dance event	3	96.5	535.7	92.3	100.0	90.0
024	F	3 day festival	16	101	8000.0	104.0	941.2	106.2
023	M	3 day festival	16	102.7	12307.7	105.9	1230.8	108.1

Sound level measurements collected via app and duration of exposure as per participant report.

the summed performance across the 35-word lists is shown in **Figures 5A,E**, and the total change within each dB S/B conditions (5 words presented per ear per SNR condition, from 0 to 24 dB S/B) is shown for the more difficult SNR conditions, including 8 dB S/B (**Figures 5B,F**), 4 dB S/B (**Figures 5C,D**), and 0 dB S/B (**Figures 5D,H**) signal to babble ratios. There was significant individual variability, and the change in performance data were not normally distributed. Spearman correlation was therefore used to determine if there were any statistically significant relationships between acute noise exposure and change in WIN performance. The correlations were statistically significant for the overall change in performance the next day (maximum possible change in score = −35 words if performance went from 100% correct to 0% correct) and within the 4 dB S/B condition (maximum possible change in score = −10 words if performance for both ears went from 5 words correct to 0 words correct). At other SNRs, there were similar trends in which performance on the WIN the day after exposure appeared to decrease as a function of increasing recreational noise exposure, but the *P*-values for the other dB S/B conditions did not meet the criterion of $P < 0.05$. The predicted change in overall performance on the WIN 35-word list as a function of noise exposure at the next day test session shown in **Figure 5A** was: change in performance on WIN $= 11.511 + (-0.150 \times \text{TWA})$. There were no statistically significant relationships between WIN score shifts and noise exposure at 1-week post-noise on the overall test or within dB S/B conditions. None of the individual participants met the clinically significant change criteria derived by Wilson and McArdle (2007) at the 1-week post-noise test time.

Acute Noise-Induced Changes in Distortion Product Otoacoustic Emission (DPOAE) Amplitude

Change in DPOAE amplitude was calculated as the difference between pre-noise DPOAE amplitude (see **Figure 1C**) and post-noise DPOAE amplitude at each test frequency. Change in DPOAE amplitude as a function of the acute noise dose is shown in **Figure 6**. The data were normally distributed at all frequencies for the next day data set, and for all but 1 and 6 kHz at the next week test. Pearson correlation was therefore used to determine if there were any statistically significant relationships between OSHA TWA and change in DPOAE amplitude except at 1 and 6 kHz at the next week test session, for which Spearman correlation was assessed. There were no statistically significant correlations.

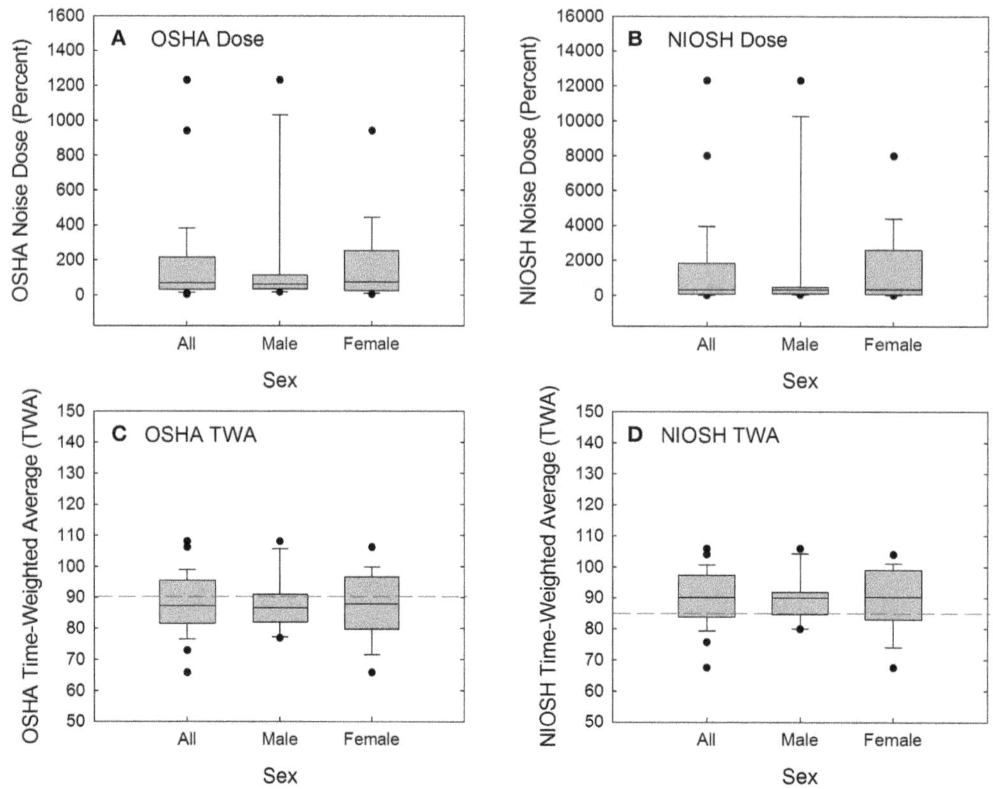

FIGURE 3 | Acute noise exposure dose was calculated per 29 CFR 1910.95 (OSHA, 1983) **(A)** and per the recommended procedures suggested by NIOSH (1998) **(B)**. Calculated dose was converted to time-weighted average (8-h equivalent level) per 29 CFR 1910.95 **(C)** and the NIOSH recommended criteria **(D)**. By converting from dose to TWA, the effects of two outliers are reduced and the distribution is normalized. OSHA TWA is calculated based on 100% dose being equivalent to 8 h exposure to 90-dBA noise (dashed line in **C**). NIOSH TWA is calculated based on 100% dose being equivalent to 8 h exposure to 85-dBA noise (dashed line in **D**).

Acute Noise-Induced Changes in Auditory Brainstem Response Amplitude Post-Exposure

Because there were statistically significant differences between males and females with respect to AP amplitude (see **Figures 1E–G**), changes in AP amplitude after noise exposure were analyzed separately for males and females. There was no statistically significant evidence of noise-induced decreases in AP amplitude, and there was no change at the individual level even in the two participants with the highest noise doses (see **Figure 7**). Noise exposure (TWA) and changes in AP amplitude data were both normally distributed within Female participants. Pearson correlation was used to assess whether there was any relationship between TWA and change in AP amplitude within Females. The TWA data was normally distributed within Male participants; the changes in AP amplitude were normally distributed at 2 and 4 kHz, and for clicks, but not for 3 kHz data. Therefore, Spearman correlation was used to assess whether there was any relationship between dose and change in AP amplitude within Males at 3 kHz, and Pearson correlation was used for the other analyses. There were no statistically significant relationships between noise exposure and changes in AP amplitude within males or females.

Relationship between Temporary Threshold Shift and Other Acute Noise-Induced Changes

Across audiometric measures (see **Figures 4–7**), there was significant individual variability with respect to the effects of noise on auditory function. Some participants had seemingly more "tender" ears, with larger changes in function after relatively lower noise doses. Other participants had seemingly "tougher" ears, with smaller changes in function, despite relatively larger noise doses. Based on this, additional analyses were performed in which changes in performance on the WIN (**Figures 8A–E**), changes in DPOAE amplitude (**Figures 8F–J**), and changes in AP amplitude (**Figures 8K–N**) were assessed as a function of the maximum TTS measured at any frequency the day after the noise exposure. Because maximum TTS at any frequency was not normally distributed, Spearman Rank Order correlation was used to assess all potential relationships.

The only statistically significant relationship between TTS the day after the exposure and other metrics was DPOAE amplitude at 6 kHz (see **Figure 8I**). As TTS increased, there were increasing deficits in DPOAE amplitude at 6 kHz. Taken together, the data may suggest that in the participants that had the most severe

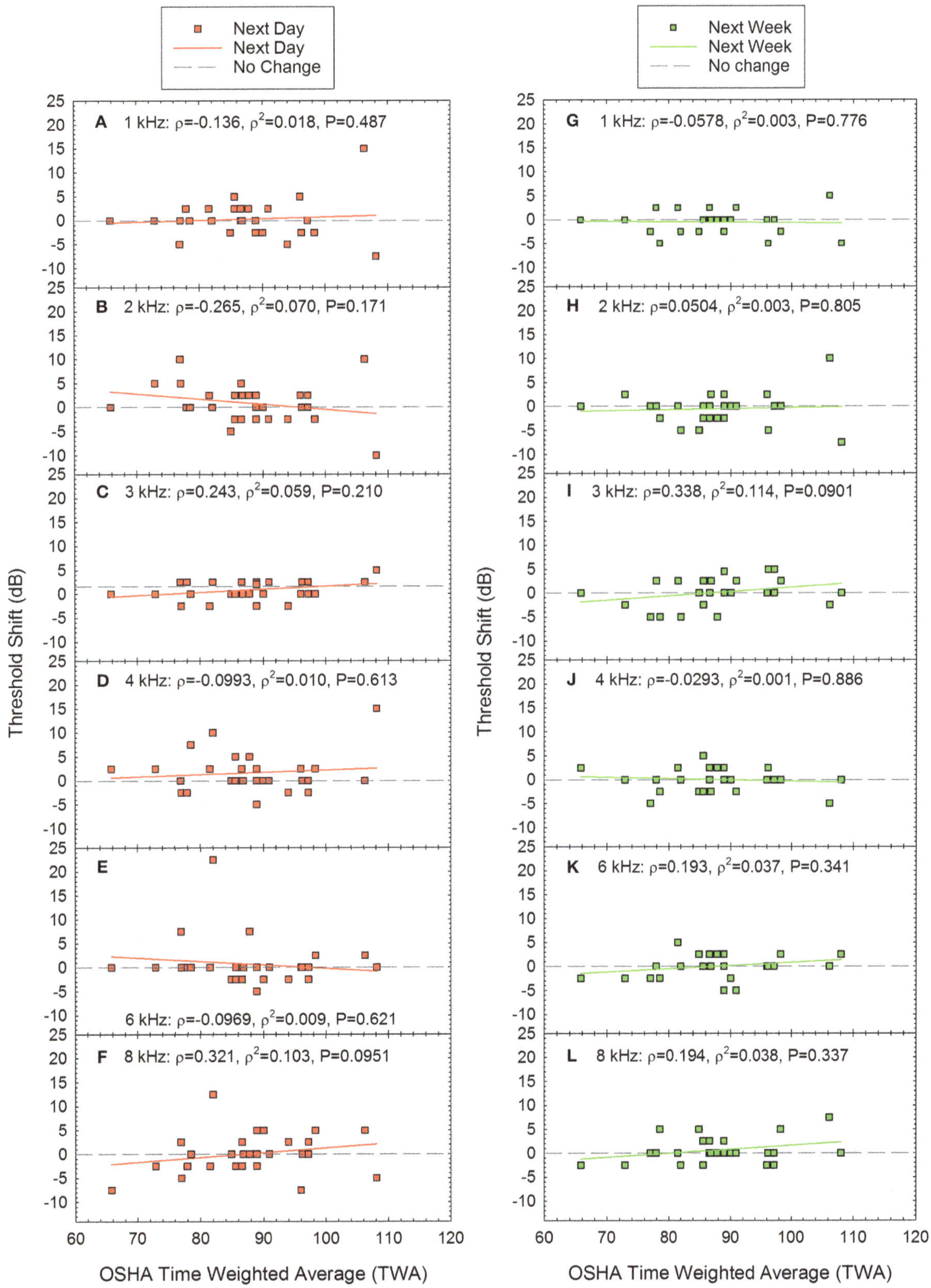

FIGURE 4 | There were no statistically significant correlations between time-weighted-average (TWA) and threshold shift at any of the frequencies tested either the day after the loud event **(A–F)** or one week later **(G–L)**. Next day data are shown for **(A)** 1 kHz, **(B)** 2 kHz, **(C)** 3 kHz, **(D)** 4 kHz, **(E)** 6 kHz, and **(F)** 8 kHz. Next week data are shown for **(G)** 1 kHz, **(H)** 2 kHz, **(I)** 3 kHz, **(J)** 4 kHz, **(K)** 6 kHz, and **(L)** 8 kHz. Lines of best fit are shown.

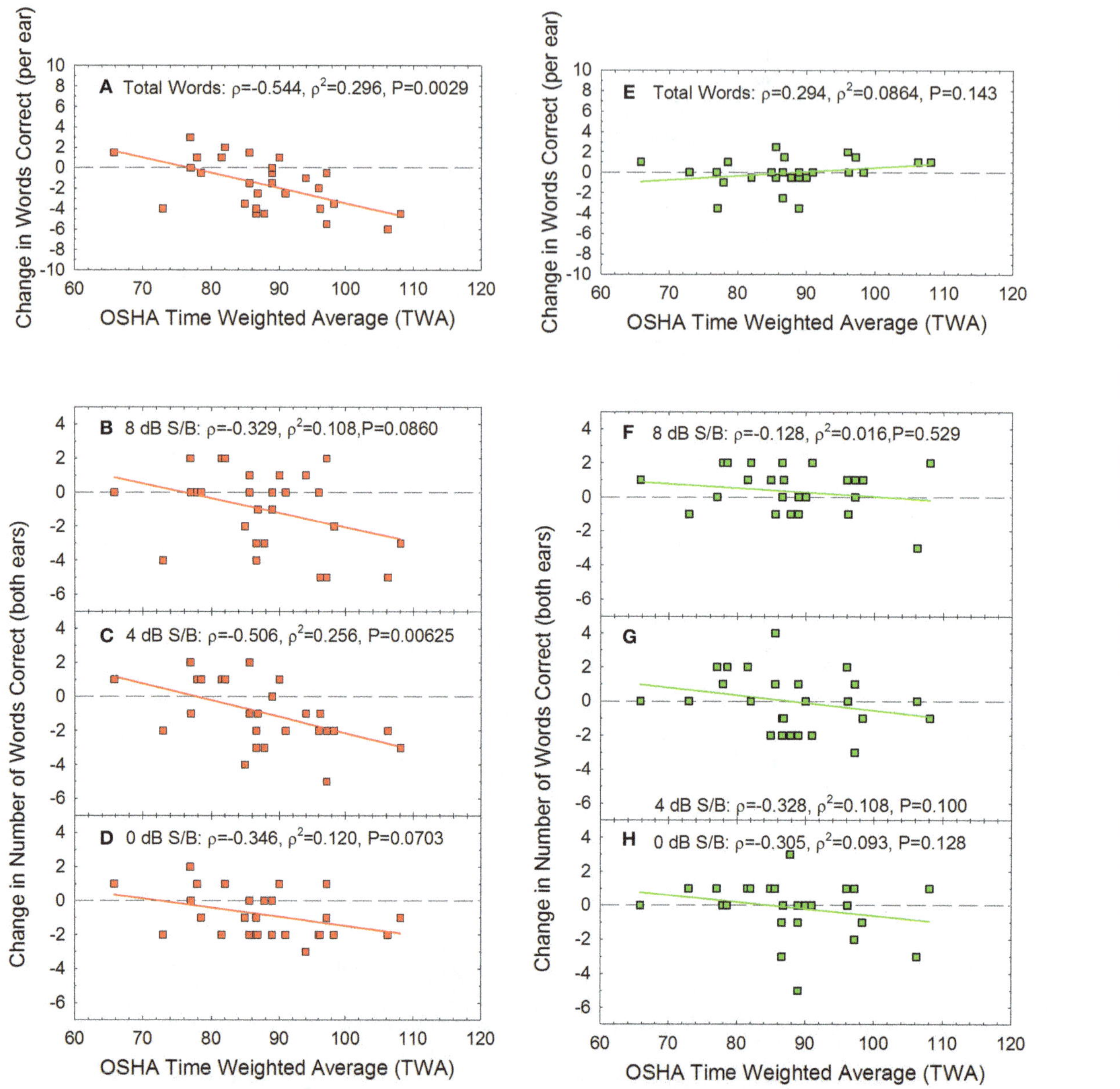

FIGURE 5 | For the Words-in-Noise (WIN) test, the summed change in performance was calculated as the total number of additional words correct (positive scores) or incorrect (negative scores) at the post-tests, relative to baseline, the "next day" (red) and "next week" (green). There was a statistically significant correlation between noise exposure (TWA) and the number of words missed the day after the noise exposure **(A)**, with the largest changes being approximately 6 words per ear out of the 35-word test lists. There were no statistically significant decreases in performance at the 1-week test time **(E)**, with the greatest deficits being approximately 3 words out of the 35 word lists; this is not a clinically significant change in speech-in-noise performance. The biggest temporary changes in performance were observed at the most difficult listening conditions. There was a statistically significant correlation between noise dose and change in performance the day after exposure within the 4 dB S/B condition **(C)**, with the largest changes being approximately 6 words out of the 10 words total that were presented to the two ears. There were similar trends for temporarily poorer performance as a function of noise exposure at other signal to noise conditions including **(B)** 8 dB/SB and **(D)** 0 dB S/B, but these were not statistically significant relationships. No statistically significant changes were evident at the one-week post noise test within **(F)** 8 dB S/B, **(G)** 4 dB S/B, or **(H)** 0 dB S/B conditions. Lines of best fit are shown.

TTS, the OHCs were the most vulnerable element, based on the data showing statistically significant decreases in OHC function at 6 kHz. Because these changes were limited to 6 kHz, and noise is expected to broadly affect the entire 3–6 kHz region, additional research will be necessary to more fully understand any underlying temporary damage to the cochlea. There were no statistically significant reductions in AP amplitude as a function of increasing TTS. Moreover, there were no reductions in AP amplitude within the small subset of individuals with TTS of 10 dB or more. Thus, while OHCs may have possibly been damaged in participants with the greatest TTS, there was no evidence of neural injury.

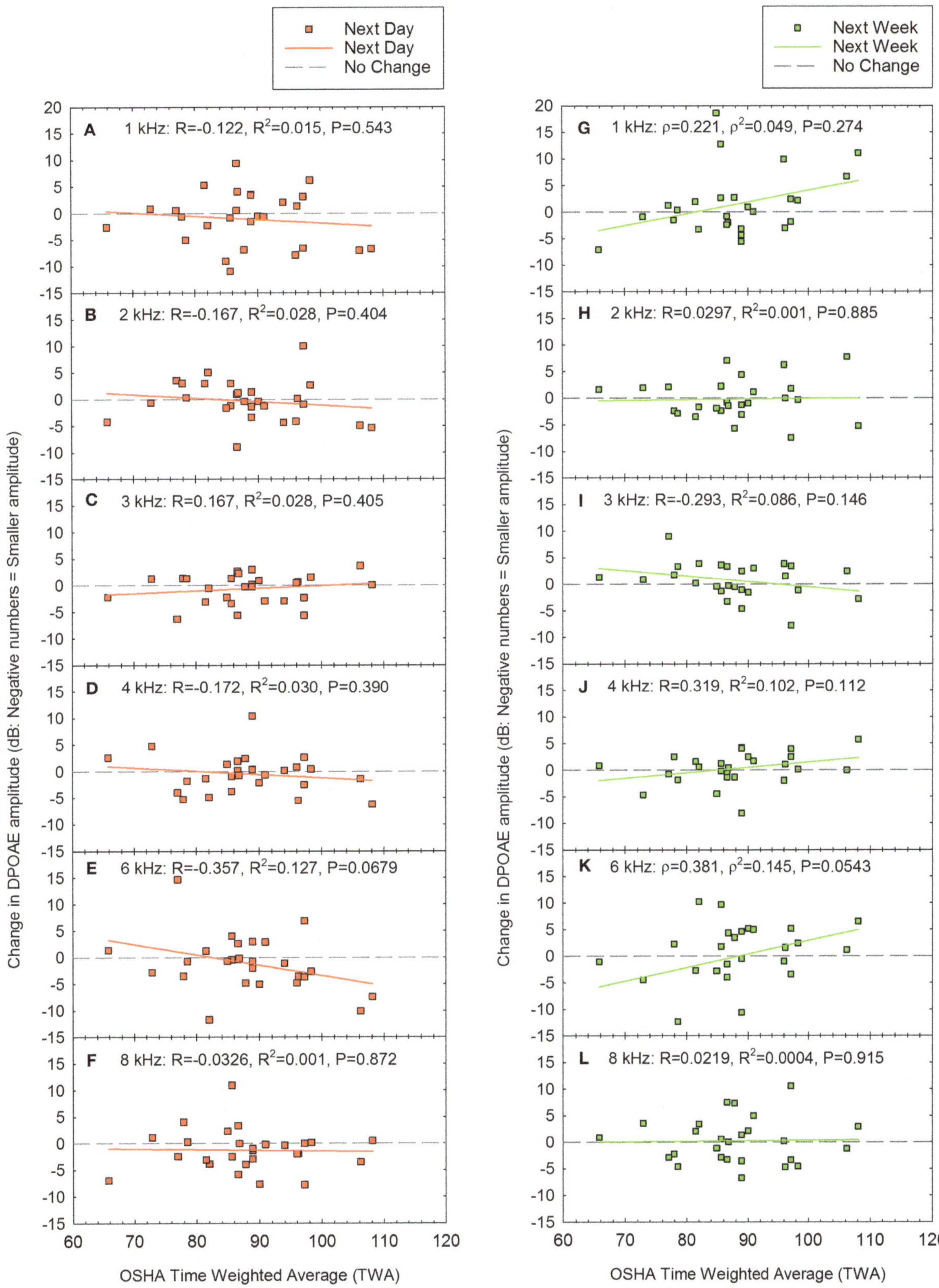

FIGURE 6 | There were no statistically significant correlations between noise exposure (TWA) and changes in DPOAE amplitude either the day after the loud event **(A–F)** or one week later **(G–L)**. Next day data are shown for **(A)** 1 kHz, **(B)** 2 kHz, **(C)** 3 kHz, **(D)** 4 kHz, **(E)** 6 kHz, and **(F)** 8 kHz. Next week data are shown for **(G)** 1 kHz, **(H)** 2 kHz, **(I)** 3 kHz, **(J)** 4 kHz, **(K)** 6 kHz, and **(L)** 8 kHz. Although there was a trend for decreased amplitude at 6 kHz **(E)**, this was not statistically significant ($P = 0.0679$). Lines of best fit are shown.

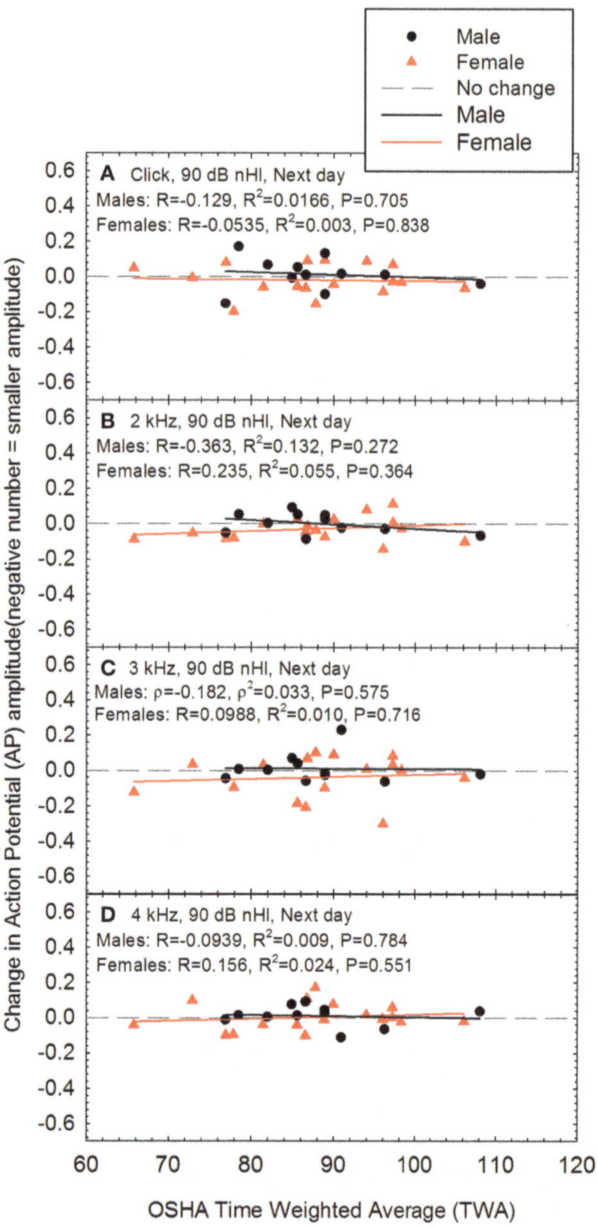

FIGURE 7 | There was no evidence of a noise-induced decrease in sound-evoked AP amplitude regardless of whether the stimuli were **(A)** clicks, **(B)** 2 kHz tone bursts, **(C)** 3 kHz tone bursts, or **(D)** 4 kHz tone bursts; all data are for 90 dB nHL stimuli, as measured the day after the noise exposure. None of the relationships were statistically significant within males or females. Lines of best fit are shown.

DISCUSSION

In the first part of this investigation, a retrospective analysis in which noise survey responses were used to compare previous noise exposure history to current auditory function, there was no evidence that a history of self-reported common recreational exposures resulted in audiometric, functional, or electrophysiological deficits. These data parallel Prendergast et al. (2017), Fulbright et al. (in press), and Spankovich et al. (2017), who evaluated three different normal-hearing young adult cohorts with varying amounts of recreational noise exposure history. In contrast to these four studies, ABR Wave-I amplitude was reported to be reduced in young adults (or, at least in young adult females) as a function of recreational noise exposure by Stamper and Johnson (2015a,b). Of note, none of these populations had significant occupational noise exposure histories or systematic exposure to loud music as rehearsing or performing musicians.

In contrast to the negative results from the above studies, Liberman et al. (2016) described statistically significant differences in extended high frequency (EHF) threshold sensitivity, word recognition performance in difficult listening conditions, SP amplitude, and the SP/AP ratio when high risk participants (15M, 7F; largely, college students enrolled in a music conservatory) were compared to low risk participants (4M, 8F; largely, college students enrolled in a communication sciences program). Bramhall et al. (2017) has also described deficits in ABR Wave-I amplitude as a function of noise exposure; they compared the amplitude of ABR Wave-I in civilians and military personnel without significant noise exposure to civilians who use firearms and military personnel with significant noise exposure (including firearm use). Taken together, the majority of data across retrospective studies now appear to be generally consistent in revealing no statistically significant relationships between common recreational noise exposure histories and ABR Wave-I (or AP) amplitude, whereas statistically significant relationships between firearm, blast, and other significant noise exposure and ABR Wave-I amplitude have emerged (Bramhall et al., 2017).

It is possible that statistically significant associations between AP (or, ABR Wave-I amplitude) and recreational noise history would emerge if larger cohorts were studied, which would increase power to detect subtle relationships. However, based on the observed Pearson R and Spearman Rho values of 0.15 or less across stimulus conditions (see **Figure 2**), new, prospective power analysis indicates that a sample size of 400 participants would be necessary to achieve 85% power to detect relationships of the size (i.e., $R = 0.15$) obtained in this retrospective analysis. Even if a large study with the power to detect small associations was conducted, it is not clear that the weak relationships indicated by R values of 0.15 would be clinically significant. As an alternative, study power presumably would be increased if additional higher-risk participants were included, assuming that the hypothesis that the strength of the observed relationships will increase as participants with increasing exposure are added is true. It is not yet clear if risk will increase relatively linearly along some graded continuum as noise exposure increases, or if there is some critical boundary at which risk of injury suddenly increases in an "all or nothing" fashion; a better understanding of this relationship is critically important with respect to the design of future studies and the eventual development of evidence-based risk criteria. Systematic manipulation of noise exposure using rodent models may provide some insight into these relationships and inform the design of human translational studies. Data from non-human primates are also likely to be necessary in order to

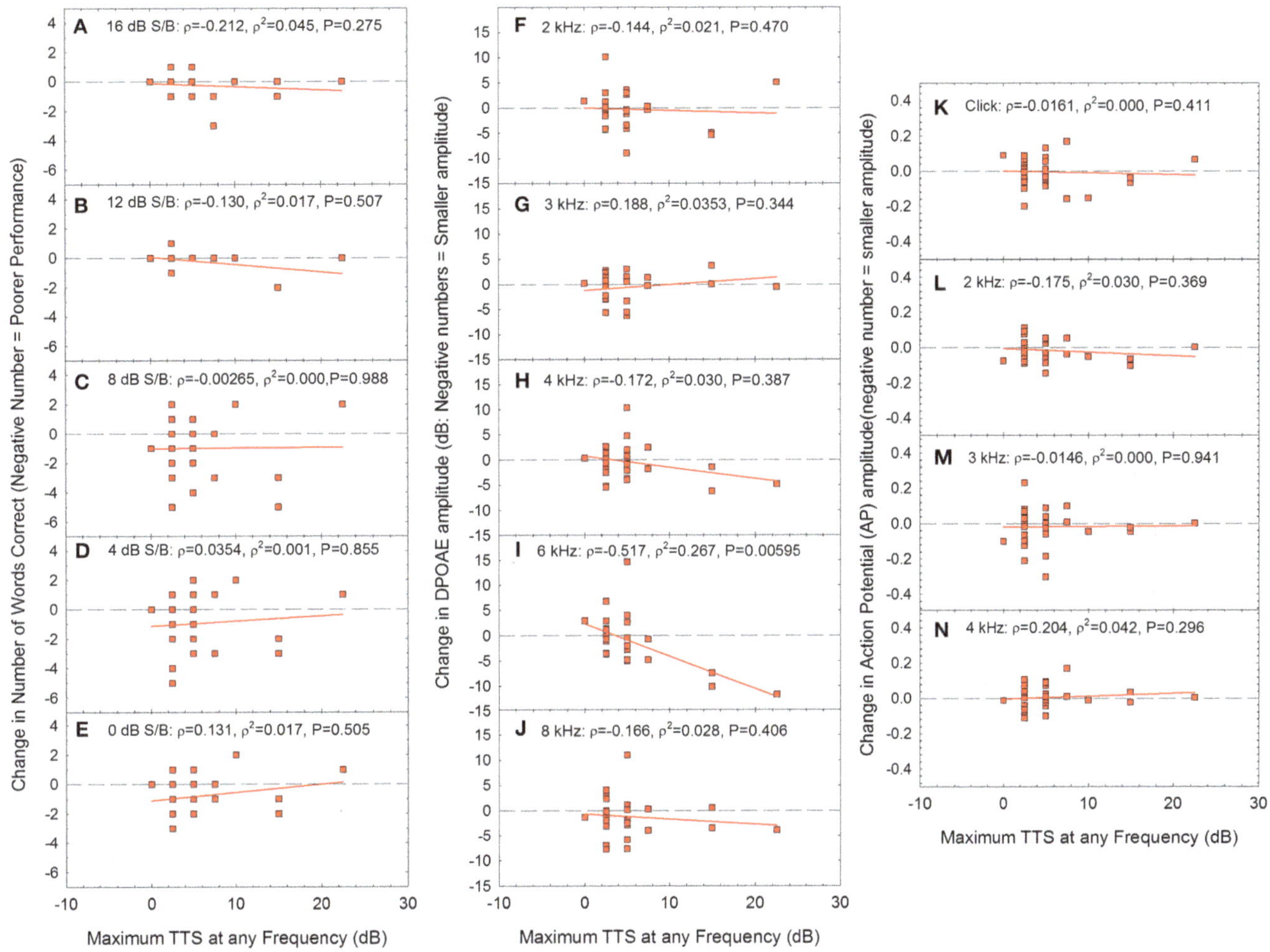

FIGURE 8 | There were no statistically significant correlations between maximum TTS at any frequency and change in performance within any of the signal-to-babble conditions (**A**: 16 dB S/B; **B**: 12 dB S/B; **C**: 8 dB S/B; **D**: 4 dB S/B; **E**:0 dB S/B). There was a statistically significant correlation between maximum TTS at any frequency and change in DPOAE amplitude at 6 kHz **(I)** with no statistically significant relationships at other frequencies (**F**: 2 kHz; **G**: 3 kHz; **H**: 4 kHz; **J**: 8 kHz). There was no statistically significant relationship between maximum TTS at any frequency and change in AP amplitude. (**K**: click; **L**: 2 kHz; **M**: 3 kHz; **N**: 4 kHz). Lines of best fit are shown in all panels.

understand risk across species, and would support additional inference related to human risk.

Most investigations assessing the potential for hidden hearing loss in humans have used NEQ-based approaches. These studies rely on an assumption that reports of noise exposure within the past 12-months provide information that is relevant and accurate. These studies further assume that exposure over the past 12-months is representative of previous lifetime noise history. If there was significantly more or less noise exposure within the past 12-months than in earlier years, the previous 12-month $L_{Aeq8760}$ metric would provide limited utility for comparisons with current functional status. Fulbright (2016) used a variety of surveys to assess both $L_{Aeq8760}$ and lifetime noise. No notable differences in outcomes were observed when current audiometric function was assessed as a function of $L_{Aeq8760}$ or lifetime noise; however, in this young adult population, lifetime noise estimates tended to be reduced relative to previous year estimates. In other words, noise exposure as a young adult was increased relative to noise exposure in earlier childhood years. Thus, it cannot be assumed that every participant in every study has a 12-month noise history (and $L_{Aeq8760}$) that is representative of their lifetime noise exposure history; careful interview is necessary to assure that there was no significant noise exposure in earlier years that would suggest a participant is at higher risk than their current $L_{Aeq8760}$ might suggest.

We did not survey self-reported difficulties in noise. It is tempting to assume that self-reported difficulty listening in noise may be a useful measure, as this approach is now being used in large epidemiological studies that rely on survey data to assess hearing problems (see for example Curhan et al., 2012). The use of surveys may also resolve challenges related to the ceiling effects observed for some speech-in-quiet and speech-in-noise tests. Certainly, there is a lack of consensus regarding an accepted "gold standard" for speech-in-noise testing (for discussion, see Le Prell and Lobarinas, 2015; Le Prell and Brungart, 2016; Le Prell and Clavier, 2017). The data collected here used the WIN test, while Bramhall et al. (2015) collected data using the QuickSin, and Liberman et al. (2016) used the widely available NU6 words within a custom hearing-in-noise test which included the addition of time compression and reverberation to NU6 words to increase the difficulty of the standardized test. There is a need for standardized, quantitative speech-in-noise performance data; as background noise levels increase, every participant (and patient) will have relatively increased difficulty understanding speech in background noise at some point. Some people may qualitatively rate their difficulties as more significant than others, even if their quantitative speech-in-noise test scores (and actual performance in real-world noise backgrounds) are equivalent. In other words, someone who self-reports difficulty understanding speech in noise, but has normal hearing thresholds and normal speech-in-noise test scores, may be functionally equivalent to others who do not report as much difficulty. Thus, a normal hearing person who self-reports difficulty understanding speech in noisy backgrounds may not necessarily have an abnormality or pathology (i.e., they may have normal hearing and speech-in-noise test scores), but could instead have different expectations regarding their performance across listening environments of varying difficulty (e.g., a one on one conversation in a co-worker's office vs. happy hour drinks with half the office staff at a busy restaurant). Such cases may potentially result in an opportunity for counseling of realistic speech-in-noise expectations and listening strategies, rather than a diagnosis of auditory dysfunction. The challenges of rehabilitation of deficits when patients do not meet the criteria for amplification were recently discussed by Kraus and White-Schwoch (2016), in their discussion of "Not-So-Hidden" Hearing Loss. This challenge of self-assessed perceptual difficulty directly parallels challenges related to the issue of tinnitus, as the self-assessed "bothersomeness" of tinnitus varies significantly from patient to patient, with no clear relationship to psychophysical parameters determined during pitch or level matching (for additional discussion, see Le Prell and Lobarinas, 2016).

There is an urgent need for validated, clinical tests that can be used to quantify patient self-report of difficulty understanding speech in noisy backgrounds. The ideal test will be sensitive to differences in performance within normal hearing listeners. For the WIN, a change of 3.5 dB-S/B (corresponding to a difference of approximately 4 words out of the 35 words presented) has been described as clinically meaningful (Wilson and McArdle, 2007). Many individual participants had changes of at least 4 words the day after noise exposure (**Figure 5A**), but not 1-week later (**Figure 5E**). The WIN should be considered for use in future studies not only based on the availability of the validated test as part of the NIH Toolbox (Zecker et al., 2013), but also based on the sensitivity of the test to acute, noise-induced changes in study participants. It may be the case that even greater sensitivity could be achieved in tests completed with higher background noise levels, or perhaps modifications (such as those of Liberman et al., 2016) that more appropriately reflect and reproduce the difficult listening environments found in real-world noisy and reverberative environments, such as restaurants, gymnasiums, bars, clubs, and other common venues with significant background noise.

The second part of this investigation was a prospective study measuring changes in audiologic function after new, acute recreational noise exposure. Audiometric, electrophysiological, and functional measures were monitored subsequent to noise exposure. There was no evidence that common recreational exposures resulted in permanent audiometric, functional, or electrophysiological deficits. Selective cochlear synaptopathy, resulting in an accompanying reduction in ABR Wave-I amplitude, has been clearly demonstrated in animals in association with noise exposures that induce a robust TTS the day after the noise exposure (for reviews, see Kujawa and Liberman, 2015; Liberman and Kujawa, 2017). The common, real-world recreational noise exposures that our participants experienced at concerts, multi-day music festivals, loud bars, etc. (see **Figure 3**), did not result in robust TTS the day after the exposure (most TTS < 15 dB, see **Figure 8**), nor did they result in decreases in AP amplitude (see **Figure 7**). Thus, they did not produce any evidence that would be interpreted as consistent with new, noise-induced cochlear synaptopathy following common, recreational noise exposure.

TTS was highly variable across individuals, which is a major challenge for studies such as these. The variability in TTS was consistent with that reported by others, as individual variability is significant after free-field exposures (Mills et al., 2001; Strasser et al., 2003) as well as controlled exposures delivered via personal music player devices (Le Prell et al., 2012, 2016; Kil et al., 2017). Across music player studies, a 100% noise dose (based on 29 CFR 1910.95) has resulted in highly variable TTS across participants, ranging from 0 dB to approximately 20 dB at 4 kHz, but with largely complete recovery the following day. Most, if not all, assessments of the effects of recreational noise have been completed immediately post exposure, with changes frequently being on the order of 8–10 dB as participants exit concerts (Opperman et al., 2006; Derebery et al., 2012; Ramakers et al., 2016) or clubs (Kramer et al., 2006); thus, the current data contribute further insight to the potential for changes in audiologic function the day after recreational exposure.

Our study found no statistically significant reduction in AP amplitude the day after exposure to common, loud, recreational events (see **Figure 7**). Although some participants had TTS exceeding typical test-retest of ±5 dB, there were no statistically significant relationships between changes in audiometric threshold sensitivity and noise dose (see **Figure 4**). There was a temporary statistically significant decrease in performance on the WIN test as a function of noise exposure in the overall analysis the day after the noise exposure (see **Figure 5A**), and for a small number of participants, the temporary deficits met the definition of clinically significant decrease in performance. However, due to a lack of a statistically significant decrease in either DPOAE amplitude (see **Figure 6**) or AP amplitude (see **Figure 7**) as a function of increasing noise exposure, it is not possible to directly attribute changes in performance on the WIN to specific OHC or synaptic injuries. It is possible to speculate that OHC injuries are more likely to underlie changes in performance on the WIN, based on the decreasing DPOAE amplitude at 6 kHz that was observed with increasing TTS (see **Figure 8I**), but these changes were limited to one frequency and it is not clear why 3 and 4 kHz failed to show similar noise-induced changes.

All of the evidence from animal models to date indicates that if noise-induced synaptopathy develops, it is immediate, and it is permanent. Thus, data from this prospective study showing temporary noise-related changes in performance on the WIN, in the absence of relationships between noise-exposure and changes in DPOAE and AP amplitude the day after noise exposure, cannot be interpreted as consistent with or otherwise suggesting synaptopathic damage in these human participants. In live human participants, cochlear synaptopathy cannot be directly measured, as synapse counts require *ex vivo* extraction of the temporal bone. The only direct evidence of synaptopathy in human cochlear tissues comes from Viana et al. (2015), who provided preliminary evidence of an age-related synaptopathy based on differences across five temporal bones. Those data are supplemented by Makary et al. (2011), who documented an age-related decrease in spiral ganglion survival which could be secondary to an age-related loss of their synaptic targets. Temporal bones may be a resource for new tissues, but unfortunately, noise history data are not always available for these tissues.

Human studies to date have generally relied on the amplitude of ABR Wave-I or the AP as an indirect proxy for potential synaptopathy (Stamper and Johnson, 2015a,b; Liberman et al., 2016; Bramhall et al., 2017; Prendergast et al., 2017; Spankovich et al., 2017; Fulbright et al., in press). ABR Wave-I amplitude has been highly correlated with synaptopathy in the animal studies thus far (Liberman and Kujawa, 2017); however, ABR measurements in anesthetized animals are much "cleaner" than ABR measurements in awake, resting humans.

At this time, there are no functional consequences that have been reliably associated with decreases in ABR Wave-I amplitude in normal hearing listeners. Bramhall et al. (2015) showed a statistically significant relationship between ABR Wave-I amplitude and performance on the QuickSin, but only in the presence of overt hearing loss; no statistically significant relationship was demonstrated between ABR Wave-I amplitude and performance on the QuickSin in participants with normal hearing. Data from rats showed that the functional deficits associated with decreases in ABR Wave-I amplitude were limited to the frequencies at which ABR Wave-I amplitude was decreased, and functional deficits were observed only in the most difficult listening condition (poorest signal to noise ratio) tested (Lobarinas et al., 2017). Although it is not clear how directly these results will translate to humans, it remains reasonable to hypothesize that speech-in-noise tests have the potential to reveal noise-induced deficits prior to the development of overt hearing loss in humans.

There are a variety of suggestions for other electrophysiological and psychophysical tools that might be considered for detection of hidden hearing loss in humans; various proposed metrics include the envelope following response (EFR) (Shaheen et al., 2015; Paul et al., 2017), middle ear muscle reflex (Valero et al., 2016), psychophysical manipulation of amplitude modulation in detection tasks (Paul et al., 2017), ABR Wave-V latency changes during forward masking (Mehraei et al., 2017), and binaural detection (Bernstein and Trahiotis, 2016). There are also suggestions to consider normalizing the amplitude of ABR Wave-I relative to the amplitude of ABR Wave-V (a measure of central response that does not appear to be affected by synaptopathy) (Verhulst et al., 2016), or relative to the amplitude of the summating potential (i.e., SP/AP ratio) (Liberman et al., 2016).

The argument that the SP/AP ratio is useful in revealing selective neural damage is based on the premise that SP is dominated by the OHC receptor potential (which is not expected to be affected by damage to the IHC/AN synapses), whereas AP is generated by the cochlear nerve. Early work by Durrant et al. (1998) attempted to resolve controversy over the relative contributions of the IHC and OHC populations to the SP; they concluded that while the OHCs made a significant contribution, the IHCs had a relatively greater contribution to the SP. Additional arguments that SP is appropriate for use normalizing AP are based on the observation that SP is more stable than AP after a variety of insults (for discussion see Liberman et al., 2016). However, the stability of SP may, in part, rely on the use of stimuli that are matched with respect to sensation level (i.e., the dB amount above individual threshold), as SP amplitude was constant across mice only when signal levels were equal sensation level (Sergeyenko et al., 2013). Furthermore, we point to data from Nam and Won (2004), who measured SP and AP after inducing TTS in human participants. They found that SP amplitude increased, but AP amplitude was unchanged, resulting in an increase in the SP/AP ratio. This finding parallels the increase in SP reported by Liberman et al. (2016) and, like Liberman et al. (2016), evidenced noise-induced changes in the SP/AP ratio to be driven by increased SP amplitude. If the SP is the measure relatively more affected by noise exposure, then the AP is essentially being normalized against a moving target, which seems counter-intuitive to the identification of selective neural deficits. Taken together, the noise-induced changes in SP and corresponding changes in SP/AP ratio (given that AP was unchanged) in those studies may be more appropriately interpreted as consistent with OHC based dysfunction, rather than synaptic neural dysfunction. Increasing OHC dysfunction as a function of increasing TTS was detected here (at least at 6 kHz), and noise-induced OHC dysfunction would be consistent with new work from Hoben et al. (2017) which importantly suggests that OHC loss or dysfunction may drive speech-in-noise deficits. Of note, the SP waveform is generally more difficult to resolve (Roland and Roth, 1997), and is highly variable across normal hearing listeners (Ferraro et al., 1994). In the current study, SP data were collected, as per the methods section, to permit calculation of SP/AP ratios following Liberman et al. (2016). Approximately 45% of the right and left ears had scorable SPs across the stimulus conditions. We initially included this ratio in the retrospective regression models, and found no statistically significant relationships detected for the subset of participants with reliable SPs. However, based on the above general concerns regarding the use of SP/AP ratios to identify selective neural damage, we did not assess potential changes in this ratio as a function of acute recreational noise exposure. Regardless, there was no relationship between AP amplitude and retrospective noise history (**Figure 2**), AP amplitude and acute recreational noise exposure (**Figure 7**), or change in AP amplitude and maximum observed TTS (**Figure 8**).

Other approaches that have been presented at recent scientific meetings include the normalization of ABR Wave-I amplitude for 4 kHz signals relative to ABR Wave-I amplitude for 1 kHz signals (Earl et al., 2017), and ABR Wave-I latency based comparisons instead of amplitude based comparisons (Skoe et al., 2017). As these different metrics and measures make their way through the peer-review process, it will hopefully become possible to begin to define the most informative strategies for those seeking evidence of hidden hearing loss in humans. If metrics selected for use in future studies include high level tone pips, some caution may be warranted with respect to interpretation of the frequency-specific effects; it is possible that high level tone bursts will activate relatively broader regions of the cochlea, perhaps even resembling the response to a click stimulus. The lack of agreed on metrics is clearly a major issue for translational human studies on hidden hearing loss (Le Prell and Lobarinas, 2016; Hickox et al., 2017; Kobel et al., 2017; Liberman and Kujawa, 2017).

SUMMARY AND CONCLUSIONS

The current investigation provided no evidence of noise-induced decreases in human AP amplitude in the retrospective analyses of noise exposure history, nor in the prospective analyses following common recreational noise exposure. The current data indicate that intra-participant changes in AP (ABR Wave-I) amplitude can be reliably monitored longitudinally; response waveforms were reliable and repeatable within individual participants, within and across sessions.

In animal models, the gold standard for identification of cochlear synaptopathy is the post-mortem counting of synaptic ribbons. Reductions in synapse count are highly correlated with the amplitude of Wave-I of the ABR (Sergeyenko et al., 2013). Liberman and Kujawa (2017) have therefore suggested that when DPOAE amplitude has returned to baseline (after noise exposure), or has not yet deteriorated (in the case of aging), the amplitude of ABR Wave-I is highly predictive of cochlear synaptopathy. In humans, there is a search for supra-threshold evoked potential metrics that will be sensitive to and specific for cochlear synaptopathy. The clinical (i.e., functional, "real-world") relevance of reduced ABR Wave-I amplitude (AP amplitude) remains to be determined, despite much speculation. Even if a permanent noise-induced reduction of human ABR Wave-I amplitude is found following noise exposure in human participants, a meaningful, real-world functional effect must be identified in order for the ABR Wave-I amplitude reduction to serve as a clinically relevant finding in audiology. Here, the correlation analyses revealed a statistically significant relationship between noise dose/TWA and change in performance on the WIN, with statistically significant growth in deficits as TWA increased. For the majority of the participants, the individual noise-induced changes in WIN performance were small (1–3 word deficits at the test session the day after recreational noise exposure) but there were some participants with deficits of 4–6 words, which meets the criteria set by Wilson and McArdle (2007) for clinically significant change.

To be successful in the identification of noise-induced synaptopathic deficits in humans, it may ultimately be the case that future studies will need to include human populations exposed to noise insults that result in the magnitude of TTS minimally necessary to observe synaptopathic injury in animals. Such TTS changes appear to be unlikely to be produced from common recreational noise exposure, but are perhaps likely to be observed within military cohorts or safety officers, based on the data of Bramhall et al. (2017). Weapons training may provide more controlled access to noise-exposed participants, but enrollment in hearing conservation studies can influence the use of hearing protection devices (HPDs) that prevent the deficits of interest (see for example Le Prell et al., 2011). Regardless of the boundary at which risk begins, or the specific relationship between TTS and "hidden hearing loss," it may ultimately prove difficult to identify a human cohort exposed to noise that is loud enough and long enough to cause neural damage, but leaves OHC function unaltered. This specific challenge was recently discussed in detail by Hickox et al. (2017), who point to the prevalence of mixed pathologies in human populations. A major remaining unknown is the extent to which repetition of noise exposure has the potential to result in a synaptopathic injury over time if smaller TTS changes are induced at each exposure (for additional discussion see Dobie and Humes, 2017; Murphy and Le Prell, 2017).

It is possible to imagine changes in conventional test batteries and/or metrics used for monitoring the effects of noise exposure if there were both compelling evidence of ABR Wave-I amplitude changes and accompanying functional deficits following noise exposure. Further research will be needed to more carefully assess the effects of noise exposures that have the potential to result in more severe TTS. Ethical practices for educating participants about the potential for auditory injury will need to be carefully considered, as per the recent commentary on TTS studies by Maison and Rauch (2017). Participants should be provided with HPDs if the investigator has reason to believe that the participant may be at risk for acoustic trauma resulting in permanent functional changes on threshold or suprathreshold measures of function. Such studies will also need to carefully assess OHC function and threshold sensitivity (including EHF threshold assessment) in order to systematically differentiate between OHC damage and potential neural synaptic damage, and document both overt and relatively more hidden supra-threshold hearing deficits.

AUTHOR CONTRIBUTIONS

SG: contributed to study design, data collection, data interpretation, and writing the manuscript. KW: contributed to study design, data collection, statistical analysis, data interpretation, and writing the manuscript. JB: contributed to study design, data collection, data interpretation, and reviewed the manuscript. CL: contributed to study design, statistical analysis, data interpretation, and writing the manuscript.

ACKNOWLEDGMENTS

This study was funded by the Emily and Phil Schepps Professorship in Hearing Science at the University of Texas at Dallas. We thank graduate student research assistants Katie Palmer and Tess Zaccardi for their contributions to data extraction, and we thank Dr. Jeffrey Martin for helpful conversations about ECochG protocols. We thank Andrew Smith of Studio 6 Digital for donating download codes for the "SPL Graph" smartphone app used by study participants.

REFERENCES

Atcherson, S. R., and Stoody, T. M. (2012). "Chapter 2: Basic instrumentation, acquisition, and recording considerations," in *Auditory Electrophysiology: A Clinical Guide*, eds S. R. Atcherson and T. M. Stoody (New York, NY: Thieme), 19–21.

Bernstein, L. R., and Trahiotis, C. (2016). Behavioral manifestations of audiometrically-defined "slight" or "hidden" hearing loss revealed by measures of binaural detection. *J. Acoust. Soc. Am.* 140:3540. doi: 10.1121/1.4966113

Bramhall, N. F., Konrad-Martin, D., McMillan, G. P., and Griest, S. E. (2017). Auditory brainstem response altered in humans with noise exposure despite normal outer hair cell function. *Ear Hear.* 38, e1–e12. doi: 10.1097/AUD.0000000000000370

Bramhall, N., Ong, B., Ko, J., and Parker, M. (2015). Speech perception ability in noise is correlated with auditory brainstem response Wave I amplitude. *J. Am. Acad. Audiol.* 26, 509–517. doi: 10.3766/jaaa.14100

Brungart, D. S., Sheffield, B. M., and Kubli, L. R. (2014). Development of a test battery for evaluating speech perception in complex listening environments. *J. Acoust. Soc. Am.* 136, 777–790. doi: 10.1121/1.4887440

Curhan, S. G., Shargorodsky, J., Eavey, R., and Curhan, G. C. (2012). Analgesic use and the risk of hearing loss in women. *Am. J. Epidemiol.* 176, 544–554. doi: 10.1093/aje/kws146

Derebery, M. J., Vermiglio, A., Berliner, K. I., Potthoff, M., and Holguin, K. (2012). Facing the music: pre- and postconcert assessment of hearing in teenagers. *Otol. Neurotol.* 33, 1136–1141. doi: 10.1097/MAO.0b013e31825f2328

Dirks, D. D., Kamm, C. A., Bower, D., and Betsworth, A. (1977). Use of performance-intensity functions for diagnosis. *J. Speech Hear. Res.* 42, 408–415. doi: 10.1044/jshd.4203.408

Dobie, R. A., and Humes, L. E. (2017). Commentary on the regulatory implications of noise-induced cochlear neuropathy. *Int. J. Audiol.* 56, 74–78. doi: 10.1080/14992027.2016.1255359

Dobie, R. A., and Sakai, C. S. (2001). "Estimation of hearing loss severity from the audiogram," in *Noise Induced Hearing Loss: Basic Mechanisms, Prevention and Control*, eds D. Henderson, D. Prasher, R. Kopke, R. J. Salvi, and R. Hamernik (London: Noise Research Network), 351–363.

Durrant, J. D., Wang, J., Ding, D. L., and Salvi, R. J. (1998). Are inner or outer hair cells the source of summating potentials recorded from the round window? *J. Acoust. Soc. Am.* 104, 370–377. doi: 10.1121/1.423293

Earl, B. R., Reeg, H., Schweinzger, I., and Roggia, S. M. (2017). Using signal-in-noise electrococleography to assess the integrity of high-threshold auditory nerve fibers. *Abs. Assoc. Res. Otolaryngol.* 40:337.

Fernandez, K. A., Jeffers, P. W., Lall, K., Liberman, M. C., and Kujawa, S. G. (2015). Aging after noise exposure: acceleration of cochlear synaptopathy in "recovered" ears. *J. Neurosci.* 35, 7509–7520. doi: 10.1523/JNEUROSCI.5138-14.2015

Ferraro, J. A., Blackwell, W. L., Mediavilla, S. J., and Thedinger, B. S. (1994). Normal summating potential to tone bursts recorded from the tympanic membrane in humans. *J. Am. Acad. Audiol.* 5, 17–23.

Fulbright, A. N. C. (2016). *Normal Hearing? What Functional Hearing Tests, Noise Exposure History and ABR Wave-I Amplitude Reveal* [Dissertation]. Ph.D, Gainesville, FL: University of Florida.

Fulbright, A. N. C., Le Prell, C. G., Griffiths, S. K., and Lobarinas, E. (in press). Effects of recreational noise on threshold and supra-threshold measures of auditory function. *Sem. Hear.* doi: 10.1055/s-0037-1606325

Furman, A. C., Kujawa, S. G., and Liberman, M. C. (2013). Noise-induced cochlear neuropathy is selective for fibers with low spontaneous rates. *J. Neurophysiol.* 110, 577–586. doi: 10.1152/jn.00164.2013

Gallun, F. J., Diedesch, A. C., Kubli, L. R., Walden, T. C., Folmer, R. L., Lewis, M. S., et al. (2012a). Performance on tests of central auditory processing by individuals exposed to high-intensity blasts. *J. Rehabil. Res. Dev.* 49, 1005–1025. doi: 10.1682/JRRD.2012.03.0038

Gallun, F. J., Lewis, M. S., Folmer, R. L., Diedesch, A. C., Kubli, L. R., McDermott, D. J., et al. (2012b). Implications of blast exposure for central auditory function: a review. *J. Rehabil. Res. Dev.* 49, 1059–1074. doi: 10.1682/JRRD.2010.09.0166

Gelfand, S. A. (2001). *Essentials of Audiology, 2nd Edn.* New York, NY: Thieme.

Grinn, S., Palmer, K., Zaccardi, T., and Le Prell, C. G. (2017). "Accuracy of "SPL Graph" and "SPL Meter" sound level meter Apps for iPhone," in *2017 Annual National Hearing Conservation Conference-The River of Aural Serenity, NHCA Spectrum*, Vol. 34 (San Antonio, TX), 40.

Hall, J. W. I. (1992). *Handbook of Auditory Evoked Responses.* Boston, MA: Allyn and Bacon.

Helfer, T. M., Jordan, N. N., Lee, R. B., Pietrusiak, P., Cave, K., and Schairer, K. (2011). Noise-induced hearing injury and comorbidities among postdeployment U.S. Army soldiers: April 2003-June 2009. *Am. J. Audiol.* 20, 33–41. doi: 10.1044/1059-0889(2011/10-0033)

Henderson, E., Testa, M. A., and Hartnick, C. (2011). Prevalence of noise-induced hearing-threshold shifts and hearing loss among US youths. *Pediatrics* 127, e39–e46. doi: 10.1542/peds.2010-0926

Hickox, A. E., Larsen, E., Heinz, M. G., Shinobu, L., and Whitton, J. P. (2017). Translational issues in cochlear synaptopathy. *Hear. Res.* 349, 164–171. doi: 10.1016/j.heares.2016.12.010

Hickox, A. E., and Liberman, M. C. (2014). Is noise-induced cochlear neuropathy key to the generation of hyperacusis or tinnitus? *J. Neurophysiol.* 111, 552–564. doi: 10.1152/jn.00184.2013

Hoben, R., Easow, G., Pevzner, S., and Parker, M. A. (2017). Outer hair cell and auditory nerve function in speech recognition in quiet and in background noise. *Front. Neurosci.* 11:157. doi: 10.3389/fnins.2017.00157

Jensen, J. B., Lysaght, A. C., Liberman, M. C., Qvortrup, K., and Stankovic, K. M. (2015). Immediate and delayed cochlear neuropathy after noise exposure in pubescent mice. *PLoS ONE* 10:e0125160. doi: 10.1371/journal.pone.0125160

Johnson, T. A., Cooper, S., Stamper, G. C., and Chertoff, M. (2017). Noise Exposure Questionnaire: A tool for quantifying annual noise exposure. *J. Am. Acad. Audiol.* 8, 14–35. doi: 10.3766/jaaa.15070

Kil, J., Lobarinas, E., Spankovich, C., Griffiths, S. K., Antonelli, P. J., Lynch, E. D., et al. (2017). Safety and efficacy of Ebselen for the prevention of noise-induced hearing loss: a randomized, double-blind, placebo-controlled, phase 2 clinical trial. *Lancet.* doi: 10.1016/S0140-6736(17)31791-9. [Epub ahead of print].

Kim, M. G., Hong, S. M., Shim, H. J., Kim, Y. D., Cha, C. I., and Yeo, S. G. (2009). Hearing threshold of Korean adolescents associated with the use of personal music players. *Yonsei Med. J.* 50, 771–776. doi: 10.3349/ymj.2009.50.6.771

Kobel, M., Le Prell, C. G., Liu, J., Hawks, J. W., and Bao, J. (2017). Noise-induced cochlear synaptopathy: past findings and future studies. *Hear. Res.* 349, 148–154. doi: 10.1016/j.heares.2016.12.008

Kramer, S., Dreisbach, L., Lockwood, J., Baldwin, K., Kopke, R. D., Scranton, S., et al. (2006). Efficacy of the antioxidant N-acetylcysteine (NAC) in protecting ears exposed to loud music. *J. Am. Acad. Audiol.* 17, 265–278. doi: 10.3766/jaaa.17.4.5

Kraus, N., and White-Schwoch, T. (2016). Not-So-Hidden Hearing Loss. *Hear. J.* 69, 38–40. doi: 10.1097/01.HJ.0000483269.59643.1a

Kujawa, S. G., and Liberman, M. C. (2006). Acceleration of age-related hearing loss by early noise exposure: evidence of a misspent youth. *J. Neurosci.* 26, 2115–2123. doi: 10.1523/JNEUROSCI.4985-05.2006

Kujawa, S. G., and Liberman, M. C. (2009). Adding insult to injury: cochlear nerve degeneration after "temporary" noise-induced hearing loss. *J. Neurosci.* 29, 14077–14085. doi: 10.1523/JNEUROSCI.2845-09.2009

Kujawa, S. G., and Liberman, M. C. (2015). Synaptopathy in the noise-exposed and aging cochlea: Primary neural degeneration in acquired sensorineural hearing loss. *Hear. Res.* 330(Pt. B), 191–199. doi: 10.1016/j.heares.2015.02.009

Le Prell, C. G., and Brungart, D. S. (2016). Speech-in-noise tests and supra-threshold auditory evoked potentials as metrics for noise damage and clinical trial outcome measures. *Otol. Neurotol.* 37, e295–e302. doi: 10.1097/MAO.0000000000001069

Le Prell, C. G., and Clavier, O. H. (2017). Effects of noise on speech recognition: challenges for communication by service members. *Hear. Res.* 349, 76–89. doi: 10.1016/j.heares.2016.10.004

Le Prell, C. G., Dell, S., Hensley, B. N., Hall, J. W. I., Campbell, K. C. M., Antonelli, P. A., et al. (2012). Digital music exposure reliably induces temporary threshold shift (TTS) in normal hearing human subjects. *Ear Hear.* 33, e44–e58. doi: 10.1097/AUD.0b013e31825f9d89

Le Prell, C. G., Fulbright, A., Spankovich, C., Griffiths, S., Lobarinas, E., Campbell, K. C. M., et al. (2016). Dietary supplement comprised of β-carotene, vitamin C, vitamin E, and magnesium: failure to prevent music-induced temporary threshold shift. *Audiol. Neurootol. Extra* 6, 20–39. doi: 10.1159/000446600

Le Prell, C. G., Johnson, A.-C., Lindblad, A.-C., Skjönsberg, A., Ulfendahl, M., Guire, K., et al. (2011). Increased vitamin plasma levels in Swedish military personnel treated with nutrients prior to automatic weapon training. *Noise Health* 13, 432–443. doi: 10.4103/1463-1741.90317

Le Prell, C. G., and Lobarinas, E. (2015). "Strategies for assessing antioxidant efficacy in clinical trials," in *Oxidative Stress in Applied Basic Research and Clinical Practice: Free Radicals in ENT Pathology*, eds J. M. Miller, C. G. Le Prell, and L. P. Rybak (New York, NY: Humana Press), 163–192.

Le Prell, C. G., and Lobarinas, E. (2016). "Clinical and translational research: Challenges to the field," in *Translational Research in Audiology and the Hearing Sciences, Springer Handbook of Auditory Research*, eds C. G. Le Prell, E. Lobarinas, R. R. Fay, and A. N. Popper (New York, NY: Springer), 241–265.

Liberman, M. C. (2015). Hidden hearing loss. *Sci. Am.* 313, 48–53. doi: 10.1038/scientificamerican0815-48

Liberman, M. C., Epstein, M. J., Cleveland, S. S., Wang, H., and Maison, S. F. (2016). Toward a differential diagnosis of hidden hearing loss in humans. *PLoS ONE* 11:e0162726. doi: 10.1371/journal.pone.0162726

Liberman, M. C., and Kujawa, S. G. (2017). Cochlear synaptopathy in acquired sensorineural hearing loss: manifestations and mechanisms. *Hear. Res.* doi: 10.1016/j.heares.2017.01.003

Lin, H. W., Furman, A. C., Kujawa, S. G., and Liberman, M. C. (2011). Primary neural degeneration in the guinea pig cochlea after reversible noise-induced threshold shift. *J. Assoc. Res. Otolaryngol.* 12, 605–616. doi: 10.1007/s10162-011-0277-0

Lobarinas, E., Salvi, R., and Ding, D. (2013). Insensitivity of the audiogram to carboplatin induced inner hair cell loss in chinchillas. *Hear. Res.* 302, 113–120. doi: 10.1016/j.heares.2013.03.012

Lobarinas, E., Spankovich, C., and Le Prell, C. G. (2017). Evidence of "hidden hearing loss" following noise exposures that produce robust TTS and ABR wave-I amplitude reductions. *Hear. Res.* 349, 155–163. doi: 10.1016/j.heares.2016.12.009

Maison, S. F., and Rauch, S. D. (2017). Ethical considerations in noise-induced hearing loss research. *Lancet.* doi: 10.1016/S0140-6736(17)31875-5. [Epub ahead of print].

Makary, C. A., Shin, J., Kujawa, S. G., Liberman, M. C., and Merchant, S. N. (2011). Age-related primary cochlear neuronal degeneration in human temporal bones. *J. Assoc. Res. Otolaryngol.* 12, 711–717. doi: 10.1007/s10162-011-0283-2

Martin, F., Armstrong, T., and Champlin, C. (1994). A survey of audiological practices in the United States. *Am. J. Audiol.* 3, 20–26. doi: 10.1044/1059-0889.0302.20

McArdle, R., and Hnath-Chisolm, T. (2014). "Speech audiometry," in *Handbook of Clinical Audiology, 7th Edn.*, eds J. Katz, M. Chasin, K. English, L. Hood, and K. Tillery (Philadelphia, PA: Wolters Kluwer), 61–75.

Megerson, S. C. (2010). *Development of a Screening Tool for Identifying Young People at Risk for Noise-Induced Hearing Loss.* Ph.D Dissertation, University of Kansas.

Mehraei, G., Gallardo, A. P., Shinn-Cunningham, B. G., and Dau, T. (2017). Auditory brainstem response latency in forward masking, a marker of sensory deficits in listeners with normal hearing thresholds. *Hear. Res.* 346, 34–44. doi: 10.1016/j.heares.2017.01.016

Mills, J. H., Schulte, B. A., Boettcher, F. A., and Dubno, J. R. (2001). "A comparison of age-related hearing loss and noise-induced hearing loss," in *Noise Induced Hearing Loss: Basic Mechanisms, Prevention and Control*, eds D. Henderson, D. Prasher, R. Kopke, R. J. Salvi, and R. Hamernik (London: Noise Research Network), 497–511.

Murphy, W. J., and Le Prell, C. G. (2017). Making sound waves: selected papers from the 2016 annual conference of the National Hearing Conservation Association. *Int. J. Audiol.* 56, 1–3. doi: 10.1080/14992027.2016.1271145

Nam, E. C., and Won, J. Y. (2004). Extratympanic electrocochleographic changes on noise-induced temporary threshold shift. *Otolaryngol. Head Neck Surg.* 130, 437–442. doi: 10.1016/j.otohns.2003.12.016

Neitzel, R., Seixas, N., Goldman, B., and Daniell, W. (2004). Contributions of non-occupational activities to total noise exposure of construction workers. *Ann. Occup. Hyg.* 48, 463–473. doi: 10.1093/annhyg/meh041

NIOSH (1998). *Criteria for a Recommended Standard, Occupational Noise Exposure.* DHHS (NIOSH) Publication No. 98–126.

Niskar, A. S., Kieszak, S. M., Holmes, A., Esteban, E., Rubin, C., and Brody, D. J. (1998). Prevalence of hearing loss among children 6 to 19 years of age: the Third National Health and Nutrition Examination Survey. *JAMA* 279, 1071–1075. doi: 10.1001/jama.279.14.1071

Opperman, D. A., Reifman, W., Schlauch, R., and Levine, S. (2006). Incidence of spontaneous hearing threshold shifts during modern concert performances. *Otolaryng Head Neck* 134, 667–673. doi: 10.1016/j.otohns.2005.11.039

OSHA (1983). *Occupational Noise Exposure; Hearing Conservation Amendment*; 29 CFR 1910.95, Final Rule.

Paul, B. T., Bruce, I. C., and Roberts, L. E. (2017). Evidence that hidden hearing loss underlies amplitude modulation encoding deficits in individuals with and without tinnitus. *Hear. Res.* 344, 170–182. doi: 10.1016/j.heares.2016.11.010

Plomp, R., and Mimpen, A. (1979). Speech-reception threshold for sentences as a function of age and noise level. *J. Acoust. Soc. Am.* 66, 1333–1342. doi: 10.1121/1.383554

Prendergast, G., Guest, H., Munro, K., Hall, D., Kluk, K., Léger, A., et al. (2017). Effects of noise exposure on young adults with normal audiograms I: Electrophysiology. *Hear. Res.* 344, 68–81. doi: 10.1016/j.heares.2016.10.028

Ramakers, G. G. J., Kraaijenga, V. J. C., Cattani, G., van Zanten, G. A., and Grolman, W. (2016). Effectiveness of earplugs in preventing recreational noise-induced hearing loss: a randomized clinical trial. *JAMA Otolaryngol.* 142, 551–558. doi: 10.1001/jamaoto.2016.0225

Remenschneider, A. K., Lookabaugh, S., Aliphas, A., Brodsky, J. R., Devaiah, A. K., Dagher, W., et al. (2014). Otologic outcomes after blast injury: the Boston Marathon experience. *Otol. Neurotol.* 35, 1825–1834. doi: 10.1097/MAO.0000000000000616

Roland, P. S., and Roth, L. (1997). Interinterpreter variability in determining the SP/AP ratio in clinical electrocochleography. *Laryngoscope* 107, 1357–1361. doi: 10.1097/00005537-199710000-00012

Ryan, A. F., Kujawa, S. G., Hammill, T., Le Prell, C., and Kil, J. (2016). Temporary and permanent noise-induced threshold shifts: a review of basic and clinical observations. *Otol. Neurotol.* 37, e271–e275. doi: 10.1097/MAO.0000000000001071

Saunders, G. H., Frederick, M. T., Arnold, M., Silverman, S., Chisolm, T. H., and Myers, P. (2015). Auditory difficulties in blast-exposed Veterans with clinically normal hearing. *J. Rehabil. Res. Dev.* 52, 343–360. doi: 10.1682/JRRD.2014.11.0275

Schaette, R., and McAlpine, D. (2011). Tinnitus with a normal audiogram: physiological evidence for hidden hearing loss and computational model. *J. Neurosci.* 31, 13452–13457. doi: 10.1523/JNEUROSCI.2156-11.2011

Sekhar, D. L., Rhoades, J. A., Longenecker, A. L., Beiler, J. S., King, T. S., Widome, M. D., et al. (2011). Improving detection of adolescent hearing loss. *Arch. Pediatr. Adolesc. Med.* 165, 1094–1100. doi: 10.1001/archpediatrics.2011.188

Sergeyenko, Y., Lall, K., Liberman, M. C., and Kujawa, S. (2013). Age-related cochlear synaptopathy: an early-onset contributor to auditory functional decline. *J. Neurosci.* 33, 13686–13694. doi: 10.1523/JNEUROSCI.1783-13.2013

Serra, M. R., Biassoni, E. C., Richter, U., Minoldo, G., Franco, G., Abraham, S., et al. (2005). Recreational noise exposure and its effects on the hearing of adolescents. Part I: an interdisciplinary long-term study. *Int. J. Audiol.* 44, 65–73. doi: 10.1080/14992020400030010

Shah, S., Gopal, B., Reis, J., and Novak, M. (2009). Hear today, gone tomorrow: an assessment of portable entertainment player use and hearing acuity in a community sample. *J. Am. Board Fam. Pract.* 22, 17–23. doi: 10.3122/jabfm.2009.01.080033

Shaheen, L. A., Valero, M. D., and Liberman, M. C. (2015). Towards a diagnosis of cochlear neuropathy with envelope following responses. *J. Assoc. Res. Otolaryngol.* 16, 727–745. doi: 10.1007/s10162-015-0539-3

Shargorodsky, J., Curhan, S. G., Curhan, G. C., and Eavey, R. (2010). Change in prevalence of hearing loss in US adolescents. *JAMA* 304, 772–778. doi: 10.1001/jama.2010.1124

Skoe, E., Tufts, J. B., Hare, C., Husereau, M., Masi, R., and Camera, S. (2017). Neurophysiological, behavioral, and dosimetric indices of noise exposure in musicians with normal audiometric thresholds. *Abs. Assoc. Res. Otolaryngol.* 40:38.

Soli, S. D. (2008). Some thoughts on communication handicap and hearing impairment. *Int. J. Audiol.* 47, 285–286. doi: 10.1080/14992020802060656

Spankovich, C., Griffiths, S. K., Lobarinas, E., Morgenstein, K. E., de la Calle, S., Ledon, V., et al. (2014). Temporary threshold shift after impulse-noise during video game play: laboratory data. *Int. J. Audiol.* 53 (Suppl. 2), S53–S65. doi: 10.3109/14992027.2013.865844

Spankovich, C., Le Prell, C. G., Hood, L. J., and Lobarinas, E. (2017). Noise history and auditory function in young adults with and without type-1 diabetes. *Ear Hear.* doi: 10.1097/AUD.0000000000000457. [Epub ahead of print].

Stamper, G. C., and Johnson, T. A. (2015a). Auditory function in normal-hearing, noise-exposed human ears. *Ear Hear.* 36, 172–184. doi: 10.1097/AUD.0000000000000107

Stamper, G. C., and Johnson, T. A. (2015b). Letter to the Editor: Examination of potential sex influences in auditory function in normal-hearing, noise-exposed human ears, *Ear Hear.* 36, 172–184, 738–740.

Strasser, H., Irle, H., and Legler, R. (2003). Temporary hearing threshold shifts and restitution after energy-equivalent exposures to industrial noise and classical music. *Noise Health* 5, 75–84. Available online at: http://www.noiseandhealth.org/article.asp?issn=1463-1741;year=2003;volume=5;issue=20;spage=75;epage=84;aulast=Strasser

Valero, M. D., Hancock, K. E., and Liberman, M. C. (2016). The middle ear muscle reflex in the diagnosis of cochlear neuropathy. *Hear. Res.* 332, 29–38. doi: 10.1016/j.heares.2015.11.005

Verhulst, S., Jagadeesh, A., Mauermann, M., and Ernst, F. (2016). Individual differences in auditory brainstem response wave characteristics: relations to different aspects of peripheral hearing loss. *Trends Hear.* 20, 1–20. doi: 10.1177/2331216516672186

Viana, L. M., O'Malley, J. T., Burgess, B. J., Jones, D. D., Oliveira, C. A., Santos, F., et al. (2015). Cochlear neuropathy in human presbycusis: Confocal analysis of hidden hearing loss in post-mortem tissue. *Hear. Res.* 327, 78–88. doi: 10.1016/j.heares.2015.04.014

Wang, Y., and Ren, C. (2012). Effects of repeated "benign" noise exposures in young CBA mice: shedding light on age-related hearing loss. *J. Assoc. Res. Otolaryngol.* 13, 505–515. doi: 10.1007/s10162-012-0329-0

Wilson, R. H. (2011). Clinical experience with the words-in-noise test on 3430 veterans: comparisons with pure-tone thresholds and word recognition in quiet. *J. Am. Acad. Audiol.* 22, 405–423. doi: 10.3766/jaaa.22.7.3

Wilson, R. H., Abrams, H. B., and Pillion, A. L. (2003). A word-recognition task in multitalker babble using a descending presentation mode from 24 dB to 0 dB signal to babble. *J. Rehabil. Res. Dev.* 40, 321–327. doi: 10.1682/JRRD.2003.07.0321

Wilson, R. H., Carnell, C. S., and Cleghorn, A. L. (2007a). The Words-in-Noise (WIN) test with multitalker babble and speech-spectrum noise maskers. *J. Am. Acad. Audiol.* 18, 522–529. doi: 10.3766/jaaa.18.6.7

Wilson, R. H., and McArdle, R. (2007). Intra- and inter-session test, retest reliability of the Words-in-Noise (WIN) test. *J. Am. Acad. Audiol.* 18, 813–825. doi: 10.3766/jaaa.18.10.2

Wilson, R. H., McArdle, R. A., and Smith, S. L. (2007b). An Evaluation of the BKB-SIN, HINT, QuickSIN, and WIN Materials on Listeners With Normal Hearing and Listeners With Hearing Loss. *J. Speech. Lang. Hear. Res.* 50, 844–856. doi: 10.1044/1092-4388(2007/059)

Zecker, S. G., Hoffman, H. J., Frisina, R., Dubno, J. R., Dhar, S., Wallhagen, M., et al. (2013). Audition assessment using the NIH Toolbox. *Neurology* 80 (11 Suppl. 3), S45–S48. doi: 10.1212/WNL.0b013e3182872dd2

Permissions

All chapters in this book were first published by Frontiers; hereby published with permission under the Creative Commons Attribution License or equivalent. Every chapter published in this book has been scrutinized by our experts. Their significance has been extensively debated. The topics covered herein carry significant findings which will fuel the growth of the discipline. They may even be implemented as practical applications or may be referred to as a beginning point for another development.

The contributors of this book come from diverse backgrounds, making this book a truly international effort. This book will bring forth new frontiers with its revolutionizing research information and detailed analysis of the nascent developments around the world.

We would like to thank all the contributing authors for lending their expertise to make the book truly unique. They have played a crucial role in the development of this book. Without their invaluable contributions this book wouldn't have been possible. They have made vital efforts to compile up to date information on the varied aspects of this subject to make this book a valuable addition to the collection of many professionals and students.

This book was conceptualized with the vision of imparting up-to-date information and advanced data in this field. To ensure the same, a matchless editorial board was set up. Every individual on the board went through rigorous rounds of assessment to prove their worth. After which they invested a large part of their time researching and compiling the most relevant data for our readers.

The editorial board has been involved in producing this book since its inception. They have spent rigorous hours researching and exploring the diverse topics which have resulted in the successful publishing of this book. They have passed on their knowledge of decades through this book. To expedite this challenging task, the publisher supported the team at every step. A small team of assistant editors was also appointed to further simplify the editing procedure and attain best results for the readers.

Apart from the editorial board, the designing team has also invested a significant amount of their time in understanding the subject and creating the most relevant covers. They scrutinized every image to scout for the most suitable representation of the subject and create an appropriate cover for the book.

The publishing team has been an ardent support to the editorial, designing and production team. Their endless efforts to recruit the best for this project, has resulted in the accomplishment of this book. They are a veteran in the field of academics and their pool of knowledge is as vast as their experience in printing. Their expertise and guidance has proved useful at every step. Their uncompromising quality standards have made this book an exceptional effort. Their encouragement from time to time has been an inspiration for everyone.

The publisher and the editorial board hope that this book will prove to be a valuable piece of knowledge for researchers, students, practitioners and scholars across the globe.

List of Contributors

Adrian Dalbert, Flurin Pfiffner, Marco Hoesli, Dorothe Veraguth, Christof Roosli and Alexander Huber
Department of Otorhinolaryngology - Head and Neck Surgery, University of Zurich, University Hospital of Zurich, Zurich, Switzerland

Kanthaiah Koka, Aniket A. Saoji and Leonid M. Litvak
Department of Research and Technology, Advanced Bionics LLC, Valencia, CA, United States

Spencer B. Smith and Barbara K. Cone
Department of Speech, Language, and Hearing Sciences, University of Arizona, Tucson, AZ, USA

Jeremy Hornibrook
Department of Otolaryngology-Head and Neck Surgery, Christchurch Hospital, University of Canterbury and University of Otago, Christchurch, New Zealand

Jae-Ryong Kim
Department of Communication Sciences and Disorders, University of Iowa, Iowa City, IA, USA
Department of Otolaryngology-Head and Neck Surgery, Inje University College of Medicine, Busan, South Korea

Viral D. Tejani, Paul J. Abbas and Carolyn J. Brown
Department of Communication Sciences and Disorders, University of Iowa, Iowa City, IA, USA
Department of Otolaryngology-Head and Neck Surgery, University of Iowa Hospitals and Clinics, Iowa City, IA, USA

Elizabeth A. Strickland
Department of Speech, Languages, and Hearing Sciences, Purdue University, West Lafayette, IN, United States

Nicolas Verhaert
ExpORL Research Group, Department of Neurosciences, University of Leuven, Leuven, Belgium

Eric Verschooten and Philip X. Joris
Laboratory of Auditory Neurophysiology, Department of Neurosciences, University of Leuven, Leuven, Belgium

Karolina K. Charaziak
Caruso Department of Otolaryngology, Keck School of Medicine, University of Southern California, Los Angeles, CA, USA
Roxelyn and Richard Pepper Department of Communication Sciences and Disorders, Hugh Knowles Center, Northwestern University, Evanston, IL, USA

Christopher A. Shera
Caruso Department of Otolaryngology, Keck School of Medicine, University of Southern California, Los Angeles, CA, USA

Jonathan H. Siegel
Roxelyn and Richard Pepper Department of Communication Sciences and Disorders, Hugh Knowles Center, Northwestern University, Evanston, IL, USA

Shuman He
Center for Hearing Research, Boys Town National Research Hospital, Omaha, NE, United States

Holly F. B. Teagle
Department of Otolaryngology—Head and Neck Surgery, University of North Carolina at Chapel Hill, Chapel Hill, NC, United States

Craig A. Buchman
Department of Otolaryngology/Head and Neck Surgery, Washington University School of Medicine in St. Louis, St. Louis, MO, United States

Richard Salvi, Wei Sun, Dalian Ding, Guang-Di Chen, Kelly Radziwon and Benjamin D. Auerbach
Center for Hearing and Deafness, University at Buffalo, Buffalo, NY, USA

Edward Lobarinas
Callier Center, University of Texas at Dallas, Dallas, TX, USA

Jian Wang
School of Human Communication Disorders, Dalhousie University, Halifax, NS, Canada

Christofer W. Bester and Stephen J. O'Leary
Department of Otolaryngology, University of Melbourne, Melbourne, VIC, Australia
Royal Victorian Eye and Ear Hospital, Melbourne, VIC, Australia

Luke Campbell, Adrian Dragovic and Aaron Collins
Department of Otolaryngology, University of Melbourne, Melbourne, VIC, Australia

Brendan P. O'Connell, Marc L. Bennett, Alejandro Rivas, George B. Wanna and David S. Haynes
Department of Otolaryngology, Vanderbilt University Medical Center, Nashville, TN, United States

Jourdan T. Holder and Robert T. Dwyer
Department of Hearing and Speech Sciences, Vanderbilt University Medical Center, Nashville, TN, United States

René H. Gifford
Department of Otolaryngology, Vanderbilt University Medical Center, Nashville, TN, United States

Jack H. Noble and Robert F. Labadie
Department of Otolaryngology, Vanderbilt University Medical Center, Nashville, TN, United States
Department of Computer Science and Electrical Engineering, Vanderbilt University, Nashville, TN, United States

Alison M. Cook and Greg A. O'Beirne
New Zealand Institute of Language Brain and Behaviour, University of Canterbury, Christchurch, New Zealand
Eisdell Moore Centre, Auckland, New Zealand

Ashleigh J. Allsop
New Zealand Institute of Language Brain and Behaviour, University of Canterbury, Christchurch, New Zealand

Jeffery T. Lichtenhan, Choongheon Lee, Farah Dubaybo and Kaitlyn A. Wenrich
Department of Otolaryngology Washington University School of Medicine, Saint Louis, MO, United States

Uzma S. Wilson
Department of Communication Sciences and Disorders, Northwestern University, Evanston, IL, United States

Joseph Attias
Research and Technology, Advanced Bionics, Valencia, CA, USA
Schneider Children's Medical Center of Israel and Rabin Medical Center, Petach Tikva, Israel

Richard Hoben, Gifty Easow and Sofia Pevzner
Department of Otolaryngology, Steward St. Elizabeth's Medical Center, Boston, MA, USA

Mark A. Parker
Department of Otolaryngology, Steward St. Elizabeth's Medical Center, Boston, MA, USA
Department of Otolaryngology, Head and Neck Surgery, Tufts University School of Medicine, Boston, MA, USA

William J. Riggs, Michael S. Harris and Oliver F. Adunka
Department of Otolaryngology/Head and Neck Surgery, Ohio State University College of Medicine, Columbus, OH, United States

Joseph P. Roche
Lab Department of Otolaryngology/Head and Neck Surgery, University of Wisconsin School of Medicine, Madison, WI, United States

Christopher K. Giardina, Zachary J. Bastian, Tatyana E. Fontenot, Kevin D. Brown and Douglas C. Fitzpatrick
Department of Otolaryngology/Head and Neck Surgery, The University of No rth Carolin a at Chapel Hill School of Medicine, Chapel Hill, NC, United States

Craig A. Buchman
Department of Otolaryngology/Head and Neck Surgery, Washington University School of Medicine in St. Louis, St. Louis, MO, United States

Alana E. Kennedy and Wafaa A. Kaf
Department of Communication Sciences and Disorders, Missouri State University, Springfield, MO, United States

John A. Ferraro
Department of Hearing and Speech, University of Kansas Medical Center, Kansas City, KS, United States

Rafael E. Delgado
Department of Biomedical Engineering, University of Miami, Coral Gables, FL, United States

Sarah K. Grinn
School of Behavioral and Brain Sciences, University of Texas at Dallas, Dallas, TX, United States
College of Public Health and Health Professions, University of Florida, Gainesville, FL, United States

Kathryn B. Wiseman, Jason A. Baker and Colleen G. Le Prell
School of Behavioral and Brain Sciences, University of Texas at Dallas, Dallas, TX, United States

Index